Activate your access today!

This text comes with access to the complete contents online, fully searchable, plus other valuable features.

Three simple steps to gain instant access...
1) Visit **www.dermforpcp.com**
2) Click on Register Now
3) Follow the instructions and then enter your access code found below when prompted

This website is for individual use only. If you are interested in multi-user access, please contact customer service. For technical assistance, email customerservice@lww.com or call 1-800-468-1128 (inside the US) or 1-410-528-4000 (outside the US).

*Disclaimer: Your online access is valid for the life of the print product. It is the discretion of the publisher to deactivate or modify the site at any given time.

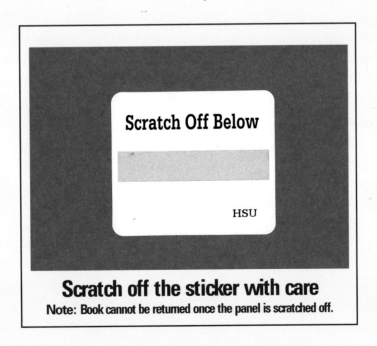

Scratch Off Below

HSU

Scratch off the sticker with care
Note: Book cannot be returned once the panel is scratched off.

Wolters Kluwer | Lippincott Williams & Wilkins
Health

Lippincott's Primary Care

Dermatology

EDITED BY

Peter C. Schalock, MD
Assistant Professor of Dermatology, Harvard Medical School
Assistant Dermatologist, Massachusetts General Hospital
Boston, Massachusetts

Jeffrey T.S. Hsu, MD
Adjunct Associate Professor of Medicine (Dermatology)
Dartmouth Medical School
Hanover, New Hampshire
Co-Director of Dermatologic, Laser & Cosmetic Surgery
The Dermatology Institute of DuPage Medical Group
Naperville, Illinois

Kenneth A. Arndt, MD
Skin Care Physicians
Chestnut Hill, Massachusetts
Clinical Professor of Dermatology, Emeritus
Harvard Medical School, Boston, Massachusetts
Clinical Professor of Dermatology
Yale Medical School, New Haven, Connecticut
Adjunct Professor of Medicine (Dermatology)
Dartmouth Medical School, Hanover, New Hampshire

 Wolters Kluwer | Lippincott Williams & Wilkins
Health

Philadelphia · Baltimore · New York · London
Buenos Aires · Hong Kong · Sydney · Tokyo

Acquisitions Editor: Sonya Seigafuse
Product Manager: Kerry Barrett
Production Manager: Bridgett Dougherty
Senior Manufacturing Manager: Benjamin Rivera
Marketing Manager: Kim Schonberger
Design Coordinator: Doug Smock
Production Service: Aptara, Inc.

© 2011 by LIPPINCOTT WILLIAMS & WILKINS, a WOLTERS KLUWER business
Two Commerce Square
2001 Market Street
Philadelphia, PA 19103 USA
LWW.com

Printed in China

Library of Congress Cataloging-in-Publication Data

Lippincott's primary care dermatology / edited by Peter C. Schalock,
Jeffrey T.S. Hsu, Kenneth A. Arndt.
  p. ; cm.
  Other title: Primary care dermatology
  Includes bibliographical references and index.
  Summary: "This book will help family practitioners, internists, nurse practitioners, and physician assistants understand, diagnose, and treat dermatologic problems commonly seen in the primary care setting. Emphasis on day-to-day outpatient office practice distinguishes Lippincott's Primary Care Dermatology from other dermatology textbooks. Coverage includes adult, geriatric, and ethnic skin. Each diagnosis begins with a realistic case and includes detailed discussions of pathogenesis, diagnostic methods, and therapy. An "at a glance" therapy section summarizes primary and secondary treatments to make treatment decisions easier. The book includes over 300 full-color images of skin lesions, numerous patient handouts, and a folded-in anatomical chart for the office. A companion website will include the fully searchable text and an image bank"—Provided by publisher.
  ISBN-13: 978-0-7817-9378-0 (hardback)
  ISBN-10: 0-7817-9378-5 (hardback)
1. Dermatology. 2. Primary care (Medicine) I. Schalock, Peter C.
II. Hsu, Jeffrey T. S. III. Arndt, Kenneth A., 1936- IV. Title: Primary care dermatology.
  [DNLM: 1. Skin Diseases—therapy. 2. Primary Health Care—methods.
3. Skin Diseases—diagnosis. WR 140 L768 2011]
  RL71.L635 2011
  616.5—dc22

2010024568

To purchase additional copies of this book, call our customer service department at (800) 638-3030 or fax orders to (301) 223-2320. International customers should call (301) 223-2300.

Visit Lippincott Williams & Wilkins on the Internet: at LWW.com. Lippincott Williams & Wilkins customer service representatives are available from 8:30 am to 6 pm, EST.

CCS0810

10 9 8 7 6 5 4 3 2 1

Dedication and Acknowledgements

First and foremost, I would like to thank my wife, Anneli, for her nonstop support and assistance while preparing this textbook. Without her, I could not have finished this project. I am greatly appreciative to the Harvard Medical School Dermatology Interest Group, the residents/faculty of the Harvard/Massachusetts General Hospital Dermatology program and Dartmouth Hitchcock Medical Center for their support and assistance in preparing the text. Lastly, Kerry Barrett at LWW has been a pleasure to work with.

PCS

For all the teachers in my life, especially my father.

JTSH

To Anne, David, Jennifer, Alexander and Benjamin,
and,
To the many fellows, residents, students, and colleagues with whom I've had the pleasure of sharing time, tales, teaching, and fun.

KAA

Contributors

Katrina Abuabara, MA
Harvard Medical School
Boston, Massachusetts

Fátima Akrouh, BA
Harvard Medical School & School of Public
    Health
Boston, Massachusetts

Falguni Asrani, MD
Wellman Laboratories
Massachusetts General Hospital
Boston, Massachusetts

Lynn Baden, MD
Centre Dermatology
Newton, Massachusetts

Jane Barry, MD
Hermitage Medical Clinic
Dublin, Ireland

Juliana Basko-Plluska, MD
Department of Medicine
McGaw Medical Center Northwestern
Chicago, Illinois

Tracie Chong, BA
John A. Burns School of Medicine at the
    University of Hawaii
Honolulu, Hawaii

Shraddha Desai, MD
Clinical Research Fellow
Dermatology Institute of DuPage Medical Group
    in Naperville
Naperville, Illinois

Jennifer L. Greenman
Harvard Medical School
Boston, Massachusetts

Jeffrey T.S. Hsu, MD
Adjunct Associate Professor of Medicine
    (Dermatology)
Dartmouth Medical School
Hanover, New Hampshire
Co-Director of Dermatologic, Laser & Cosmetic
    Surgery
The Dermatology Institute of DuPage
    Medical Group
Naperville, Illinois

Stephanie Hu, MD
Harvard Medical School
Boston, Massachusetts

Susan J. Huang, MD
Harvard Medical School
Boston, Massachusetts

Abel Jarell, MD
Chief Resident in Dermatology
Harvard Medical School Combined Residency in
    Dermatology
Boston, Massachusetts

Daniela Kroshinsky, MD
Instructor of Dermatology
Harvard Medical School
Assistant in Dermatology
Massachusetts General Hospital
Boston, Massachusetts

Lilla Landeck, MD
Department of Dermatology
Harvard Medical School
Massachusetts General Hospital
Boston, Massachusetts

Chao Li, BS
Harvard Medical School
Boston, Massachusetts

Evelyn Lilly, BA
Harvard Medical School
Boston, Massachusetts

Vinod E. Nambudiri, AB
Harvard Medical School
Boston, Massachusetts

Andrew A. Nelson, MD
Division of Dermatology
University of California—Los Angeles
Los Angeles, California

Ilka Netravali, BS
Harvard Medical School, MD-PhD Program
Boston, Massachusetts

My-Linh T. Nguyen, BS
Harvard Medical School
Boston, Massachusetts

Nina Otberg, MD
Skin and Laser Center
Potsdam, Germany

Mahendra Pancholi, MD
Nairobi, Kenya

Pranav Pancholi, MD
Nairobi, Kenya

Sam Rodriguez, MD
Resident in Anesthesia/Critical Care
Massachusetts General Hospital
Boston, Massachusetts

Ellen K. Roh, MD
Instructor of Dermatology
Harvard Medical School
Assistant in Dermatology
Massachusetts General Hospital
Boston, Massachusetts

Arturo Saavedra-Lauzon, MD
Instructor of Dermatology
Harvard Medical School
Assistant in Dermatology
Brigham and Women's Hospital/Dana Farber
   Cancer Institute
Boston, Massachusetts

Greg K. Sakamoto, MD
Kaiser Permanente Hawaii
Honolulu, Hawaii

Peter C. Schalock, MD
Assistant Professor of Dermatology
Harvard Medical School
Assistant Dermatologist
Massachusetts General Hospital
Boston, Massachusetts

Jennifer K. Tan-Billet, MD
Chief Resident in Dermatology
Harvard Medical School Combined Residency in
   Dermatology
Boston, Massachusetts

Khanh P. Thieu, MD
Resident in Dermatology
New York Presbyterian Hospital–Columbia
New York, New York

Jacob P. Thyssen, MD, PhD
Department of Dermatology
Gentofte Hospital
University of Copenhagen
Copenhagen, Denmark

Thanh-Nga T. Tran, MD
Instructor of Dermatology
Harvard Medical School
Assistant in Dermatology
Massachusetts General Hospital
Boston, Massachusetts

Jennifer Villaseñor, MD, PhD
Resident in Dermatology
Department of Dermatology
University of Pennsylvania School of Medicine
Philadelphia, Pennsylvania

James Y.T. Wang, BS
Harvard Medical School
Boston, Massachusetts

Molly Wanner, MD, MBA
Instructor of Dermatology
Harvard Medical School
Assistant in Dermatology
Massachusetts General Hospital
Boston, Massachusetts

Gregory L. Wells, MD
Adjunct Professor of Medicine (Dermatology)
Dartmouth Medical School
Hanover, New Hampshire

Preface

Primary Care Dermatology is designed to be a useful review of the most commonly seen cutaneous conditions. As well, some of the rarer skin diseases that should not be missed in the primary care setting are covered. The first four chapters of the book discuss basics of dermatology—descriptions of skin lesions, types of topical therapy, basics of outpatient dermatologic procedures, and finally a discussion of maintenance of normal skin. The following chapters discuss basic skin conditions that we all often see.

Each diagnosis starts with a realistic case, often taken from histories of actual clinic patients. Pathogenesis, diagnostic methods, and therapy are all covered in detail. To make treatment decisions easier, options are summarized in an "At a Glance" Treatment section.

It is impossible to cover all topics within dermatology in this text. This book is meant to be a quick reference and synopsis of commonly seen skin conditions. We attempt to give broad differential diagnoses and useful treatment suggestions for each discussed disease. We hope you find this text useful and informative.

Contents

Introduction to Lippincott's Primary Care Series

Welcome to Lippincott's Primary Care Series. The intended goal of this series is to help assist you in all of the use-case scenarios that you might encounter each day.

In this product, <u>Primary Care Dermatology</u>, you will find:

1. **Book:** The book contains both bulleted points for quick look-up access when you need an answer right away, as well as longer text for the occasions when you need a little more information.

   Additionally we have included pedagogy to highlight certain aspects of the text. These elements include:

 Not to Be Missed—Things to watch out for or possible diagnoses to keep in mind during the examination

 When to Refer—When to suggest further options to your patient

2. **Website** that includes:
   - Fully searchable text of the book
   - Image bank that can be downloadable into PowerPoint for presentations
   - PDF downloadable Patient Information Sheets

3. **Anatomical Chart for Your Office**

We certainly hope this product is useful and meets your needs.

Please look for other titles in the Lippincott's Primary Care Series.

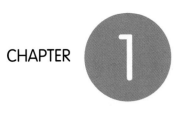
Basic Definitions and Differential Diagnosis

Shraddha Desai and Jeffrey T.S. Hsu

Introduction

Primary care providers (PCPs) must understand multiple aspects of medicine. From headaches to foot pain, the physician must be prepared to address all of these conditions in an appropriate and timely manner. As more patients are being limited from seeing specialists, they turn to their PCP with more complex issues. This is especially true for dermatologic conditions. Often, dermatoses appear similar and are difficult to describe, resulting in delayed diagnosis. However, by understanding basic terminology and common presentations, PCPs can effectively diagnose skin conditions. It is our hope that this text will help PCPs deal with common dermatologic presentations.

Before one can accurately diagnose dermatologic conditions, learning the descriptive terminology is helpful. Being able to accurately describe skin lesions allows concise communication between providers, especially by telephone or electronic communication. This chapter attempts to summarize the common vocabulary of dermatology and to present that information in a usable format.

General Terms

- A lesion is an area of altered skin. All dermatologic descriptions should include a primary and/or secondary lesion descriptor.
  - Primary lesion—the physical change in skin that is caused directly by the disease
  - Secondary lesion—the changes that occur in the skin after the evolution of the disease or resulting appearance after scratching or infection
- Dermatosis: skin disease
- "Dermatitis" and "eczema" are synonyms. In common usage, "dermatitis" is often used for acute rashes and "eczema" for more chronic rashes. Also, "eczema" is often used as a synonym for atopic dermatitis
- Morphology: form or structure of a lesion
- Maculopapule or "maculopapular": There is no such thing as a maculopapule. This term is often used as a description for hypersensitivity-related dermatitis. A better descriptor in many cases would be "morbilliform."

Primary Skin Lesions

Macule—a flat area of color change that cannot be detected by touch (Fig. 1-1A)
Patch—a flat area greater than 1 cm (Fig. 1-1B)

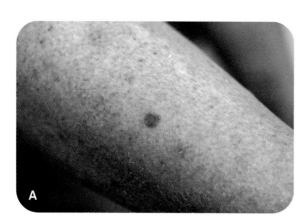
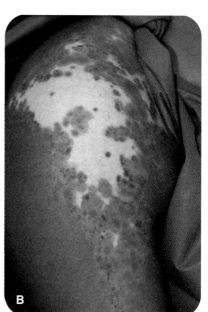

Figure 1-1 A Macule. Blue nevus on the shin. **B** Patch. Vitiligo.

Papule—a solid raised lesion less than 1.0 cm that can have a variety of shapes (acuminate, dome-shaped, etc.) and may be associated with secondary lesions like scale and crust (Fig. 1-2)

Nodule—a raised solid lesion that is more firm than a papule or plaque and often deeper (Fig. 1-3)

Tumor—a solid mass of the skin or subcutaneous tissue that is larger than a nodule (Fig. 1-4)

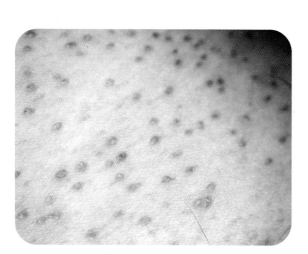
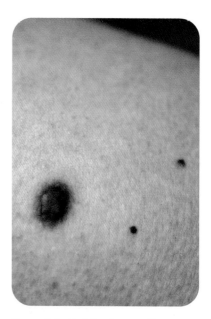

Figure 1-2 Papule. Lichen nitidus on the inner arm.

Figure 1-3 Nodule. Dermatofibroma on the shoulder (note two macular nevi adjacent and lateral).

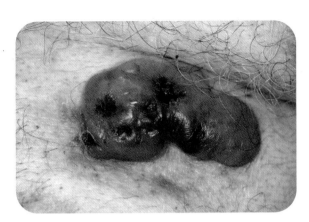

Figure 1-4 Tumor. B-cell lymphoma on the upper abdomen of a 70-year-old male.

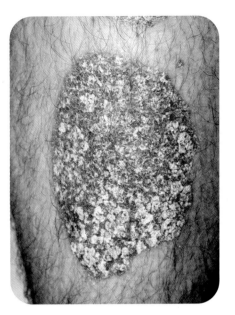

Figure 1-5 Plaque. Psoriasis on the shin.

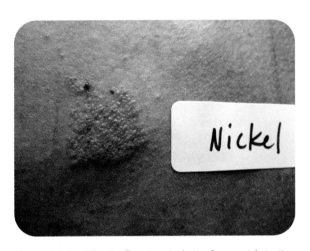

Figure 1-6 Vesicle. Confluent vesiculation from patch testing (ACD—nickel).

Plaque—a solid lesion greater than 1.0 cm, which is often elevated or thickened and formed by the confluence of papules (Fig. 1-5)

Vesicle—a small circumscribed collection of free fluid less than 1.0 cm in diameter (Fig. 1-6)

Bulla—a large circumscribed collection of free fluid greater than 1.0 cm in diameter (Fig. 1-7)

Pustule—a circumscribed elevated lesion (less than 1.0 cm) that contains purulent material (protein-rich and filled with neutrophils); an abscess is a larger collection of pus (Fig. 1-8)

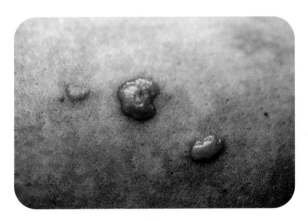

Figure 1-7 Bulla. Three linear bullae from poison ivy.

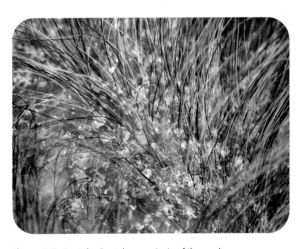

Figure 1-8 Pustule. Pustular psoriasis of the scalp.

CHAPTER 1 Basic Definitions & DDx

Figure 1-9 Wheal. Urticarial plaque, note follicular accentuation.

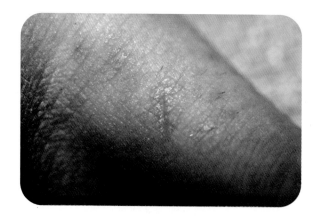

Figure 1-10 Burrow. Scabies burrow on the finger.

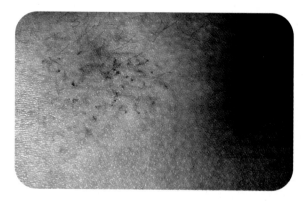

Figure 1-11 Telangiectasia. Patch of telangiectasia on the lower back.

Wheal—an area of swelling in the epidermis; transient (Fig. 1-9)

Burrow—a raised tortuous channel produced by a parasite (scabies) (Fig. 1-10)

Telangiectasia—a permanently dilated superficial blood vessel in the skin; this can be isolated or part of a larger condition such as ataxia telangiectasia (Fig. 1-11)

Secondary Skin Lesions

Scale—compact desquamated layers of stratum corneum that look like plates and flakes; these are caused by abnormal keratinization and shedding (Fig. 1-12)

Crust—the result of drying plasma and exudate on the skin (Fig. 1-13)

Atrophy—the thinning of epidermis or subcutaneous fat resulting in a depression of the skin (Fig. 1-14)

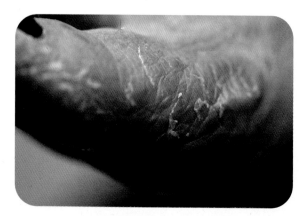

Figure 1-12 Scale. Tinea pedis.

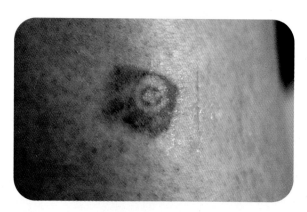

Figure 1-13 Crust. A thermal burn resulting in crust in the distribution of the burn.

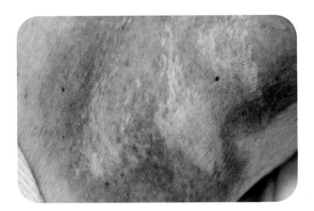

Figure 1-14 Atrophy. Cutaneous lichen sclerosus.

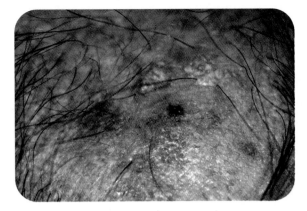

Figure 1-15 Hypertrophy. Hypertrophic actinic keratosis on the forehead.

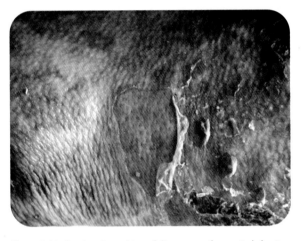

Figure 1-16 Erosion. Pemphigus foliaceus on the central chest.

Hypertrophy—thickening of the skin (Fig. 1-15)

Erosion—a slightly depressed appearance of skin due to the loss of epidermis; this heals without scarring because it does not penetrate below the dermoepidermal junction (DEJ) (Fig. 1-16)

Ulceration—focal loss of epidermis and dermis; heals with scarring (Fig. 1-17)

Scar—dermal damage resulting in an abnormal connective tissue pattern; can also result in pigmentary changes (Fig. 1-18)

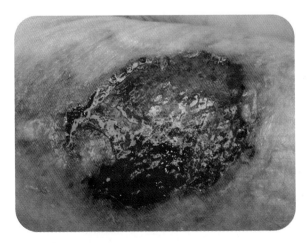

Figure 1-17 Ulceration. Chronic ulceration on the arm, possibly self-inflicted.

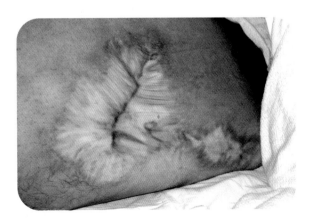

Figure 1-18 Scar. Scar 1 year after Coumadin necrosis on thigh.

CHAPTER 1 Basic Definitions & DDx

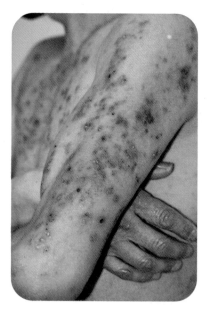

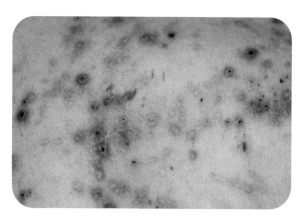

Figure 1-19 Lichenification. Lichenification and skin erosions due to allergic dermatitis.

Figure 1-20 Excoriations. Prurigo nodules, erosions, and linear excoriations on the back.

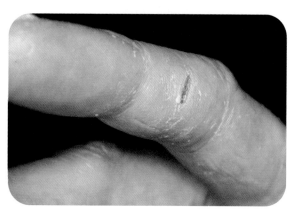

Figure 1-21 Fissure. Full-thickness fissure on the finger secondary to hand eczema.

Lichenification—area of thickened epidermis with exaggerated skin lines due to chronic scratching or rubbing (Fig. 1-19)

Excoriation—traumatized area of skin often caused by scratching; excoriations often appear linear (Fig. 1-20)

Fissure—a linear cleavage of skin that extends into the dermis (Fig. 1-21)

Keloid—an exaggerated connective tissue response to injury that extends beyond the original borders of the wound (Fig. 1-22)

Petechiae, purpura, and ecchymoses—bleeding in the skin that does not blanch when pressed; petechiae are smaller than 1.0 cm, while purpura and ecchymoses are larger (Figs. 1-23, 1-24)

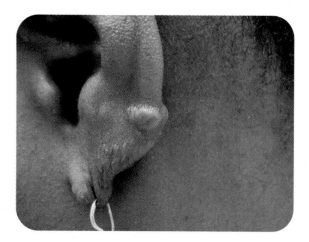

Figure 1-22 Keloid. On the helix following a surgical procedure.

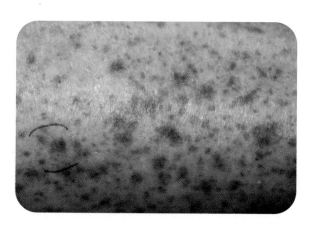

Figure 1-23 Petechiae/purpura on shins of a 75-year-old man with hypocomplementemic urticarial vasculitis.

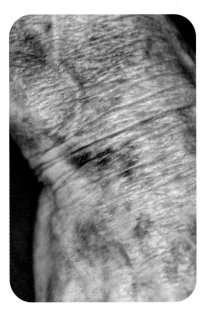

Figure 1-24 Ecchymosis. Senile ecchymoses on the lower extensor forearm.

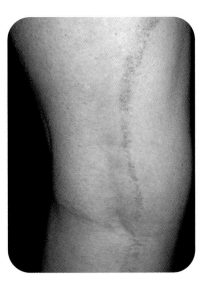

Figure 1-25 Linear. Lichen striatus on the posterior leg.

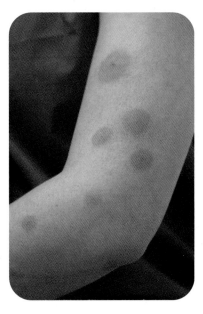

Figure 1-26 Target. Erythema multiforme.

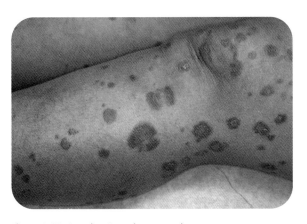

Figure 1-27 Annular. Granuloma annulare.

Configuration: Shape of Lesions

Linear—line or bandlike lesion often due to an external cause such as scratching (Fig. 1-25)

Target—concentric rings similar to a bull's eye (Fig. 1-26)

Annular—ring-shaped lesions (tinea corporis, erythema migrans, and granuloma annulare) (Fig. 1-27)

Discrete—lesions remain separate from each other (*Varicella*) (Fig. 1-28)

Clustered—lesions that are grouped together (*Herpes simplex* or insect bites) (Fig. 1-29)

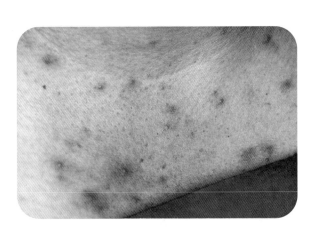

Figure 1-28 Discrete. Primary varicella.

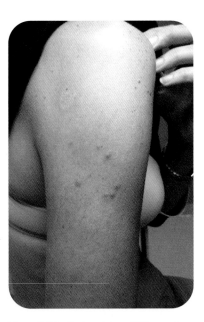

Figure 1-29 Clustered. Insect bite reaction.

CHAPTER 1 Basic Definitions & DDx

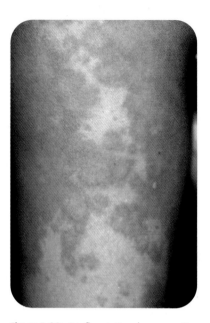

Figure 1-30 Confluent. Drug hypersensitivity reaction.

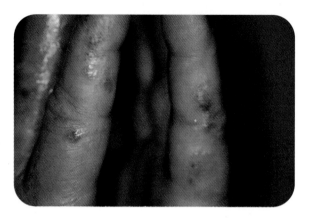

Figure 1-31 Eczematous. Allergic contact dermatitis secondary to the rubber accelerator thiuram.

Confluent—lesions that run together (drug hypersensitivity reaction) (Fig. 1-30)

Eczematous—inflamed lesions that tend to cluster, ooze, and crust (atopic or allergic contact dermatitis) (Fig. 1-31)

Guttate—lesions appear droplike on the skin (guttate psoriasis) (Fig. 1-32)

Multiform—lesions that have a variety of shapes

Morbilliform—appearance of lesions is similar that of the measles rash: macular lesions that are red and are usually 2–10 mm in diameter but may be confluent in places (Fig. 1-33)

Serpiginous—snakelike appearance of lesions (Fig. 1-34)

Reticular—lacelike pattern of lesions, often found in newborns or in vascular disorders (Fig. 1-35)

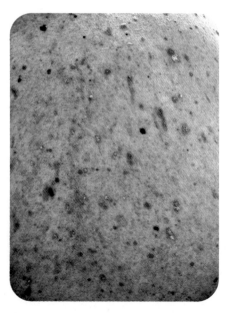

Figure 1-32 Guttate. Guttate psoriasis.

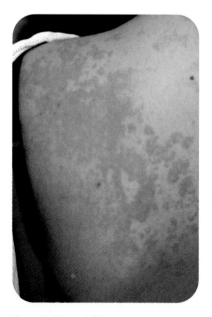

Figure 1-33 Morbilliform. Drug hypersensitivity reaction.

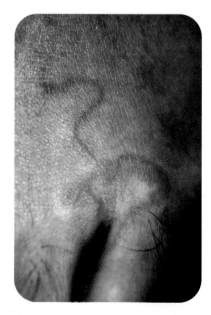

Figure 1-34 Serpiginous. Cutaneous larva migrans.

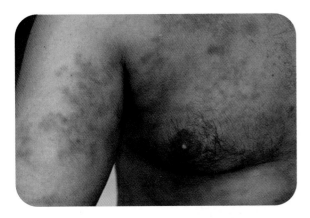

Figure 1-35 Reticular. Cutaneous polyarteritis nodosa.

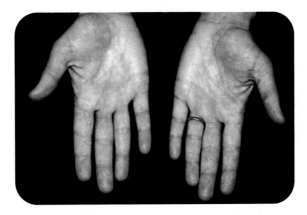

Figure 1-36 Acral skin. Palmar.

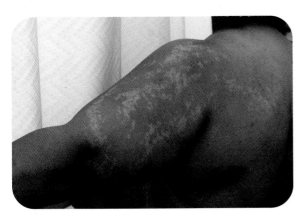

Figure 1-37 Blaschkoid distribution of hypopigmentation.

Distribution: Patterns of Spread

Acral—distal portions of limbs (hand, foot) (Fig. 1-36)

Blaschko lines—follow a roughly linear, segmental pattern described by Blaschko (Fig. 1-37)

Dermatomal/zosteriform—lesions follow a dermatome which corresponds with nerve root distribution (*Herpes zoster* shingles) (Fig. 1-38)

Extensor/flexor—involves outer (extensor) and inner (flexor) surfaces of limbs (Figs. 1-39, 1-40)

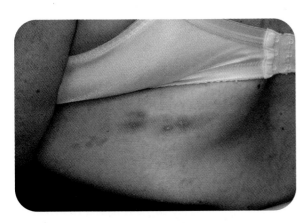

Figure 1-38 Herpes zoster on the trunk.

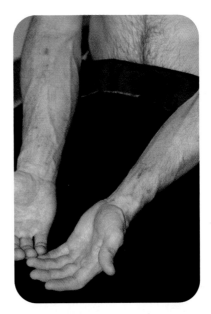

Figure 1-39 Flexor surface of the forearm.

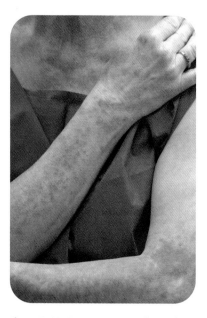

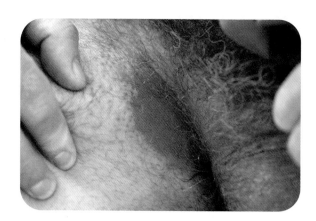

Figure 1-40 Extensor arms. Polymorphous light eruption.

Figure 1-41 Flexural. Candidal intertrigo.

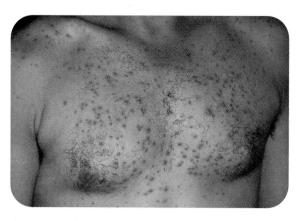

Figure 1-42 Folliculitis on the chest from *Pityrosporum* infection.

Flexural—involving skin flexures (intertriginous areas) (Fig. 1-41)

Follicular—lesions arising from hair follicles (Fig. 1-42)

Generalized—universal distribution, may be scattered or diffuse (Fig. 1-43)

Herpetiform—grouped umbilicated vesicles (Fig. 1-44)

Koebnerized—the appearance of lesions arising in a wound or scar; this is also known as the Koebner phenomenon or isomorphic response (warts, lichen planus, pyoderma gangrenosum) (Fig. 1-45)

Symmetrical—affects same region in a similar way on both left and right sides (Fig. 1-46)

Truncal—prone to trunk; rarely affects limbs (Fig. 1-47)

Unilateral—affects one side only (Fig. 1-48)

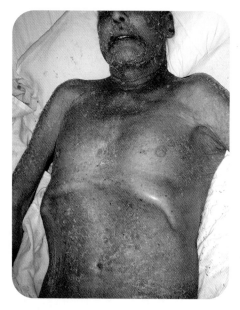

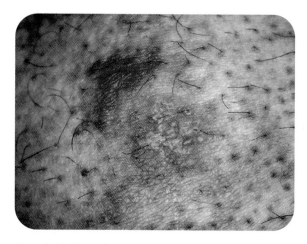

Figure 1-43 Generalized. Erythroderma secondary to psoriasis.

Figure 1-44 Herpetiform. Grouped umbilicated vesicles in acute herpes simplex.

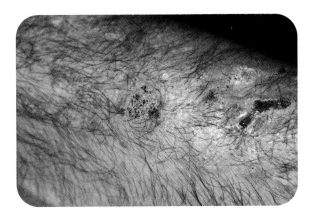

Figure 1-45 Koebnerized verruca vulgaris in self-inflicted prurigo.

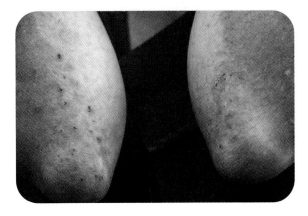

Figure 1-46 Symmetric. Dermatitis herpetiformis on the extensor forearms.

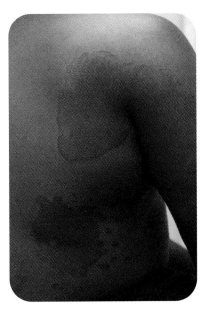

Figure 1-47 Truncal. Confluent and reticulated papillomatosis.

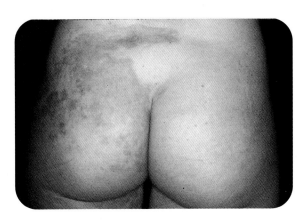

Figure 1-48 Unilateral. Morphea on the buttock.

Conclusion

Although a multitude of skin conditions and variations exist, understanding the basic terminology and descriptors for lesions cannot only help PCPs develop a good set of differential diagnoses, but also aid in determining the correct diagnosis. Furthermore, taking into consideration the distribution and shape of lesions, as well as the patient's age, will additionally narrow down possibilities. This, in turn, will not only make PCPs more efficient when dealing with dermatologic issues, but also make seeing patients with these conditions a more enjoyable experience.

CHAPTER 2 Topical Therapy

Peter C. Schalock

For many diseases of the skin, topical application of medications is the mainstay of therapy. A thorough understanding of how the base of the topical medicaments is produced and the therapeutic benefits and pitfalls in choosing a particular base are essential for those desiring successful topical treatment of cutaneous disease. In many cases, the choice of an ointment versus the use of a cream or lotion may be the difference between successful therapy and failure.

Vehicles

The vehicle for many topical medicaments is white petrolatum. Petrolatum is derived from petroleum distillation and is made up of long-chain aliphatic hydrocarbons. There are two forms, white and yellow petrolatum, with the difference being the amount of refining/impurities present. White petrolatum is the most refined and most commonly is used as a skin protectant and moisturizing agent, as well as the base for creams and lotions. In its pure form, white petrolatum does not require preservatives and is not a cause of allergic contact dermatitis (ACD). Yellow petrolatum is a rare cause of ACD. The different vehicle types are discussed below and are also summarized in Table 2-1.

White petrolatum is used most often as a base for ointments. Many topical medicaments, in addition to the white petrolatum base, add humectants such as propylene glycol (PG) or glycerin. Other lipophilic bases are sometimes used for topical medicaments. Beeswax, lanolin, and natural oils (jojoba, sweet almond, peanut oil, and others) are infrequently used as a base for delivery of medicaments. PG is the base for water-soluble products and is also added to lipophilic ointments and creams to increase potency and penetration of the epidermis, as well to act as a humectant. Corticosteroid preparations often add PG. Lipophilic ointments are an effective barrier for water loss for 4 to 6 hours after application. They are occlusive, provide excellent hydration, and increase penetration of the epidermis if a medication such as a corticosteroid is part of the ointment system.

Creams, at their simplest, are white petrolatum or other oil with added water. This addition makes the cream less greasy and more easily rubbed/absorbed into the skin, making creams much more accepted by patients compared to ointments. Because of the added water content, addition of a preservative agent to prevent spoilage is necessary. These agents prevent microbial overgrowth, but also may cause allergic sensitization. Common additives are summarized in Table 2-2. Creams are most commonly used in clinical practice due to their

Table 2-1 Bases for Topical Therapy

BASE	DESCRIPTION	EXAMPLE
Ointment	Lipophilic base	White petrolatum/ Aquaphor
Cream	Lipophilic base with added water	Eucerin
Lotion	Lipophilic base with even more water	Nivea
Gel	Glycerin or PG base, rubs in easily	
Foam	Gas bubbles trapped in liquid; easy application on hair-bearing areas	Hair mousse or betamethasone diproprionate foam
Solution	Alcohol or water base, liquid; applied in dropwise fashion	Fluocinonide solution
Shampoo	Blend of surfactants, fragrances; may include medication	Clobetasol or coal tar shampoo
Emulsion	Particulate added to solution, will settle out of solution	Calamine lotion

Table 2-2 Additives to Topical Products Causing Allergic Contact Dermatitis

CHEMICAL	CLASS	% OF PATIENTS ALLERGIC (NACDG 03-04)*
2-bromo-2-nitropropane (Bronopol)	Formaldehyde-releasing preservative	2.3%
Cocamidopropyl betaine	Surfactant	1.8%
Diazolidinyl urea	Formaldehyde-releasing preservative	3.5%
dl-alpha-tocopherol (vitamin E)	Antioxidant	1.1%
DMDM hydantoin	Formaldehyde-releasing preservative	2.3
Fragrance	Fragrance	9.1%
Imidazolidinyl urea	Formaldehyde-releasing preservative	2.9%
Iodopropynyl butylcarbamate	Preservative	0.5%
Lanolin (wool alcohol)	Naturally derived (sheep sebum)	2.2%
Methylchloroisothiazolinone/ methylisothiazolinone	Preservative	2.2%
Methyldibromoglutaronitrile/ Euxyl K400	Preservative	6.1%
Parabens	Preservative	1.1%
Propylene glycol	Preservative/humectant	3.3%
Quaternium 15	Formaldehyde-releasing preservative	8.9%

*Warshaw EM, Belsito DV, DeLeo VA, et al. North American Contact Dermatitis Group Patch-Test Results, 2003–2004 Study Period. *Dermatitis* 2008;19(3):129–136.

great patient acceptance. They are less hydrating compared to ointments and are poorly tolerated on hair-bearing skin such as the scalp or thicker trunk hair due to matting of the hair.

Lotions are thick liquids, composed of water or alcohol bases with added ingredients. A lotion may simply be an oil-in-water emulsion, basically a cream with further added water for even easier application. A "shake lotion" is a powder-in-water suspension, the most common being Calamine lotion. This is composed of zinc oxide, talc, glycerin, water, ferric oxide, bentonite magma, and calcium hydroxide. Shake lotions are excellent for use in areas to which application is challenging, such as hair-bearing skin or scalp. Shake lotions traditionally have been useful in exudative, inflammatory processes to which creams are challenging to apply. In addition, lotions are useful in conditions where drying of the affected skin is desirable, such as in an exudative intertrigo. Lotions with an alcohol base are helpful for pruritic skin as they are cooling and astringent. A common example of such a lotion is the commercially available Sarna lotion.

Gels are vehicles that are commonly used on sebaceous areas of the body such as the face and chest or for hair-bearing areas such as the scalp. The main component of a gel is water, acetone, alcohol, or propylene glycol with organic polymers suspended with substances such as agar, gelatin, hydroxypropylcellulose, carbomer methylcellulose, pectin, and/or polyethylene glycol. Gels are semi-solid on application but then melt due to body heat and are absorbed into the skin without leaving a film. This base enhances penetration and absorption through the epidermis for the medicament contained in the gel (often a corticosteroid or retinoid preparation). In some individuals, gels may cause mild xerosis of the skin.

Powders are finely particulate, hygroscopic substances that are used to dry moist skin areas and minimize friction between opposing surfaces. A common location for the use of a powder would be in intertriginous areas such as the inguinal crease, axillae, or under skin folds in larger individuals. Common bases include zinc oxide, zinc or magnesium stearate, talc, cornstarch, or precipitated calcium carbonate. Some powders contain added medication, often an antibacterial or antimycotic agent.

Pastes are powder mixed with an ointment. The most common dermatologic paste is zinc oxide compounded in white petrolatum. Pastes are useful for skin protection such as in a diaper or other areas where irritant contact dermatitis can occur, or as a sunscreen. Zinc oxide paste is opaque when applied and is a broad-spectrum ultraviolet (UV) blocker. Micronized zinc oxide is more cosmetically acceptable as visible light passes through, but UVA and UVB are blocked.

Choice of Bases and Application Techniques

Application techniques and choice of base depend on the type of condition being treated and body site on which the medication will be applied (Table 2-3). The most basic distinction is whether the area to be treated is exudative or xerotic. For dry skin or conditions where moisturization is desired, the best base to choose is an ointment. Use after bathing/showering helps to seal moisture in the skin and the occlusive effect of the ointment helps retain the moisture. If a medicated ointment is used, absorption through the epidermis is greater than for a cream of the same potency. Creams are useful as less sticky/messy variants of ointments. Many patients will not use an ointment or will use it too sparingly due to its long-lasting stickiness and potential to stain clothing. Due to the increased water content, creams will absorb readily into the skin. For exudative lesions/conditions, use of a lotion or gel is useful, as they have drying properties. Another factor to keep in mind is the amount of hair in the area of application.

Table 2-3 Choice of Steroid Class by Site

SITE	COMMON STEROID CLASS	EXAMPLE
Scalp	Class I or II	Clobetasol or fluocinonide solution
Face/neck/ periorbital	Class V or VI	Desonide
Trunk/ extremities	Moderate inflammation: Class II–IV Recalcitrant/severe inflammation: Class I–II	Moderate: triamcinolone Severe: clobetasol
Genitalia	Class IV–VII	Acute treatment: class IV or less Chronic: not recommended
Acral	Up to Class I	Clobetasol/halobetasol

For patients with significant amounts of body hair or for scalp/pubic application, lotions, solutions, or foams are much more acceptable. Creams and ointments will mat the hair and will be challenging to apply.

The amount of a topical medicament to prescribe is an important factor in the success of topical therapy. Many patients come to the dermatologist using steroids of adequate potency, but are not applying enough of the medication to improve the condition. This may be due to concern of side effects, lack of understanding of how to apply a medication, or simply receiving too little medication for the body surface area to be treated. Guidelines for amounts of topical steroid based on body areas suggested by Long and Finaly are presented in Table 2-4. These suggestions are the minimum necessary for treatment of the given area, and in some cases more will be necessary for adequate treatment, especially of active dermatitis. These amounts can also be generalized to other classes of topical therapy such as retinoids, vitamin D derivatives, or topical immunotherapy. When counseling patients on the amount of a topical medicine to apply, the fingertip unit is a helpful way to describe the amount to use.

Table 2-4 Amounts of Topical Corticosteroid to Prescribe

AREA OF BODY	GRAMS REQUIRED FOR 1 APPLICATION	MINIMUM WEIGHT REQUIRED FOR ADULT MALE TO TREAT BID × 1 WEEK	FINGERTIP UNITS NEEDED FOR 1 APPLICATION
Face/neck	1.25	17.5	2.5
Trunk (single side)	3.5	49	7
Single arm	1.5	21	3
Single hand (one side)	0.25	3.5	1
One leg	3	42	6
One foot	1	15	2

Long CC, Finaly AY. The finger-tip unit—a new practical measure. *Clin Exp Dermatol.* 1991;16(6):444–447; Ference JD, Last AR. Choosing topical corticosteroids. *Am Fam Physician.* 2009;79(2):135–140; Hengge UR, Ruzicka T, Schwartz RA, et al. Adverse effects of topical glucocorticosteroids. *J Am Acad Dermatol.* 2006;54(1):5.

One fingertip unit is the amount of ointment that is applied from the tip of the finger to the distal interphalangeal joint on the index finger. This gives a rough standard amount to recommend. Table 2-4 describes the average number of fingertip units needed to treat any given body area.

Topical Medicaments

The majority of medications used in dermatology are used topically. The most commonly used classes of topical therapy are summarized in Table 2-5. While this table will not encompass every topical therapy, the most often used classes will be outlined. Specific therapies will be discussed in the appropriate chapters.

Probably the most commonly prescribed skin medications are corticosteroid preparations used for inflammatory conditions. These will be discussed in greater detail here, as this class of medication is by far the most often used medication in dermatology. There are multiple classification systems for describing the potency of a steroid. The basic assay to determine potency is the vasoconstrictor potency assay. In this test, the amount of skin blanching following application of a corticosteroid agent is measured. From this data, classifications of corticosteroids have been assigned. Some are based on the potency assay, and others are based on the chemical structure; these are summarized in Table 2-6. An alternate classification system is by the chemical structure of the molecule. This is mostly used for classification of corticosteroid allergic contact dermatitis (A, B, C, D1, and D2) and is not otherwise clinically helpful. If a patient is suspected of having a corticosteroid allergy, choosing a topical from group C may be helpful.

While a steroid cream may have the same percentage of medication (i.e., betamethasone dipropionate 0.05%, mometasone furoate 0.1%, or triamcinolone acetonide 0.1%), the actual potency of the medication may vary. The vehicle that the medication is contained in determines that actual potency. For instance, betamethasone dipropionate 0.05% in an ointment base in Diprolene ointment is class I potency, but the exact same medication in Diprosone lotion is class V. In general, a given corticosteroid is stronger in an ointment due to increased penetration of the epidermis and occlusion effect. Additionally, propylene glycol is also added to corticosteroid preparations, which will further increase the potency/effect of a given steroid preparation compared to the same agent without PG added in the preparation. There are many potential side effects from topical steroid application. The most common are application site skin irritation (66% of patients), atrophy (15%), and striae (15%). These potential side effects are summarized in Table 2-7.

When prescribing topical corticosteroids or any other topical agent, dispensing enough of the medication is important for successful therapy. If a generalized dermatitis is being treated with an adequate potency steroid such as triamcinolone 0.1% cream, but only 30 grams is dispensed, this therapy will not be successful despite an appropriate steroid being given. Minimum amounts based on body area are summarized in Table 2-4.

Another very commonly used topical medicament is topical antibiotics, both physician- and self-prescribed. Who has not met a patient using a "triple antibiotic" or neomycin ointment on a cut or wound? The common practice for many years following skin biopsies or surgery has been the application of a topical antibiotic. Recent evidence suggests this is unnecessary.

For uninfected clean surgical wounds or traumatic cuts/scrapes, dressing with plain white petrolatum is adequate and preferable. Use of an occlusive ointment for dressing is desirable as it keeps the wound bed moist and allows for faster wound healing. If there is no infection, use of an antibacterial only increases the risk for developing an allergic contact dermatitis to the antibacterial agent. Also, in patients treated with a topical antibacterial following

Table 2-5 Nonsteroidal Therapeutic Agents

CLASS OF MEDICATION	MECHANISM	INDICATIONS
Anti-inflammatory (noncorticosteroid)		
Tacrolimus	Inhibition of calcineurin	Atopic dermatitis (eczema), facial/genital psoriasis
Pimecrolimus	Inhibition of calcineurin	Atopic dermatitis (eczema), facial/genital psoriasis
Antineoplastic		
Diclofenac	Nonsteroidal anti-inflammatory	Actinic keratoses (AK)
Imiquimod	Toll-like receptor (TLR)-7 agonist	AK, superficial basal cell carcinoma, condyloma acuminatum
5-Fluorouracil	Pyrimidine analog, inhibits DNA and RNA synthesis	AK
Vitamin D analog Calcipotriene	Vitamin D3 derivative, mechanism unknown	Psoriasis
Antibiotics (rosacea)		
Metronidazole	Unknown (for rosacea)	Rosacea
Sodium sulfacetamide	Bacteriostatic sulfonamide; inhibits dihydropteroate synthetase	Rosacea, acne
Antibiotics (impetigo/SITL)		
Mupirocin	Bacterial isoleucyl transfer-RNA synthetase inhibitor	Methicillin-resistant *Staphyllococcus aureus* (MRSA) infections, impetigo, secondarily infected traumatic lesions (SITL)
Retapamulin	Pleuromutilin antibiotic, inhibits bacterial protein synthesis (50S ribosome)	Methicillin-sensitive *S. aureus* (MSSA) infections, impetigo, SITL
Neomycin	Bactericidal, binds to bacterial 30S ribosome	MSSA infections, impetigo, SITL
Bacitracin	Dephosphorylation of the C55-isoprenyl pyrophosphate; interferes with cell wall synthesis	MSSA infections, impetigo, SITL
Polymyxin	Increases permeability of cell membrane, gram-negative activity	MSSA infections, impetigo, SITL
Fusidic acid	Bacteriostatic; prevents translocation of elongation factor G; gram-positive activity	MSSA infections, impetigo, SITL
Combination therapy		
Betamethasone diproprionate/calcipotriene	Corticosteroid/vitamin D3 analog	Psoriasis
Benzoyl peroxide (BP)/clindamycin	Bactericidal through generation of reactive oxygen species/antibiotic	Acne
BP/tretinoin	Bactericidal through generation of reactive oxygen species/exact mechanism not known	Acne
BP/adapalene	Bactericidal through generation of reactive oxygen species/exact mechanism not known	Acne

CHAPTER 2 Topical Therapy

(Continued)

Table 2-5 Nonsteroidal Therapeutic Agents (*Continued*)

CLASS OF MEDICATION	MECHANISM	INDICATIONS
Combination therapy		
Keratolytics (salicylic acid, lactic acid, urea)	Keratolytic	Psoriasis, palmoplantar keratoderma
Retinoids (tretinoin, adapalene, tazarotene)	Exact mechanism not known; binds retinoic acid receptors, antiproliferative	Acne, psoriasis, lichen planus
Antifungals		
Terbinafine	Allylamine; reduces ergosterol synthesis; inhibits squalene epoxidase	Dermatophyte fungal infection
Econazole and other azoles	Interferes with the synthesis of ergosterol, increases membrane permeability	Dermatophyte fungal infection
Ciclopirox	Fungicidal, mechanism unknown	Dermatophyte fungal infection
Coal tars	Inhibits cell mitosis; mechanism unknown.	Psoriasis, seborrheic dermatitis
Anthralin	Inhibits T-cell lymphocytes; exact mechanism unknown	Psoriasis

biopsies, the infections that developed tended to be harder and more costly to treat than gram-negative infections.

For treatment of superficial bacterial infections of the skin, such as impetigo or a secondarily infected traumatic lesion, a topical agent such as bacitracin, neomycin, or retapamulin ointment is appropriate. Although not available in the United States, a common antibacterial used in Europe is fusidic acid. These agents all have excellent gram-positive coverage, though are not

Table 2-6 Corticosteroid Potency and Classification

CLASS	CLASS	ACTIVE INGREDIENT EXAMPLES	BRAND NAME EXAMPLES
I	Super-potent	clobetasol proprionate 0.05% halobetasol proprionate 0.05% diflorasone diacetate 0.05% betamethasone dipropionate 0.05%	Temovate o/c Clobex s/l Ultravate o/c Psorcon o Diprolene o/AF c
II	Intermediate	betamethasone dipropionate 0.05% triamcinolone acetonide 0.5% fluocinonide 0.05% mometasone furoate 0.1%	Diprosone ointment Kenalog Lidex o/c/s/g Elocon o
III	Moderate	betamethasone dipropionate 0.05%	Diprosone c
IV	Moderate	triamcinolone acetonide 0.1% mometasone furoate 0.1%	Kenalog Elocon c/l
V	Low	betamethasone dipropionate 0.05%	Diprosone l
VI	Low	desonide 0.05%	DesOwen c
VII	Over-the-counter	hydrocortisone acetate	

o, ointment; c, cream; l, lotion; s, spray/solution; g, gel

Table 2-7 Potential Side Effects of Topically Applied Corticosteroids

Cutaneous

Local irritation

Atrophy

Striae

Rosacea

Folliculitis

Facial/genital erythema and burning following steroid withdrawal

Worsening of bacterial skin infections

Worsening of fungal infections (including causing Majocchi granulomas)

Allergic contact dermatitis (steroid or preservative)

Telangiectasia

Systemic

Hypothalamal-pituitary-adrenal suppression

Glaucoma

Hypertension

Hyperglycemia

Septic necrosis of femoral head

Ocular cataracts

used for methicillin-resistant strains of *Staphylococcus aureus* (MRSA) infection. Mupirocin is approved and effective for use against topical MRSA infections, though bacterial resistance is increasing.

There are many other topical therapeutic agents used in dermatology. These agents are summarized in Table 2-5. Further discussion of each agent and for the respective indications are found in later chapters.

Conclusion

The choice between an ointment, cream, gel, or lotion may make the difference between resolution of a troubling condition and continued irritation. Topical steroids are very useful medications for treatment of inflammatory conditions. Choosing the right strength and base allows successful therapy and minimization of potential side effects. Many dermatologic conditions are successfully treated topically. Understanding the use of topical medications is key to successful nonsystemic therapy.

Suggested Reading

Ference JD, Last AR. Choosing topical corticosteroids. *Am Fam Physician*. 2009;79(2):135–140.

Hengge UR, Ruzicka T, Schwartz RA, et al. Adverse effects of topical glucocorticosteroids. *J Am Acad Dermatol*. 2006;54(1):5.

Long CC, Finaly AY. The finger-tip unit—a new practical measure. *Clin Exp Dermatol*. 1991;16(6):444–447.

Smack DP, Harrington AC, Dunn C, et al. Infection and allergy incidence in ambulatory surgery patients using white petrolatum vs bacitracin ointment. A randomized controlled trial. *JAMA*. 1996 Sep 25;276(12):972–977.

Tam CC, Elston DM. Allergic contact dermatitis caused by white petrolatum on damaged skin. *Dermatitis*. 2006;17(4):201–203.

Warshaw EM, Belsito DV, DeLeo VA, et al. North American Contact Dermatitis Group Patch-Test Results, 2003–2004 Study Period. *Dermatitis*. 2008;19(3):129–136.

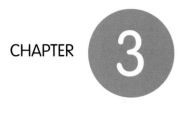

Procedures in Dermatologic Diagnosis and Therapy

Abel Jarell and Peter C. Schalock

There are many procedures commonly used by dermatologists that can be incorporated into the practice of all medical providers. Most dermatologic procedures require only a handful of supplies, and the techniques are relatively easy to master without extensive training. This chapter details the indications and techniques for the procedures most commonly used on the skin such that any provider can feel confident to perform them.

KOH Preparation for Examination for Fungal Elements

For the many dermatologic conditions that produce scale, superficial dermatophytosis should be considered. This question can be readily addressed with a potassium hydroxide (KOH) preparation. A 10% potassium hydroxide solution will digest the keratin in the tissue but leave most fungal forms intact for visualization under a microscope. This diagnostic method is used to confirm the presence or absence of fungal forms, including hyphae, spores, and pseudospores. It is important to note that even though certain fungi have characteristic appearances on microscopic examination, the exact species cannot be determined without a culture. When determination of a species is necessary, the organism can be cultured. Be aware that results may take 3 to 4 weeks for fungal growth to occur.

To obtain a specimen for examination, cleanse the surface of the skin with either an alcohol prep or soap and water. Allow the skin to dry. A #15 Bard-Parker blade is optimal for scraping to lift scale off the surface of the skin, taking care to scrape in a horizontal movement without cutting into the skin. See Figure 3-1 for an illustrated depiction of the procedure. The scale can either be swept onto a microscope glass slide with the blade, or the scale that is adherent to the edge of the blade can be directly wiped onto the slide. Alternatively, in especially robust flaky and dry scale, one microscope slide may be used to scrape the scale onto another microscope slide. In specimens that are moist owing to maceration of the area, for instance, in the toe web spaces, smear the moistened scale onto the slide.

After an amount of scale that can be visualized under the microscope has been obtained, use a coverslip to sweep all of the scale onto the center of the slide into a pile. The coverslip should be gently placed over the scale and a drop of KOH 10% solution is applied to the outer edge of the coverslip on the slide and allowed to spread throughout the underside of the coverslip by capillary action. An additional drop or two may be necessary, as well as slight pressure applied to various points on the coverslip to effect a complete spreading of the

KOH Preparation for microscopic analysis of scale for fungal forms

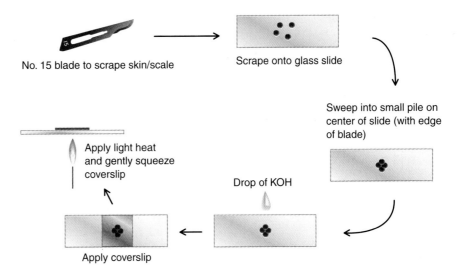

No. 15 blade to scrape skin/scale

Scrape onto glass slide

Sweep into small pile on center of slide (with edge of blade)

Drop of KOH

Apply light heat and gently squeeze coverslip

Apply coverslip

Figure 3-1 KOH preparation. Step-by-step depiction begins with scraping of skin using a No. 15 blade to obtain specimen.

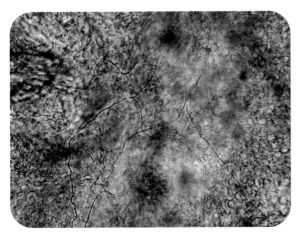

Figure 3-2 Positive KOH preparation. This slide demonstrates fungal forms. Note that they are often subtle and can be easily confused with cellular parts and other debris.

KOH solution, thereby enveloping the pile of scale. Stains such as methylene blue may be added to aid visualization. It is helpful to flatten the scale by applying moderate pressure with a fingertip to the coverslip. A small flame from a lit match or a lighter helps hasten the chemical reaction. The amount of heat should be enough to warm the underside of the glass slide but not enough to cause boiling of the KOH solution. This usually takes less than 5 seconds. It is best to allow 3 to 5 minutes for the chemical reaction to complete before viewing. Wipe the underside of the slide to remove any blackened carbon if it has been created by the heating flame, and place the slide on the microscope stage for viewing. To the novice, the microscopic exam can be an exercise in patience. Thoroughly and methodically scan the slide, sometimes focusing up and down to distinguish edges and shapes. A positive KOH preparation is demonstrated in Figure 3-2.

Scabies Preparation

The suspicion of scabies infestation is often high when a patient presents with a persistent itchy rash, often subtle with only few scattered red papules and excoriations. The index of suspicion is elevated when the patient reports a worsening of symptoms at night, when there has been a previous infestation either in the patient or a close contact, and when the patient is a nursing home resident. The diagnosis of scabies infestation can often be easily confirmed with the scabies preparation. However, false-negative results are common owing to poor technique or improper lesion selection.

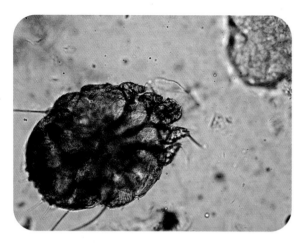

Figure 3-3 Positive scabies preparation. Note the organism of *Sarcoptes scabei var. hominis.*

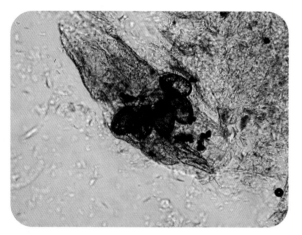

Figure 3-4 Scabies eggs from scraping of skin burrow.

The scabies preparation is a simple technique only requiring mineral oil, a scalpel or small curette (2 to 4 mm), glass slide, coverslip, and a light microscope. The cutaneous finding of a burrow, which is the tunnel that the female mite excavates within the epidermis to dwell and lay her eggs, is an ideal lesion to examine for scabies identification. Clinically, a burrow is typically in the range of 0.1 cm to 1.0 cm and appears as a wavy, sometimes thread-like lesion that is often white or somewhat gray. The preparation is performed by scraping away this lesion, often located in the web space of the fingers or sometimes on the scrotum in men or areolae in women. Local anesthetic with lidocaine is not necessary as the lesions are not typically tender, and the overlying burrow skin is without sensation. The scraping in this case is more aggressive than for KOH preparation, often drawing blood. The lesion is then wiped onto a glass microscope slide, engulfed in a drop of mineral oil, and finally mounted with a coverslip. This specimen can be examined under low power for either adult mites, eggs, or fecal pellets, also known as scybala. Any of these findings confirms the diagnosis, as in Figures 3-3 and 3-4.

The following procedures in this chapter generally require written consent from the patient; however, this requirement may vary by institution and by local regulations. It should be explained to the patient that when the procedure is performed, there are risks that include, but are not limited to, bleeding, infection, nerve damage, scar formation, danger to underlying structures, failure to make the diagnosis, lesion recurrence, and pain. The risks are low, but vary by patient, procedure site, and reason for performing the procedure. Table 3-1 presents suggestions for type of biopsy to perform based on the suspected type of lesion being sampled.

Shave Biopsy

Establishing the diagnosis by shave or tangential biopsy is appropriate for a variety of lesions, especially lesions that are raised, pedunculated, or easily palpable. It can be used for flat, macular, or very rarely subcuticular nodules, but more care is required. Because of its relative ease, it is the procedure most frequently used for obtaining tissue.

The shave biopsy, along with all of the following procedures, should be performed with a "clean technique." This does not require the use of sterile gloves or a sterile field; however, take precautions to prevent infection. The clean procedure is one in which a quick wipe-down of the area to be shaved is performed (usually with an alcohol swab, Betadine prep, or chlorhexidine-soaked gauze). The provider performing the procedure should wear clean gloves that need not be sterile.

The procedure begins by choosing the site to be biopsied. Local anesthesia is obtained with lidocaine with or without epinephrine, often less than 1 to 2 cc around and under the lesion. Flatter lesions can be elevated and made more accessible for shaving by simply infiltrating underneath the lesion with local anesthetic, thereby creating a wheal underneath the lesion. For a raised lesion, enough of the lesion should be surrounded by blade so as to sharply remove it from its base. Typical cutting devices for the shave biopsy include the No. 10 or

Table 3-1 Suggested Procedure by Lesion Type

SUSPECTED LESION TYPE	PROCEDURE SUGGESTED
Neoplasm	
Basal cell carcinoma	Shave
Actinic keratosis	Shave
Squamous cell carcinoma in situ (Bowen)	Shave
Squamous cell carcinoma	Shave
Keratoacanthoma	Shave
Atypical/dysplastic nevus (<5 mm)	Punch or shave
Atypical/dysplastic nevus (<5 and >10 mm)	Shave
Atypical/dysplastic nevus (10 mm or greater)	Excision
Melanoma (nonfacial)	Excision or multiple punch biopsies
Melanoma (facial)	Multiple punch biopsies
Other benign neoplasm (superficial morphology, i.e., seborrheic keratosis)	Punch/shave
Other benign neoplasm (deep nodular, i.e., lipomas or cyst)	Punch biopsy
Inflammatory	
Dermatitis of any type	Punch
Psoriasis	Punch
Infection (i.e., cellulitis/ impetigo/deep fungal)	Punch

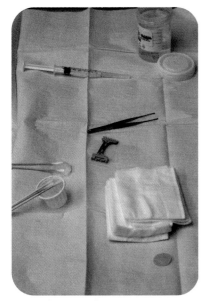

Figure 3-5 A typical tray used for shave excision or biopsies. The shave biopsy technique is simple to master with little experience. Take care when biopsying pigmented lesions as transecting the base of the melanoma makes histologic evaluation of the true depth of the lesion impossible.

15 blade scalpel or a flat razor. Either of these cutting tools is appropriate for the shave biopsy and selection is user dependent. Most will agree that the highly malleable straight flat razor blade on a handle (i.e., Dermablade) is much easier to use in general, but a No. 15 blade offers better accessibility to lesions in tighter locations, i.e., the medial canthus.

An appropriate specimen is one in which there is sampling down to the dermis. Too often the shave biopsy is too superficial to render an accurate diagnosis. The specimen may be stabilized using a forceps, especially if removal of the lesion requires any amount of sawing of the specimen. If a forceps is used for traction, one should be extra careful not to crush the specimen, as this may result in artifacts that interfere with histologic evaluation. This can best be avoided by using a toothed forceps as opposed to one with flat tongs. Hemostasis is obtained by manual pressure and chemical cautery, such as 20% aluminum chloride solution. Place the specimen in a 10% formaldehyde solution for transport and processing. A typical shave biopsy set-up is shown in Figure 3-5.

Punch Biopsy

The punch biopsy is another technique frequently performed in the office that requires very little equipment and modest technical expertise. This technique can be used to obtain tissue in which one suspects that pathology lies in the dermis or deeper. Most inflammatory conditions manifest their pathology at this depth, as do many tumors of the skin, including melanoma.

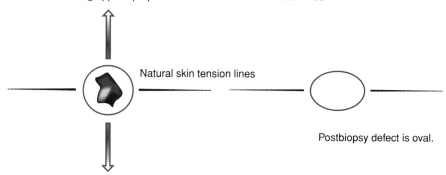

Skin stretching applied perpendicular to natural skin tension lines

Natural skin tension lines

Postbiopsy defect is oval.

Figure 3-6 Punch biopsy technique for optimal defect closure. If tension is applied in the axis perpendicular to the natural skin tension lines (left side, prebiopsy with lesion present), then after the punch procedure is performed, the final defect will be in the shape of an oval that is oriented in a direction parallel to the skin tension lines (right side of figure with lesion removed).

Successful performance of this technique entails laying out all of the necessary tools in advance, including the punch biopsy device, forceps, scissors, specimen container with fixative (usually 10% formaldehyde solution), gauze, bandage, ointment (white petrolatum), and needle driver with suture material if necessary (see below). Punch biopsy devices vary in size from 1.5 mm to 12 mm. The most commonly used biopsy tool and one that usually provides adequate tissue for analysis is the 4-mm tool. As with the shave biopsy preparation above, identify the site, wipe it clean with an alcohol swab or sterile cleaning agent of choice, and anesthetize with local anesthetic. For optimal closure, the tissue around the biopsy specimen should be forcefully stretched in a direction that is perpendicular to the natural skin tension lines. The circular biopsy plunger can then be pressed and twisted into the skin, often to the hilt depending on site, and when the device is removed and the forceful stretching is relaxed, the created defect will naturally fall into an oval that has its axis parallel to the natural skin tension lines. Understanding of the surgical anatomy is critical, because the underlying vasculature and nerves must be avoided. Care should be taken not to excessively disrupt the tissue of interest (Figs. 3-6, 3-7). A pair of forceps should be used to gently grasp the tissue, preferably near the base or absolute lowest point of the specimen, usually in the subcutaneous tissue, and the tissue specimen is cut with scissors as low as possible. For punch biopsies 1.5 mm or 2 mm, it is generally not necessary to place a suture for closure. Gentle pressure on the site for 1 to 4 minutes will often give hemostasis. Various types of suture materials and their uses are discussed in Table 3.2. For punch biopsies of 3 mm or larger, most clinicians will use a suture, although it is debatable whether or not a suture is necessary for defects less than 4 mm. Instead of sutures, some prefer to pack the wound with hemostatic gelatin sponge (Gelfoam). One to two single interrupted stitches are usually all that are required, oriented perpendicular to the natural skin tension lines (Fig. 3-8). Apply white petrolatum and a bandage over the defect. For the smaller biopsies, less than or equal to 3 mm, the scar is nearly imperceptible several months after the procedure regardless of whether sutures are used for closure. When sutures are used on the face, it is best to remove them in 5 to 7 days. For other sites on the body sutures are generally removed in 12 to 14 days. For punch biopsies more than 4 mm, buried vertical mattress sutures are recommended in addition to epidermal sutures to achieve acceptable cosmesis. Punch biopsies larger than 8 mm are not recommended; these lesions are best removed by elliptical excision.

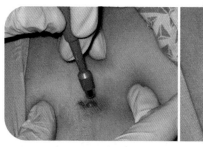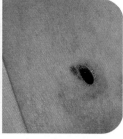

Figure 3-7 Punch biopsy for optimal closure, 6-mm trephine. Left-hand dominant procedure—right middle finger and thumb are used to stretch the skin perpendicular to the natural skin tension lines. A circular punch performed with the left hand results in an oval-shaped defect, which will close with minimized redundant/puckered skin ("dog ears").

Table 3-2 Suture Types

BRAND NAME	MATERIAL	ABSORBS?	TIME TO ABSORB (DAYS)	SITE USED
Dexon	Polyglycolic acid	Yes	90	Subcutaneous
Vicryl	Polyglactin 910	Yes	80	Subcutaneous
PDS	Polydioxanone	Yes	180	Subcutaneous
Monocryl	Poliglecaprone	Yes	~100	Subcutaneous
	Catgut	Yes	90	Subcutaneous
	Steel	No		Orthopedic/cardiac
Mersilene/Dacron	Polyester	No		Epidermal closure
Ethibond/Dermalon	Nylon monofilament	No		Epidermal closure
Surgilon	Nylon braided	No		Epidermal closure
Prolene	Polypropylene	No		Epidermal closure
	Silk	No		Epidermal closure–often eyelids

Elliptical Excision

An elliptical excision requires more advanced surgical techniques. The risks of surgical excision include scar formation, pain, nerve and underlying anatomical structure damage, bleeding, and infection, among others. Indications for surgical excision include both complete histopathologic analysis and surgical cure by complete removal. Excisions are generally performed for benign lesions including epidermal inclusion and pilar cysts, lipomas, dermatofibromas, and melanocytic nevi, as well as to remove malignant lesions such as basal and squamous cell carcinoma or malignant melanoma.

Unlike the previously described techniques, elliptical excision should be performed by establishing a sterile field as opposed to a "clean" field. Before setting up the sterile field, infiltrate local anesthetic subcutaneously into the area that will be excised. Prep and drape the area of the excision using sterile technique. This entails first performing a chlorhexidine or Betadine scrub. Surgical drapes or towels are then placed around the lesion to be excised, giving about 2 to 3 cm of clearance in all directions. Throughout the set-up, take care to not contaminate the field. Before the procedure begins, ensure all of the necessary equipment is laid out and kept sterile on an easily accessible tray. A surgical excision

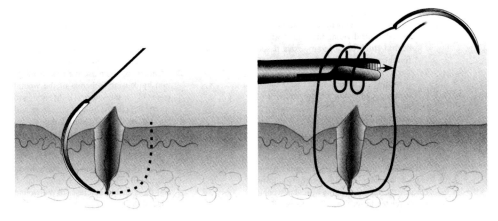

Figure 3-8 Simple interrupted skin suture secured with instrument tie. Reprinted with permission from Fleischer GR, Ludwig S, Henretig FM, et al., eds. *Textbook of Pediatric Emergency Medicine,* 5th ed. Philadelphia: Lippincott Williams & Wilkins, 2005.

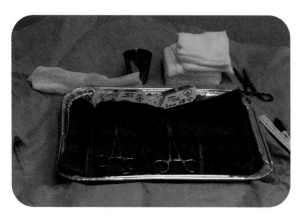

Figure 3-9 A typical excision tray set-up.

tray should contain at a minimum: scissors; toothed forceps; suture material (absorbable suture for the dermal layers and nonabsorbable suture for the epidermal layer); needle driver; and scalpel (usually fitted with No. 15 blade) (Fig. 3-9). There should be two types of scissors, one for cutting sutures and another, either a Kay or curved baby Metzenbaum based on personal preference, for undermining. Optionally, skin hooks may be used.

The technique is performed by first outlining the lesion to be excised, with margins if necessary. For basal cell carcinomas, for example, a 4-mm margin all around the clinically apparent tumor can expect to produce a cure rate of greater than 90%. A football-shaped ellipse with 30-degree angle tips, oriented with the long axis parallel to natural skin tension lines is then outlined around the lesion. The scalpel is used to sharply trace the outline and cut down to the level of the superficial subcutaneous tissue. Care should be taken to cut precisely perpendicular to the surface of the skin and to not bevel the edges. The entire ellipse is then removed by cutting sharply along the bottom of the specimen in a single plane either with scissors or scalpel. The specimen can then be submitted *in toto* for histological analysis. Hemostasis should be obtained with electrocautery or electrodessication. Ensure the skin edges are not burned. Use a minimum amount of electrocautery to prevent extensive tissue necrosis. Because cutaneous excisions rarely involve the violation of any major vessel, hemostasis should typically be achieved with minimal effort.

To begin the closure, either Kay or Metzenbaum scissors are used in both blunt and sharp fashion for undermining of the tissue surrounding the ellipse. The importance of undermining cannot be overstated. Undermining is necessary for both tissue reapproximation for ease of tissue movement, as well as for improved final cosmetic appearance. The deep dermal layers are reapproximated using inverted interrupted vertical mattress absorbable sutures, followed by the epidermal layer using a running suture or simple interrupted stitches (Fig. 3-10). While the entire procedure can be performed without an assistant, having an assistant present increases the overall efficiency of the procedure.

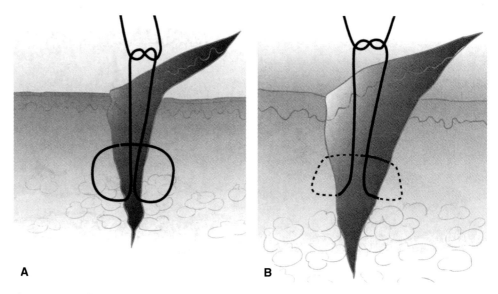

A   **B**

Figure 3-10 A: The buried subcutaneous suture. **B:** The horizontal dermal stitch. Reprinted with permission from Fleischer GR, Ludwig S, Henretig FM, et al., eds. *Textbook of Pediatric Emergency Medicine,* 5th ed. Philadelphia: Lippincott Williams & Wilkins, 2005.

Cryosurgery

Cryosurgery is a treatment modality that has become a mainstay in dermatological procedures for the purpose of destroying benign, premalignant, and malignant conditions. It is a technique that is mobile, expedient, and effective. With proper technique, it can be utilized with an excellent cosmetic result. Without proper employment, however, it can be dangerous, as the local destruction is nondiscriminating of adjacent tissue. Cryosurgery is most frequently used to treat such entities as verruca, actinic keratoses, molluscum contagiosum, lentigines, dermatofibromas, and some nonmelanoma skin cancers.

The goal of cryosurgery is selective necrosis of targeted tissues, while leaving the surrounding tissue intact without injury. Maximum destructive effect can be accomplished with multiple freeze-thaw cycles. Liquid nitrogen, which has a boiling point of approximately −196° C, is the typically used agent. It can be applied to the selected lesion using a hand-held firing canister device or with a cotton-tip applicator. For lesions such as actinic keratoses, warts, and mollusca, cryotherapy is applied to the lesion until the lesion is completely frozen. It should take approximately 15 seconds before completely thawing. It is important to note that the cryotherapy should not be applied for a full 15 seconds, rather, it only takes generally 3 to 5 seconds of cryotherapy application to achieve a 15-second ice ball. This is generally a safe amount of time for an ice ball to form that will not cause any damage to the surrounding tissue. For recalcitrant warts, the time of application can be extended to 7 to 8 seconds, which will produce a thaw time of up to 30 seconds. Patients should be extensively counseled on the risks. Short-term reactions include burning/itching and pain at the application site, erythema lasting hours to days, and crusting lasting 1 to 2 weeks. A blister may form at the site. Long-term side effects include hyper- and/or hypopigmentation, as well as scar formation. Again, these risks can usually be avoided with less aggressive cryotherapy, which stays within the time frames outlined above.

Conclusion

In this chapter, the common dermatologic procedures are reviewed. In general, they are simple to learn and require only a small number of supplies. Choosing the appropriate procedure based on the lesion type is essential (i.e., performing a punch biopsy for dermatitis and not a shave biopsy). As the provider becomes more comfortable with the techniques described, they can be incorporated into the care of dermatologic patients.

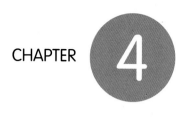

Care and Maintenance of Normal Skin

Falguni Asrani and Molly Wanner

The skin serves a variety of important functions including regulation, defense, and protection. The skin protects us from the elements: from wind, cold, heat, and ultraviolet (UV) light, and is a first line of defense again infection. It is an organ of temperature regulation, sensation, and excretion, and allows us to prevent water loss to the environment.

The efficacy of the skin barrier will affect skin's ability to protect. Eczema patients have a deficiency of their skin barrier that makes them more susceptible to infection and inflammation. Although patients with normal skin may not have an internal predisposition to a poor skin barrier, the environment has external forces that influence the skin barrier. As a result, even normal skin requires care and maintenance.

This chapter will review the cleansing, moisturizing, and sun protection routine that normal skin requires. It will review how different environments create different needs, how skin through the years changes in its requirements, and it will present ways to protect and preserve the skin barrier.

Skin Barrier

The care and maintenance of normal skin begins with an understanding of the skin barrier. The skin's barrier is at the outermost surface of the skin and is called the stratum corneum. The role of the stratum corneum is to prevent water loss, and minimizing water loss is crucial for normal skin functioning. Water and the water gradient within the stratum corneum drive the function of enzymes necessary for normal skin turnover. Internal and external conditions can affect the water-retaining ability of the stratum corneum, and routine skin care can enhance the efficacy of the stratum corneum.

The stratum corneum is comprised of skin cells and intercellular lipid material. These two components form the "brick and mortar" structure of the skin that surrounds and protects our internal organs. Inside the skin cells of the stratum corneum, there is a substance called the "natural moisturizing factor" (NMF) that in combination with intracellular lipids prevents water loss.

SKIN BARRIER CORNEOCYTES

The bricks of the skin barrier are called the corneocytes of the stratum corneum. The corneocytes start as undifferentiated skin cells called keratinocytes in the basal layer of the epidermis; these are gradually pushed outward as they undergo changes ultimately designed to create the skin barrier that protects us. Corneocytes do not have intracellular organelles and rather, contain the NMF. Corneocytes are surrounded by a strong, protective shell called the cornified cell envelope, which protects the corneocytes from mechanical damage, and are linked by corneodesmosomes, which hold the cells together.

The NMF is a potent attractor of water that keeps the skin hydrated, corneocytes plump and healthy, and the skin barrier tight and flexible. The NMF is also critical for creating the aqueous environment important for normal skin turnover or desquamation. The NMF draws water from the deeper layers of the skin and may draw water from the environment as well.

An insoluble protein called profilaggrin is dephosphorylated to form filaggrin, which is subsequently altered in the outmost layers of the skin to form the NMF. The NMF is comprised of amino acids, organic acids, urea, inorganic acids, and ions such as calcium and magnesium.

SKIN BARRIER INTERCELLULAR LIPIDS

The mortar of the skin barrier is comprised of ceramides, cholesterol, and free fatty acids. These lipids are bipolar, and when combined, form alternating hydrophilic and hydrophobic lipid bilayers. It is not only the presence of these lipids, but their ratios that determine the efficacy of the mortar. Cholesterol is thought to provide the structure and stabilize the bulk of the material, which is comprised of ceramides.

The strength of the skin barrier depends on the quantity and quality of the materials, and disease states such as atopic dermatitis or congenital disorders called ichthyoses are characterized by compromised building blocks. Patients with atopic dermatitis have been found to have mutations in filaggrin and low levels of ceramides, which in part explains the ineffective skin barrier seen in these patients.

SKIN BARRIER AND THE ENVIRONMENT

Even in patients with "normal" skin, a variety of exogenous factors can affect the skin barrier. Environmental conditions such as temperature, humidity, seasonal change, and UV light alter the skin barrier, with UV light being particularly harmful. Temperature, too hot or cold, but particularly too cold, can be problematic. Cold air holds less moisture than warm air and cold reduces the mobility and flexibility of the skin. Dry environments are not detrimental to the skin barrier, per se, as the skin will accommodate. However, shifting from a humid to a dry environment can delay barrier recovery. Thus, a patient who lives year-round in a dry climate like Arizona will have better barrier function than a patient who travels to different climates or who lives in an environment with seasonal changes from humid to dry.

Efforts to cleanse the skin can damage the skin barrier; even routine cleansing can remove much of the soluble NMF from the skin. Cleansing can also harm the skin barrier because many cleansers have a high pH, which triggers breakdown of the corneodesmosomes that hold corneocytes together. Aging decreases the NMF, and the skin barrier becomes less effective over time. Conditions of stress, which lead to elevated glucocorticoids or even medications that lower cholesterol, can alter the skin barrier. Thus, the care and maintenance of normal skin will vary with environmental conditions, the type of cleansing required, the age of the patient, and even medications.

Cleansers

Cleansing is accomplished using surfactants, which are molecules with hydrophilic and hydrophobic moieties. Surfactants such as sodium tallowate and sodium cocoate are present in soap. Synthetic surfactants such as sodium cocoyl isethionate are used in synthetic cleansers, called syndets. These molecules remove dirt and bacteria from the skin, but also have the secondary effect of damaging the skin barrier. These secondary effects are due to alteration of the skin's normal pH (5.5), alteration in ability of proteins in the skin to bind water after cleansing, a decrease of the NMF, damage to the lipid layers, or reduction of lipids in the skin.

The type of cleansing required depends on the amount of dirt and bacteria to remove as well as on environmental and patient characteristics. Aggressive surfactants may be needed to remove heavy dirt. On the other hand, in conditions of cool temperatures or low humidity, gentle cleansing is recommended. Gentle cleansing is also more appropriate in older patients who are predisposed to a less effective skin barrier.

Soaps such as Ivory or soap detergent combinations such as Irish Spring and Dial are alkaline lipid formulations with a pH of 9 to 10 that can effectively solubilize dirt or other materials from the skin. Because soaps are equally efficacious at stripping the natural lipids and moisturizers of the skin as well, soaps are best reserved when the removal of dirt, environmental pollutants, bacteria, or oil is required. Even glycerin-based transparent soaps, while milder, have an alkaline pH that can be irritating. If aggressive cleaning is needed, it should be used in combination with moisturizers to replace lost moisture to avoid damaging the skin barrier.

When heavy cleaning is not required, patients are advised to use gentle cleansers that are pH balanced similarly to the skin. These syndet cleansers, such as Dove, Olay, or Cetaphil have a pH of 5.5 to 7. Syndets are formulated using synthetic surfactants, most commonly sodium cocoyl isethionate. The formulation of a cleanser as a liquid, instead of a bar, may further facilitate gentle cleansing.

Liquid body washes are formulated either as a solution of surfactants or in some cases, in combination with emollients as a moisturizing wash. Moisturizing washes deposit lipids to protect the skin barrier during the cleansing process and are the mildest type of cleanser. Moisturizing cleansers are especially useful during the winter season for older patients.

Facial cleansers tend to have gentler ingredients than body washes and can be formulated as foaming or nonfoaming cleansers. Foaming cleansers use mild surfactants, while nonfoaming cleansers use emollient cleansers instead of surfactants and are the mildest of all. Nonfoaming cleansing lotions or milks can even be wiped off (instead of rinsed) to further enhance gentleness. Nonfoaming cleansers are best reserved for older patients. Foaming cleansers may be preferred by younger patients who may not like or need an emollient residue left on the skin after cleansing. Cleansers can be combined with materials to remove make-up as well.

Moisturizers

A moisturizer is necessary if the skin barrier has been altered through the normal aging process or via exogenous factors such as a cleansing routine. A moisturizer can repair the skin barrier and lead to decreased bacterial colonization. Recall that the skin barrier is formed by corneocytes filled with NMF and an intercellular lipid bilayer comprised of ceramides, cholesterol, and free fatty acids. Moisturizers simulate the NMF and/or the lipid bilayer to enhance skin barrier repair. Although moisturizers can hydrate the skin somewhat, moisturizers primarily function through prevention of water loss, which facilitates the body's own barrier repair mechanisms.

The NMF is a potent attractor of water; the NMF corollary in moisturizers is called a humectant. Like the NMF, humectants such as glycerin, sorbitol, urea, and alpha hydroxyl acids pull water into the outmost layer of the skin. 2-Pyrrolidone-5-carboxylic acid is reported to be a particularly effective humectant. Humectants such as alpha hydroxyl acids may also increase skin elasticity.

Ingredients that mimic the effects of the lipid bilayer are emollients and occlusives, which seal the skin and decrease water loss. Moisturizers can occlude the skin and/or interact with intercellular lipids in the stratum corneum to facilitate "moisture," that is, water retention in the skin. Occlusives such as petrolatum, lanolin, mineral oil, dimethicone, beeswax, and silicone form an occlusive barrier to prevent water loss. Emollients such as cholesterol, squalene, and fatty acids fill in spaces between desquamating corneocytes to seal the skin. Physiologic lipids such as cholesterol, fatty acids, and ceramides penetrate to deeper layers of the skin, whereas petroleum only penetrates the very superficial layers of the stratum corneum.

Most moisturizers utilize a combination of humectants and emollients or occlusives. Creating an occlusive barrier is more effective in combination with a humectant to bring water to the stratum corneum. Using a humectant alone will draw water to the outer surface of the skin, which will be lost to the environment with an impaired barrier. However, moisturizers without humectants may also make skin more susceptible to irritation.

The ingredients of a moisturizer and the proportions of these ingredients can affect outcome. A study of the effect of moisturizer use on normal skin showed that moisturizers can increase or decrease transepidermal water loss depending on the components of the moisturizer. When physiologic lipids of the skin barrier (cholesterol, ceramides, and fatty acids) are used as emollients, all three components must be present, or barrier repair is impaired. Moisturizers can also be created with a positive (cationic), negative (anionic), or neutral charge. A cationic lotion can bind to the slightly negative keratin proteins in the stratum corneum and may offer long-lasting moisture.

Moisturizers can be formulated as creams, lotions, ointments, oils, pastes, and gels. In a simple classification, moisturizers can be described as oil-in-water emulsions (lotions); water-in-oil emulsions (creams); or oil-only moisturizers (petrolatum). A more detailed description of moisturizer formulations has been described elsewhere (Chapter 2). In general, creams (water-in-oil emulsions) provide more effective hydration than oil-in-water emulsions; however, patients often prefer oil-in-water lotions for ease of application.

In terms of efficacy, petroleum jelly is the most effective moisturizer and reduces transepidermal water loss by 99%, followed by creams, and then lotions. Lotions are best suited for use in the summer. Lotions may not provide enough moisture during the winter, particularly in climates characterized by low humidity and low temperatures. Traveling on airplanes in low-humidity environments or from humid to dry places may require the use of a cream. For older patients, who have less natural moisturizer in the skin and may be on cholesterol-lowering agents, petroleum jelly may be necessary. The aggressiveness of the cleansing routine will also influence the type of moisturizer required.

Sun Protection

Sunlight emits mainly infrared, visible, and ultraviolet (UV) light, although other wavelengths are also present. Consisting of UVA (315 to 400 nm), UVB (280 to 315 nm), and UVC (100 to 280 nm), ultraviolet radiation is instrumental in the development of skin cancer and photoaging. UVA comprises the majority of UV light, about 96.5%, reaching the earth. UVB represents the remainder as UVC is absorbed by the ozone layer. UV light in general is affected by geographical location on the earth, time of day, and weather conditions, although UVA light, in particular, is affected less so than other wavelengths.

Table 4-1   American Academy of Dermatology Be Sun Smart^{SM} Guidelines

- **Generously apply a broad-spectrum, water-resistant sunscreen** with a sun protection factor (SPF) of at least 15 to all exposed skin. "Broad-spectrum" provides protection from both ultraviolet A (UVA) and ultraviolet B (UVB) rays. Reapply approximately every 2 hours, even on cloudy days, and after swimming or sweating.

- **Wear protective clothing,** such as a long-sleeved shirt, pants, a wide-brimmed hat, and sunglasses, where possible.

- **Seek shade** when appropriate, remembering that the sun's rays are strongest between 10 AM and 4 PM. If your shadow is shorter than you are, seek shade.

- **Protect children** from sun exposure by playing in the shade, using protective clothing and applying sunscreen.

- **Use extra caution near water, snow, and sand** as they reflect the damaging rays of the sun, which can increase your chance of sunburn.

- **Get vitamin D safely** through a healthy diet that may include vitamin supplements. Don't *seek* the sun.

- **Avoid tanning beds.** Ultraviolet light from the sun and tanning beds can cause skin cancer and wrinkling. If you want to look like you've been in the sun, consider using a sunless self-tanning product, but continue to use sunscreen with it.

- **Check your birthday suit on your birthday.** If you notice anything changing, growing, or bleeding on your skin, see a dermatologist. Skin cancer is very treatable when caught early.

http://www.aad.org/public/sun/smart.html

UVA rays, the longest UV waves, penetrate deep into the skin to enter the dermis. UVA 2 (320 to 340 nm) represents 95% of UVA rays reaching the earth. UVA 1 (340 to 400 nm) comprises the remainder. UVA causes immunosuppression and DNA damage by reactive oxygen species that can lead to skin cancer. UVA rays are constantly present throughout the day and can penetrate the normal window glass surfaces.

UVB rays are the major contributors to sunburn and most sunscreens are targeted to protect against UVB, unless specified otherwise. Like UVA, UVB causes immunosuppression and DNA damage. UVB is absorbed by DNA and causes damage by cross-linking adjacent pyrimidines in the DNA. The strength of UVB rays changes with weather conditions and times of the day. UVB rays are the strongest at midday, and sun avoidance at peak hours is recommended (Table 4-1). Window glass protects against UVB.

SUN PROTECTION RECOMMENDATIONS

Because UV light is a known carcinogen, blockage of UVA and UVB is central to the prevention of skin cancer and photoaging changes such as wrinkling and pigmentary changes. All races, irrespective of ethnicity, should apply sunscreen. Although patients with skin of color will have natural sun protection, protection against UVA and UVB is incomplete, and patients are still susceptible to skin cancer. All age groups, including children and the elderly, should use sun protection. Very young children, under 6 months of age, should not use sunscreens as the sun protection modality. Two concerning issues in infants are their increased body surface to volume ratio and sunscreens inherent decrease in production of perspiration and thus the potential to cause overheating in young infants who rely on perspiration for heat loss.

Sun avoidance is the most effective means to protection. Sunbathing should be avoided, and tanning beds should not be used. Sunscreens and physical barriers are important additional modalities in the practice of sun safety. Those who practice sun safety may be susceptible to low vitamin D. Adequate vitamin D obtained through diet or supplementation is recommended by the American Academy of Dermatology.

SUNSCREENS

Sunscreens filter UVA, UVB, or both UVA and UVB light. Both chemical and physical sunscreens exist. Physical sunscreens reflect and/or absorb light depending on the sunscreen particle size. They are best for sensitive skin. Titanium dioxide and zinc oxide are examples of physical sunscreens. Chemical sunscreens absorb light. Chemical sunscreens are often unstable and are combined together to improve stability. They are not recommended for children less than 2 years of age, due to the potential for systemic absorption.

The American Academy of Dermatology recommends that all patients, of all races, use a broad spectrum sunscreen with UVA and UVB protection and SPF 30 throughout the year. The sunburn protection factor (SPF) is primarily a measure of UVB and UVA II (320 to 340 nm), but not UVA I (340 to 400 nm). SPF is defined as: the ratio of UV radiation dose required to produce recognizable redness on skin that has been protected with a sunscreen to the UV radiation dose required to produce the same redness on unprotected skin.

In other words, a person who applies a sunscreen of SPF 15 should be able to stay 15 times longer in the sun without encountering erythema. The difference between an SPF 15 and an SPF 30 is that SPF 15 filters out 94% of UVB radiation while SPF 30 filters 97%. It cannot be emphasized enough that SPF is a measure of protection against sunburn not sun damage, and as a result, other sun safe behaviors are required to prevent sun damage. Sunscreens, which prevent sunburn, should not be used to allow sun overexposure as such behavior could potentially lead to an increase in sun damage. It has been demonstrated that exposure to UV at suberythema doses can induce DNA damage. Chemical sunscreens that block UVB include Padimate O (octodimethyl PABA), octyl methoxycinnamate, cinoxate, octyl salicylate, homosalate, octocrylene, camphor derivatives, and ensulizole. Physical sunscreens such as titanium dioxide and zinc oxide protect against UVB rays, and in some cases against UVA rays.

The assessment of UVA protection is less well defined and varies world wide. The situation is further complicated by the fact that many sunscreens that claim to protect against UVA do not protect against UVA 1. A four-star rating system in the United States has been proposed to aid in determining which sunscreens have adequate UVA protection. Ingredients with known UVA blocking effects include butyl methoxydibanzoylmethane (avobenzone, Parsol 1789), menthyl anthranilate; terephthalydene dicamphor sulphonic acid (Mexoryl SX, Ecamsule), drometrizole trisiloxane (Mexoryl XL), oxybenzone; Tinosorb, titanium dioxide, and zinc oxide. Some of these filters also block UVB. Mexoryl XL is not available in the United States. Oxybenzone, titanium dioxide, and zinc oxide have the disadvantage of having relatively low UVA 1 (> 340 nm) efficacy. Avobenzone is limited by its inherent instability, although it can be stabilized if combined with other sunscreens such as octocrylene, Tinosorb, or micronized zinc oxide or titanium dioxide. Look at labels for avobenzone combined with octocrylene, Helioplex by Neutrogena, or Active Photobarrier Complex by Aveeno to ensure that avobenzone is stabilized.

Even if the correct ingredients are chosen, the sunscreen must be applied appropriately. The SPF is based on the use of a sunscreen layer that is 2 mg/cm^2. However, patients routinely apply less than 25% to 50% of this amount. This underapplication results in SPF that is far less than that on the bottle. The application of a sunscreen layer that is 1 mg/cm^2 will lead to an actual SPF that is the square root of the original SPF and an application that is 0.5 mg/cm^2 will lead to an SPF that is the fourth root of the original SPF. Thus, if a 0.5 mg/cm^2 is applied SPFs of 4, 8, and 16 become 1.4, 1.7, and 2.0. If SPF 100 is underapplied by 50%, the SPF becomes 10. So, even a high SPF will not compensate for under-application. Nevertheless, some argue that sunscreens with higher SPF prevent more suberythemal effects.

The American Academy of Dermatology recommends the application of 1 ounce, which is about enough to fill a shot glass, to cover the exposed areas of the body properly. Sunscreen should be applied 15 to 30 minutes before going in the sun and reapplied every 2 hours. Use of a sunscreen daily, rather than intermittently, better protects against UV damage. After swimming or sweating, even water-resistant sunscreens should be reapplied. The SPF of water-resistant sunscreens reflects the sun protection factor achieved after a total of 40 minutes of water contact. Very water-resistant corresponds to a total of 80 minutes of water contact, and very, very resistant corresponds to a total of 160 minutes of water contact.

PHYSICAL BARRIERS

Sun protection clothing, hats, sunglasses, and window filters all provide physical barriers to sun exposure. Clothing provides more UVB than UVA protection. The degree of protection depends on the weave, thickness, and color of the fabric. Sun protection provided by clothing is known as UPF, or "UV protection factor" and is equivalent to SPF. UPF increases after washing due to shrinkage of the clothing after the wash and decreases if clothing is stretched. If clothing is worn close to the skin, there is less scattering of light and therefore, less protection. Cotton t-shirts provide a UPF of 5 to 9, and even less when wet. In contrast to cotton, wool clothing has a UPF greater than 15. Black stockings have a UPF of 1.5 to 3 depending on the thickness. UPF of clothing can be increased by washing clothing with UV absorbers such as Tinosorb.

Sun protection offered by hats also depends on the material, weave, and brim. If a hat is held to the light, and light passes easily through the hat, the protection is unlikely to be effective. Wide-brimmed hats with tight weaves are recommended; however, even a wide-brimmed hat (>7.5 cm) has SPF as little as 2 for the chin and 3 for the cheeks. Sunglasses that absorb UVB and UVA light are recommended, and expensive brands do not guarantee protection. Look for glasses that protect against UV absorption up to 400 nm or that meet the American National Standards Institute (ANSI) UV requirements. Clear window glass provides protection against wavelengths below 320 nm, while tinted glass protects against UVA and visible light. Plastic film can be purchased to block UVA.

Conclusion

Sun protection, cleansers, and moisturizers affect the health of the skin. Good skin care depends on both patient characteristics and environmental conditions. Cleansing and moisturizing choices will change throughout the year and over time. Sun protection, on the other hand, should remain a constant part of the daily routine of all patients at all times of the year.

Suggested Reading

Abbas S, Goldberg JW, Massaro M. Personal cleanser technology and clinical performance. *Dermatol Ther.* 2004;17:35–42.

American Academy of Dermatology and AAD Association 2008. Position Statement on Vitamin D. http://www.aad.org/Forms/Policies/Uploads/PS/PS-Vitamin%20D.pdf

American Academy of Dermatology. Facts about sunscreens. http://www.aad.org/media/background/fact_sheets/fact_sunscreen.html

American Cancer Society. How do I protect myself from UV? http://www.cancer.org.

Ananthapadmanabhan KP, Moore DJ, Subramanyan K, et al. Cleansing without compromise: The impact of cleansers of the skin barrier and the technology of mild cleansing. *Derm Ther.* 2004;17:16–25.

Baranda L, Gonzalez-Amaro R, Torres-Alverez R, et al. Correlation between pH and irritant effect of cleansers marketed for dry skin. *Int J Dermatol.* 2002;41:494–499.

Baumann L, Avashia N, Castanedo-Tardan MP. Sunscreens. In: Baumann L, ed. *Cosmetic Dermatology.* New York: McGraw-Hill; 2009.

Baumann L. *Cosmetic Dermatology.* New York: McGraw-Hill; 2002.

Baumann L. Cosmetics and skin care in dermatology. In: Freedberg IM, Eisen AZ, Wolff K, et al. *Fitzpatrick's Dermatology in General Medicine.* New York: McGraw-Hill.

Buraczewska I, Berne B, Lindberg M, et al. Changes in skin barrier function following long term treatment with moisturizers, a randomized controlled trail. *British J Dermatol.* 2007;156:492–498.

Carolyn B, Lyde R, Bergstresser PR. Ultraviolet protection for sun avoidance. *Dermatol Ther.* 1997;4:72–78.

Chatelain E, Gabard B. Photostabilization of butyl methoxydibenzoylmethane (Avobenzone) and ethylhexyl methoxycinnamate by bisethylhexyloxyphenol triazine (Tinosorb S), a new UV broadband filter. *Photochem Photobiol.* 2001;74:401–406.

Davis S, Capjack L, Kerr N, et al. Clothing as protection from ultraviolet radiation: which fabric is most effective? *Int J Dermatol.* 1997;36:374–379.

Denda M, Sato J, Masuda Y, et al. Exposure to a dry environment enhances epidermal permeability barrier function. *J Invest Dermatol.* 1998;111:858–863.

Denda M, Sokabe T, Fukumi-Tominaga T, et al. Effects of skin surface temperature on epidermal permeability barrier homeostasis. *J Invest Dermatol.* 2007;127:654–733.

Denda M, Tsuchiya T, Elias PM, et al. Stress alters cutaneous permeability barrier homeostasis. *Am J Physiol.* 2000;278:R367–R372.

Denda M. Epidermal proliferative response induced by sodium dodecyl sulphate varies with environmental humidity. *Br J Dermatol.* 2001;145:525–528.

Diffey B. Spectral uniformity: a new index of broad spectrum (UVA) protection. *Int J Cos Sci.* 2009; 31:63–68.

Diffey BL. People do not apply enough sunscreen for protection. *British Med J.* 1996;313:942.

Diffey BL. What is light? *Photodermatol Photoimmunol Photomed.* 2002;18:68–74.

Draelos ZD. Cosmetics and Cosmeceuticals. In: Bolognia JL, Jorizzo JL, Rapini RP. *Dermatology* 2nd ed. New York: Mosby Elsevier; 2008.

Elias PM, Feingold KR, Fluhr JW. Skin as an organ of protection. In: Freedberg IM, Eisen AZ, Wolff K, et al., eds. *Fitzpatrick's Dermatology in General Medicine.* New York: McGraw-Hill 2003:107–118.

Elwood JM, Jopson J. Melanoma and sun exposure: an overview of published studies. *Int J Cancer.* 1997;73:198–203.

Faurschou A, Wulf HC. The relation between sun protection factor and amount of sunscreen applied in vivo. *British J Dermatol.* 2007:156:716–719.

FDA Consumer Health Information. FDA Aims to upgrade sunscreen labeling. http://www.fda.gov/consumer/updates/sunscreen082307.html.

Fluhr J, Holleran WM, Berardesca E. Clinical effects of emollients on skin. In: Leyden JJ, Rawlings AV, eds. *Skin Moisturization.* New York: Marcel-Dekker; 2002:223–244.

Fluhr JW, Elias PM. Stratum corneum pH: formation and function of the acid mantle. *Exog Dermatol.* 2002;1:163–175.

Gallagher CH, Canfield PJ, Greenoak GE, et al. Characterization and histogenesis of tumors in the hairless mouse produced by low-dosage incremental ultraviolet radiation. *J Invest Dermatol.* 1984; 83:169–174.

Gasparro FP, Brown D, Diffey BL, et al. Sun protective agents: formulations, effects, and side effects. In: Freedberg IM, Eisen AZ, Wolff K, et al., eds. *Dermatology in General Medicine.* New York: McGraw-Hill;2003:2344–2352.

Ghadially R, Brown B, Sequiera-Martin SM, et al. The aged epidermal permeability barrier: structural, functional, and lipid biochemical abnormalities in humans and a senescent murine model. *J Clin Invest.* 1995;95:2281–2290.

Ghadially R, Halkier-Sorensen L, Elias PM. Effects of petrolatum on stratum corneum structure and function. *J Am Acad Dermatol.* 1992;26:387–396.

Gil EM, Kim TH. UV-induced immune suppression and sunscreen. *Photodermatol Photoimmunol Photomed.* 2000;16:101–110.

Gloster HM, Neal K. Skin cancer in skin of color. *J Am Acad Dermatol.* 2006;55:741–760.

Goddard ED. Substantivity through cationic substitution. *Cosmetics Toiletries.* 1987;102:71–80.

Grunewald AM, Gloor M, Gehring W, et al. Damage to the skin by repetitive washing. *Contact Dermatitis.* 1995;32:225–232.

Harding C. The stratum corneum: structure and function in health and disease. *Dermatol Ther.* 2004;17:6–15.

Harding CR, Scott IR. Histidine-rich proteins (filaggrins). Structural and functional heterogeneity during epidermal differentiation. *J Mol Bio.* 1983;170:651–673.

Hayden CG, Roberts MS, Benson HA. Systemic absorption of sunscreen after topical application. *Lancet.* 1997;350:863–864.

Holick MF. Vitamin D deficiency. *N Engl J Med.* 2007;357:266–281.

Jacobi O. About the mechanism of moisture regulation in the horny layer of the skin. *Proc Scient Sect Toil Goods Assoc.* 1959;31:22–26.

Johnson AW. Overview: fundamental skin care-protecting the barrier. *Dermatol Ther.* 2004; 7:1–5.

Johnson AW. The skin moisturizer marketplace. In: Leyden JJ, Rawlings AV, eds. *Skin Moisturization.* New York: Marcel-Dekker;2002:61–80.

Kaidbey KH. The photoprotective potential of the new superpotent sunscreens. *J Am Acad Dermatol.* 1990;22:449–452.

Katagiri C, Sato J, Nomura J, et al. Changes in environmental humidity affect the water-holding property of the stratum corneum and its free amino acid content, and the expression of filaggrin in the epidermis of hairless mice. *J Dermatol Sci.* 2003;31:29–35.

Kimyai-Asadi A, Jih MH, Freedberg IM. Epidermal cell kinetics, epidermal differentiation, and keratinization. In: Freedberg IM, Eisen AZ, Wolff K, et al., eds. *Dermatology in General Medicine.* New York: McGraw-Hill;2003:89–98.

Kullavanijaya P, Lim HW. Photoprotection. *J Am Acad Dermatol.* 2005;52:937–958.

Lavker RM, Gerberick GF, Veres D, et al. Cumulative effects from repeated exposure to suberythemal doses of UVB and UVA in human skin. *J Am Acad Dermatol.* 1995:32:53–62.

Leiter U, Garbe C. Epidemiology of melanoma and nonmelanoma skin cancer—the role of sunlight. *Adv Exp Med Biol.* 2008;624:89–103.

Levy SB. Sunscreens for photoprotection. *Dermatol Ther.* 1997;4:59–71.

Loden M. Do moisturizers work? *J Cosmet Dermatol.* 2004;2:141–149.

Loden M. The clinical benefit of moisturizers. *J Eur Acad Dermatol Venereol.* 2005;19:672–688.

Loden M. Urea-containing moisturizers influence barrier repair properties of normal skin. *Arch Dermatol Res.* 1996;288:103–107.

Lynde C. Moisturizers for treatment of inflammatory skin conditions. *J Drugs Dermatol.* 2008;7:1038–1043.

Madison KC. Barrier function of the skin: "la raison d'etre" of the epidermis. *J Inves Dermatol.* 2003; 121:231–241.

Man MQ, Feingold KR, Elias PM. Exogenous lipids influence permeability barrier recovery in acetone treated murine skin. *Arch Dermatol.* 1993;129:728–738.

Matsumura Y, Ananthaswamy HN. Toxic effects of ultraviolet radiation in the skin. *Toxicol Appl Pharmacol.* 2004;195:298–308.

Menon GK, Norlen L. Stratum corneum ceramides and their role in skin. In: Leyden JJ, Rawlings AV, eds. *Skin Moisturization.* New York: Marcel-Dekker;2002:31–60.

Menzies SW, Lukins PB, Greenoak GE, et al. A comparative study of fabric protection against ultraviolet-induced erythema determined by spectrophotometric and human skin measurements. *Photodermatol Photoimmunol Photomed.* 1991;8:157–163.

Nash J, Tanner T, Grosick T, et al. Sunscreen market analysis: the evolution and use of UVA-1 actives. *J Am Acad Dermtol.* 2004;50 (suppl 3):34.

Nemes Z, Steinert PM. Bricks and mortar of the epidermal barrier. *Exp Mol Med.* 1999;31:5–19.

Nopper AJ, Horii KA, Sookdeo-Drost S, et al. Topical ointment therapy benefits premature infants. *J Pediatr.* 1996;128:660–669.

Palmer CN, Irvine AD, Terron-Kwiatkowski A, et al. Common loss-of-function variants of the epidermal barrier protein filaggrin are a major predisposing factor for atopic dermatitis. *Nat Genet.* 2006;38:441–446.

Phillips TJ, Bhawan J, Yaar M, et al. Effect of daily versus intermittent sunscreen application on solar stimulated UV radiation-induced skin response in humans. *J Am Acad Dermatol.* 2000;43:610–618.

Rawlings AV, Canestrari DA, Dobkowski B. Moisturizer technology versus clinical performance. *Dermatol Ther.* 2004;17:49–56.

Rawlings AV, Harding CR. Moisturization and skin barrier function. *Dermatol Ther.* 2004;17:43–46.

Rawlings AV, Scott IR, Harding CR, et al. Stratum corneum moisturization at the molecular level. *J Invest Dermatol.* 1994;103:731–740.

Rogers JS, Harding CR, Mayo A, et al. Stratum corneum lipids: the effect of aging and the seasons. *Arch Dermatol Res.* 1996;288:765–770.

Sayre RM, Hughes SN. Sun protective apparel: advancements in sun protection. *Skin Cancer J.* 1993;8:41–47.

Semes L. UV-A absorbing characteristics of commercial sunglasses intended for recreational and general use. *J Am Optom Assoc.* 1991;62:754–758.

Sinclair SA, Diffey BL. Sun protection provided by ladies stockings. *Br J Dermatol.* 1997;136:239–241.

Stanford DG, Georgouras KE, Pailthorpe MT. Sun protection by a summer-weight garment: the effect of washing and wearing. *Med J Aust.* 1995;162:422–425.

Stewart MI, Bernhard JD, Cropley TG, et al. The structure of skin lesions and fundamentals of diagnosis. In: Freedberg IM, Eisen AZ, Wolff K, et al., eds. *Fitzpatrick's Dermatology in General Medicine.* New York: McGraw-Hill; 2003:11–30.

Tabachnick J, Labadie JH. Studies on the biochemistry of the epidermis. IV. The free amino acids, ammonia, urea, and pyrrolidone carboxylic acid content of conventional and germ free albino guinea pig epidermis. *J Invest Dermatol.* 1970;54:24–31.

Tezuka T. Electron-microscopic changes in xerosis senilis epidermis. Its abnormal membrane-coating granule formation. *Dermatologica.* 1983;166:57–61.

Van Weelden H, van der Putte SC, Toonstra J, et al. UVA-induced tumours in pigmented hairless mice and the carcinogenic risks of tanning with UVA. *Arch Dermatol Res.* 1990;282:289–294.

Walker SL, Hawk JLM, Young AR. Acute and chronic effects of ultraviolet radiation on the skin. In: Freedberg IM, Eisen AZ, Wolff K, A, et al., eds. *Fitzpatrick's Dermatology in General Medicine.* New York: McGraw-Hill; 2003:1275–1282.

Wang SQ, Kopf AW, Marx J, et al. Reduction of ultraviolet transmission through cotton T-shirt fabrics with ultraviolet protection by various laundering methods and dyeing: Clinical implications. *J Am Acad Dermatol.* 2001:44:767–774.

Wang SQ, Setlow R, Berwick M, et al. Ultraviolet light and melanoma: A review. *J Am Acad Dermatol.* 2001:44:837–846.

Wang SQ, Stanfield JW, Osterwalder U. In vitro assessments of UVA protection by popular sunscreens available in the United States. *J Am Acad Dermatol.* 2008;59:934–942.

Wenger CB. Thermoregulation. In: Freedberg IM, Eisen AZ, Wolff K, et al, eds. *Fitzpatrick's Dermatology in General Medicine.* New York: McGraw-Hill; 2003:119–127.

CHAPTER 4 Normal Skin Care/Maintenance

CHAPTER 5 Bacterial Diseases

Greg K. Sakamoto, Tracie Chong, and Jacob P. Thyssen

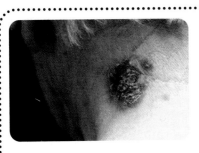

A 64-year-old woman presents to the clinic with a 2-week history of crusted erosions on the posterior neck. Upon examination, there is a 3-cm crusted plaque with honey-colored crusts (Fig. 5-1). She otherwise feels well with no local or systemic symptoms. She has no blisters on her skin or mucous membranes. What is the most likely diagnosis? What diagnostic tests should be done? What should the treatment be?

Exposure to bacteria is ubiquitous in the human experience, with millions of organisms being present in and on the body. In many cases, the relationship between bacteria and the human being is commensal but in some important cases, infection is pathogenic. These bacterial skin infections are important to recognize, diagnose correctly, and treat promptly. In this chapter, common skin infections will be discussed.

Impetigo

BACKGROUND/EPIDEMIOLOGY

Impetigo is a highly contagious superficial skin infection. It is the most common bacterial skin infection in children between the ages of 2 and 5. Although mainly affecting children, adults are also susceptible to infection, especially those with diabetes mellitus, AIDS, and the otherwise immunosuppressed. The incidence tends to increase during the summer months. Infections are typically prevalent among nurseries, day care centers, and elementary schools.

Patients are able to autoinoculate themselves, leading to spread of the infection to other areas of the body. The organism is transmitted through direct skin contact and enters through any breach in the skin barrier. Once it invades, it causes an infection of the superficial epidermis that can manifest as two different subtypes: nonbullous and bullous impetigo. Bullous impetigo tends to occur more commonly in neonates.

PATHOGENESIS

Impetigo is among one of several cutaneous infections caused by *Staphylococcus aureus* and to a lesser extent, group A β-hemolytic streptococci. The nonbullous type accounts for 70% of the cases and is an immune-mediated condition. The bullous form is toxin-mediated and the cleavage of the epidermis is mediated by exfoliative toxins A and B, which disrupt cellular adhesion. Exfoliative toxin A and B are known to target desmoglein I, which is a desmosomal cadherin that is a key structure in intercellular adhesion in the epidermis. The result is a split in the granular layer of the epidermis with the formation of a thin-roofed blister.

KEY FEATURES

- There are two forms of impetigo: bullous and nonbullous.

- Impetigo is primarily caused by infection by *Staphylococcus aureus* and group A β-hemolytic streptococci.

- The most commonly affected group is children. Adults at risk for impetigo are those with diabetes mellitus, acquired immunodeficiency syndrome (AIDS), and the homeless. Bullous impetigo tends to occur more commonly in neonates.

- Treat with topical mupirocin initially (at least 7 days), in widespread cases or when clinically necessary, add appropriate systemic therapy.

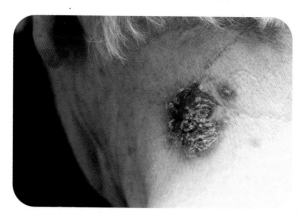

Figure 5-1 Characteristic honeycomb crust of impetigo on the posterior neck of an adult woman.

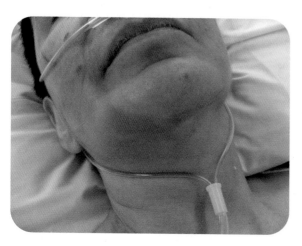

Figure 5-2 Impetigo in a hospitalized adult with fragile bulla on the submental region filled with yellow fluid.

CLINICAL PRESENTATION

Nonbullous impetigo usually begins as a macule or papule that quickly becomes vesicular or pustular. The vesicle is easily ruptured and leads to the characteristic "honey-colored" or "golden" crust overlying the erosions of the skin (Fig. 5-1). Skin surfaces such as the perioral region and nares are frequently affected. Autoinoculation can lead to a linear or grouped arrangement of these vesicles. Most patients have skin lesions only, without systemic symptoms. In a minority of cases, regional lymphadenopathy may occur. Impetigo is usually a self-limited process that resolves in about 2 weeks without scarring or postinfectious sequelae. Five to ten percent of the cases are caused by *S. pyogenes* and can result in an acute poststreptococcal glomerulonephritis. Use of systemic antibiotics does not prevent nephritis.

Bullous impetigo typically begins as large, flaccid bullae on the trunk or extremity with no surrounding erythema as seen in Figure 5-2. It favors the intertriginous regions such as the axillae, crural folds, and neck folds. When the bullae are ruptured, they ooze yellow serous fluid that forms the characteristic yellow, "honeycombed" crust. Because the bullae are fragile, erosions are often seen in place of ruptured bullae. The erosions usually have a collarette of scale at the periphery signifying previous bullae that have been unroofed. Similar to nonbullous impetigo, most cases are self-limited and resolve in 1 to 2 weeks without scarring. Systemic symptoms when seen include fever, weakness, and diarrhea. In rare cases, bullous impetigo has been associated with meningitis, pneumonia, sepsis, and even death.

DIAGNOSIS

Most cases are diagnosed on the basis of clinical presentation. When the diagnosis is in question, a Gram stain and culture of the blister fluid may reveal the pathogenic bacteria. Sensitivities to antibiotics may also be required to identify methicillin-resistant *S. aureus* (MRSA) strains and determine appropriate antibiotic coverage.

DIFFERENTIAL DIAGNOSIS
- Nonbullous impetigo:
  - Contact dermatitis
  - Herpes simplex
  - Varicella
  - Dermatophytosis

- Bullous impetigo:
  - Bullous erythema multiforme
  - Bullous pemphigoid
  - Pemphigus vulgaris
  - Stevens-Johnson syndrome

THERAPY

Although impetigo is thought to be a self-limited condition, treatment is usually instituted to prevent the progression of lesions and systemic involvement as well as prevent the spread to others. If the area of involvement is limited, topical antibiotics remain the mainstay of treatment. Mupirocin is the most effective topical antibiotic and should be applied twice daily for at least 7 days. It was found to be effective in clearing MRSA strains and is routinely used in decolonizing patients who harbor MRSA. Systemic antimicrobials are the treatment of choice for widespread infections and infections with systemic symptoms. Beta-lactamase resistant antibiotics such as cephalexin, dicloxacillin, and amoxicillin/clavulanate should be used. Azithromycin and clarithromycin are also efficacious, but more costly. If the strains are methicillin resistant, then vancomycin, linezolid, and quinupristin/dalfopristin should be used. Other antibiotics that are effective against MRSA include trimethoprim-sulfamethoxazole, minocycline, and clindamycin. In case of MRSA, supplementary treatments should be initiated (e.g., hot washing of all towels, bed sheets, and clothes the patient has used).

"AT A GLANCE" TREATMENT

- First-line therapy for isolated lesions: mupirocin ointment or cream twice daily for at least 7 days
- First-line therapy for widespread infections and infections with systemic symptoms: beta-lactamase resistant antibiotics such as cephalexin, dicloxacillin, and amoxicillin/clavulanate azithromycin or clarithromycin
- MRSA outpatient: based on sensitivities, empirically—minocycline, clindamycin, or trimethoprim-sulfamethoxazole
- MRSA inpatient: vancomycin, linezolid, and quinupristin/dalfopristin

COURSE AND COMPLICATIONS

Impetigo is usually acute and self-limited to 1 to 2 weeks. The lesions usually resolve without any complications or evidence of scarring. However, neonates have a higher incidence of developing a generalized infection as well as pneumonia and meningitis. If no improvement is seen while on antibiotic therapy, antibiotic sensitivities should be obtained to rule out drug-resistant strains. Other potential complications include endocarditis, cellulitis, guttate psoriasis, toxic shock syndromes, and staphylococcal scalded skin syndrome.

ICD9 Codes	
684	Impetigo

WHEN TO REFER

- When the diagnosis is not clear or the possibility of another more serious infection or blistering disorder is being entertained, the patient should be referred to a dermatologist for evaluation. This may include a bacterial Gram stain and culture, direct immunofluorescence antibody testing, viral culture, or skin biopsy. In severe cases with bullous lesions, frozen section biopsies may be indicated.

- In widespread/severe cases where Stevens-Johnson syndrome (SJS), toxic epidermal necrolysis (TEN) or staphylococcal scalded skin syndrome (SSSS) is a possibility, emergent inpatient evaluation and care is indicated. These conditions can be life threatening and progress rapidly. See Chapter 23 for further discussion of SJS/TEN.

NOT TO BE MISSED

- MRSA infection should always be ruled out by bacterial culture and sensitivities.
- In widespread cases, consider SSSS or SJS/TEN.

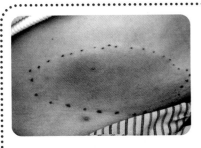

A 28-year-old woman presents with a lower abdomen lesion with ill-defined, non-palpable borders; erythema (Fig. 5-3); warmth; pain; and swelling. Regional lymph nodes are palpable. She is not diabetic or immunocompromised. History includes recent shaving of the pubic hair prior to a 2-day history of fever, chills, and malaise. We tell her that clinical diagnosis points toward a skin infection. What organism is the most likely cause in this case?

Cellulitis

BACKGROUND/EPIDEMIOLOGY

Cellulitis, a painful spreading infection in the deep dermis or subcutaneous tissue, is one of the most common bacterial skin infections. By definition, it does not involve muscle or deeper structures. It can occur anywhere on the body, but most commonly affects the lower limbs and digits, followed by the face, feet, hands, torso, neck, and buttocks. It frequently occurs in the settings of minor trauma, alcoholism, diabetes mellitus, intravenous drug use, peripheral vascular disease, and damage to the lymphatic

KEY FEATURES

- Common bacterial infection of the dermis, most often due to *Streptococcus pyogenes* (group A β-hemolytic streptococci) or *Staphylococcus aureus* in immunocompetent adults.
- Lower limbs and digits most commonly affected.
- Treat with oral antibiotics with gram-positive coverage.

system. Those with interdigital tinea pedis, onychomycosis, or impetigo are more susceptible to chronic lower extremity cellulitis.

PATHOGENESIS

Cellulitis is most often due to *Streptococcus pyogenes* (group A β-hemolytic streptococci) or *Staphylococcus aureus* in immunocompetent adults. Most cellulitis in childhood is associated with *S. aureus*, because infection by *Haemophilus influenza* has become less common since vaccine implementation. Cellulitis in diabetic patients (generally surrounding diabetic ulcers) is polymicrobial, caused by gram-positive cocci and gram-negative aerobes and anaerobes. Damage to the skin barrier is often the mechanism of infection in immunocompetent patients, while a hematogenous route is likely the source in the immunocompromised.

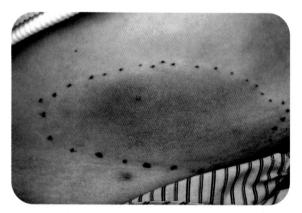

Figure 5-3 An erythematous plaque of cellulitis. The leading edge was marked to help assess the progression of the infection.

CLINICAL PRESENTATION

Cellulitis generally follows a period of systemic symptoms such as fever, chills, and malaise. The area exhibits induration and typical signs of inflammation (erythema, warmth, pain, and swelling). Upon examination, the lesion has ill-defined, advancing, nonpalpable borders such as that seen in Figure 5-3. Severe cases may present with vesicles, bullae, pustules, or necrotic tissue. Infection may progress to include ascending lymphangitis and regional lymph node involvement. Location of cellulitis varies by age and demographics: children usually show involvement of the head and neck, while the extremities are often affected in adults. Cellulitis in intravenous drug abusers commonly presents in the upper extremities.

DIAGNOSIS

Diagnosis of cellulitis is generally based on clinical presentation. Leukocyte count is typically normal or slightly elevated, and blood cultures are nearly always negative (except in immunocompromised individuals). The exception is infection with *H. influenza*, which presents with an elevated leukocyte count with left shift and positive blood cultures. Atypical organisms are common in children and the immunocompromised. Such cases may necessitate needle aspiration and skin biopsy for routine pathology and tissue culture.

Histopathologic analysis is usually not required but will typically show inflammatory infiltrate of lymphocytes and neutrophils throughout the dermis, which may extend into the subcutaneous fat. There may also be edema and dilation of lymphatics and small blood vessels, and subepidermal bullae may be noted in cases of severe dermal edema. Special stains may elucidate the causative organism, but organisms are rarely found in cellulitic lesions because immunocompetent cells rapidly eliminate most viable bacteria by the time of clinical presentation. Involvement simultaneously of both lower extremities ("bilateral cellulitis") is exceedingly rare and other diagnoses such as stasis dermatitis or allergic contact dermatitis must be considered.

THERAPY

Treatment includes immobilization, elevation, wet dressings, and analgesics. Antibiotic treatment is aimed against *S. pyogenes* and *S. aureus*. The majority of cases may be given a 10-day course of an oral antibiotic with gram-positive coverage. More serious cases or patients with facial cellulitis may require hospitalization and parenteral antibiotics. Parenteral antibiotic therapy should include penicillin along with a penicillinase-resistant penicillin such as cloxacillin to cover *S. aureus*. Broad-spectrum coverage such as an aminoglycoside plus clindamycin or an advanced-generation cephalosporin is needed in diabetic or decubitus ulcers complicated by cellulitis.

If there is no improvement following 24 to 36 hours of treatment, cultures and sensitivities should be ordered and antibiotics may be adjusted appropriately. Although anti-inflammatory agents may enhance resolution of the infection, NSAIDs are generally avoided in the treatment of cellulitis as they may mask the signs and symptoms of deeper necrotizing infections.

"AT A GLANCE" TREATMENT

- First-line: recommended basic care such as immobilization, elevation, wet dressings, and analgesics
- For uncomplicated cellulitis, consider a course of oral antibiotic with gram-positive coverage such as cephalexin or dicloxacillin
- Facial cellulitis or cases with rapidly spreading disease/constitutional illness may require inpatient care

COURSE AND COMPLICATIONS

Cases of superficial cellulitis generally improve within several days, but some patients with dermal thickening may take several days of parenteral antibiotics for significant improvement to occur. Although complications are infrequent, acute glomerulonephritis, lymphadenitis, and bacterial endocarditis may result. Damage to lymphatic vessels may lead to lymphedema and increased risk of recurrent infection.

WHEN TO REFER

- Consider referral when the diagnosis is uncertain or if the cellulitis fails to respond to antibiotics within the expected time period.
- Severe blistering should be emergently evaluated.

NOT TO BE MISSED

- Deep vein thrombosis.
- Stasis dermatitis.
- Superficial thrombophlebitis.
- Panniculitis.
- Allergic or irritant contact dermatitis.
- Lupus erythematosus.
- Stevens-Johnson syndrome or toxic epidermal necrolysis.

ICD9 Codes

681.00	Unspecified cellulitis and abscess of finger
681.01	Felon
681.02	Onychia and paronychia of finger
681.10	Unspecified cellulitis and abscess of toe
681.11	Onychia and paronychia of toe
681.9	Cellulitis and abscess of unspecified digit
682.0	Cellulitis and abscess of face
682.1	Cellulitis and abscess of neck
682.2	Cellulitis and abscess of trunk
682.3	Cellulitis and abscess of upper arm and forearm
682.4	Cellulitis and abscess of hand, except fingers and thumb
682.5	Cellulitis and abscess of buttock
682.6	Cellulitis and abscess of leg, except foot
682.7	Cellulitis and abscess of foot, except toes
682.8	Cellulitis and abscess of other specified sites
682.9	Cellulitis and abscess of unspecified sites

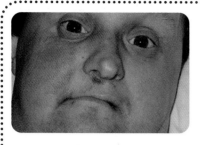

A 60-year-old man presents with a rapidly expanding fiery red rash on the face (Fig. 5-4). The rash was preceded by 1 day of high fever, chills, and malaise. He does not recall a history of trauma or any other inciting event. On physical examination, there is a well-circumscribed red, indurated shiny plaque extending across both cheeks in a butterfly distribution. The plaques are well-circumscribed and are warm and tender to palpation. There is mild regional lymphadenopathy. You suspect erysipelas. How do you differentiate erysipelas from classic cellulitis? What treatment should by instituted?

Erysipelas

BACKGROUND/EPIDEMIOLOGY

Erysipelas is an acute bacterial infection of the dermis and the subcutaneous tissues. It was once referred to as "St. Anthony's Fire." In the Middle Ages, people who ingested fungi that produced ergot alkaloids developed bright red extremities that led to gangrene, and it was believed that only the shrine of St. Anthony provided a cure. Classically, erysipelas involved the face, but in recent times, the distribution has shifted to the legs. It affects all age groups, although infants and the elderly are at a higher risk. Females are affected more than males. It tends to occur more commonly in the summer months.

PATHOGENESIS

Erysipelas is caused mainly by group A β-hemolytic *Streptococcus* and rarely by *S. agalactiae* and *S. dysgalactiae sp. equisimilis*. The bacteria have protective and virulence factors that allow tissue invasion. Inoculation of a site where the skin has been breached initially sets off a cascade that leads to the characteristic clinical findings. Risk factors for development of erysipelas include stasis ulcerations, inflammatory dermatoses, dermatophyte infections, surgical incisions, and traumatized skin (e.g., following vein stripping). Additional risk factors include alcoholism, human immunodeficiency virus (HIV), diabetes, and immunosuppression.

In most cases (90%), the leg is affected. The portal of entry is thought to be due to tinea pedis or onychomycosis. Other sites of predilection include the arms and the face. Most patients develop a prodrome of symptoms including fever which tends to be higher than the fever of cellulitis, chills, and malaise. Some patients report symptoms of pharyngitis that began several days or weeks before the onset of the rash.

KEY FEATURES

- Erysipelas is a common bacterial infection of the dermis, due to *Streptococcus pyogenes* (group A β-hemolytic streptococci) or *S. agalactiae* and *S. dysgalactiae sp. equisimilis*.

- The lower limbs (typically unilateral affection) and face are most commonly affected.

- Treat with oral antibiotics with gram-positive coverage.

CLINICAL PRESENTATION

Usually within 24 hours, a tender, erythematous, well-demarcated plaque develops. The plaque advances rapidly, extending 2 to 10 cm per day. In cases of extremity involvement, it typically affects only one extremity and both extremely rarely. On palpation, the plaques are warm, tender, and very edematous, as noted by the shiny appearance with occasional peau d'orange skin changes (Figs. 5-4, 5-5). The rash has a very distinct raised border, unlike cellulitis, where the border should not be sharply raised. With time, the erythema becomes duskier, but maintains its bright red color on the leading edge. About a week after the onset of the rash, the erythematous zones show central clearing, and the skin may begin to exfoliate. Some of the areas may heal with postinflammatory pigmentary changes.

DIAGNOSIS

In most cases, erysipelas is diagnosed based on the clinical findings. Laboratory findings include leukocytosis, increased erythrocyte sedimentation rate (ESR), and positive blood cultures in a small fraction of patients. Cultures from the nasopharynx are often positive for *Streptococcus* spp. and help confirm the diagnosis.

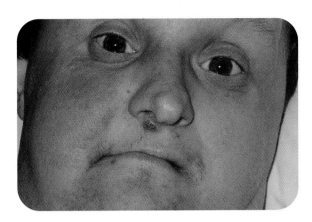

Figure 5-4 Erysipelas. Reprinted with permission from Berg D, Worzala K. *Atlas of Adult Physical Diagnosis*. Philadelphia: Lippincott Williams & Wilkins, 2006.

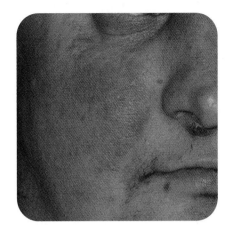

Figure 5-5 Erysipelas on the face of a man with Down syndrome. Reprinted with permission from Berg D, Worzala K. *Atlas of Adult Physical Diagnosis*. Philadelphia: Lippincott Williams & Wilkins, 2006.

CHAPTER 5 Bacterial Diseases

THERAPY

Rest and elevation of the leg can help with reducing swelling and pain. *Streptococcus* continues to be sensitive to beta-lactam antibiotics and penicillin still remains a first-line therapy. This should be given for 10 to 14 days or until the plaque completely resolves. A macrolides antibiotic can be given to those patients that are penicillin allergic. To monitor the initial course, one may mark the extension of cutaneous symptoms with a pen upon initiation of treatment. Predisposing conditions such as tinea pedis or stasis ulcers should be treated aggressively to prevent secondary and superinfections from occurring. Hospitalization and intravenous antibiotics are warranted for the immunocompromised, infants, and the elderly and in severe cases of erysipelas.

"AT A GLANCE" TREATMENT

- First-line: recommended basic care such as immobilization, elevation, wet dressings, and analgesics
- Oral antibiotics are recommended; in most cases, penicillins are first-line therapy
- Hospitalize for monitoring and intravenous (IV) antibiotics for all severe cases and consider hospitalization for infants, the elderly, and immunocompromised individuals

COURSE AND COMPLICATIONS

The prognosis for patients with erysipelas is excellent. The infection usually responds rapidly to antibiotic therapy and resolves with mild exfoliation of the skin and with occasional hyperpigmentation. There is a 10% recurrence rate within 6 months after the first episode. In selected patients with recurrent erysipelas, prophylactic antibiotic therapy should be considered. More importantly, for those patients who suffer from repeated instances of erysipelas due to dry skin or recurrent fungal toe infections, thorough instruction and treatment remedies (topical moisturizing lotions and antifungal remedies, respectively) should be offered. The most common complications are thrombophlebitis, legs ulcers, and gangrene. Rare cases can progress to septicemia, endocarditis, and glomerulonephritis.

WHEN TO REFER

- Referral to a dermatologist is warranted if the rash is unresponsive to antibiotic therapy.
- Infectious disease specialists should also be consulted in cases of antibiotic-resistant disease.

NOT TO BE MISSED

- *H. influenza* cellulitis.
- Allergic contact dermatitis.
- Herpes zoster.
- Necrotizing fasciitis.

ICD9 Codes

035   Erysipelas

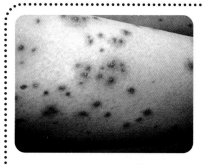

A 35-year-old woman comes to the clinic complaining of small raised areas on her legs that are red and itching (Fig. 5-6). She has a recent medical history of topical corticosteroid use, and states that she first noticed the lesions when the weather became more hot and humid. We prescribe an antibacterial wash containing chlorhexidine and bacitracin ointment.

KEY FEATURES

- Folliculitis is a benign infection (typically *Staphylococcus aureus*) of the hair follicle.

- It may occur on any hair-bearing skin surface.

- Antibacterial washes, topical antibacterial preparations, and occasionally oral therapy should be considered.

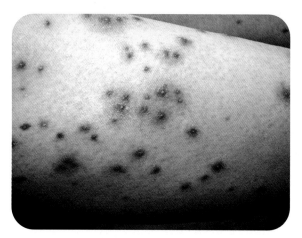

Figure 5-6 Folliculitis on the calf.

Folliculitis

BACKGROUND/EPIDEMIOLOGY

Bacterial folliculitis is a common and benign infection of the hair follicle, often caused by *Staphylococcus aureus*. Risk factors include hyperhydration of the skin, maceration, depilation, occlusion, topical corticosteroid use, humid weather, and diabetes mellitus.

PATHOGENESIS

Pseudomonas folliculitis is linked to contamination of undertreated water in hot tubs and whirlpools. Acne vulgaris patients on long-term oral antibiotics (particularly tetracyclines) may develop folliculitis due to gram-negative bacteria including *Enterobacter, Klebsiella, Escherichia coli,* and *Proteus.* Immunocompromised patients may acquire folliculitis due to commensal organisms. A rarer variant of folliculitis is caused by follicular infection with the yeast *Malassezia furfur* (Pityrosporum folliculitis). *Propionibacterium acnes* is the cause of acne vulgaris and in some cases folliculitis on other body areas, such as the scalp.

CLINICAL PRESENTATION

Folliculitis may occur on any skin surface bearing hair, and typically affects the head/neck, chest, back, buttocks, or extremities (Fig. 5-6). Appearance of lesions varies depending on the depth of follicular involvement. Superficial folliculitis presents with small (1 to 4 mm) clustered pustules or crusted papules sitting on an erythematous base. It may be either tender or painless. In contrast, large, erythematous papules with a central pustule that are tender and/or pruritic suggest deep folliculitis.

DIAGNOSIS

Diagnosis is often made on the basis of clinical examination. Identification of the causative organism(s) is made via Gram stain and bacterial/fungal cultures. Skin biopsy is rarely indicated, other than in cases of treatment recalcitrant folliculitis such as Pityrosporum folliculitis.

THERAPY

Superficial cases are treated with antibacterial washes containing chlorhexidine or triclosan. In some cases, alcohol-based cleansing gels applied once or twice daily to the affected areas may be quite helpful. Another effective method consists of applying antibacterial gels or lotions (erythromycin, clindamycin, etc.) for 7 to 10 days. Deep folliculitis may be treated with oral antibiotics, such as doxycycline or minocycline. Second-line agents include first-generation cephalosporins, penicillinase-resistant penicillins, macrolides, and fluoroquinolones. Nonbacterial folliculitis (Pityrosporum) requires oral antifungal therapy. Oral ketoconazole 200 mg PO QD × 2 weeks is often successful.

"AT A GLANCE" TREATMENT

- Treat superficial cases with antibacterial washes containing chlorhexidine or triclosan or use an alcohol-based gel

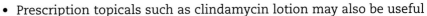

- Prescription topicals such as clindamycin lotion may also be useful
- Deep/extensive folliculitis: treat with a doxycycline or minocycline first line. Usually 3 to 4 weeks at 100 mg BID will be effective
- Nonbacterial folliculitis (Pityrosporum) requires oral antifungal therapy. Oral ketoconazole 200 mg PO QD × 2 weeks is often successful

COURSE AND COMPLICATIONS

The condition is self-limited and typically heals without sequelae. Superficial folliculitis generally does not result in scarring, whereas lesions of the deep subtype may resolve with residual scars.

> ***ICD9 Codes***
> *704.8   Other specified diseases of hair and hair follicles*
> *695.3   Rosacea*
> *706.1   Other acne*

WHEN TO REFER

Referral is appropriate in the case of questionable diagnosis or when lesions remain unresponsive to the above treatment.

NOT TO BE MISSED

- Acne vulgaris.
- Rosacea.
- Chloracne.
- Pseudofolliculitis barbae.
- Keratosis pilaris.

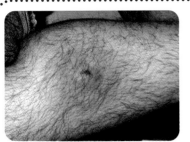

A 21-year-old man presents with a hard, tender, red nodule on his right medial calf that he says has enlarged and become painful (Fig. 5-7). He recently returned from a 1-year military service in Iraq. Rupture of the lesion expels pus and alleviates the pain.

KEY FEATURES

- Cutaneous abscess. Furuncle—1 hair follicle involved; carbuncle—multiple follicles.
- *Staphylococcus aureus* is the most common cause.
- Pain is a significant component, often relieved by drainage of the lesion.
- Therapy include incision and drainage when necessary and oral antibiotics.

Furuncles and Carbuncles

BACKGROUND/EPIDEMIOLOGY

A furuncle (boil) is an accumulation of pus that is sealed from surrounding tissue, otherwise known as a cutaneous abscess. Furuncles develop as a follicular infection that progresses deeper and extends out from a single hair follicle. The term carbuncle refers to an adjoining collection of infected and multiple inflamed follicles. They may occur anywhere on the skin, although they are generally found only in hair-bearing skin. Common areas for furuncles are the face, neck, axillae, buttocks, and thigh. Sites exposed to friction or minor trauma are especially predisposed. Carbuncles tend to occur in locations with thicker skin, such as the nape of the neck, back, and thigh.

Furuncles most commonly affect adolescents and young adults. Risk factors include chronic *Staphylococcus aureus* carriage, immunodeficiency, diabetes mellitus, obesity, and poor hygiene. Furunculosis, or multiple or recurrent furuncles, may develop from chronic S. *aureus* carriage.

PATHOGENESIS

The usual organism responsible is S. *aureus*, although it may also be caused by anaerobic bacteria (anogenital furuncles). A small percentage of cutaneous abscesses may also be sterile, due to a foreign body reaction such as a ruptured epidermal inclusion or pilar cyst.

CLINICAL PRESENTATION

The typical appearance consists of a subcutaneous, inflamed, erythematous nodule, which may have fluctuant collections of pus upon palpation (Fig. 5-7). Rupture lessens the pain. The skin surface may show multiple draining sinus tracts and ulceration may be present. Unlike furuncles, systemic symptoms

CHAPTER 5 Bacterial Diseases

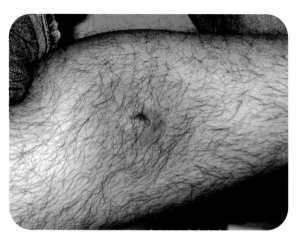

Figure 5-7 Methicillin-resistant *Staphylococcus aureus* (MRSA) furuncle on the calf of a 21-year-old veteran.

such as fever and malaise are usually present with carbuncles. These lesions heal rather slowly and scar formation often results.

DIAGNOSIS

Furuncles and carbuncles are diagnosed clinically. Confirmative tests include Gram stain and cultures from the lesion(s). Severe cases may include an increased leukocyte count and systemic symptoms such as fever/malaise.

THERAPY

Mild cases may not require treatment, although warm compresses can encourage maturation and drainage and alleviate the symptoms. Incision and drainage may be effective in the case of fluctuant lesions. Many cases are caused by *S. aureus* infection. When choosing an oral antibiotic, using an agent that covers both sensitive and resistant strains may be beneficial. For sensitive strains of *S. aureus*, use a penicillinase-resistant penicillin or a cephalosporin. For community-acquired methicillin resistant strains of *S. aureus*, treatment with clindamycin, trimethoprim-sulfamethoxazole, doxycycline, or rifampin may be indicated. Serious cases of non-MRSA infection may call for use of parenteral antibiotics such as cloxacillin (Tegopen) or a first-generation cephalosporin such as cefazolin (Ancef).

"AT A GLANCE" TREATMENT

- Mild cases: warm compresses, analgesia, and surgical incision/drainage as appropriate
- Oral antibiotics are useful in more involved cases:
  - MSSA: penicillinase resistant penicillin (dicloxacillin) or a cephalosporin (cephalexin)
  - MRSA: consider clindamycin, trimethoprim-sulfamethoxazole, doxycycline, or Rifampin
- Severe cases: hospitalize for IV antibiotics. Consider cloxacillin (Tegopen) or cefazolin (Ancef)

WHEN TO REFER

- Referral to dermatology should be considered if lesions worsen or fail to clear upon therapy.

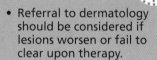

NOT TO BE MISSED

- Ruptured epidermoid or pilar cyst.
- Hidradenitis suppurativa ("acne inversa").
- Cystic acne.

COURSE AND COMPLICATIONS

Furuncles and carbuncles are usually self-limited and treatment is generally successful at eradicating the lesions. Some scarring may occur in the case of carbuncles.

ICD9 Codes	
680.0	Carbuncle and furuncle of face
680.1	Carbuncle and furuncle of neck
680.2	Carbuncle and furuncle of trunk
680.3	Carbuncle and furuncle of upper arm and forearm
680.4	Carbuncle and furuncle of hand
680.5	Carbuncle and furuncle of buttock
680.6	Carbuncle and furuncle of leg, except foot
680.7	Carbuncle and furuncle of foot
680.8	Carbuncle and furuncle of other specified sites
680.9	Carbuncle and furuncle of unspecified site

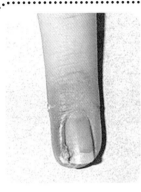

A 30-year-old woman presents with a 1-day history of intense swelling and pain of the proximal nail fold of the right second digit (Fig. 5-8). She has a history of ony-chophagia (nail biting) and admits to recently traumatizing the nail fold after incessant nail biting. Examination reveals erythema and edema affecting only the digit mentioned above. In addi-tion, there is an accumulation of purulent material on the proximal and lateral nail folds. The finger is tender to palpa-tion and there is no nail dystrophy. You tell the patient that she has an acute infection of the nail fold and you decide to drain the purulent material.

Acute Bacterial Paronychia

BACKGROUND/EPIDEMIOLOGY

Acute paronychia is an infection of the nail folds. It is usually preceded by trauma to the cuticle or the nail fold, allowing bacterial inoculation. Examples of such trauma include nail-biting, splinters, dishwashing, hangnails, or manicuring. It can also occur as a mani-festation of other diseases such as psori-asis and pemphigus vulgaris that result in dystrophy.

Acute paronychia is one of the most common causes of infections occurring on the hands. It occurs in persons of all ages and is three times more common in women than men. Predisposing condi-tions include diabetes, hyperhidrosis, and immunosuppression. Occupations that pose a higher risk include florists, bartenders, chefs, and those that require frequent and prolonged water contact. Patients usually complain of intense pain and swelling of one of the nail folds.

KEY FEATURES

- Paronychia is an acute nail fold infection most com-monly caused by *S. aureus*.
- Chronic infections are most commonly caused by *C. albicans*.
- Treatment is drainage of accumulated pus, appro-priate topical antimicro-bials, and, if indicated, systemic antibiotics.

PATHOGENESIS

The most common pathogen is *Staphylococcus aureus*, although *Streptococcus pyogenes*, *Proteus vulgaris*, and *Pseudomonas pyocyanea* have also been known to cause infection. The chronic form is usually associated with presence of the yeast *Candida albicans*, but there may be acute deterioration, which is typically caused by *S. aureus*.

CLINICAL PRESENTATION

The infection mainly affects the nail folds of the fingers, although the toes can also be involved. It is usually limited to one digit and characterized by the rapid onset of erythema and swelling with tenderness of the nail folds (Figs. 5-8, 5-9). In darker-skinned patients, only swelling may be observed and

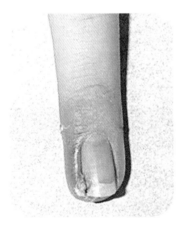

Figure 5-8 Acute bacterial parony-chia. Courtesy of Mary L. Brandt, MD.

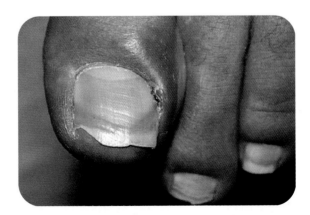

Figure 5-9 Acute bacterial paronychia. Reprinted with permis-sion from Goodheart HP. *Goodheart's Photoguide to Common Skin Disorders,* 3rd ed. Philadelphia: Lippincott Williams & Wilkins, 2009.

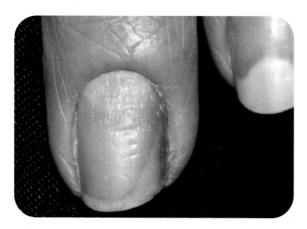

Figure 5-10 Chronic paronychia. Reprinted with permission from Goodheart HP. *Goodheart's Photoguide to Common Skin Disorders*, 3rd ed. Philadelphia: Lippincott Williams & Wilkins, 2009.

it may be useful to use the same finger from the other hand for reference. Occasionally, purulent material will accumulate under the nail fold leading to pus drainage with compression of the nail. If left untreated, the infection can lead to a subungual abscess and may cause dystrophy of the nail. If the purulent material collects subungually, the nail plate can separate from the nail bed, leading to loss of the nail. This can be compared to a chronic paronychia (Fig. 5-10), in which, in addition to erythema and edema, you can also observe nail dystrophy and the absence of a cuticle.

DIAGNOSIS

The diagnosis is usually suggested in patients with a history of periungual trauma and is most often clinical. Biopsy is not indicated in most cases. If the infection is severe or an abscess has formed, a culture should be obtained to rule out methicillin-resistant *Staphylococcus aureus*. Potassium hydroxide examination for fungal elements may be helpful to evaluate for yeast/fungal infection. Also, if any vesicles are present, send a direct fluorescent antibody (DFA) scraping and viral culture to evaluate for herpetic whitlow. Other conditions to consider include malignant melanoma, squamous cell carcinoma, syphilitic chancres, granulomas, and viral warts.

THERAPY

The treatment of choice depends on the severity of the paronychia. For acute paronychial infections without abscess formation, hot compresses may be effective. Topical antibiotics alone or potent topical steroids can be used. If the infection persists, oral antistaphylococcal antibiotics can be used. Broad-spectrum antibiotics such as amoxicillin/clavulanate or clindamycin can be used if there is history of exposure to the oral flora due to possible anaerobic infection. If the infection does not improve despite antibiotic therapy, surgical intervention may be needed. In the case of a less-developed paronychial abscess, simply lifting the eponychial fold from the nail with a blunt instrument may be all that is needed to evacuate the pus. If this does not work, then incision of the proximal nail can be performed to allow drainage. The wound should be irrigated and the patient should still receive a course of oral antibiotics for at least 7 days. With more advanced paronychias, incision and drainage of the lesion is often required.

Treatment of chronic paronychia begins with avoidance of the inciting irritant exposures such as prolonged water exposure, glove use, and/or frequent hand washing. Encourage the patient to refrain from picking/manipulating the affected areas. For mild cases, warm water soaks followed by application of a topical antifungal agent such as miconazole can be effective. For more severe cases, addition of an oral antifungal such as ketoconazole or fluconazole may be warranted.

"AT A GLANCE" TREATMENT

- Acute paronychia:
  - Mild cases: hot soaks/compresses, +/− topical antibiotic (mupirocin) or potent topical corticosteroid (clobetasol)
  - Persistent/more severe cases: mild treatment plus addition of an oral antistaphylococcal antibiotic (amoxicillin/clavulanate or clindamycin)
  - Consider incision and drainage in cases with obvious abscess formation

WHEN TO REFER

- Referral to dermatology is warranted when the paronychia is unresponsive to antimicrobial therapy.
- In cases of complex abscess formation requiring surgical drainage, consider consulting a hand surgeon or surgically oriented dermatologist.

NOT TO BE MISSED

- Herpetic whitlow.
- Systemic retinoids may cause chronic, multiple finger paronychia.
- A rare finding of the paraneoplastic syndrome acrokeratosis neoplastica (see Chapter 17) is acute paronychias on multiple fingers.

COURSE AND COMPLICATIONS

Most cases of acute paronychia resolve with antibiotic or surgical treatment. In rare cases, especially in the immunocompromised, the paronychia can evolve into more serious infections such as osteomyelitis and a tenosynovitis.

> *ICD9 Codes*
>
> *681.02   Onychia and paronychia of finger*
> *681.11   Onychia and paronychia of toe*

Suggested Reading

Bernard P, Beden C, Mounier M, et al. Causes of erysipelas and cellulitis in adults. *Arch Dermatol.* 1989;125:779–782.

Bisno AL, Stevens DL. Streptococcal infections of skin and soft tissues. *N Engl J Med.* Jan 25 1996;334:240–245.

Bonnetblanc JM, Bédane C. Erysipelas: recognition and management. *Am J Clin Dermatol.* 2003;4:157–163.

Bratton RL, Nesse RE. St. Anthony's fire: diagnosis and management of erysipelas. *Am Fam Physician.* 1995;51:401–404.

Brook I, Fiengold S. Aerobic and anaerobic bacteriology of cutaneous abscesses in children. *Pediatrics.* 1981;67:891–895.

Brown J, Shriner D, Schwartz RA, et al. Impetigo: an update. *Int J Dermatol.* 2003;42:251–255.

Chartier C, Grosshans E. Erysipelas: an update. *Int J Dermatol.* Nov 1996;35:779–781.

Cole C, Gazewood J. Diagnosis and treatment of impetigo. *Am Fam Physician.* 2007;75(6):859–864.

Darmstadt G, Lane A. Impetigo: an overview. *Pediatr Dermatol.* 1994;11:293–303.

Davison A, Rotstein O. The diagnosis and management of common soft-tissue infections. *Can J Surg.* 1988;31:333–336.

Falagas M, Vergidis P. Narrative review: Diseases that masquerade as infectious cellulitis. *Ann Intern Med.* 2005;142:47–55.

Jebson PJ. Infections of the fingertip. Paronychias and felons. *Hand Clin.* 1998;14:547–555.

Koning S, Verhagen AP, van Suijlekom-Smit LW, et al. Interventions for impetigo. *Cochrane Database Syst Rev.* 2004. CD003261.

Ladhani S, Garbash M. Staphylococcal skin infections in children: rational drug therapy recommendations. *Paediatr Drugs.* 2005;7:77–102.

Lewis R. Soft tissue infections. *World J Surg.* 1998;22:146–151.

Meislin H, Lerner S, Graves M. Cutaneous abscesses: anaerobic and aerobic bacteriology and outpatient management. *Ann Intern Med.* 1977;87:145–149.

Plewig G, Jansen T. Acneiform dermatoses. *Dermatology.* 1998;196:102–107.

Rigopoulos D, Larios G, Gregoriou S. Acute and chronic paronychia. *Am Fam Physician.* 2008;77:339–346.

Sachs M. Cutaneous cellulitis. *Arch Dermatol.* 1991;127:493–500.

Shriner D, Schwartz R, Janniger C. Impetigo. *Cutis.* 1994;45:30–32.

Stulberg D, Penrod M, Blatny R. Common bacterial skin infections. *Am Fam Physician.* 2002;66:119–124.

Wickboldt L, Fenske N. Streptococcal and staphylococcal infections of the skin. *Hosp Pract.* 1986;3:41–47.

Wollina U. Acute paronychia: comparative treatment with topical antibiotic alone or in combination with corticosteroid. *J Eur Acad Dermatol Venereol.* 2001;15:82–84.

CHAPTER **6** Acne and Related Disorders

Jennifer Villaseñor and Daniela Kroshinsky

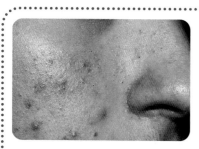

A 15-year-old boy presents with pleomorphic lesions on the central face consisting of papules, pustules, and open comedones (Fig. 6-1). These began following puberty and have become progressively worse, leaving scars and red macules/patches on his face. What is the most likely diagnosis?

The chapter is divided into five sections: acne vulgaris, acne rosacea, hidradenitis suppurativa and the follicular occlusion tetrad, perioral dermatitis, and acne keloidalis. Each section contains a discussion of the clinical features, current and potential treatment alternatives, the clinical course, and prognosis for each disorder.

Acne Vulgaris

BACKGROUND

Arguably the most common cutaneous disorder, acne vulgaris is a self-limited inflammatory reaction involving the pilosebaceous unit that often presents among adolescents. Lesions are often pleomorphic and include comedones, papules, pustules, and nodules with a range in severity of disease. Although most cases are self-limiting, a significant number of patients present with psychiatric comorbidity, especially as a result of the permanent sequelae of acne vulgaris. In rare cases, mortality due to suicide has been associated with patients with severe cases of acne vulgaris. Treatment of acne vulgaris has been associated with significant improvement of self-esteem. Effective treatment is, therefore, essential for both the resolution of acne vulgaris and remediation of associated psychiatric comorbidity.

EPIDEMIOLOGY

The impact of acne vulgaris encompasses a large proportion of the patient population, accounting for over 10% of all patient encounters and over 4.8 million visits per year. In the majority of cases, acne vulgaris becomes a significant problem after the onset of puberty and is thought to be an early manifestation of puberty. Following puberty, the incidence steadily declines with age. Many cases of acne persist beyond adolescence, particularly in women. Genetics is likely to influence the occurrence of acne vulgaris as there is often a familial association observed in many cases.

PATHOGENESIS

Acne vulgaris evolves through a series of events that include follicular keratinocyte hyperproliferation resulting in microcomedo formation, excess

KEY FEATURES

- Follicular epidermal hyperproliferation and excess sebum production lead to follicular clogging and inflammation.

- Characteristic lesions are comedones.

- Common findings are comedones, papules, pustules, nodules on face, chest, and back.

- Treatment includes combinations of oral and topical antimicrobials, retinoids, and hormonal agents.

sebum production, inflammation, and the presence and activity of *Propionibacterium acnes*. Keratinocyte hyperproliferation due to increased proliferation and decreased desquamation of keratinocytes lining the follicular orifice within the pilosebaceous unit is the earliest event. Increased cohesion between proliferative keratinocytes results in the formation of a plug within the follicular ostium and downstream concretions of keratin, sebum, and bacteria that eventually lead to the dilation of the upper hair follicle and microcomedo formation. Androgen stimulation via the production of dihydrotestosterone (DHT) is thought to play an important role in the formation of acne. Follicular keratinocytes convert dehydroepiandrosterone sulfate (DHEAS) to DHT. Increased production of DHT is thought to play a role in keratinocyte proliferation.

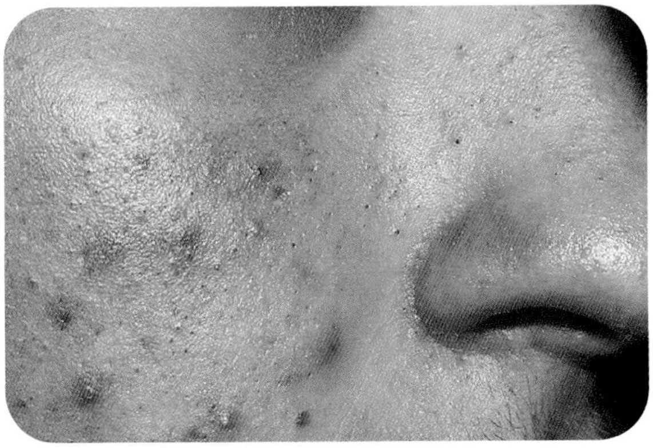

With the onset of puberty, androgen hormones bind and influence sebocyte activity, resulting in enlargement of sebaceous glands and increased sebum production. This provides a rich source of fatty acids for *Propionibacterium acnes*, an anaerobic gram-positive diphtheroid that is a normal component found in the sebaceous follicle, and results in the increased proliferation, clumping, and colonization of *P. acnes*. Proliferation of *P. acnes* and increased keratin and sebum production lead to enlargement of the microcomedo, eventually resulting in follicular wall rupture and extrusion of its contents into the dermis, triggering a brisk inflammatory response. The presence of *P. acnes* is an important trigger for inflammatory response.

CLINICAL PRESENTATION

The onset of acne typically occurs gradually after the onset of puberty. Acne vulgaris usually presents as an isolated cutaneous disease; abrupt onset is concerning for hormonal dysregulation including hyperandrogenism, especially in the setting of a female presenting with associated hirsutism and irregular menstrual periods. The presence of morphologically homogenous acneiform lesions should also prompt further investigation for the use of medications such as anabolic steroids, corticotropin, corticosteroids, isoniazid, vitamin B complexes, phenytoin, and lithium.

The typical lesions of acne vulgaris consist of pleomorphic lesions found on the areas of the body with the highest concentration of sebaceous glands including the face, chest, shoulders, and back. Lesions are either noninflammatory or inflammatory in nature (Fig. 6-1). Noninflammatory lesions include closed and open comedones (Fig. 6-2). The closed comedone, or whitehead, is usually a small, approximately 1-mm papule with no follicular opening or erythema. Open comedones, or blackheads, are flat or slightly raised, dome-shaped papules with a dilated follicular opening containing an inspissated core of shed keratin. Melanin deposition and lipid oxidation of the debris cause the black coloration found within open comedones. Inflammatory lesions include a range of lesions including erythematous papules, pustules, and nodules (Fig. 6-3). Scarring is a consequence of both noninflammatory and inflammatory acne.

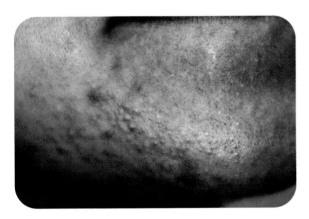

Figure 6-1 Acne vulgaris. Typical acne showing papules, pustules and open comedones on the central face. From Goodheart HP. *Goodheart's Photoguide to Common Skin Disorders,* 3rd ed. Philadelphia: Lippincott Williams & Wilkins, 2009.

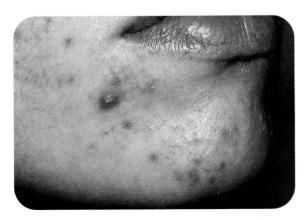

Figure 6-2 Open and closed comedones of acne vulgaris.

Figure 6-3 Inflammatory acne. From Goodheart HP. *Goodheart's Photoguide to Common Skin Disorders,* 3rd ed. Philadelphia: Lippincott Williams & Wilkins, 2009.

Table 6-1 Variants of Acne Vulgaris

Acne fulminans	Most severe form of cystic acne; abrupt onset of nodular and suppurative acne with associated systemic manifestations; osteolytic bone lesions (clavicle, sternum) associated with systemic features (fever, arthralgias, myalgias, hepatosplenomegaly)
Acne conglobata	Severe nodulocystic acne without systemic manifestations; part of the follicular occlusion tetrad
SAPHO syndrome	Synovitis, acne, pustulosis, hyperostosis, and osteitis
PAPA syndrome	Sterile pyogenic arthritis, pyoderma gangrenosum and acne; autosomal dominant inheritance; associated history of sterile cutaneous abscesses, inflammatory bowel disease, and pancytopenia
Acne excoriee des jeunes filles	Often women who pick at their skin; mild acne with excoriations; systematically excoriated leaving crusted erosions that scar; often with psychiatric comorbidity
Acne mechanica	Acneiform eruptions following physical trauma to skin from clothing, sports equipment, adhesive tape
Acne with solid facial edema	Mid-facial edema with accompanying erythema and acne; severity of edema fluctuates without spontaneous resolution
Acne associated with endocrine abnormalities	Polycystic ovarian syndrome, congenital adrenal hyperplasia
Drug-related acneiform eruptions	Glucocorticoids, phenytoin, lithium, isoniazid, high-dose vitamin B complex, halogenated compounds, epidermal growth factor receptor inhibitors (erlotinib, cetuximab, panitumumab, gefitinib)
Chloracne/Occupational	Exposure to chlorinated and halogenated compounds cause characteristic acne with prominent open comedones on posterior auricular skin

Acne vulgaris is classified according to the number and types of lesions and whether scarring is present (Table 6-1). Mild acne is characterized by a predominance of comedones and occasional small, inflamed papules or pustules. Comedones, papules, and pustules are more prevalent and involve the face, back, chest, and shoulders in those with moderate acne. Additionally, mild scarring and occasional cysts and nodules are often present. Severe acne is characterized by the predominance of large cysts on the face, neck, and upper trunk with the presence of severe scarring.

DIAGNOSIS

Differential Diagnosis

Acne vulgaris is often clinically apparent and distinguished by the presence of pleomorphic lesions including comedones. The presence of comedones is what distinguishes acne vulgaris from other cutaneous disorders. The most common acne mimics are rosacea, perioral dermatitis, and folliculitis. Rosacea and perioral dermatitis are part of the differential diagnosis of inflammatory acne.

Diagnostic Methods

Acne vulgaris is usually diagnosed clinically by the presence of a pleomorphic collection of lesions including papules and pustules. The presence of comedones is required for the clinical diagnosis of acne vulgaris. In general, the diagnosis of acne vulgaris does not require laboratory testing. However, a thorough evaluation of a patient presenting with acne should include a complete history to rule out a systemic etiology of disease. Rapid onset of acne associated with virilization should prompt laboratory testing of hormonal levels and imaging studies to rule out an underlying adrenal or ovarian tumor. Elevated serum androgens are found in patients with severe cystic acne and in association with endocrine abnormalities or neoplastic processes. The majority of patients with acne have normal levels of serum androgens. Additionally, a complete medication list should be obtained to rule out medication-induced acne. Physical examination should focus on the type and location of lesions, scarring, keloids, and postinflammatory pigmentary changes.

THERAPY

Treatment for acne vulgaris is guided by the severity of the acne and is aimed at correcting the altered pattern of follicular keratinization, decreasing sebaceous gland activity, decreasing the follicular bacterial population, and providing an anti-inflammatory effect. Treatment modalities include both local and systemic therapies and may include combinations of both types of therapies. Most patients with mild to moderate acne respond to benzoyl peroxide, a topical antibiotic, or a combination of both drugs. Combination therapy is especially useful for patients with acne that includes both comedonal acne and inflammatory lesions. Some suggestions for treatment regimens and therapy options are presented in Tables 6-2 and 6-3.

Table 6-2 Step-wise Suggestions for Acne Therapy

Mild inflammatory acne
- Step 1: OTC benzoyl peroxide 5%–10% wash to use when showering and/or salicylic acid solution OTC for the evening. Alternately prescription clindamycin 1% gel or lotion may be substituted once daily (morning or evening)
- Step 2: Prescription clindamycin 1%/benzoyl peroxide 5% (Duac or BenzaClin) gel QAM and a retinoid such as tretinoin 0.05% or adapalene 0.3% QHS
- Recommend use of a mild cleanser such as Cerave and stress that the face should not be scrubbed. Lesions should not be picked unless absolutely necessary.

Mild comedonal acne
- Step 1: Prescription retinoids topically are the therapy of choice as they help prevent comedone formation

Moderate to severe inflammatory and/or comedonal acne
- Step 1: Prescription clindamycin 1%/benzoyl peroxide 5% (Duac or BenzaClin) gel QAM and a retinoid such as tretinoin 0.05% or adapalene 0.3% QHS.
- Step 2: Oral antibiotic therapy. In some cases starting one of the agents along with topicals is desirable.
  - First-line: doxycycline or minocycline 100 mg PO BID × 2 months, then taper PRN
  - Second-line: amoxicillin 500 PO QD, trimethoprim/sulfamethoxazole 160 mg TMP/800 mg SMZ PO q12h (adult dosing), azithromycin (dosing controversial; some recommend 500 mg PO 3× weekly.

Severe inflammatory/nodulocystic/scarring acne
- First-line: oral and topical therapy appropriate for moderate/severe acne above
- If those fail, have a low threshold to refer the patient to an IPLEDGE registered physician for oral retinoid therapy (isotretinoin)
- Intralesional triamcinolone acetonide 3.3 mg/cc ~0.1–0.2 cc per lesion is helpful for discreet nodulocystic lesions

Table 6-3 Medications Used in Acne Therapy

TOPICAL AGENTS	CLASS	THERAPY TIER/NOTES
Salicylic acid	Keratolytic	First-line; mild to moderate
Benzoyl peroxide	Antibacterial	First-line; mild to moderate
Clindamycin	Antibacterial	First-line; mild to moderate
Sodium sulfacetamide	Antibacterial	Second-line; mild to severe
Azelaic acid	Antibacterial/Keratolytic/ Anti-inflammatory	Second-line; mild
Adapalene	Retinoid	First-line; mild to severe
Tazarotene	Retinoid	Second-line; moderate to severe
Tretinoin	Retinoid	First-line; mild to severe
SYSTEMIC AGENTS		
Doxycycline	Antibacterial/ Anti-inflammatory	First-line; mild to moderate
Minocycline	Antibacterial/ Anti-inflammatory	First-line; mild to moderate
Erythromycin/ Azithromycin	Antibacterial	Second-line; mild to moderate
Trimethoprim/ sulfamethoxazole	Antibacterial	Second-line; mild to severe
Amoxicillin	Antibacterial	Second-line; mild to severe
Isotretinoin	Retinoid	First-line; severe treatment-resistant nodulocystic
Spironolactone	Antiandrogen	Second-line for female patients; second-line, mild to moderate
Yaz/Ortho-tricyclen	Antiandrogen	Second-line for female patients; second-line, mild to moderate

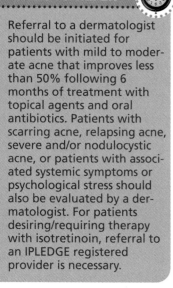

WHEN TO REFER

Referral to a dermatologist should be initiated for patients with mild to moderate acne that improves less than 50% following 6 months of treatment with topical agents and oral antibiotics. Patients with scarring acne, relapsing acne, severe and/or nodulocystic acne, or patients with associated systemic symptoms or psychological stress should also be evaluated by a dermatologist. For patients desiring/requiring therapy with isotretinoin, referral to an IPLEDGE registered provider is necessary.

NOT TO BE MISSED

- Scarring acne should be aggressively treated. If there is no response to conservative therapy, consider referral for systemic isotretinoin.

- Women with virilization should be evaluated for hormonal dysfunction.

- Ensure female patients are not pregnant before initiating topical or systemic retinoids.

One of the most effective therapies for acne vulgaris is oral isotretinoin. This medication is Food and Drug Administration (FDA) approved for therapy of treatment-resistant scarring nodulocystic acne. As with all retinoids, isotretinoin is teratogenic with pregnancy category X. The FDA has mandated a pregnancy prevention program for all providers desiring to prescribe isotretinoin (IPLEDGE). This requires extensive patient education and consent, monthly monitoring/ pregnancy tests, two forms of birth control (or complete sexual abstinence), with safeguards at the office level and at the pharmacist. Males, and females not capable of becoming pregnant (hysterectomy or after menopause), are also enrolled in the IPLEDGE program, though the requirements are not as strict.

"AT A GLANCE" TREATMENT

- Topical and systemic acne therapies are summarized in Tables 6-2 and 6-3.

COURSE AND COMPLICATIONS

Acne vulgaris is typically a self-limited disease with a variable course that may continue for several years up to the third and fourth decades. It may include periods of remission. The overall prognosis is generally favorable; however, treatment should be initiated early during the course of the disease to prevent the permanent sequelae of the disease. Some of the complications of acne vulgaris may be as benign as transient macular erythema to more persistent or permanent sequelae such as postinflammatory hyperpigmentation or scarring. Scarring acne should be treated aggressively. Additionally, it is estimated that up to 50% of patients with acne have psychiatric comorbidities and experience similar levels of social, psychological, and emotional impairments as those suffering from asthma or epilepsy.

> *ICD9 Codes*
> *706.1   Other acne*

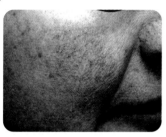

A 35-year-old white female presents with complaints of persistent erythema of her cheeks with papules and pustules resembling acne (Fig. 6-4). She reports a long history of sensitivity to various facial lotions and astringents.

Upon closer inspection, there are telangiectasias present without evidence for comedones. She reports flushing/blushing with alcohol consumption and hot/spicy foods. Her mother has had similar eruptions. What is the most likely diagnosis? What test can be done to confirm the diagnosis?

Acne Rosacea

BACKGROUND

Rosacea is a chronic acneiform disorder of unknown etiology affecting approximately 14 million adults and found most frequently among the white population. The most characteristic feature of rosacea is persistent erythema of the central face involving the nose, cheeks, chin, and forehead. Primary clinical features include flushing/transient erythema, nontransient erythema, papules, pustules, and telangiectasias. Secondary features include facial burning or stinging, edema, plaques, dryness, phyma, peripheral flushing, and ocular manifestations. The presentation of rosacea is quite variable and four distinct sub-types have been described.

KEY FEATURES

- Rosacea presents with persistent erythema of the central face: nose, cheeks, chin, and forehead.

- Primary clinical features include flushing (transient erythema), papules, pustules, telangiectasias.

- Secondary features include facial burning or stinging, edema, plaques, dryness, phyma, peripheral flushing, and ocular manifestations.

- Hot or cold temperature, sunlight, alcohol, exercise, spicy foods, emotional stress, topical irritants, and medications are triggers of rosacea.

- Prevention of rosacea involves sun protection and avoidance of triggers of rosacea.

- Treat using ultraviolet (UV) protection, topical and oral antibiotics, topical retinoids, intense pulsed light, vascular laser modalities.

PATHOGENESIS

The etiology and pathogenesis of acne rosacea is still unclear. However, factors affecting facial vascular reactivity, changes in dermal connective tissue structure or composition, matrix composition, pilosebaceous structure, microbial colonization, or a combination of these factors have been attributed to the development of rosacea.

CLINICAL PRESENTATION

Rosacea is a chronic disorder characterized by periods of exacerbation and remission that can be triggered or worsened by various stimuli including hot or spicy foods, alcohol, and temperature changes. Facial erythema, particularly on the nose and cheeks, and telangiectasias are typical presenting symptoms of rosacea. Severe sebaceous gland growth with associated papules, pustules, cysts, and nodules may also be present and appear very similar to the lesions of acne vulgaris. However, the lack of comedones distinguishes rosacea from acne vulgaris. Ocular symptoms associated with the typical skin lesions of rosacea may develop and are characterized by foreign body sensation and burning, telangiectasia and irregularity of lid margins, meibomian gland dysfunction, keratitis, conjunctivitis, and episcleritis. Another characteristic feature associated with rosacea is rhinophyma, which results from hyperplasia of the soft tissues of the nose.

Sub-types of Rosacea

Erythematotelangiectatic rosacea (ETR). Erythematotelangiectatic rosacea (ETR) is characterized by persistent facial erythema and flushing lasting longer than 10 minutes. The most intense color involves the central portion of the face and the periocular skin is typically spared. Telangiectasias, central face edema, burning or stinging, roughness, or scaling are also typical features of ETR (Fig. 6-4). Patients with ETR often have a lower threshold for irritation from topically applied substances and often experience associated stinging, burning, or itching. The skin of patients with ETR is usually fine in texture, lacks a sebaceous quality or oiliness, and may have associated roughness and scaling around affected sites. Particular stimuli that have been associated with the onset of ETR symptoms include emotional stress, hot drinks, alcohol, spicy foods, exercise, or temperature extremes.

Papulopustular rosacea (PPR). Papulopustular rosacea is also known as classic rosacea or pink papular rosacea. The most prominent clinical feature of PPR is persistent or episodic erythema of the central portion of the face with a predominance of small papules and pustules (Fig. 6-5). Edema can be mild or severe, with severe edema presenting similarly to solid facial edema. There is usually sparing of the periocular and perioral skin with intense redness at adjacent sites. A history of flushing may be present; however, irritation from external stimuli is not as prominent or persistent compared to those with ETR. Additionally, scaling and roughness are usually absent and there may be subtle telangiectasias.

Phymatous rosacea. Skin thickening and irregular surface nodularities, particularly of the nose (rhinophyma) and chin (gnathophyma) are the most common clinical features of phymatous rosacea. For a typical example, see Figures 6-6 and 6-7. Other areas of prominent skin thickening include the forehead (metophyma); one or both ears (otophyma); and the eyelids (blepharophyma).

Ocular rosacea. The clinical features of ocular rosacea include blepharitis and conjunctivitis, inflammation of the lids with recurrent chalazion and inflammation of meibomian glands. Interpalpebral conjunctival hyperemia, conjunctival telangiectasias, and watery or dry, irritated eyes may also occur. Patients may also complain of burning or stinging, itching, light sensitivity,

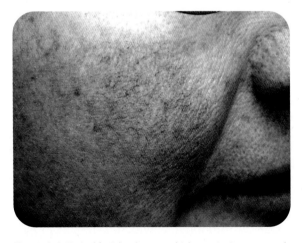

Figure 6-4 Typical facial redness and telangectasias commonly seen in erythematotelangiectatic rosacea.

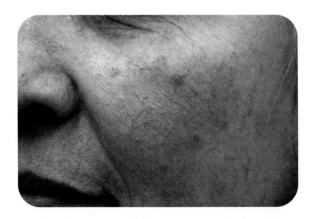

Figure 6-5 Mild papulopustular rosacea. This woman also has a prominent telangiectatic component.

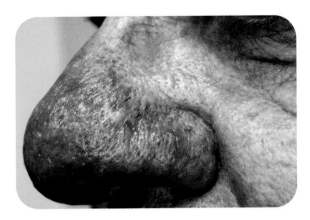

Figure 6-6 Early rhinophymatous rosacea.

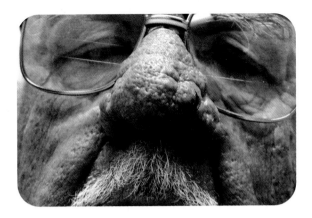

Figure 6-7 Later stage rhinophymatous rosacea.

KEY FEATURES

- Characterized by blepharitis and conjunctivitis, often in conjunction with or following other skin findings.

or a foreign body sensation. In rare instances, keratitis, scleritis, or iritis may develop. Ocular rosacea may precede other cutaneous signs of rosacea in up to 20% of affected individuals. Fifty percent of affected individuals will develop ocular symptoms after skin symptoms. Simultaneous development of skin and eye symptoms occurs in a minority of affected individuals. However, the severity of ocular rosacea does not generally correlate with the severity of skin symptoms.

DIAGNOSIS

Differential Diagnosis

Conditions that resemble rosacea include systemic diseases such as polycythemia vera; connective tissue disorders (e.g., lupus erythematosus, dermatomyositis); carcinoid syndrome; mastocytosis; and neurologic causes of flushing. A thorough history including a list of medications may be useful for differentiating between rosacea and medication-induced flushing (Table 6-4). Although rosacea may occur in the presence of acne vulgaris, the primary differentiating feature between the two are the presence of comedones in acne alone.

Diagnostic Methods

The diagnosis of rosacea is often made clinically. The presence of one or more of the following features makes the diagnosis of rosacea more likely: flushing (transient erythema); nontransient erythema; papules and pustules; and telangiectasia. Additionally, the presence of one or more of the following secondary

Table 6-4 Medications Known to Cause Flushing

Amyl and butyl nitrite	Nicotinic acid (niacin)
Bromocriptine	Systemic steroids
Calcium channel blockers	Tamoxifen
Cholinergic drugs	Thyroid releasing hormone
Cyclosporine	Vasodilators
Cyproterone acetate	
Morphine	

features may appear independently or in combination with other features of rosacea: burning or stinging, plaque formation, edema, ocular manifestations, and phymatous changes.

THERAPY

Effective treatment for all types of rosacea requires careful identification of specific factors that trigger symptoms in each individual and emphasis should be placed on avoidance of these triggers. Avoidance of harsh products and ingredients including astringents, toners, menthol, camphor, and sodium lauryl sulfate should be emphasized in individuals with ETR or PPR because these individuals tend to be particularly sensitive to these chemicals. Additionally, use of gentle, broad-spectrum sunscreen and avoidance of direct sunlight should be emphasized.

In general, current treatments for rosacea are focused on symptom control rather than cure. Mild topical antimicrobials, photoprotection, low-dose isotretinoin, oral tetracyclines, vascular laser, intense pulsed light, topical retinoid maintenance, and tretinoin cream plus emollient are recommended treatments for ETR and PPR. More aggressive treatment modalities such as mid- to high-dose isotretinoin, spironolactone, and surgical and laser debulking and contouring techniques are used for phymatous and glandular rosacea in addition to topical and/or oral microbials and topical retinoids. Ophthalmologic assessment should be performed for those presenting with ocular rosacea and use of gentle cleansers, ophthalmic ointments, and oral tetracyclines are indicated.

Topical Treatments

Topical metronidazole and azelaic acid are the most effective treatments for rosacea. However, other topical treatments that have been shown to be effective include clindamycin, erythromycin, calcineurin inhibitors, and retinoids. "Manual therapy" or facial massage may decrease dermal inflammation via mechanical mobilization of edema. Studies have also shown beneficial effects with the use of tretinoin cream, which is thought to promote connective tissue remodeling and to decrease dermal inflammation with long-term use. However, 4 to 6 months may be required in order to see any significant changes.

Oral Treatments

Treatment with the tetracycline family analogs is the most common and most helpful oral therapy. There are two dosing regimens commonly used. Some begin therapy with medications such as doxycycline at 100 mg PO twice daily for 1 to 2 months until the flare has resolved, then refill the medication as necessary for flares. Some require chronic maintenance dosing. Others start at a much lower dose of medication, below the antimicrobial threshold at 40 mg per day (Oracea). Isotretinoin is quite helpful in recalcitrant/extensive cases. For those patients unwilling/unable to take systemic retinoids, Dapsone may be beneficial.

"AT A GLANCE" TREATMENT

- Topical therapy:
  - Azelaic acid 15% gel
  - Metronidazole 0.75% or 1%, available in cream, gel, and lotion vehicles
  - Sodium sulfacetamide 10% with 5% sulfur, available in cleanser, cream, suspension, and lotion vehicles
  - Benzoyl peroxide, 2.5% once or twice daily, increasing to 5% to 10%; not for use in patients with sensitivity to benzoyl peroxide or those who experience dryness with use

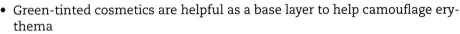

- Green-tinted cosmetics are helpful as a base layer to help camouflage erythema
- Oral therapy:
  - First-line oral therapy: doxycycline or minocycline 100 mg PO BID × 1 to 2 months, then taper. In some cases, lower dose therapies are helpful (Oracea)
  - Recalcitrant rosacea responds well to oral retinoids (isotretinoin)
  - Ocular rosacea is treated commonly with oral doxycycline or minocycline as well as daily lid hygiene (hot compresses and gentle cleansing).
- Surgical/cosmetic therapy:
  - Vascular lasers and intense pulsed light may help treat the redness component
  - Phymatous rosacea may be successfully reduced surgically

COURSE AND COMPLICATIONS

Acne rosacea is a chronic disorder with variable periods of exacerbation and remission. Symptom control is the goal of treatment with absolute cure an unlikely scenario. Ideally, early treatment and control of facial erythema, telangiectasias, and inflammatory lesions should be initiated before the occurrence of advanced manifestations that require more aggressive treatment.

ICD9 Codes

695.3	Rosacea
448.0	Hereditary hemorrhagic telangiectasia
448.1	Nevus, non-neoplastic
448.9	Other and unspecified capillary diseases

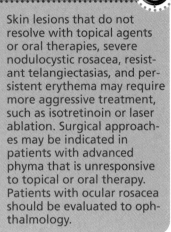

A 40-year-old woman presents with persistent tender and erythematous nodules in her axillae and inframammary areas (Fig. 6-8). She reports that these lesions recur every month and occasionally produce a malodorous discharge. On physical examination, there are various 0.5 to 2.0 mm deep-seated erythematous nodules in the axillary and inframammary regions that are tender to palpation. Ropelike scars also surround the active lesions. What is the most likely diagnosis? What should the treatment be?

Hidradenitis Suppurativa

BACKGROUND

The HS encompasses hidradenitis suppurativa (HS), acne conglobata, dissecting cellulitis of the scalp. In this section, we will primarily discuss HS. The other components are discussed elsewhere. When first described, HS was considered a disorder of the apocrine glands. The term "hidradenitis suppurativa" was based on the clinical features of the first reported cases of the condition, which involved the presence of superficial abscess formation in the axillary, mammary, and perianal regions with an associated suppurative process with the sweat glands. Further histopathologic characterization of this disorder revealed the prominence of follicular occlusion, inflammation, fibrosis, and scarring. However, there was a lack of apocrine gland involvement.

EPIDEMIOLOGY

Based on objective clinical findings, the point prevalence of this order has been reported to be up to 4.1%. The disorder affects all races equally. However, there is a female predilection with reported sex ratios of 3:1.

ASSOCIATED FACTORS

Genitofemoral lesions are featured more prominently among females; however, axillary involvement affects males and females equally. A genetic association of HS is still unclear. Several diseases have been associated with HS. Crohn's disease, particularly with perianal involvement, has been reported to be associated with HS. Obesity has also been associated with the HS; however, it is unlikely to be the primary cause of the disease. Other associated factors in the pathogenesis of HS include bacterial infections, particularly *Staphylococcus aureus* and coagulase-negative staphylococci, and use of tobacco products.

CLINICAL PRESENTATION

Affected individuals with HS often initially present with tender papules or deep-seated nodules in apocrine-bearing intertriginous areas such as the axilla (Fig. 6-8), perineum, mammary and inframammary regions, buttocks, pubic region, chest, and scalp. The axillae, groin, and inframammary regions are the most common areas affecting women whereas the perineal and perianal skin are more commonly involved in men. Abscesses that develop may resolve or rupture spontaneously, producing purulent discharge. When healing occurs, the lesion develops scarring with fibrosis forming dermal contractures and ropelike elevation of the skin. Additionally, sinus tracts may develop involving deep tissue, including muscle and fascia, urethra, and bowel.

The Hurley system characterizes the disease in three clinical stages. The primary stage is defined by the presence of abscess without evidence of sinus tracts or scarring (Fig. 6-9). Nodules expand and merge to form abscesses in isolated locations and may eventually rupture and release purulent discharge. The secondary stage of the disease involves the development of sinus tracts with scars bridging individual lesions and the formation of discrete recurrent abscesses (Fig. 6-10). Diffuse involvement, coalescing lesions with scarring and sinus tract formation, inflammation, and chronic discharge characterize the tertiary stage of the disease (Fig. 6-11). The progression of the disease usually occurs through these stages with repetition of the cycle and extension of disease into neighboring areas. About 75% of patients are in the primary stage, 24% in the secondary stage, and 1% in the tertiary stage.

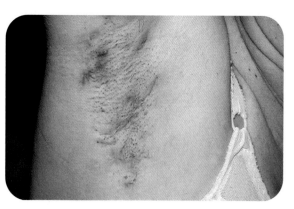

Figure 6-8 HS of the axilla. From Goodheart HP. *Goodheart's Photoguide to Common Skin Disorders,* 3rd ed. Philadelphia: Lippincott Williams & Wilkins, 2009.

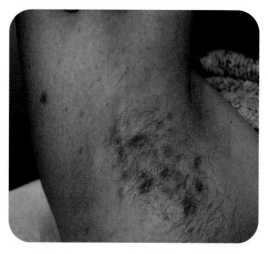

Figure 6-9 Primary stage HS. From Goodheart HP. *Goodheart's Photoguide to Common Skin Disorders,* 3rd ed. Philadelphia: Lippincott Williams & Wilkins, 2009.

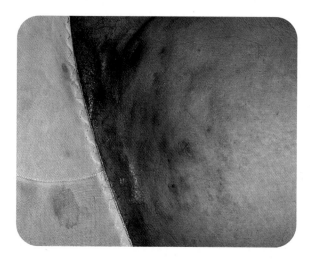

Figure 6-10 Secondary stage HS. From Goodheart HP. *Goodheart's Photoguide to Common Skin Disorders,* 3rd ed. Philadelphia: Lippincott Williams & Wilkins, 2009.

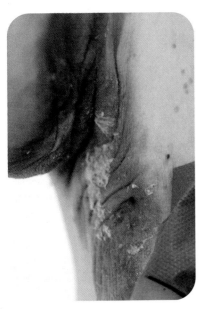

Figure 6-11 Ulcerations, scarring, and cordlike fibrosis seen in Tertiary stage HS.

DIAGNOSIS

The diagnosis of HS is based on characteristic clinical manifestations and biopsy is rarely needed. Although no specific diagnostic criteria exist, there are three main diagnostic features of the disorder:

1. The typical lesions include deep-seated nodules, comedones and/or fibrosis
2. A characteristic distribution involving the axillae, groin and inframammary areas
3. Recurrence

The diagnosis is made if the patient has either (a) active disease with one or more primary lesions in a typical site in addition to a history of three or more discharging or painful lumps in designated sites since the age of 10 years; or (b) inactive disease with a history of five or more discharging or painful lumps in designated sites since age 10 years.

Differential Diagnosis

Other disorders similar to HS include abscesses, furuncles/carbuncles, actinomycosis, cat scratch disease, donovanosis, lymphogranuloma venereum, lymphadenitis, infected Bartholin cyst, Crohn's disease, ulcerative colitis, tuberculosis, tularemia, and a ruptured epidermal cyst.

Diagnostic Methods

In order to determine the best treatment, several studies may be considered during the evaluation of the patient.

Laboratory studies. The following initial studies may help guide treatment: (a) aerobic culture swabs of lesions; (b) aerobic and anaerobic skin aspirate of lesions; (c) baseline complete blood count (CBC) with differential, basic metabolic panel including magnesium, liver function tests (LFTs), glucose-6 phosphate dehydrogenase (G6PD) level, and fasting lipids. Patients with acute lesions may have increased erythrocyte sedimentation rate or C-reactive protein. Deep cultures taken at different depths in the lesions should be performed if there is a concern for infection and should be submitted for bacterial, tuberculosis, and fungal cultures. If a female patient presents with hirsutism, consider checking levels of dihydroepiandrosterone sulfate, total and free levels of testosterone, sex-hormone-binding globulin, and progesterone. Histopathology may be helpful.

TREATMENT

The HS is a chronic disease with variable periods of remission and recurrence. Many of the options for treatment do not provide significant remission from the disease. Surgical treatment may provide more rapid resolution of symptoms and longer periods of remission. Combined medical and surgical treatment may be indicated for some cases. However, there is no cure for the disease. The main objectives are (a) the prevention or the reduction of primary lesions; and (b) resolution, amelioration, or regression of secondary disease features such as scarring or sinus tract formation.

Initial treatment measures include:

- Practicing local hygiene
- Reduction of further trauma to involved areas through avoidance of heat and humidity, friction from clothing, and perspiration; weight loss; or use of loose, breathable clothing may also be helpful
- Use of gentle antimicrobial cleansers and avoidance of washcloths
- Encourage cessation of smoking

Medical treatment. This includes use of antibiotics, antiandrogens, and retinoids, all of which effectively treat early lesions of the disease and may be effective in prevention of new lesions.

Topical treatment. Treatment with topical antibiotics such as clindamycin, benzoyl peroxide, or chlorhexidine may result in improvement of lesions.

Systemic treatment

- *Antibiotics.* The anti-inflammatory actions of antibiotics may beneficial. Although the disease is not a primary infectious disease, antibiotic use may diminish odor and reduce pain from lesions. However, there is no data to support that use of antibiotics alters the course of the disease or prevents recurrence.
- *Antiandrogens.* Only a few reports show effective treatment with antiandrogen therapy. In one study, finasteride 5 mg once a day resulted in improvement by 8 weeks and remission from 8 to 18 months. Use of ethinyl estradiol/drospirenone and the antiandrogen spironolactone (50 to 100 mg) may prevent recurrent groin and vulvar lesions.
- *Immunosuppression.* The inflammatory component of HS may be reduced with use of immunosuppressive treatment. However, the effectiveness of these treatments have only been demonstrated in a few case reports, many of which report rebound following withdrawal of treatment.
- *Retinoids.* There may be little benefit with treatment with systemic retinoids.
- *TNF-alpha inhibitors.* The newer antitumor necrosis alpha agents such as infliximab and etanercept are being used for HS with success, though the use is off-label. Patients with severe/recalcitrant disease may benefit from these agents.

Surgical treatment. Surgical excision is the treatment of choice for early disease and for definitive treatment. For severe disease, both medical and surgical treatments are required to stop development of new lesions and to effectively control inflammation.

"AT A GLANCE" TREATMENT

- A treatment regimen based on the Hurley staging is presented in Table 6-5.

COURSE AND COMPLICATIONS

Onset of HS is typically at or following puberty. The average duration of the disease is 20 years. Early diagnosis of disease is essential for effective treatment as patients with primary disease can be effectively controlled. Secondary and tertiary disease becomes increasingly difficult to treat, requiring a multi-modal treatment approach and making cure less likely. In patients with severe disease, recurrence rates of greater than 25% have been reported even after extensive surgery.

Local complications of the disease include extensive scarring that may limit mobility. Anal, urethral, or rectal strictures may develop from chronic genitofemoral inflammation. In severe disease, urethral fistulas may also occur. Systemic complications have also been reported and include septicemia and, in rare cases, lumbosacral epidural abscesses. In addition to the physical complications of the disease, patients with severe disease report very low quality of life as measured by the Dermatology Life Quality Index. Quality of life was affected by disease severity and progression of disease, disease-associated pain, and prolonged duration.

WHEN TO REFER

Skin lesions that do not resolve with topical agents and oral therapies may require more aggressive treatment. Patients with severe disease may require surgical treatment with wide excision. Patients desiring anti-TNF agents should be referred to a dermatologist or rheumatologist actively using these agents for consultation and management.

NOT TO BE MISSED

- Surgical treatment by wide excision is often helpful for severely affected patients.

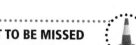

ICD9 Codes

705.83   *Hidradenitis*

Table 6-5 Treatment Recommendations for HS

HURLEY STAGE	THERAPY

Primary	Topical antibiotics
	  Clindamycin 1% solution BID
	  Benzoyl peroxide 5%–10% solution or wash BID
	  Chlorhexidine 4% solution BID

Secondary	Topical antibiotics +
	Systemic antibiotics:
	  Doxycycline 50–100 mg BID or minocycline
	    50–100 mg BID
	  Amoxicillin 250–500 mg BID
	  Sulfamethoxazole/trimethoprim DS BID
	  Clindamycin 300 mg BID
	Antiandrogen (Females PRN):
	  Spironolactone 50–200 mg QD

Tertiary	Topical antibiotics + systemic antibiotics
	Other therapies:
	  Dapsone, finasteride, isotretinoin
	Immunomodulators:
	  Systemic steroids, infliximab, etanercept, cyclosporine
	Antiandrogen PRN

Independent of severity	Adjunctive therapy (weight loss, smoking cessation,
	  sitz bath, warm compresses, intralesional steroids)
	Pain management (nonsteroidal anti-inflammatories,
	  opiates)
	Surgical excision

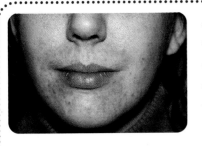

A 27-year-old woman presents with persistent erythematous papules and pustules with surrounding scale distributed around her mouth, sparing the vermillion edge (Fig. 6-12). She reports that her only medication is inhaled steroids for asthma. What is the most likely diagnosis? What should the treatment be?

Perioral Dermatitis

BACKGROUND

Perioral dermatitis is characterized by the presence of small discrete papules, vesicles, and pustules in a perioral, periorbital, and perinasal distribution. Historically, it has been described in young women between the ages of 15 and 25 years. However, it is increasingly recognized in children between 7 months and 13 years of age. No predilection for males or females or a particular race has been described in affected children. A rare granulomatous form of perioral dermatitis is found mostly in prepubertal children.

PATHOGENESIS

The pathogenesis of perioral dermatitis is related to the use of topical corticosteroids on the face in some cases. Some experts suggest it may be a subtype of rosacea or severe seborrheic dermatitis. Typically the patient will reveal an acute eruption around the mouth, nose, and/or eyes. In some cases this follows the use of topical corticosteroids and worsens when it is discontinued. Although there is an established link between perioral dermatitis and corticosteroid use, not all cases are the result of corticosteroid use or misuse. Other potential causes in these cases have been linked to photosensitivity; microbiologic causes (e.g., candidal, fusiform bacteria, or *Demodex folliculorum* infections); or allergenic

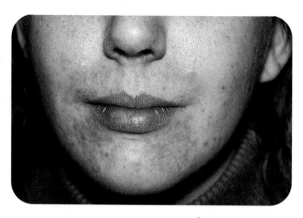

Figure 6-12 Multiple acneiform papules with characteristic sparing around the lips. From Goodheart HP. *Goodheart's Photoguide to Common Skin Disorders,* 3rd ed. Philadelphia: Lippincott Williams & Wilkins, 2009.

contact with fluorides in toothpaste and dentrifices. Other cases seem to be a subtype of rosacea, responding to similar therapies as discussed above. However, many of these associations have not been substantiated by other studies.

CLINICAL PRESENTATION

The primary lesions of perioral dermatitis include discrete or grouped erythematous papules, vesicles, and pustules in an erythematous background with surrounding scale as shown in Figure 6-12. The lesions are usually symmetrically distributed along the perioral, perinasal, and periorbital areas; however, lesions may also be unilaterally distributed. There is often sparing at the vermilion edge around the lips. Associated symptoms may include a sensation of burning or tension. Pruritus is rare. The lesions of the granulomatous variant of perioral dermatitis are small flesh-colored, erythematous, or yellow-brown papules, some with confluence, and distributed periorally. Blepharitis or conjunctivitis may be associated with the granulomatous variant in rare cases.

DIAGNOSIS

The diagnosis is made clinically with no expected laboratory abnormalities.

Differential Diagnosis

Nongranulomatous perioral dermatitis may mimic other diseases such as acne rosacea; acne vulgaris; seborrheic dermatitis; allergic (often cinnamon flavorants) and irritant contact dermatitis (fluoride in toothpaste); gram-negative folliculitis; angular cheilitis; and lip-licking cheilitis. Unlike perioral dermatitis, rosacea tends to involve the nose and facial convexities with presence of persistent erythema and telangiectasias.

THERAPY

First-line therapy includes concurrent use of topical and systemic antibiotics. Topical metronidazole or azelaic acid twice a day is combined with either oral doxycycline 100 mg BID or minocycline 50 to 100 mg BID for a course of 8 to 10 weeks with a taper of the last 2 to 4 weeks. Second-line therapy includes topical erythromycin or clindamycin twice daily combined with oral erythromycin 400 mg three times daily. Oral erythromycin is best reserved for patients who are under 8 years of age, nursing mothers, and patients who do not tolerate tetracycline.

KEY FEATURES

- Perioral dermatitis is an inflammatory skin disorder related to rosacea.

- It presents with stinging/burning papules, vesicles, and pustules in perioral, periorbital, and perinasal distribution.

- Presentation is predominantly in young women between 15 to 25 years and children between 7 months and 13 years.

- Treatment includes cessation of topical corticosteroid use; systemic antibiotics, topical metronidazole, and/or sulfur preparations.

WHEN TO REFER

Skin lesions that do not resolve with topical and systemic agents as outlined above or patients with associated systemic symptoms may benefit from an evaluation by a dermatologist.

NOT TO BE MISSED

- Allergic contact dermatitis to flavorants (often cinnamon) or irritant reactions to fluoride in toothpastes may cause perioral flares.

"AT A GLANCE" TREATMENT

- First-line therapy:
  - Topical metronidazole or azelaic acid twice a day AND
  - Oral doxycycline 100 mg BID or minocycline 50 to 100 mg BID for a course of 8 to 10 weeks with a taper of the last 2 to 4 weeks
- Second-line therapy:
  - Topical erythromycin or clindamycin BID combined with oral erythromycin 400 mg three times daily

COURSE AND COMPLICATIONS

The clinical course of perioral dermatitis is usually self-limited, lasting a few weeks with resolution within months. In rare cases, the disease may span years. Upon resolution of the disease, scarring may occur on rare occasions.

ICD9 Codes	
695.3	Rosacea

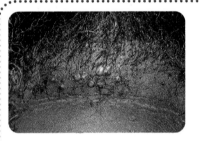

A 25-year-old African-American male presents for treatment of persistent nodules on the back of his head (Fig. 6-13). Initially, they began as small nodules that were asymptomatic. They have progressively enlarged and are now pruritic and painful. He became very concerned because he has developed bandlike areas that do not grow hair. What is the most likely diagnosis? What should the treatment be?

Acne Keloidalis Nuchae

BACKGROUND

Acne keloidalis nuchae (AKN) is characterized by the presence of keloid-like papules and plaques on the occiput and nape of the neck. It occurs almost exclusively in African-American men, although there have been cases reported in Hispanics and Asians. Rarely, the disorder occurs in whites. The reported male-to-female ratio is approximately 20:1. The disease begins in early adulthood, but some cases develop during adolescence. The disorder represents nearly 0.5% of all dermatologic cases in the black population.

KEY FEATURES

- Acne keloidalis nuchae is a chronic scarring folliculitis characterized by fibrotic papules and nodules of the nape of the neck and occiput.

- It is predominantly in young men of African descent, rare in women.

- Treatment should be initiated are early as possible to prevent scarring and includes intralesional injections of corticosteroids, potent topical steroids, and topical or oral antibiotics; for recalcitrant disease, surgery or laser hair removal may be effective.

PATHOGENESIS

The etiology of AKN is still unclear. Several causative factors have been proposed and include constant irritation due to shirt collars; a low-grade bacterial infection; injury during haircuts (especially when the posterior hairline is shaved with a razor, a common practice in African-American men); curved hair and hair follicles; and a dysregulated autoimmune process. However, none of these theories have been proven and all are based on anecdotal evidence. Ingrown hairs, the causative factor in pseudofolliculitis barbae, was once associated with acne keloidalis. However, this has not been proven. Other causative factors may include antiepileptics drugs, cyclosporine, and an increased number of mast cells in the occipital region.

CLINICAL PRESENTATION

Early papular lesions are usually asymptomatic and begin as firm, dome-shaped follicular papules 2 to 4 mm in diameter at or below the occipital hairline that enlarge as the disease progresses and coalesce into hairless keloid-like plaques that are usually arranged in a band-like distribution (Fig. 6-13). Pustular lesions may be pruritic and painful. Larger lesions are often painful and contain abscesses and sinus that may emit a malodorous discharge.

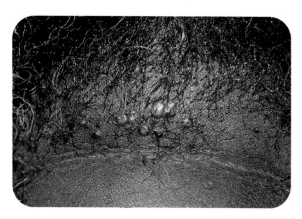

Figure 6-13 Acne keloidalis on the posterior scalp. From Goodheart HP. *Goodheart's Photoguide to Common Skin Disorders*, 3rd ed. Philadelphia: Lippincott Williams & Wilkins, 2009.

DIAGNOSIS

The diagnosis is made clinically. Features of AKN include the disappearance of follicular ostia, concomitant epidermal atrophy or the presence of pustules, scaling, and other signs of inflammatory skin changes. Bacterial culture and sensitivity from any pustular or draining lesion should be taken in order to help guide antibiotic treatment. Biopsy is essential for confirmation of clinical diagnosis and in all suspected cases of scarring alopecia.

Differential Diagnosis

The differential diagnosis for AKN includes acne vulgaris, acneiform eruptions, folliculitis, hidradenitis suppurativa, nevus sebaceous, perifolliculitis capitis abscedens et suffodiens, and seborrheic dermatitis. Folliculitis decalvans, dissecting cellulitis, pediculosis capitis, and pseudofolliculitis barbae should also be considered.

THERAPY

Preventative measures including avoidance of razors at the occipital hairline and avoidance of tight-fitting shirts or other clothes that may cause mechanical irritation. Treatment for early papular lesions of acne keloidalis should be initiated as early as possible to prevent enlargement of lesions. This includes intralesional injections of corticosteroids, potent topical steroids, and topical or oral antibiotics. Combination therapy with tretinoin and a class 2 or 3 corticosteroid cream or gel twice daily may alleviate symptoms and reduce existing lesions. Use of a foam formulation of clobetasol propionate 0.05% twice daily in a pulsed-dose regimen for 8 weeks followed by betamethasone valerate 0.12% foam for an additional 4 weeks resulted in reduced papule count and reduced symptoms in studies. Lesions with evidence of inflammation including crust formation or drainage can be treated with topical antibiotics twice daily following culture and sensitivities from lesions. Intralesional steroid injections (triamcinolone 10 to 40 mg/mL) are helpful.

Surgical treatment and laser hair removal are alternatives to lesions recalcitrant to medical treatment. Individual papules may be punch excised while larger plaques may be removed by elliptical excision. However, recurrence is likely, and the risk may be reduced with postoperative regimen consisting of topical or intralesional corticosteroids and antibiotics. Long-term benefit from laser hair removal using diode or long pulse Nd:YAG followed by intralesional triamcinolone injections 10 mg/mL every 2 to 3 weeks has been reported to prevent disease progression and recurrence. Cryotherapy has some reported benefits; however, the morbidity is greater than other treatment alternatives and the treated site often becomes hypopigmented and may remain so for 12 to 18 months.

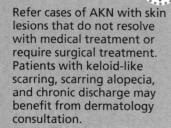

WHEN TO REFER

Refer cases of AKN with skin lesions that do not resolve with medical treatment or require surgical treatment. Patients with keloid-like scarring, scarring alopecia, and chronic discharge may benefit from dermatology consultation.

"AT A GLANCE" TREATMENT

- Preventative measures including avoidance of razors at the occipital hairline and avoidance of mechanical irritation.
- Treatment for early papular lesions of acne keloidalis should be initiated as early as possible to prevent enlargement of lesions.
  - Potent topical steroids such as clobetasol propionate solution BID combined with tretinoin 0.05% gel daily is synergistic
  - Topical antibiotics: benzoyl peroxide 5% to 10% wash daily, clindamycin lotion twice daily
- More advanced cases may respond to intralesional injections of corticosteroids (triamcinolone 10 to 40 mg/cc)

NOT TO BE MISSED

- Discontinuation of shaving or hair trimming in affected areas is essential as is avoidance of mechanical/shearing trauma to the affected area.

- Combination topical therapy with a superpotent steroid and retinoid is synergistic.

- Surgical treatment and laser hair removal are alternatives to lesions recalcitrant to medical treatment.
- Individual papules may be punch excised or curetted, while larger plaques may be removed by elliptical excision. Recurrence is likely.

COURSE AND COMPLICATIONS

The prognosis of AKN is relatively good if lesions are treated early. Treatment becomes more difficult and morbidity increased once scarring develops. Complications include keloid-like scarring, scarring alopecia, and chronic discharge.

ICD9 Codes

706.1	Other acne

Suggested Reading

Chia CY, Lane W, Chibnall J, et al. Isotretinoin therapy and mood changes in adolescents with moderate to severe acne: a cohort study. *Arch Dermatol.* 2005;141:557–560.

Crawford GH, Pelle MT, James WD. Rosacea: I. Etiology, pathogenesis, and subtype classification. *J Am Acad Dermatol.* 2004;51:327–341; quiz 342–324.

Danby FW. Diet and acne. *Clin Dermatol.* 2008;26:93–96.

Harries MJ, Sinclair RD, Macdonald-Hull S, et al. Management of primary cicatricial alopecias: options for treatment. *Br J Dermatol.* 2008;159:1–22.

James WD. Acne. *N Engl J Med.* 2005;352:1463–1472.

Laude TA, Salvemini JN. Perioral dermatitis in children. *Semin Cutan Med Surg.* 1999;18:206–209.

Mekkes JR, JDB. Long-term efficacy of a single course of infliximab in hidradenitis suppurativa. *Br J Dermatol.* 2008;158:370–374.

Nguyen V, Eichenfield LF. Periorificial dermatitis in children and adolescents. *J Am Acad Dermatol.* 2006;55:781–785.

Quarles FN, Brody H, Badreshia S, et al. Acne keloidalis nuchae. *Dermatol Ther.* 2007;20:128–132.

Ritz JP, Runkel N, Haier J, et al. Extent of surgery and recurrence rate of hidradenitis suppurativa. *Int J Colorectal Dis.* 1998;13:164–168.

Rompel R, Petres J. Long-term results of wide surgical excision in 106 patients with hidradenitis suppurativa. *Dermatol Surg.* 2000;26:638–643.

Schwarz T, Kreiselmaier I, Bieber T, et al. A randomized, double-blind, vehicle-controlled study of 1% pimecrolimus cream in adult patients with perioral dermatitis. *J Am Acad Dermatol.* 2008;59:34–40.

Slade DE, Powell BW, Mortimer PS. Hidradenitis suppurativa: pathogenesis and management. *Br J Plast Surg.* 2003;56:451–461.

Sperling LC, Homoky C, Pratt L, et al. Acne keloidalis is a form of primary scarring alopecia. *Arch Dermatol.* 2000;136:479–484.

van Zuuren EJ, Gupta AK, Gover MD, et al. Systematic review of rosacea treatments. *J Am Acad Dermatol.* 2007;56:107–115.

Zaenglein AL, Thiboutot DM. Expert Committee Recommendations for Acne Management. *Pediatrics.* 2006;118:1188–1199.

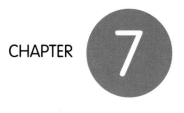
Premalignant and Malignant Skin Lesions

Thanh-Nga T. Tran

Squamous cell carcinoma (SCC), basal cell carcinoma (BCC), melanoma, and Merkel cell carcinoma (MCC) are among the most common cutaneous malignancies encountered by primary care physicians as well as dermatologists. Primary skin malignancies account for more than 50% of all malignancies in the United States. There are more than 1 million cases of nonmelanoma skin cancers (NMSCs) as well as more than 60,000 cases of malignant melanoma diagnosed annually (melanoma in situ will account for an additional 46,000 cases). Approximately 75% to 80% of NMSCs are basal cell carcinomas (BCCs) and up to 25% are squamous cell carcinoma (SCCs). Although BCCs rarely metastasize and hence, rarely cause death, they can result in significant morbidity due to local invasion if not diagnosed and treated appropriately. SCCs, on the other hand, have a metastatic potential and can be locally aggressive, creating significant morbidity as well as mortality for the patient. Actinic keratoses (AKs) are the most commonly treated neoplasm of the skin, and are thought to be a precursor to SCCs. Melanoma, on the other hand, has remained one of the deadliest skin malignancies, and its incidence is on the rise, possibly related to the pattern of sun exposure. Therefore, it is imperative to recognize the cutaneous signs of melanoma and refer patients appropriately. Merkel cell carcinoma (MCC), while a relatively rare tumor of neuroendocrine origin, is also important due to its high rate of recurrence and relatively poor prognosis. The treatment and diagnosis of many cutaneous tumors are continually changing, and the role of clinicians (e.g., primary care providers, dermatologists, plastic surgeons, pathologists) focuses on an accurate diagnosis and a thorough understanding of the clinical sequelae. In addition, these rare cutaneous tumors are often difficult to diagnose based solely on the physical examination findings, and the proper diagnosis relies on excisional biopsy with histologic studies. This chapter focuses mainly on nonmelanoma skin cancers, with an emphasis on skin cancer precursors and Merkel cell carcinoma.

Pathogenesis

Ultraviolet radiation (UVR) is the major cause of NMSCs and AKs and has also been linked to MCC development. The sun emits UVR that is subdivided into UVA (400 to 320 nm); UVB (320 to 290 nm); and UVC (290 to 200 nm). More than 95% of the sun's UVR that reaches the earth's surface is UVA and about 1% to 10% of radiation that reaches the earth is UVB. Most UVC is absorbed by the ozone layer and oxygen in the atmosphere and is thus a very small source of adverse human health effects. UVR targets nucleic acids, proteins, lipids, and other macromolecules. The biologic consequences for DNA structure are particularly striking with formation of "signature" mutations in the p53 gene. These are found frequently in human cancer and in more than 90% of skin cancer, specifically in SCC. P53 is a tumor suppressor gene that is a central factor in cellular stress response, and governs response to such insults as DNA damage, hypoxia, nucleotide imbalance, oxidative stress, and spindle damage. Modification of p53 occurs in a dose-dependent manner after exposure to UVR and the loss of p53 confers a survival advantage to UV-damaged cells. However, the role of p53 in melanoma is still unclear. The exact cause of MCC is unknown, but it appears to be linked to sun exposure and immunosuppression, with most cases occurring on sun-exposed areas of the body.

Risk Factors and Epidemiology

Although several associations have been established for skin cancer risk, such as skin phototype, immune response, viral infection, and genetic background, solar UVR is broadly accepted to be the main initiator and promoter of skin cancer, particularly basal cell carcinoma (BCC) and squamous cell carcinoma (SCC). For SCC, the weight of evidence points toward "chronic" or total exposure. However, for BCCs, intermittent intense exposures as well as burning appear to have a greater influence on subsequent skin cancer risk. Most skin cancers cause a large immune response that is suppressed with continued actinic exposure, leading to reduced immune surveillance for mutated cells. Melanoma incidence has most strongly and consistently been associated with reported "intermittent sun exposure" that is mostly accrued through recreational activities. Among other risk factors are the use of tanning equipment, exposure to therapeutic UV sources such as psoralen plus UVA (PUVA) or narrow-band UVB for skin diseases; exposure to ionizing radiation; chemical exposure such as arsenic, pesticides, asphalt, and tar; infection with human papilloma virus (HPV), especially of the anogenital region in organ transplant patients, etc. Other possible risk factors include residence at high altitudes, dietary fat intake, tobacco abuse, thermal burns, and chronic ulcers.

The development of skin cancers can be influenced by genetics, such as in xeroderma pigmentosum (XP), a disorder of DNA repair mechanisms or in oculocutaneous albinism, a group of autosomal recessive disorders in which there is a variable degree of pigmentary dilution of the skin, eyes, and hair, leading to increased risk in development of skin cancers. BCC is associated with mutations that activate the proto-oncogene SMOOTHENED or that inactivate the tumor-suppressor PATCHED. Nevoid basal cell carcinoma syndrome (NBCCS) is a rare, autosomal dominant disorder, in which the underlying genetic defect is a mutation in the human PATCHED (PTCH) gene. Mutation in PTCH leads to loss of control of several genes known to play a role in both organogenesis and carcinogenesis, and this may explain both the congenital anomalies and cancer predisposition seen in NBCCS. BCCs can number from a few to thousands, making treatment decisions difficult.

One of the more important risk factors for the development of skin cancers, particularly SCCs, is immunosuppression. Several years after transplantation, AKs and SCCs begin to appear with increasing frequency. In organ transplantation patients, the risk of developing BCCs is 5 to 10 times that of the general population, whereas the risk for SCCs is 40 to 250 times greater, influenced by skin type, cumulative UV light exposure, age at transplantation, direct carcinogenic effects of immunosuppressive medications, HPV infection, and the degree and the length of immunosuppression. Of the two cancers, SCCs can cause significant morbidity and mortality in transplant patients, as the lesions tend to be more numerous, especially in sun-exposed areas with greater risk of local and regional recurrences. HPV DNA is found in approximately 70% to 90% of transplant-associated SCCs.

MCCs have been linked to sun exposure, with most cases occurring on sun-exposed areas of the body, as well as to immunosuppression, exposure to other sources of ultraviolet light, and certain conditions such as HIV infection, chronic lymphocytic leukemia, Hodgkin lymphoma, ectodermal dysplasia, and Cowden disease. Other possible causes include exposure to arsenic and treatment for psoriasis that uses psoralens and ultraviolet-A light (PUVA).

Among women under 40, the rate of BCC has tripled in the past 30 years, while that of SCC has quadrupled. At current rates, 1 in 5 people in the United States will develop a skin cancer of some sort during their lifetime, with more than 1 million new cases appearing in 2008 alone. The lifetime risk in the United States of invasive melanoma has increased from 1:1,500 in 1935 to 1 in 63 for invasive melanomas and 1 in 33 if in situ melanoma is included, in 2007. In the United States, melanoma is the most common form of cancer in young adults 25 to 29 years old and the second most common cancer in adolescents and young adults 15 to 29 years old. One American dies from melanoma almost every hour (every 62 minutes). Although melanoma accounts for only 5% of total cutaneous malignancy, it is responsible for approximately 75% to 80% of skin cancer-related deaths. Approximately 1,200 new cases of MCCs are diagnosed in the United States each year with the incidence rising, with a 3-fold increase between 1986 and 2001.

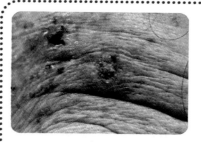

A 65-year-old patient with skin phototype I who spent his childhood on the beach came in to the office due to rough, scaly spots on his scalp and forehead (Fig. 7-1). None has bled or grown rapidly. However, they just "do not go away." He seeks diagnosis and treatment. What is the most likely diagnosis? What test can be done to confirm the diagnosis?

PREMALIGNANT SKIN LESION

Actinic Keratosis

BACKGROUND

Actinic keratoses (AK) are some of the most frequently encountered lesions in clinical practice. Individuals most at risk include the elderly, those with lighter skin types, and those with a history of chronic sun exposure. They have historically been characterized as being "precancerous" or "premalignant" because the atypical keratinocytes within these lesions are confined to the epidermis, not yet reaching full thickness invasion characteristic of carcinomas. The likelihood of an invasive SCC evolving from a given AK has been estimated to occur at a rate of 0.075% to 0.096% per lesion per year, and the rate of development of SCCs for a typical average number of 7.7 AKs per person can range anywhere from 10% to 20% over 10 years if lesions are left untreated.

PATHOGENESIS

AKs are induced by UV radiation, occurring more frequently in fair, red-haired, or blonde patients who burn frequently and tan poorly (Fitzpatrick's skin phototype I and II; Table 7-1). Increased sun exposure and higher-intensity exposure increase the chance of AK development as well as immunosuppression following organ transplantation.

CLINICAL PRESENTATION

Most often, the primary lesion is a rough, erythematous patch or papule with gritty white to yellow scale that may be associated with tenderness and may range in size from a few millimeters to large confluent patches several centimeters in diameter, especially in heavily sun-exposed individuals. A typical

KEY FEATURES

- The actinic keratosis is one of the most frequently encountered lesions in clinical practice.

- They are most commonly present on sun-exposed areas of face, ears, scalp, dorsal hands, forearms.

- These lesions represent in-situ dysplasia (precancer) resulting from sun exposure.

- Clinically, they are discrete, flat or elevated, gritty lesions that can have associated erythema, pigmentation or an adherent scale.

FITZPATRICK'S SKIN PHOTOTYPE	TYPICAL FEATURES	TANNING ABILITY
Table 7-1 Fitzpatrick's Skin Phototypes		
I	Pale white skin, blue/hazel eyes, blond/red hair	Always burns, never tans
II	Fair skin, blue eyes	Mostly burns, sometimes tans
III	Darker white skin	Tans after initial burn
IV	Light brown skin	Burns minimally, tans easily
V	Brown skin	Rarely burns, tans darkly easily
VI	Dark brown or black skin	Always tans darkly, never burns

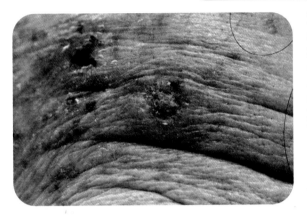

Figure 7-1 Rough, scaly papules on the forehead; note the background dermatoheliosis.

hypertrophic AK is shown in Figure 7-1. On palpation, the surface is rough, sandpaper-like, and could be more easily felt than seen due to their rough, gritty texture. One of the earliest signs is slight erythema with almost imperceptible adherent scale usually on a background of solar damage such as dyspigmentation, telangiectasia, and wrinkling. More advanced lesions are typically thicker with more visible hyperkeratosis and erythema or even a cutaneous horn. Sun-exposed areas are most often involved. Sites such as the tops of the ears, upper forehead, nasal bridge, malar eminences, dorsal hands, extensor forearms, and scalp in bald individuals must be examined. Lesions larger than 6 mm are suspicious for squamous cell carcinoma and should be biopsied.

DIAGNOSIS

Differential Diagnosis

The differential for AK must include the possibility of invasive squamous and basal cell carcinoma, although these lesions tend to be more indurated and nodular, with more rapid growth and often eroded and ulcerated surface. Other diseases to consider include:

- Discoid lupus erythematosus, which has more dyspigmentation, dilated follicles, and atrophy
- Seborrheic keratosis: greasy, brown crusts; sharply demarcated borders; but does not have an erythematous scaly base; may occur in non sun-exposed areas
- Bowen disease: a larger plaque with a sharp outline
- Warts: tend to be more verrucous with punctate red dots representing thrombosed capillaries
- Porokeratosis: a premalignant lesion characterized by small, light brown, keratotic papule or plaque that forms irregularly shaped, annular plaque with a raised, ridgelike border. The risk of malignant degeneration is ~10% with large, long-standing lesions being at highest risk. Most lesions can be followed clinically unless atypical features are seen.

Diagnostic Methods

Visualization and palpation is helpful for the diagnosis of AKs. However, in the case that malignancy is suspected, a biopsy is recommended.

THERAPY

It is impossible to predict the fate of AKs as they may remain unchanged, spontaneously resolve, or progress to invasive SCC. Although the risk of progression of any one AK to invasive SCC is small, a patient may have many lesions, increasing the risk of malignant progression. Because therapy is generally well tolerated and simple, treatment is warranted.

First and foremost in management of AKs is medical education regarding chronic sun exposure, especially during the hours from 10:00 AM to 4:00 PM when sunlight is more intense. Adequate use of sunscreen of a sun-protection factor (SPF) of 30 or above is recommended. There are two broad categories of treatments, medical therapy and surgical therapy.

MEDICAL THERAPY

Medical therapy or field therapy is useful in patients with numerous AKs on a background of severe sun damage where individual lesion therapy is difficult. This has the advantage of being able to treat large areas with many lesions, although it is often associated with lengthy treatment course as well as prolonged discomfort and irritation. Currently, the U.S. Food and Drug Administration (FDA) has approved four medications for the treatment of AKs. These are topical 5-fluorouracil (5-FU), 5% imiquimod cream, topical diclofenac gel, and photodynamic therapy (PDT) with topical delta-aminolevulinic acid (ALA-PDT).

- 5-FU has been used more extensively before the development of imiquimod. Several formulations are available, including a 5% cream or solution, a 2% solution, a 1% cream or solution, and, most recently, a micronized 0.5% cream with relatively little difference among the various formulations. The most popular is the 5% cream, which is applied twice daily for 1 month. Patient must be warned that the lesions will likely become increasingly erythematous, leading to possible significant discomfort and can be temporarily disfiguring, with erythematous ulcerations and crust formation. However, if the patient completes the treatment, the lesions usually heal within 2 weeks of stopping treatment, resulting in improved texture of the skin (smoother) as well as reduction in number and size of AKs.
- Imiquimod is a topical medication that up-regulates a variety of cytokines, invoking a nonspecific immune response (interferons, macrophages, natural killer cells) and a specific immune response (T lymphocytes). It is applied 2 to 3 times a week for up to 4 months. Reaction to the medication can range from barely perceptible erythema to exudative inflammation, including reaction of subclinical lesions. For patients with a brisk inflammatory response, the dose can be reduced to one to twice a week without significant change in therapeutic efficacy.
- Topical diclofenac is a nonsteroidal anti-inflammatory drug with unclear mechanism of action against AKs. It is an effective therapy when applied twice a day for 3 months with the chief advantage in that it produces little to no inflammation and thus is very well tolerated.
- ALA-PDT uses delta-aminolevulinic acid, a light-sensitizing compound that preferentially accumulates in dysplastic AK cells, converting intracellularly via enzymatic processes to protoporphyrin IX, a potent photosensitizer. Upon exposure to light at an appropriate wavelength, oxygen free radicals are generated and cell deaths results. The side effect can be similar to topical 5-FU, with intense erythema and irritation, as well as pain, although only one treatment is needed usually.

SURGICAL CARE

Surgical management of AKs often involves physical destruction with limited to no damage to surrounding normal tissue. When the diagnosis is unclear and invasive tumor is possible, biopsy is indicated. The most common method of physical destruction involves cryosurgery, where a cryogen—most often liquid nitrogen with a temperature of −195.8°C—is sprayed precisely on an AK lesion. Keratinocytes die when exposed to approximately −40 to −50°C, whereas other structure in the skin, such as collagen, blood vessels, and nerves, are more resistant to the lethal effects of cold than keratinocytes. Melanocytes are much more cold sensitive, and hence can also be destroyed during this process, leaving a white spot. Overall, the clearance rate is 67%.

If malignancy is suspected, a lesion can be treated with curettage, shave excision, or conventional excision, and the tissue can be sent for histologic examination. Side effects include possible reaction to local anesthesia, wound infection, and scarring.

Other methods include ablative laser resurfacing procedures where the entire epidermis is removed (such as in carbon dioxide laser resurfacing) can also be effective though almost never performed. Less invasive resurfacing procedures include medium and deep chemical peels as well as dermabrasion. All of these are cosmetic procedures unlikely to be covered by insurance; all carry the risk of scarring and postinflammatory hyperpigmentation or hypopigmentation, especially in darker-skinned individuals.

"AT A GLANCE" TREATMENT

- Medical care:
  - Imiquimod cream: used applied 2 to 3 times a week for up to 4 months
  - 5-fluorouracil cream: often 0.5% prescribed at once daily to the affected field and/or discreet lesions for 4 weeks
  - Diclofenac cream and ALA-PDT are less commonly used.
- Surgical care:
  - Cryosurgery with liquid nitrogen
  - Less commonly used: chemical peels, photodynamic therapy

COURSE AND COMPLICATIONS

Complications are most often seen in patients with severe actinic damage treated aggressively with cryotherapy or medical therapy. In these patients, blisters may form and exudative inflammation may cause pain, discomfort, and pruritus, as well as increase the risk for infection. Untreated lesions may progress into invasive squamous cell carcinomas especially nodular, indurated, or unresponsive lesions, where a biopsy is warranted.

ICD9 Codes

702.0   *Actinic keratosis*

WHEN TO REFER

Refer patients with significant sun damage and rough lesions on skins, or for skin lesions that do not resolve with cryosurgery or medical therapy, and patients with numerous skin lesions requiring comprehensive treatments such as ALA-PDT.

NOT TO BE MISSED

- Lesions that are tender to touch and/or rapidly growing should be biopsied to rule out invasive SCC.
- Field therapy for patients with multiple AKs is beneficial and worth the upfront treatment side effects of inflammation.

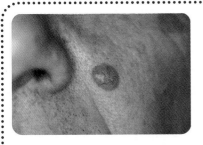

A 55-year-old construction worker who spends most of his days out in the sun develops a skin-colored pearly growth on his medial cheek (Fig. 7-2A) that has been slowly growing over the past year and occasionally bleeds with trauma. What is the most likely diagnosis? What should the treatment be?

MALIGNANT SKIN LESIONS
Basal Cell Carcinoma
BACKGROUND

Basal cell carcinoma (BCC) is the most common malignancy, primarily among white, fair-skinned population. Risk factors include chronic sun exposure, positive family history for BCC, immunosuppression, prior blistering sunburns, red hair/fair complexion, skin phototype I and II. BCC is usually slow growing and rarely metastasizes, but it can cause clinically significant local destruction and disfigurement if neglected or inadequately treated. However, prognosis is excellent with proper therapy. Many clinical variants exist and diagnosis is dependent on the clinician being aware of the many forms BCC may take. Treatment is often tailored on the histologic variant.

PATHOGENESIS

The true pathogenesis for BCCs has not exactly been elucidated, although UVR has been shown to be associated with the development of BCCs. Intermittent intense exposures as well as burning appear to have a greater influence on subsequent BCC development. UV-induced mutations in the p53 tumor-suppressor gene have been found in some cases of BCC. Activated BCL2 (an antiapoptosis proto-oncogene) also is commonly found in BCCs and may be detected immunohistochemically. Most BCCs have abnormalities in either patched (PTCH) or smoothened (SMO) genes, which are involved in the hedgehog intracellular signaling pathway, which influences differentiation of a variety of tissues during fetal development, as well as regulation of cell growth and differentiation after embryogenesis. Loss of inhibition of this pathway is associated with human malignancy, including BCC. Other associated risk factors include immunosuppression, arsenic exposure, exposure to artificial UV light such as tanning booths and UV light therapy, certain genodermatoses such as xeroderma pigmentosum, nevoid basal cell carcinoma syndrome with defects in PTCH and SMO genes, as well as history of other NMSC. The risk of developing new nonmelanoma skin cancers is reported to be 35% at 3 years and 50% at 5 years after an initial skin cancer diagnosis.

CLINICAL PRESENTATION

Most often the nodular BCC characterized by a pearly papule with surface telangiectasia (Fig. 7-2A) and rolled border (Fig. 7-2B) is the typical lesion. However, several clinical and histologic subtypes of BCC may exhibit different clinical and histologic appearance such as superficial (Fig. 7-3); morpheaform (Fig. 7-4); micronodular (Fig. 7-5); or pigmented BCC (Fig. 7-6). Good lighting and magnification is helpful, as well as palpation, and stretching of the skin may help to delineate the tumor and estimate its size and depth. Oblique illumination of the tumor can highlight surface changes, such as a rolled border. Features of BCC are reviewed in Table 7-2.

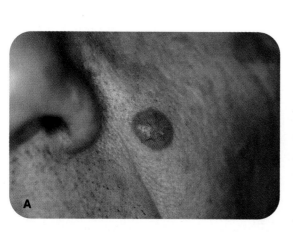
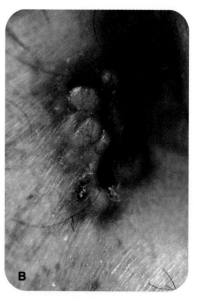

Figure 7-2 A. Nodular BCC on the medial cheek. **B.** Rolled borders of a nodular BCC.

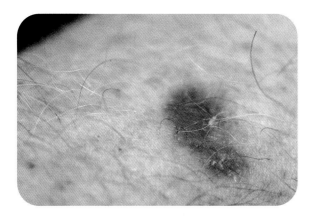

Figure 7-3 Superficial BCC on the upper back.

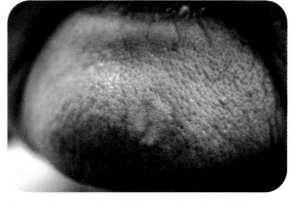

Figure 7-4 Morpheaform BCC on the chin of an elderly woman.

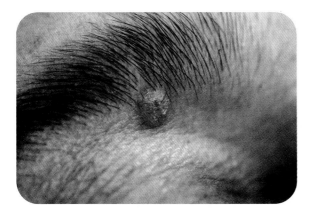

Figure 7-5 Micronodular BCC on the upper eyelid.

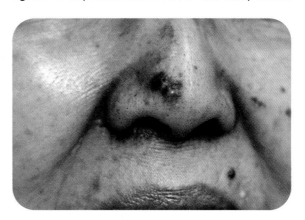

Figure 7-6 A pigmented BCC on the nose of a Vietnamese woman.

CHAPTER 7 Malignant Skin Lesions

Table 7-2 Common Types of Basal Cell Carcinoma

Nodular	This is the most common type of basal cell carcinoma accounting for 50%-80% of BCCs. Usually presents as a round, pearly, flesh-colored papule with surface telangiectases forming around a central depression that may or may not be ulcerated, crusted, and bleeding. See Figures 7-2A,B
Superficial	15.5% of BCCs, favoring the trunk (45%), head and neck (40%), or distal extremities (14%). Most frequently present as scaly patches or papules that are pink to red-brown, often with central clearing. Papules may mimic psoriasis or eczema. The lesions are slowly progressive and not prone to invasion. Numerous superficial BCCs may indicate arsenic exposure. See Figure 7-3
Morpheaform	An uncommon BCC variant (2%-6%). Presents as a white or yellow, waxy, sclerotic plaque that rarely ulcerates. 95% occurs on the head and neck. See Figure 7-4
Micronodular	Aggressive BCC subtype that is not prone to ulceration, and may appear yellow-white when stretched, and it is firm to the touch. It may have a seemingly well-defined border though the micronodular growth pattern makes it less amenable to curettage. See Figure 7-5
Pigmented	This is an uncommon variant of nodular BCC that has all the features of a nodular BCC but with brown-black macules in some or all areas, often making it difficult to differentiate from melanoma. This is usually common in more darkly pigmented individuals. See Figure 7-6

DIAGNOSIS

Clinical suspicion can be confirmed by biopsy. Usually, a shave biopsy is required to determine the nature of the lesion as well as the histologic subtype. However, in the case of a pigmented lesion where there may be difficulty distinguishing between pigmented BCC and melanoma, an excisional or punch biopsy may be indicated.

The differential diagnosis for BCC includes SCCs, actinic keratoses (especially the hypertrophic type); sebaceous hyperplasia or overgrowth of the sebaceous unit; fibrous papule; desmoplastic trichoepithelioma (a benign lesion of hair follicle origin); as well as a melanocytic lesion.

THERAPY

Medical Care

In the majority of cases, surgery is the treatment of choice as medical therapy is often suboptimal and only available for a few forms of BCCs. Generally, medical therapy yields a cure rate that is less than that of surgical modalities. However, here are a few options for patients not recommended for surgical care:

- 5% 5-fluorouracil (5-FU) applied twice daily for 2 to 12 weeks of treatment can be effective in treating superficial basal cell carcinoma, with a reported cure rate as high as 93%. For other types of BCCs, the use of 5-FU is not recommended due to poor penetration into the dermis. Side effects include irritation and crusting as well as discomfort.
- Imiquimod cream is FDA approved for the treatment of superficial BCC with cure rate up to 88% for superficial and nodular BCCs. A thin film of the medication is applied 5 times per week for about 6 weeks and advanced as tolerated to once daily and even twice daily if tolerated to maintain mild-to-moderate skin irritation. The FDA labeling suggests that this should not be used on the face, hands, or feet.

Surgical Care

Given the indolent nature of most BCCs, surgical modalities are the most studied, most effective, and most used treatments for BCCs, though the cure rates are dependent on the surgeon's skills. Modalities used include electrodessication and curettage, excisional surgery, Mohs micrographic surgery, and cryosurgery. Ionizing radiation, although a nonsurgical modality, should be considered in select patients and is discussed below. Factors determining the selected modality depend on whether the tumor is primary or recurrent, as well as on its location, size, and histologic type.

- Electrodessication and curettage (ED&C): see Chapter 3 for procedural details.
  - Advantages: this is a short procedure (<5 min) and is more than 95% effective in treating primary nodular and superficial basal cell carcinoma.
  - Disadvantages: this procedure often leaves a white atrophic scar and is highly operator-dependent. It is not as effective in treating infiltrating, micronodular, morpheaform (sclerosing), and recurrent BCCs where Mohs micrographic surgery is often the treatment of choice.
- Surgical excision: most often used on noncosmetically sensitive areas.
  - Advantages: surgical excision usually produces good-to-excellent cosmetic results and cure rates as high as 95%.
  - Disadvantages: surgical excision is operator-dependent, as tumor margins may be difficult to detect, especially in the BCC subtypes with less

distinct margins such as infiltrating, micronodular, and morpheaform (sclerosing) BCCs. This method is and is far less effective in treating recurrent BCCs than it is in treating primary BCCs.

- Mohs micrographical surgery: this is a method where the lesion and a minimal amount of tissue are removed and the edges are processed by frozen section and examined directly. The procedure is repeated if there is still persisting tumor until the margins are clear.
  - Advantages: this method offers the highest cure rate of any treatment modality (99% for primary BCC, 90% to 95% for recurrent BCC); spares as much uninvolved skin as possible; and is the treatment of choice for infiltrating, micronodular, morpheaform (sclerosing); and recurrent BCCs. It is most often used on cosmetically sensitive areas.
  - Disadvantages: time consuming, more expensive, and patients might require additional anesthesia before each stage.
- Cryosurgery: liquid nitrogen is applied to the clinically apparent tumor.
  - Advantages: good cosmetic results as well as good cure rates for tumors with well-defined margins such as nodular BCC. A good option for patients who are not surgical candidates.
  - Disadvantages: operator-dependent, as well as dependent on accurate clinical detection of tumor margins
- Ionizing radiation: superficial x-ray is usually administered as 10 treatments of 4 gray (Gy) (400 rad). Electrons (electron beam) can be used and has gained favor over superficial x-rays by many radiation oncologists.
  - Advantages: good treatment option for patients who are not surgical candidates, especially those patients who have facial tumors.
  - Disadvantages: requires multiple visits and is less effective for nonfacial tumor. Treatment results in radiation damage and, therefore, should be reserved for older patients.

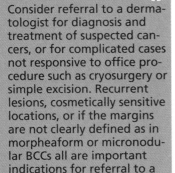

WHEN TO REFER

Consider referral to a dermatologist for diagnosis and treatment of suspected cancers, or for complicated cases not responsive to office procedure such as cryosurgery or simple excision. Recurrent lesions, cosmetically sensitive locations, or if the margins are not clearly defined as in morpheaform or micronodular BCCs all are important indications for referral to a Mohs surgeon.

"AT A GLANCE" TREATMENT

- Medical care: treat sBCC (5-FU or imiquimod) or nodular BCC (nodular) only. The other subtypes should be surgically treated.
  - 5% 5-fluorouracil (5-FU) applied twice daily for 2 to 12 weeks of treatment can be effective in treating superficial basal cell carcinoma.
  - Imiquimod cream applied 3 times per week for about 12 weeks and advanced as tolerated to once daily and even twice daily if tolerated to maintain mild-to-moderate skin irritation.
- Surgical care:
  - Modalities used include electrodessication and curettage, elliptical excision, Mohs micrographic surgery, and cryosurgery. Choosing the correct lesion type and treatment modality is essential. See the text for details.

NOT TO BE MISSED

- Micronodular BCC are subtle and often mistaken for scars.
- Infiltrating, micronodular, morpheaform (sclerosing), and recurrent BCC should be treated by Mohs surgery.

COMPLICATIONS

If left untreated, the tumor can become locally invasive, leading to significant disfigurement from ulceration, tissue invasion, and possible bacterial superinfection. Because this cancer most commonly affects the head and neck, cosmetic disfigurement is not uncommon. Loss of vision or the eye may occur with orbital involvement. Perineural spread can result in loss of nerve function and in deep and extensive invasion of the tumor. Death from BCC is extremely rare. Individuals with BCC have a 30% greater risk of having another BCC unrelated to the previous lesion within 5 years compared with the risk in the general population.

ICD9 Codes

184.1	Malignant neoplasm of labia majora
184.2	Malignant neoplasm of labia minora
184.3	Malignant neoplasm of clitoris
184.4	Malignant neoplasm of vulva, unspecified site
140.0	Malignant neoplasm of upper lip, vermilion border
140.1	Malignant neoplasm of lower lip, vermilion border
140.9	Malignant neoplasm of lip, unspecified, vermilion border
173.0	Other malignant neoplasm of skin of lip
173.1	Other malignant neoplasm of skin of eyelid, including canthus
173.2	Other malignant neoplasm of skin of ear and external auditory canal
173.3	Other malignant neoplasm of skin of other and unspecified parts of face
173.4	Other malignant neoplasm of scalp and skin of neck
173.5	Other malignant neoplasm of skin of trunk, except scrotum
173.6	Other malignant neoplasm of skin of upper limb, including shoulder
173.7	Other malignant neoplasm of skin of lower limb, including hip
173.8	Other malignant neoplasm of other specified sites of skin
173.9	Other malignant neoplasm of skin, site unspecified

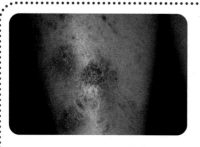

An 80-year-old female with history of renal cell carcinoma, status post organ transplantation, presents with multiple, rapidly growing, painful crusty bumps on her legs that have spontaneously bled in the past (Fig. 7-7). What is the most likely diagnosis? What should the treatment be?

Squamous Cell Carcinoma

BACKGROUND

SCC is the second most common form of skin cancer that is influenced strongly by chronic, long-term sun exposure. The incidence of SCC is related to the annual amount of UVR exposure. High-risk SCC carries a significant risk of metastasis and, as such, requires careful evaluation and treatment. Risk factors for the development of SCC includes the male sex; age over 50 years; geography (closer to the equator); fair skin (burns easily or rarely tans); high cumulative UV exposure; exposure to chemical carcinogens, such as arsenic and tar; chronic immunosuppression; ionizing radiation exposure; HPV infection; as well as chronic scarring conditions and certain genodermatoses.

PATHOGENESIS

SCCs' pathogenesis is similar to that of AKs and BCCs. Their development is strongly associated with UV radiation, occurring more frequently in fair, red-haired, or blonde patients who burn frequently and tan poorly, and can arise from a pre-existing premalignant lesion (actinic keratosis). UV targets nucleic acids, proteins, lipids, and other macromolecules and the biologic consequences for DNA structure are particularly striking, resulting in "signature" mutations in the p53 gene, which are found frequently in human cancer, and in more than 90% of skin cancer, specifically in SCC. Increased sun exposure and higher-intensity exposure increase the chance of SCCs development as well as immuno-suppression following organ transplantation. HPV DNA is found in approximately 70% to 90% of transplant-associated SCCs, including strains that occur in common benign cutaneous warts (HPV types 1 and 2); epidermodysplasia

KEY FEATURES

- Squamous cell carcinoma (SCC) is a malignant tumor of epidermal keratinocytes.

- SCC is the second most common form of skin cancer and frequently arises on the sun-exposed skin of middle-aged and elderly individuals.

- Invasive SCC is an erythematous keratotic papule or nodule that arises within a background of sun-damaged skin.

- SCC in situ is often a scaly pink patch to a thin keratotic papule or plaque similar to an AK.

- The primary cause of most SCC is cumulative lifetime sun exposure.

- Invasive SCC does carry a risk of metastasis (rate from all skin sites ranges from 0.5% to 5.2%); therefore appropriate treatment is imperative.

verruciformis (HPV 5 and others); high-risk oncogenic warts (HPV types 16 and 18); and low-risk oncogenic genital warts (HPV types 6 and 11). Sometimes, several HPV types are detected within a single tumor. Other associated risk factors include immunosuppression, arsenic exposure, exposure to artificial UV light such as tanning booths and UV light therapy, or certain genodermatoses such as xenoderma pigmentosum with defects in DNA repair.

CLINICAL PRESENTATION

SCC is typically a slow-growing malignancy, but some lesions enlarge rapidly. It often presents as a new or enlarging lesion with associated symptoms such as bleeding, weeping, pain, or tenderness, especially with larger tumors. The lesion may be indurated, rounded, or superficial and discrete with a hyperkeratotic scale and can be dull-red in color (Fig. 7-7). Invasive SCC tends to have a more nodular architecture with associated ulcer and hyperkeratotic core (Figs. 7-8, 7-9). Less commonly, SCC may manifest as a pink cutaneous nodule (Fig. 7-10). Numbness, tingling, or muscle weakness may alert the physician for possible underlying perineural involvement, which can carry a high recurrence as well as metastasis rate. SCC often arises from a background of severe sun damage such as a field of AKs or sun-exposed areas such as face and dorsal hands. With any invasive SCC, regional lymph nodes should be examined. Lymph node enlargement is an ominous sign that may indicate the presence of metastatic disease.

Perioral SCC of the lip usually arises on the vermillion border of the lower lip, close to the midline. The precursor lesion is actinic cheilitis, which manifests as xerosis, fissuring, atrophy, and dyspigmentation and which is analogous to AK of the skin. SCC in this location manifests as a new papule, erosion, or focus of erythema/induration. Intraoral SCC typically manifests as a white plaque (leukoplakia) with or without reddish reticulation (erythroplakia). Lip and ear lesions metastasize more frequently when compared to other sites. Common types of SCC are summarized in Table 7-3 (Figs. 7-7 to 7-13).

Table 7-3 Common Types of Squamous Cell Carcinoma

SCC in situ (SCCis)	Usually, presents as a scaly pink patch to a thin keratotic papule or plaque similar to an AK. Histologically, SCC-IS has atypia involving the full thickness of the epidermis but without invasion into the dermis. An example is shown in Figure 7-9. Bowen disease is a subtype of SCC characterized by a sharply demarcated, pink plaque arising on non-sun-exposed skin. Erythroplasia of Queyrat refers to Bowen disease of the glans penis, which manifests as one or more velvety red plaques.
Invasive SCC	Often presents as a raised, firm, pink-to-flesh-colored papule or plaque with hyperkeratotic scale, ulceration, or cutaneous horn on a background of actinically damaged skin. Approximately 70% of all SCCs occur on the head and neck, with an additional 15% found on the upper extremities. See Figs. 7-7–7-10
Periungual SCC	Often misdiagnosed for years as a wart, periungual SCC may mimic a verruca or resemble chronic paronychia with swelling, erythema, and tenderness of the nail fold; onychodystrophy may also be noted (Fig. 7-11)
Marjolin ulcer	Often at the site of a pre-existing scar or ulcer, this subtype of SCC appears as a new area of induration, elevation, or ulceration (Fig. 7-12).
Verrucous carcinoma	This is an aggressive tumor that has basaloid histologic features as well as eosinophilic squamoid features of SCC. See Figure 7-13

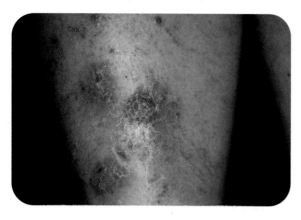

Figure 7-7 Multiple SCC on the shin of an older woman.

DIAGNOSIS

Suspected lesion should be confirmed with a skin biopsy, often with a punch biopsy to evaluate the base of the lesion for any possible invasion. Patients with lymphadenopathy or neurologic symptoms should be evaluated for metastasis, usually with CT scanning, MRI, ultrasound, or if high-risk patient, positron emission tomography (PET) scanning. Currently, no formal guidelines regarding the use of radiologic imaging in cutaneous SCC have been developed. Clinical or imaging-evident lymph nodes that are highly suspicious for malignancy should be further evaluated with lymph node biopsy or fine-needle aspiration. Differential diagnosis includes a premalignant lesion such as actinic

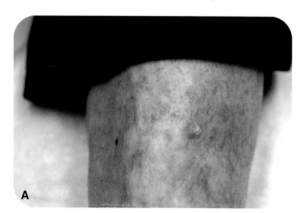

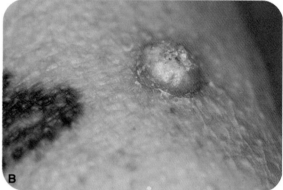

Figure 7-8 A. Invasive SCC with keratotic core. **B.** An invasive SCC of the keratoacanthoma type.

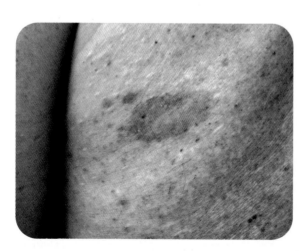

Figure 7-9 Scaly pink plaque on the upper lateral back c/w SCC-IS.

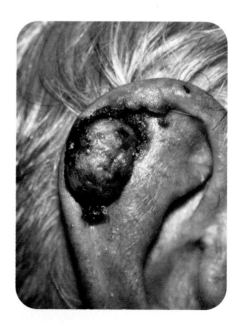

Figure 7-10 Poorly differentiated SCC on the ear of an elderly man.

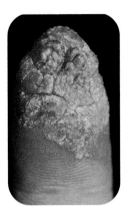

Figure 7-11 Periungual SCC-in situ. From Rassner G, trans. Burgdorf WHC. *Atlas of Dermatology,* 3rd ed. Philadelphia: Lea & Febiger, 1994.

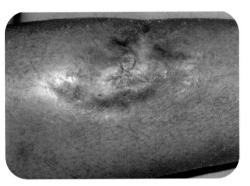

Figure 7-12 Marjolin ulcer-an SCC arising in a burn scar. From Goodheart HP. *Goodheart's Photoguide to Common Skin Disorders,* 3rd ed. Philadelphia: Lippincott Williams & Wilkins, 2009.

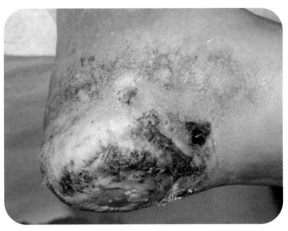

Figure 7-13 Verrucous carcinoma on the foot.

keratosis, atypical fibroxanthoma, BCC, desmoplastic melanoma, proliferating epidermoid cyst, pyoderma gangrenosum, or wart.

THERAPY

Most SCCs are treated in the physician's office with surgical or destructive method. Most medical managements are for superficial or in situ SCCs but are generally not recommended for invasive SCC. SCCs with evidence of perineural involvement or extensive local invasion may be treated with radiation therapy.

For in situ or superficial lesions topical therapy, topical immune response modifiers, or photodynamic light therapy can be useful. For patients not amenable for surgery or those with metastatic, highly invasive disease or evidence of perineural invasion, radiation therapy is an option as adjuvant therapy. Systemic chemotherapy is available for patients with metastatic disease. Reduction in immunosuppression may be helpful in organ transplant patients with aggressive SCC where tumors develop rapidly. This must be done in conjunction with a transplantation physician due to the risk of organ rejection.

"AT A GLANCE" TREATMENT

- Medical and surgical treatments for SCC are summarized in Tables 7-4 and 7-5.

COURSE AND COMPLICATIONS

For most SCCs, treatment is with intention to cure. The 3-year survival rate can approach 90% to 100% for lesions with no patient- and tumor-related high-risk factors, but decreases to 70% with at least one risk factor. Tumor-related factors include location (i.e., lips, ear, scar); size greater than 2 cm; invasion to subcutaneous fat; poor differentiation; recurrent tumor; and perineural involvement. Patient-related factors include chronic immunosuppression (including states such as human immunodeficiency virus [HIV], hematologic malignancy) and organ transplantation. It is not uncommon to have local recurrence that may subsequently lead to metastasis and death, which occurs in 2% to 6% of the patients. For patients with lymph nodes metastasis, 5-year survival rate is rather low at 25% to 35%. However, this rate can be much improved (up to 73%) for patients with nodal metastasis treated with surgery and adjuvant chemotherapy. Once the cancer has spread to distant organs, there is no effective method for cure. Hence, the emphasis is on early detection and surveillance. Across-the-board prevalence rate of metastasis for primary cutaneous

CHAPTER 7 Malignant Skin Lesions

Table 7-4 Surgical Methods for Treatment of SCC

Fusiform excision	Simple excision is most valuable in the treatment of small primary SCCs on the trunk, extremities, or neck Highly effective, well-tolerated Cure rates for T1 lesion as high as 95%–99%; this rate drops to 77% for recurrent SCC
Electrodessication and curettage	Treat superficially invasive SCCs without high-risk characteristics Lacks of histologic margin Fast, minimally invasive, well-tolerated and effective treatment for in situ and superficially invasive lesions
Cryosurgery	Cure rate for superficial lesions up to 95% Not often used for invasive SCC because deeper portions of the tumor may not be destroyed by liquid nitrogen Scar developing at the cryosurgical site might obscure a recurrence
Mohs' micrographic surgery (MMS)	Use for: 　Highly aggressive tumors with perineural invasion 　Recurrent lesions 　Cosmetically sensitive areas 　Ill-defined tumor Lesions >2 cm in size should be treated with definitive removal with MMS due to their increased potential for metastasis and recurrence Allows for 100% evaluation of the surgical margin Provides the best cure rate (94%–99%)

SCC is 2% to 6%, and higher for larger lesions. Prognosis is extremely poor for patients with a compromised immune system, with metastasis to multiple lymph nodes, or with cervical lymph nodes greater than 3 cm in diameter. The lips and ears have a much higher rate of recurrent and metastatic disease than SCC at other sites. Involvement of the nerve also has extremely poor prognosis, with local recurrence and metastasis as high as 47%.

WHEN TO REFER

Refer for suspicious lesions that have been growing rapidly and when invasive SCC is suspected.

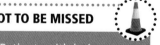

NOT TO BE MISSED

• Patients with lesions on high-risk sites (lip and ear) or with high-risk features of their tumor (size >2 cm, invasion to subcutaneous fat, poor differentiation, recurrent tumor, and perineural involvement) should be aggressively treated.

ICD9 Codes

184.1	Malignant neoplasm of labia majora
184.2	Malignant neoplasm of labia minora
184.3	Malignant neoplasm of clitoris
184.4	Malignant neoplasm of vulva, unspecified site
140.0	Malignant neoplasm of upper lip, vermilion border
140.1	Malignant neoplasm of lower lip, vermilion border
140.9	Malignant neoplasm of lip, unspecified, vermilion border
173.0	Other malignant neoplasm of skin of lip
173.1	Other malignant neoplasm of skin of eyelid, including canthus
173.2	Other malignant neoplasm of skin of ear and external auditory canal
173.3	Other malignant neoplasm of skin of other and unspecified parts of face
173.4	Other malignant neoplasm of scalp and skin of neck
173.5	Other malignant neoplasm of skin of trunk, except scrotum
173.6	Other malignant neoplasm of skin of upper limb, including shoulder
173.7	Other malignant neoplasm of skin of lower limb, including hip
173.8	Other malignant neoplasm of other specified sites of skin
173.9	Other malignant neoplasm of skin, site unspecified

Table 7-5 Medical Therapy of SCC

Topical chemotherapy	5-FU can be used to treat superficial SCCs Usual regimen is once daily on affected areas for 4 weeks
Topical immune response modifier	Imiquimod is an imidazoquinoline that enhances cell-mediated immune responses via the induction of proinflammatory cytokines via interaction with toll-like receptor 7 Effective for SCCIS as monotherapy and in combination with topical 5-FU Not approved to treat invasive SCC Regimen is twice weekly to affected areas for 16 weeks
ALA-PDT	Uses delta-aminolevulinic acid, a light-sensitizing compound that preferentially accumulates in dysplastic AK cells, converting intracellularly via enzymatic processes to protoporphyrin IX, a potent photosensitizer Upon exposure to light at an appropriate wavelength, oxygen free radicals are generated and cell deaths results Side effect similar to topical 5-FU, with intense erythema and irritation as well as pain Only one treatment is needed usually
Radiation therapy	Reserved for difficult cases where surgical and medical treatment is suboptimal Offers the potential advantage of avoiding the deformity and trauma of a surgical procedure with cure rates for T1 lesions range from 85%–95% Immediate and long-term side effects such as cutaneous atrophy, dyspigmentation, and telangiectasia in the radiation field as well as increased risk of cutaneous carcinoma such as SCC and sarcoma Nonideal first-line therapy
Systemic chemotherapy	Variety of different chemotherapeutic agents have been used to treat metastatic cutaneous SCC including capecitabine (Xeloda), an oral formation of 5-FU, which when used either alone or in combination with interferon, has shown some efficacy in the treatment of advanced cutaneous SCC

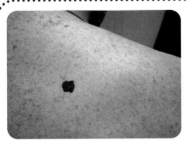

A 35-year-old male with history of growing up on the beach with multiple blistering sunburns and multiple odd-looking moles has been noticing that one of his brown spots has become more enlarged and irregular (Fig. 7-14A). He was recently married and his wife asked him to have this lesion on his back examined. He has no other symptoms related to this nevus. His father has a history of an invasive melanoma 10 years ago. What is the most likely diagnosis? What should the treatment be?

Melanoma

BACKGROUND

Melanoma is a malignant tumor arising from pigment-producing cells called melanocytes, which reside at the dermoepidermal junction. In about half of the cases, melanoma arises from pre-existing nevus, but in other cases it will develop de novo on normal appearing skin. The incidence of melanoma has increased in the past decades, possibly relating to the patterns of sun exposure, and it has become one of the most common forms of cancer in young adults. Melanoma is rare among darker races, with the acral type of melanoma accounting for the majority of the cases in darker-skinned individuals. Children rarely manifest congenital or acquired melanomas and seldom before puberty. However, children with giant congenital

KEY FEATURES

- Melanoma is a malignant tumor arising from melanocytes, which are pigment-producing cells.

- The incidence and mortality rates of melanoma have been increasing in recent decades, and it is one of the most common cancers of young adults.

- Melanoma accounts for only 3% of all skin cancers; however, it causes 80% of skin cancer–related deaths worldwide.

- Early detection is an important goal in melanoma management.

- Appropriate surgical treatment of low-risk melanoma (<1 mm Breslow depth) with 1 cm margins will cure patients in at least 90% of cases.

nevi have a 6.3% lifetime risk of developing melanoma and therefore should be closely monitored. However, the melanoma that develops in giant congenital nevi tends to be deeper and hence, more difficult to detect. Given that melanoma is an indolent, painless tumor, it may escape detection until late stages, leading up to 20% of patients to develop metastatic disease.

PATHOGENESIS

Although no precise cause has been elucidated, melanoma has been associated with a light complexion and eyes, blond or red hair, occurrence of blistering sunburns in childhood, the presence of large number of nevi or giant congenital nevi, family history of melanoma, previous history of melanoma or non-melanoma skin cancer, as well as presence of xeroderma pigmentosum or familial atypical mole melanoma syndrome; these two genodermatoses confer a 500- to 1,000-fold greater relative risk of developing melanoma. Epidemiologic studies implicate intense intermittent exposure of unacclimatized skin to sunlight as a major factor in the induction of cutaneous melanoma. However, in contrast to nonmelanoma skin cancers, in which there are often distinctive UVB-induced mutations in the p53 gene, melanomas seldom demonstrate signature UVB mutations. This has led to the supposition that UVA may play an important role in melanoma, which has implications for public health education efforts regarding the use of tanning beds (which are primarily UVA) and also use of broad-spectrum sunscreen.

CLINICAL PRESENTATION

Melanoma often is brought to the patient's attention as a new or changing mole with variation in color and/or an increase in diameter, height, or asymmetry of borders of a pigmented lesion. Less commonly, patients may note symptoms such as bleeding, itching, ulceration, and pain in a pigmented lesion, which warrant further evaluation.

The ABCDE criteria for melanoma are imperfect, but have provided a useful tool for patients to perform self-exam and report any suspicious lesions.

A—Asymmetry: half the lesion does not match the other half.
B—Border irregularity: the edges are ragged, notched, or blurred.
C—Color variegation: pigmentation is not uniform and may display shades of tan, brown, or black; white, reddish, or blue discoloration.
D—Diameter: a diameter greater than 6 mm is characteristic, although some melanomas may have smaller diameters; any growth in a nevus warrants an evaluation.
E—Evolving: changes in the lesion over time are characteristic; this factor is critical for nodular or amelanotic (nonpigmented) melanoma, which may not exhibit the classic criteria above.

Physicians may also rely on the "ugly duckling" warning sign, wherein skin examination is focused on recognition of a pigmented or clinically amelanotic lesion that simply looks different from the rest. This method may aid with detection of lesions that lack the classic ABCDE criteria (e.g., nodular, amelanotic, or desmoplastic melanomas) and in patients with large number of atypical nevi. Patients with family history of melanoma as well as numerous common or dysplastic nevi should be educated regarding the ABCDE criteria as well as the importance of frequent skin self-examination.

Primary cutaneous melanoma is broadly classified according to four different histologic subtypes that are primarily based on growth patterns. These include: (a) superficial spreading melanoma; (b) nodular melanoma; (c) lentigo maligna melanoma; and (d) acral lentiginous melanoma. These clinical subtypes, however, are not indicative of prognosis but rather the measured depth of invasion (Breslow depth) or ulceration is most linked to

Table 7-6 Different Types of Primary Cutaneous Melanoma

TYPE OF MELANOMA	FREQUENCY (%)	SITE	SPECIAL FEATURES
Superficial spreading (SSM)	60–70	Any site, preference for lower extremities (women), trunk (men and women)	Most common type of melanoma in fair-skinned individuals. It begins as an asymptomatic brown to black macule with color variations and irregular, notched borders and can arise de novo or in a pre-existing nevus. In up to two-thirds of tumors, regression (visible as gray, hypo- or depigmentation) of part of the lesion is observed, reflecting the interaction of the host immune system with the progressing tumor. See Figure 7-14A,B
Nodular	15–30	Any site, preference for trunk, head, neck More frequently in men than in women	Second most common type of melanoma in fair-skinned individuals and is diagnosed most frequently in patients in their sixth decade of life, accounting for approximately 15% to 30% of all melanomas. They usually present as a blue to black, but sometimes pink to red-colored, nodule, which may be ulcerated or bleeding and has developed rapidly over months. See Figure 7-15
Lentigo maligna	5–15	Face, especially nose and cheeks	Began as an asymmetric, brown to black macule with color variation and an irregular, indented border that slowly darkens over years. Predilection for sun-damaged skin. It has been estimated that 5% of lentigo malignas progress to invasive melanoma. See Figure 7-16
Acral lentiginous (ALM)	5–10	Palms, soles, nail unit	Most common melanoma type in patients with darker skin types. It typically presents as an asymmetric, brown to black macule with color variation and irregular borders. Melanoma of the nail matrix can present as longitudinal melanonychia or as hyperpigmentation extending onto the hyponychium or beyond the lateral or proximal nail. Suspicion for melanoma should be raised in all fair-skinned individuals with pigmented nail bands. See Figure 7-17

aggressiveness. These different subtypes of melanoma are summarized in Table 7-6 (Figs. 7-14 to 7-17).

DIAGNOSIS

When melanoma is suspected, skin biopsy should be performed, and should include the full epidermal/dermal thickness, preferably to the subcutaneous fat. For highly suspicious lesions, an excisional biopsy should be performed. In the case of suspected lentigo maligna, a broad, paper-thin shave biopsy or multiple smaller biopsies of suspicious areas may be the best technique.

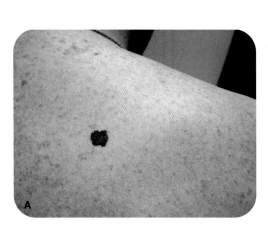
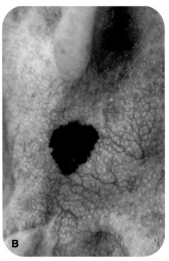

Figure 7-14 A. Superficial spreading melanoma on the back. **B.** Melanoma in situ on the jawline.

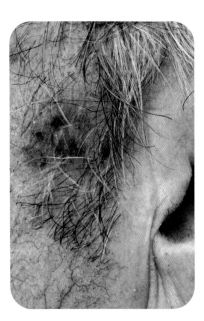

Figure 7-15 Nodular melanoma on the preauricular skin.

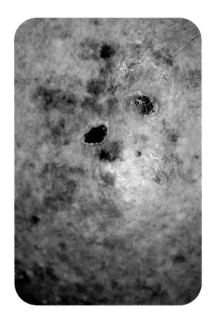

Figure 7-16 Lentigo maligna on sun damaged skin of the cheek. Note two healing biopsy sites.

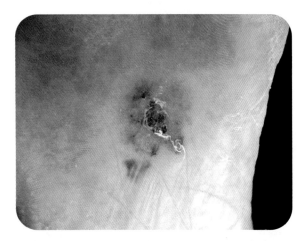

Figure 7-17 Acral lentiginous melanoma. Clark level IV, Breslow depth 2.71 mm.

Once the diagnosis of melanoma is confirmed, further studies and workup are dependent on the depth of the lesion (>1 cm depth being more concerning), the American Joint Committee on Cancer (AJCC) stage and when certain high-risk histologic features (e.g., ulceration, extensive regression, high mitotic rate, angiolymphatic invasion) are present. The most important aspects of the initial workup for patients with cutaneous melanoma are a careful history, review of systems, and physical examination.

In asymptomatic patients with primary cutaneous melanoma (AJCC stages I and II), extensive radiologic studies such as CT scanning, MRI, PET scanning, ultrasonography, and bone scanning are not recommended. Baseline metastatic staging for melanoma patients with primary tumors greater than 1 mm in depth may include

CXR, which typically is repeated every 6 to 12 months for routine surveillance (optional in the absence of signs or symptoms of metastatic disease). There is no single useful laboratory test or radiologic study that is beneficial for stage I/II cutaneous melanoma patients without signs and symptoms of metastasis.

A metastatic workup should be initiated if physical findings or symptoms suggest disease recurrence or if the patient has documented nodal metastasis based on results from the sentinel lymph node biopsy (see Therapy section below).

THERAPY

Melanoma remains one of the deadliest skin cancers with few effective medical therapies. Numerous adjuvant therapies have been investigated for the treatment of localized cutaneous melanoma following complete surgical removal though none has shown survival benefit. Other therapies include non-specific (passive) immunotherapy, radiation therapy, retinoid therapy, vitamin therapy, or biologic therapy, all of which did not improve survival. Adjuvant interferon (IFN)α-2b is the only adjuvant therapy approved by the U.S. FDA for high-risk melanoma (currently defined as stages IIB, IIC, and III), which is associated with a 40% to 80% chance of relapse and death. IFNα-2b has demonstrated limited antitumor activity in metastatic stage IV melanoma, with overall response rates of 10% to 15%. IFN-α has been most widely studied in the adjuvant setting for stage II and III disease and has been shown in some trials to improve disease-free survival, although evidence for overall survival is less clear. The potential benefits of high-dose IFN must be weighed against its substantial tolerability and toxicity issues, including the yearlong duration of therapy, constitutional (flu-like) and neuropsychiatric (depression, suicidal intention) symptoms hematologic and hepatic side effects, as well as cases of fatal rhabdomyolysis.

Surgery is therefore the mainstay of therapy. Wide excision with or without sentinel lymph node biopsy (SLNB) is the primary treatment for most types of melanoma, although there are some controversies regarding excision margins. See Table 7-7 for recommendations on surgical margins.

One of the more controversial topics in melanoma management is SLNB. SLNB is based on the finding that the cutaneous site of the melanoma drains to one or more lymph node basins and particularly to one (or two but rarely more) lymph node, the sentinel node, which is the first site of deposition of metastatic cells. This procedure is performed in conjunction with wide local excisions where a radioactive compound, 99m technetium sulfur colloid and blue dye are injected into the skin surrounding the melanoma biopsy site. A

WHEN TO REFER (?)

Refer to a dermatologist whenever melanoma is suspected.

CHAPTER 7 Malignant Skin Lesions

Table 7-7 Surgical Treatment of Primary Melanoma

THICKNESS	EXCISION MARGINS (CM)	COMMENTS
In situ	0.5	No randomized studies. For lentigo maligna, Wood's lamp examination can aid in defining the lesion and some authors suggest 1 cm surgical margins for this variant of melanoma when the primary lesion is >1 cm in diameter
<1 mm	1.0	1-cm margin for melanomas <1 mm
1–4 mm	2.0	2-cm margin for melanomas ≥4 mm
>4 mm	2.0	No randomized studies

NOT TO BE MISSED

- Changing or suspicious pigmented lesions should be evaluated by an appropriate biopsy.
- Patients with a first-degree relative with a confirmed melanoma should have (at least) yearly screening full-body skin exams.

hand-held gamma counter is subsequently used to detect any radioactivity in the possible draining lymph node basins, and an incision is made to see whether any nodes have taken up the dye. These "hot, blue" sentinel nodes are then selectively biopsied and examined by histology and immunohistochemistry. If metastatic melanoma is identified, then a complete regional lymph node dissection is undertaken. The controversy remains whether this procedure actually improves overall survival.

"AT A GLANCE" TREATMENT

- The treatment of melanoma is surgical removal with appropriate margins of normal surrounding tissue
- For lesions greater than 1 mm in depth, consider referring the patient for SLNB
- Metastatic disease has a dire prognosis and should be treated by surgical and medical oncology in conjunction with a pigmented lesion specialist within dermatology

COURSE AND COMPLICATIONS

Early detection and appropriate excision leads to a cure rate of over 90% in low-risk (<1 mm Breslow depth, a measurement of the thickness of the tumor or depth of invasion) melanoma patients. There is currently no effective cure for metastatic melanoma and therefore, this type of disease usually leads to death. Early detection is imperative.

ICD9 Codes	
172.0	Malignant melanoma of skin of lip
172.1	Malignant melanoma of skin of eyelid, including canthus
172.2	Malignant melanoma of skin of ear and external auditory canal
172.3	Malignant melanoma of skin of other and unspecified parts of face
172.4	Malignant melanoma of skin of scalp and neck
172.5	Malignant melanoma of skin of trunk, except scrotum
172.6	Malignant melanoma of skin of upper limb, including shoulder
172.7	Malignant melanoma of skin of lower limb, including hip
172.8	Malignant melanoma of other specified sites of skin
172.9	Melanoma of skin, site unspecified

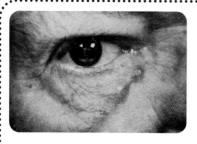

A 70-year-old male who loves to sail and golf and acquire a dark tan notices a fixed bump underneath his skin on the lower right eyelid that has doubled in size for the past several months (Fig. 7-18). *The lump is slightly blue-violet in color and is painless. His ophthalmologist first thought it was a chalazion, but it is not mobile or fluctuant. Given the rapid growth, patient is quite concerned. What is the most likely diagnosis? What should the treatment be?*

Merkel Cell Carcinoma

BACKGROUND

Merkel cell carcinoma (MCC) is a rare, aggressive type of skin cancer originating from specialized neuroendocrine cells called Merkel cells, a type of slow-acting mechanoreceptor in the basal layer of the epidermis, which are believed to play a role in making the skin sensitive to touch. The diagnosis is rarely suspected at the time of biopsy, as the appearance is rather nondescript. It is, however, an aggressive tumor with a propensity for dermal and nodal spread.

CHAPTER 7 Malignant Skin Lesions

KEY FEATURES

- Merkel cell carcinoma (MCC) is a rare, aggressive type of skin cancer that appears to be linked to sun exposure and immunosuppression, with most cases occurring on sun-exposed areas of the body.

- Most patients diagnosed with MCC are over age 50 at diagnosis (the average age is 69), with only 5% of cases diagnosed in those under age 50.

- MCC presents as a firm, painless cutaneous to subcutaneous nodule, papule, or tumor, which is pink, red to violet or reddish-brown, dome-shaped, and usually solitary. The overlying skin is often intact, but also can ulcerate.

- The prognosis for MCC is dependent on the stage of the disease with tumors less than 2 cm and no lymph node involvement yielding a 5-year survival rate of more than 90%. Recurrence is common, in about 50% of patients. Overall, 5-year survival for patients diagnosed with MCC is 64%, but half of patients with advanced MCC will live only 9 months.

- Surgery and radiation are the usual treatments for MCC.

Approximately 1,200 new cases of MCCs are diagnosed in the United States each year. The incidence of MCCs has been rising, with a 3-fold increase between 1986 and 2001. Most patients diagnosed with MCC are over age 50 at diagnosis (average age is 69), with only 5% of cases diagnosed in those under age 50. MCC is more common in white people than in other racial/ethnic groups.

CLINICAL PRESENTATION

The tumor favors the head and neck region, followed by the extremities and the buttocks. Clinically, it presents as a firm, painless cutaneous to subcutaneous nodule, papule, or tumor, which is pink, red to violet or reddish-brown, dome-shaped, and usually solitary (Fig. 7-16). The surface is often shiny with overlying telangiectasias. The behavior is that of an aggressively growing tumor, with frequent recurrences after excision. At presentation, about one-third of cases have nodal involvement and eventually, 50% of these patients develop hematogenous spread. It is therefore imperative to examine the lymph nodes for patient whose biopsy returns as Merkel cell carcinoma.

DIAGNOSIS

Diagnosis is confirmed by skin biopsy. The tumor is composed of monotonously uniform, small, round to oval cells that are about two to three times larger than mature lymphocyte and often shows an aggressive growth pattern as a poorly defined dermal mass frequently infiltrating the subcutaneous fat, fascia, and muscle.

The differential diagnosis often includes nonmelanoma skin cancer (especially BCC) and cyst. Due to the violaceous, sometime hemorrhagic appearance of the tumor, the differential diagnosis includes hemangioma, abscess, angiosarcoma, and lymphoma. Metastatic neuroendocrine tumor of the lung, lymphoma, melanoma, and poorly differentiated SCCs are among the tumors that can have similar histologic appearance. The alternative diagnosis of cutaneous metastasis from a primary small cell neuroendocrine carcinoma (oat cell carcinoma) of the lung can be ruled out via radiography of the chest. Staging CT or MRI studies are needed to assess the possibility of dissemination of primary MCC to the lymph nodes or the viscera.

THERAPY

Unfortunately, few treatment options exist. Wide local excision with at least 3-cm margins is the primary approach with adjuvant chemotherapy,

WHEN TO REFER

Refer to a dermatologist for rapidly growing lesion for further evaluation and diagnosis. For untreated, but diagnosed MCC, consultation with radiation oncology, surgical oncology, and medical oncology is helpful.

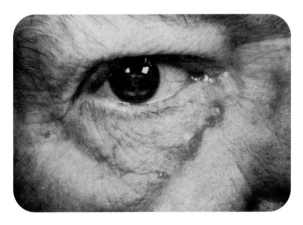

Figure 7-18 Merkel cell carcinoma on the lower eyelid. From Tasman W, Jaeger E. *The Wills Eye Hospital Atlas of Clinical Ophthalmology*, 2nd ed. Lippincott Williams & Wilkins, 2001.

NOT TO BE MISSED

- These lesions are often not suspected as MCC. Biopsy any rapidly growing skin lesion, especially those on sun damaged skin of older individuals.

immunotherapy, and radiation therapy often simultaneously administered owing to the aggressive course of the disease. Sentinel lymph node mapping has also been recommended. For metastatic disease, various chemotherapeutic regimens have been employed, but none has been proven to result in improved survival as MCC is chemosensitive but only rarely chemocurable in patients with metastasis or locally advanced tumors. Chemotherapy also can be associated with a high incidence of toxic death; therefore, its role in treatment is unclear. Radiotherapy may help to control unresectable primary or metastatic lesions, and can reduce local and regional recurrence rate, although it may not lead to improved overall survival.

"AT A GLANCE" TREATMENT

- Surgical excision with 3-cm margins
- Sentinel lymph node biopsy is recommended
- Concominant chemotherapy and/or radiation therapy should be considered

COURSE AND COMPLICATIONS

Although the prognosis for the MCC patients depends greatly on the stage of the disease at the time of diagnosis, and whether there is distant involvement, the prognosis is poor, with distant metastases develop in approximately 40% of the patients, and about 30% will die of the disease within 5 years.

ICD9 Codes

209.31	Merkel cell carcinoma of the face
209.32	Merkel cell carcinoma of the scalp and neck
209.33	Merkel cell carcinoma of the upper limb
209.34	Merkel cell carcinoma of the lower limb
209.35	Merkel cell carcinoma of the trunk
209.36	Merkel cell carcinoma of other sites

Suggested reading

Becker JC, Schrama D, Houben R.Merkel cell carcinoma. *Cell Mol Life Sci.* 2009; 66(1): 1–8.

Bolognia JL, Jorizzo, JL, Rapini RP, et al. *Dermatology.* New York: Mosby, 2007.

Brash DE, et al. A role for sunlight in skin cancer: UV-induced p53 mutations in squamous cell carcinoma. *Proc Natl Acad Sci U S A.* 1991;88(22):10124–10128.

Brash DE, et al. Sunlight and sunburn in human skin cancer: p53, apoptosis, and tumor promotion. *J Investig Dermatol Symp Proc.* 1996;1(2):136–142.

Cui R, et al. Central role of p53 in the suntan response and pathologic hyperpigmentation. *Cell.* 2007; 128(5):853–864.

Findlay GM. Ultra-violet light and skin cancer. *The Lancet.* 1928;212(5491):1070–1073.

Gailani MR, et al. Relationship between sunlight exposure and a key genetic alteration in basal cell carcinoma. *J Natl Cancer Inst.* 1996;88(6):349–354.

Hall A. Relationships of sunlight, complexion and heredity to skin carcinogenesis. *Arch Dermatol Syph.* 1950;61:589–610.

Henness S, Vereecken P. Management of Merkel tumours: an evidence-based review. *Curr Opin Oncol.* 2008; 20(3):280–286.

Ibrahim SF, Brown, MD. Tanning and cutaneous malignancy. *Dermatol Surg.* 2008;34(4):460–474.

Kraemer KH, et al. The role of sunlight and DNA repair in melanoma and nonmelanoma skin cancer. The xeroderma pigmentosum paradigm. *Arch Dermatol.* 1994;130(8):1018–1021.

Kricker A, et al. Does intermittent sun exposure cause basal cell carcinoma? A case-control study in Western Australia. *Int J Cancer.* 1995;60(4):489–494.

Marks R, Rennie G, SelwoodT. The relationship of basal cell carcinomas and squamous cell carcinomas to solar keratoses. *Arch Dermatol.* 1988;124(7):1039–1042.

Moan J, Porojnicu AC, Dahlback A. Ultraviolet radiation and malignant melanoma. *Adv Exp Med Biol.* 2008; 624:104–116.

Tai P. Merkel cell cancer: update on biology and treatment. *Curr Opin Oncol.* 2008;20(2):196–200.

Ziegler A, et al. Mutation hotspots due to sunlight in the p53 gene of nonmelanoma skin cancers. *Proc Natl Acad Sci U S A.* 1993;90(9):4216–4220.

Ziegler A, et al. Sunburn and p53 in the onset of skin cancer. *Nature.* 1994;372(6508):773–776.

CHAPTER 8 Dermatologic Reactions to Arthropods

James Y.T. Wang

While skin pathology can impact the appearance and health of the skin, external influences also cause important changes in the skin. In this chapter, the focus will be on arthropods that may cause clinically significant disease and irritation of the dermis and epidermis. In many cases, the barrier of the skin is broken via needle-like penetration of arthropod body parts used to access the blood stream. In other cases, arthropod structures release toxins or are themselves toxic to the skin and cause pathology. The chapter is divided into three sections: infestations, bites, and miscellaneous. There are many more diseases caused by arthropods, but the purpose of this chapter is to give a succinct overview of the most commonly encountered conditions caused by arthropods.

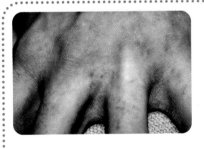

A 20-year-old woman complains of an "itchy rash" on her right arm and hand. Upon examination, it is noted that there are small excoriated papules between her fingers on her right hand and around the right elbow (Fig. 8-1). Five weeks ago, she had gone on a retreat with the volleyball team and everyone had shared bedding. Her roommate is also starting to develop similar symptoms. What is the most likely diagnosis? What test can be done to confirm the diagnosis?

INFESTATIONS

Scabies

BACKGROUND

Scabies is an ectoparasitic skin infestation with the mite *Sarcoptes scabiei var. humanus*. First described in 1687 with the organism responsible being identified in the 18th century, this intensely pruritic disease was named from the Latin word for "scratch," *scabere*. Scabies affect people of all races and age groups and the geographic distribution is worldwide. It is spread by skin-to-skin, via both sexual and nonsexual contact, and in some cases as fomites.

KEY FEATURES

- Hypersensitivity reactions to feces of scabies mite *Sarcoptes scabiei* are responsible for signs and symptoms.

(Continued)

PATHOGENESIS

The adult mite is 1/3-mm long and has a life cycle of 30 days. An infestation occurs when a fertilized female mite burrows into the stratum corneum of the host's skin. As it burrows, it lays eggs and expels fecal pellets behind it. A hypersensitivity reaction to the scybala may be responsible for skin irritation and itching because IgE titers are elevated and eosinophilia develop after initial infestation.

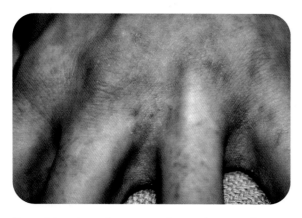

Figure 8-1 Scabies infection—papules in web spaces of hand.

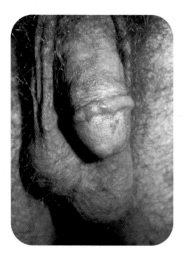

Figure 8-2 Scabies infection causing erythematous papules and nodules on the penis. From Goodheart HP. *Goodheart's Photoguide to Common Skin Disorders,* 3rd ed. Philadelphia: Lippincott Williams & Wilkins, 2009.

KEY FEATURES (Continued)

- Pruritic erythematous vesicles, papules, and/or macules are typically distributed in digit web spaces, groin, flexor folds, peri-umbilical regions.

- Diagnosis is by skin scrapings and wet mount— visualization of mites, eggs, and/or scybala under microscope.

- Treat using topical scabicides, antipruritic medications, and antibiotics (if necessary).

CLINICAL PRESENTATION

Patients with scabies infestation manifest intractable pruritus, stereotypically with nocturnal exacerbations. Lesions may be eczematous with impetiginization and are often excoriated. Those infected may be asymptomatic for one month following initial infestation by at least one scabies mite. Distribution of skin lesions includes digit web spaces (Fig. 8-1); sides of the fingers; buttocks; peri-umbilical areas; and flexor aspects of the wrists, elbows, and axillary folds. Other areas that may be affected include the penis (Fig. 8-2) and scrotum in men and areolae in women. If noticeable, visualization of a burrow (Fig. 8-3), which can be seen as a short, S-shaped, dark line on the surface of the skin, is pathognomonic for scabies. Family members of patients may also develop similar symptoms and signs. Manifestations of scabies infections are outlined in Table 8-1.

DIAGNOSIS

Differential Diagnosis

Scabies can oftentimes be confused with atopic dermatitis, papular urticaria, pyoderma, insect bites, or dermatitis herpetiformis. Subspecies of nonhuman scabies are also able to cause pruritic eruptions in humans, but these cases do

Table 8-1 Manifestations of Scabies Infection

Scabies in patients with good hygiene	Sparse lesions with subtle burrow formation
Scabies incognito	Seen in immunosuppressed patients; manifests as widespread, scaly, pruritic dermatosis
Nodular scabies	Reddish-brown, pruritic papules and nodules on covered areas
Scabies in infants and young children	Mostly in patients <2 years; distribution on face, scalp, palms, and soles with secondary eczematization and impetiginization
Scabies in elderly	Often seen in elderly group-care facilities; minimal or atypical cutaneous changes; often mistakenly attributed to "senile pruritus," xerosis, drugs, or psychogenic causes
Crusted scabies	Seen patients with advanced age, debility, developmental disability, immunosuppression; commonly hyperkeratotic, nonpruritic lesions with fissured and excoriated skin that can lead to bacteremia; serious infestations of thousands to millions of mites on the host
Scabies and HIV/AIDS	Unusual forms, including crusted scabies and atypical papular scabies
Scabies of the scalp	Mostly occurs in infants, children, elderly, nursing home patients, those residing in the tropics, and patients with crusted scabies, AIDS, dermatomyositis
Bullous scabies	Occurs usually in otherwise healthy 65+ individuals; eruptions indistinguishable from bullous pemphigoid clinically, pathologically, and immunopathologically

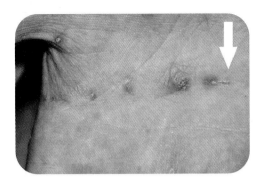

Figure 8-3 Scabies burrow on the palm. From Goodheart HP. *Goodheart's Photoguide to Common Skin Disorders,* 3rd ed. Philadelphia: Lippincott Williams & Wilkins, 2009.

not have the normal body distribution of human mites and are usually self-limited. Some of these mites include *S. scabiei var. canis, S. scabiei var. bovis, Notoedres cati, Cheyletiella yasguri, Cheyletiella blakei, Dermanyssus gallinae,* and *Ophionyssus natricis.*

Diagnostic Methods

The visualization of burrows is pathognomonic for scabies, but they may be difficult to find amid excoriations and eczematous plaques. It is generally safe to rely on the characteristic distribution of pruritic lesions seen in scabies. In males, there can also be papules, nodules, and/or ulcers on the penis (Fig. 8-2). A definitive diagnosis requires microscopic identification of mites, eggs, or fecal pellets (scybala). However, in the case that signs of *S. scabiei* cannot be found but clinical suspicion is high for scabies, it is advisable to proceed with treatment for scabies.

- Direct Examination: after applying mineral oil to a skin lesion, scrape or shave area with scalpel blade to remove tops of burrows or papules. Scrapings observed under a microscope under low power should show the scabies mite, eggs, or scybala. Small dermal curettes may also be used to obtain sample. (See Chapter 3, Figs. 3-3 and 3-4 for examples of typical scabies findings seen on scraping.)
- Dermoscopy: luminescence microscopy over skin lesions shows small, dark, triangular structures (pigmented section of mite) and a subtle linear segment behind the triangle containing air bubbles (burrow with eggs and fecal pellets).
- Potassium Hydroxide Wet Mount: mite feces may dissolve when mount is heated.
- Polymerase Chain Reaction (PCR): positive for *S. scabiei* DNA.

THERAPY

Medication is needed to both kill the mites and destroy the eggs. Scabicides must be applied thoroughly to areas behind ears and from the neck down to the soles of the feet. Regions to emphasize coverage are between the fingers and toes, the umbilicus, groin, between buttocks, and under fingernails and toenails. Topical creams ought to be washed off after the recommended time period to avoid toxicity. The morning after topical treatment, all linens, towels, and clothing in the vicinity of the affected individual should be machine-washed and dried using the hot cycles. This ensures that no mites are present to reinfest the host after treatment. Members of the affected household should also be treated with scabicides. Itching and eczema may persist for several months after treatment, even if all mites are successfully removed.

- **Topical Scabicides**
  - **Permethrin 5% cream:** apply and leave on overnight. Second application 5 to 7 days later. Not for use in infants younger than 2 months or pregnant/nursing women. Adverse reactions: burning, stinging, pruritus, contact dermatitis (rare).
  - **Lindane 1%:** apply and leave on for 8 hours, then wash off. Use for resistant cases only. Not for use in infants, young children, pregnant/nursing women, or patients with seizure disorders or neurologic diseases. Adverse reactions: over-application may lead to central nervous system (CNS) toxicity.
  - **Sulfur** (precipitated sulfur, 6%, in petrolatum): apply nightly for 3 nights and wash off thoroughly 24 hours after last application. Not for use in infants younger than 2 months of age, and women who are pregnant or lactating.

- **Ivermectin (200 mcg/kg × 1 dose, repeat in 7 days):** use with caution in elderly patients.
- **Antipruritic Medications:** sedating antihistamines (i.e., hydroxyzine, 25 to 50 mg PO q4h) or short course of topical or systemic glucocorticoids.
- **Antibiotic Therapy:** topical mupirocin or broad-spectrum antibiotics where excoriation has led to impetiginization.

In cases of crusted scabies and scabies in conjunction with human immunodeficiency virus/acquired immunodeficiency syndrome (HIV/AIDS), sequential use of two or more compounds may sometimes be necessary. The entire area of skin should be treated and patients should be isolated until treatment has been completed. The surrounding environment and personal items should be assiduously cleaned.

"AT A GLANCE" THERAPY

- **Topical Scabicides**
  - Permethrin 5% cream: apply and leave on overnight. Second application 5 to 7 days later.
  - Lindane 1%: apply and leave on for 8 hours, then wash off. **Use only for resistant cases.**
  - Sulfur (precipitated sulfur, 6%, in petrolatum): apply nightly for 3 nights and wash off thoroughly 24 hours after last application.
- **Ivermectin (200 mcg/kg × 1 dose, repeat in 7 days):** use with caution in elderly patients.
- **Antipruritic Medications**
  - hydroxyzine, 25 to 50 mg PO q4h PRN
  - topical corticosteroid: triamcinolone 0.1% BID PRN to AA
  - systemic prednisone taper
- **Antibiotic Therapy:** topical mupirocin or broad-spectrum antibiotics such as Keflex 500 mg PO QID × 10 days. Use these only with impetiginization.

COURSE AND COMPLICATIONS

Complications are most often seen in patients with atopic dermatitis. In these individuals, there is an increase in eczematous lesions during the infestation that may persist even after treatment. Excoriations from these lesions can lead to secondary pyoderma and colonization by nephritogenic strains of streptococci, which are most prevalent in tropical regions. The resulting complication is glomerulonephritis. In nonatopics, postscabetic itch can last several months.

WHEN TO REFER

Skin lesions do not resolve with scabicide treatment.

NOT TO BE MISSED

- Treat close contacts at the same time as the patient. Infections can be passed back and forth.
- Launder all bedding and personal items in hot water after treatment.

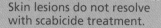

ICD9 Codes

133.0   *Scabies*

Pediculosis

BACKGROUND

Pediculosis refers to the infestation of certain body areas by head, body, or crab lice. Lice are obligate human ectoparasites that cannot live without their hosts for more than 10 days. The three types of lice, *Pediculosis humanis capitis*, *Pediculosis humanis corporis*, and *Pthirus pubis*, affect different parts of the body, but have similar life cycles and features. Generally, they are 1 to 4 mm long, flat, wingless insects with terminal claws at the end of their three pairs of legs. The legs tend to be clustered toward the anterior aspect of the body, immediately behind the head. The lice live on the hair shafts and crawl down to the

KEY FEATURES

- Lice are bloodsucking insects that reside and lay eggs near the base of hair shafts or in clothing. Each of the three main types of lice has a characteristic distribution on the body (scalp, body, and pubic area).

- Presentation is with intense pruritus, excoriations, and secondary impetiginization in affected areas.

- Diagnosed by examining plucked hairs for louse or eggs under the microscope.

- Treat using topical pediculicides.

Pediculosis capitis
- A worldwide infestation caused by bloodsucking, wingless insects, *Pediculus humanus capitis*, who live on head hair and feed on blood from the scalp.

- Diagnosis confirmed by presence of nits attached to head hairs or identification of a louse.

- Head lice is spread by head-to-head contact and fomites.

- Worldwide resistance to traditional treatments (pyrethrin, Permethrin) is increasing.

Pediculosis corporis
- Body lice is caused by an infestation of humans and their clothing by *Pediculus humanus corporis*.

- Body lice lay their eggs in clothing, not on people.

- Commonly found in those in crowded, unsanitary living conditions.

- Lice may transmit epidemic typhus, trench fever, and relapsing fever.

Pediculosis pubis
- May involve pubic as well as other hair-bearing sites such as the beard, eyelashes, axillae, and perianal regions.

- Transmission via sexual, close contact, or rarely through contaminated clothing, towels, and bedding.

skin to feed on human blood about five times a day. They pierce the skin with their claws, inject anticoagulants and other irritants into the site, and suck blood. Lice are active and travel quickly, resulting in high transmissibility of pediculosis. Most often noticeable in patients with pediculosis is the presence of nits, or eggs, laid by the female lice. Six eggs are laid by the female louse each day for about one month. The nits themselves are less than 1 mm long and are firmly attached to the base of the hair shafts or to fibers on clothing in the case of the body louse. Their proximity to the skin provides nits with the warmth needed to sustain continued growth. Nits are hard to remove, even with a fine-toothed comb.

CLINICAL PRESENTATION

The bite of the louse itself is painless, but hypersensitivity to the saliva and feces of the mite may lead to inflammation and pruritus. Immediate urticarial lesions may appear in some individuals, but most develop small macules or papules hours to days later. Intense scratching of these areas can result in trauma to the skin, excoriations, and secondary bacterial infections. Most often seen are the results of pruritus. A comparison of the different types of pediculosis is presented in Table 8-2.

PATHOGENESIS

Saliva and fecal material can induce a hypersensitivity reaction and inflammation. The resulting pruritus leads to scratching and the development of excoriations and secondary impetiginization of the affected area(s).

PEDICULOSIS CAPITIS

There are over 12 million cases per year of head lice in the United States alone. The area of infestation is limited to the human head and is commonly seen on the back of the head and neck and behind the ears. It occurs primarily in children, especially in girls. African Americans have very low incidence of head lice. Head lice are spread by close physical contact and sharing of head gear, combs, brushes, and pillows. Usually, an infestation on an individual will have less than 20 adult lice.

Clinical Features

Intense pruritus leads to scratching, resulting in inflammation and secondary bacterial infection. Common clinical features include excoriations with pustules, crusting, and *maculae ceruleae* (blue to slate-gray macule) in the head and neck region as well as conjunctivitis and cervical lymphadenopathy.

Table 8-2 Comparison of Head, Body, and Crab Lice

TYPE OF LOUSE	COMMON AREAS OF BODY AFFECTED	COMMONLY SEEN
Capitis	Back of the head, behind ears, eyes	Children, male>female
Corporis	Waistband, buttocks, thighs	Destitute, homeless, refugees, wartime soldiers
Pubis	Pubic area, perianal region, axilla, eyelashes	Sexually active individuals, MSM

Diagnosis

Differential diagnosis. Conditions that resemble head lice include the presence of seborrheic scales, hair casts, and hairspray.

Diagnostic methods. Live nits on proximal head hair shafts can often be seen with the naked eye in cases of *Pediculosis capitis* infestation. Examine plucked hairs under the microscope to determine whether the nits contain live larvae. The presence of live adult lice, immature nymphs, or viable eggs confirms the diagnosis.

PEDICULOSIS CORPORIS

The structure of body lice looks similar to head lice, but body lice tend to be larger. It is an infestation associated with poverty and poor living condition. Therefore, it is most often seen in the poor, homeless, recent refugees, and soldiers in wartime conditions. The main mode of transmission is via contaminated bedding or clothing because body lice do not lay eggs on humans, but rather in clothes that the person wears.

Clinical Presentation

The presence of *maculae ceruleae* in areas where clothing most commonly contacts a person, such as the waistband and on buttocks and thighs, is highly suspicious for body lice. The lesions may or may not be pruritic, but there will be linear excoriations, sometimes with secondary impetiginization, seen on the trunk from the intense pruritus. Adult lice are rarely seen.

Diagnosis

Diagnostic methods. Careful examination of clothing for nits, especially in the seams, is crucial. An effective method may involve shaking out the patient's clothing over a sheet of newspaper. Lice may then be seen moving on the paper.

Associated diseases. Body lice are vectors for *Rickettsia prowazekii* (epidemic typhus); *Rickettsia quintana* (trench fever); and *Borrelia recurrentis* (relapsing fever).

PEDICULOSIS PUBIS

The crab louse (*Phthirus pubis*) is physically distinctive from head and body lice. Its body is more rounded, resembling the shape of a crab, and has progressively larger claws from its front pairs of legs toward the rear pairs. This formation allows the louse to grip sparser, coarser hairs of the pubic area, eyebrows, eyelashes, thighs, and perianal regions. The incidence of crab lice is slightly higher in men, potentially due to larger amounts of coarse body hair. It is considered a sexually transmitted disease and is associated with other sexually transmitted infections. There are no racial differences in incidence of infestation, although pediculosis pubis often recurs in men who have sex with men (MSM).

Clinical Presentation

Maculae ceruleae are often present in the pubic region. Patients will present with intense itching and excoriations in the infested areas. Local lymphadenitis and fever may present concurrently due to secondary bacterial infection of those excoriations. Hairier individuals may also have infestations of hairs of the thighs, trunk, and perianal area. Even beard, moustache, and eyelashes can be affected. Infestation of eyelashes and periphery of scalp occurs mainly in children and may indicate sexual abuse. Extra-pubic infestations, such as those of the beard, moustache, and eyelashes are more common in the homeless population.

Diagnosis

Diagnostic methods. Examine plucked hairs under microscopy for louse or nits.

THERAPY

Pediculosis Capitis

- **Topical pediculicides**
  - Synergized pyrethrin creams (RID, A-200, R&C shampoo)
  - Permethrin 5% cream: hair should be combed with fine-toothed comb to remove remaining nits
  - Malathion lotion 0.5% (Ovid): kills all lice and ova in 10 minutes
  - Lindane (gamma-benzene hexachloride) 1% shampoo
  - Benzyl alcohol 5% lotion
- **Environmental control**
  - Use fine-toothed comb to remove as many nits as possible. An *8% formic acid* rinse helps to dislodge nits from their attachment to the hair.
  - Members of household should be examined. Treatment of household members up to discretion of physician.
  - Following therapy, clothing and bedding should be washed and dried using hot cycle; nonwashables should be dry cleaned, ironed, or put in the clothes dryer without washing. Wash combs and brushes in very hot water, can add pediculicides first.
  - "No nit" policies excluding children with nits from attending school are excessive.

Pediculosis Corporis

- Discarding or laundering infested clothing and restoring proper hygiene should cure the infestation because body lice lay eggs in the clothing and not on the human body.
- Bedding should be laundered with hot water, boiled, or discarded.
- Consider treating the patient head to toe with a single application of Permethrin 5% cream.

Pediculosis Pubis

- Use topical treatments (synergized pyrethrins) as in cases of *Pediculosis capitis*, but in areas affected by crab lice specifically, such as the pubic and perianal regions. A common cause of treatment failure is neglect of thighs, trunk, and axillary regions in hairier individuals. Sexual contacts should be treated simultaneously and clothing/bedding should be washed and dried using the hot cycle.
- Parasitophobia is often a consequence postinfestation.
- Specific agents: therapy for eyelash involvement is applying petrolatum twice daily for 8 days, followed by removal of nits. HIV/AIDS patients may be unresponsive to conventional therapy.

There are signs of local resistance to topical medications for treatment of pediculosis. In resistant cases, systemic therapy with ivermectin (adult dosage [for >5 years; safety in <5 not established]: 150 to 200 mcg/kg/d PO as single dose; 12 mg PO repeated in 7 to 10 days) is indicated.

"AT A GLANCE" THERAPY

Pediculosis Capitis

- Topical pediculicides
  - First-line:
    - Synergized pyrethrin creams (RID, A-200, R&C shampoo)
    - Permethrin 5% cream
  - Second-line:
    - Malathion lotion 0.5% (Ovid): kills all lice and ova in 10 minutes.
    - Lindane (gamma-benzene hexachloride) 1% shampoo
    - Benzyl alcohol 5% lotion
- Environmental control
  - Use fine-toothed comb to remove as many nits as possible.
  - *8% formic acid* rinse helps to dislodge nits from their attachment to the hair.
  - Examine and treat close contacts.
  - Following therapy, clean bedding and local environment.

Pediculosis Corporis

- Discard/launder infested clothing and restoring proper hygiene should cure the infestation.
- Bedding should be laundered with hot water, boiled, or discarded.
- Consider treating with a single application of Permethrin 5% cream.

Pediculosis Pubis

- Use topical treatments (synergized pyrethrins) as in cases of *Pediculosis capitis*.
- Sexual contacts should be treated simultaneously.
- Clothing/bedding should be washed and dried using the hot cycle.
- Eyelash involvement: petrolatum twice daily for 8 days, followed by removal of nits.
- Resistant infections
  - Systemic therapy with ivermectin
    - Adult dosage (for >5 years): 150 to 200 mcg/kg/d PO as single dose; 12 mg PO repeated in 7 to 10 d)
    - Safety in children younger than 5 years not established

ICD9 Codes	
132.0	*Pediculus capitis (head louse)*
132.1	*Pediculus corporis (body louse)*
132.2	*Phthirus pubis (pubic louse)*
132.3	*Mixed pediculosis infestation*
132.9	*Pediculosis, unspecified*

 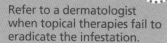
BITES

Spiders

Spiders are carnivorous arthropods with four sets of legs. They are generally not aggressive and bite humans only when threatened. They have fangs containing venom, which are usually used to catch and immobilize prey. Spider venom usually contains inflammatory factors that simply cause pain and swelling. However, some may have neuromuscular effects and can lead to significant necrosis of the skin and underlying tissues. Although some spider bites may not be felt at the time of the initial bite, most do cause pain at the instant they occur. Localized pain, swelling, itching, erythema, blisters, and necrosis may be found, along with two puncta (fang marks) in the center. The swelling appears at the bite site, expanding radially to a few centimeters, and can be significant for some species of spiders.

For most spider bites, the lesions resolve spontaneously. Treatment of itching and swelling is sufficient by applying ice and taking antihistamines. However, some spider bites are more venomous and may require further treatments.

Most spiders in the United States are not able to bite humans due to small mouth parts. There are two spiders that are able to bite and envenomate humans, the black widow (*Lactrodectus spp.*) and the brown recluse (*Loxoscelidae reclusus*) spiders, which will be examined in more detail. There are other spiders which may bite humans, but these are even rarer than these examined in this section.

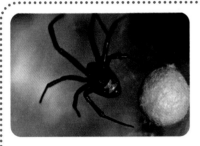

A 35-year-old man is re-stacking an old pile of wood that had fallen over during winter. After picking up a piece of firewood, he feels an acute pain on the dorsum of his right hand. He sees a black shiny spider on the ground nearby that had obviously fallen from the piece of wood (Fig. 8-4). His hand is swelling and two punctae are seen. What should he do next?

KEY FEATURES

- The black widow spider is found in all U.S. states except Alaska.

- It is identified by a red hourglass-shaped marking on abdomen and the shiny black carapace.

- Common places humans encounter this spider is in woodpiles, barns, garages, closets, and within shoes.

- Acute pain and edema noted at site of bite, sometimes bite mark can be seen.

- Symptoms similar to acute abdomen with abdominal muscle spasms, weakness, hypertension.

BLACK WIDOW SPIDER

Background

The black widow spider (*Latrodectus spp.*) is found in every state except Alaska and is especially numerous in the rural Southern United States. These spiders are identified by their large abdomen with a red hour-glass marking on their underside (Fig. 8-4). Adult female spiders can grow to a length of 4 cm and are responsible for venomous bites. Males do not produce venom and are eaten by the female after sexual encounters. Female black widow spiders are especially aggressive when protecting their egg sacs. They are normally found in woodpiles, barns, and garages, but can also be found in closets, cupboards, and within shoes.

Pathogenesis

Black widow spider venom contains alpha-latrotoxin that acts by binding to muscular motor endplates of both sympathetic and parasympathetic nerves. Its action is one of depolarization, which leads to unregulated exocytosis of neurotransmitters from the nerve terminals. The increased synaptic concentration of catecholamines leads to muscle cramping and spasm.

Clinical Presentation

Bites may produce immediate sharp pain, followed by light swelling and appearance of small, red fang marks. Within 15 minutes to 2 hours, dull muscle

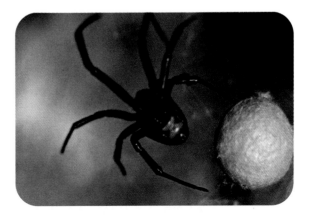

Figure 8-4 A black widow spider. Courtesy of CDC.

CHAPTER 8 Derm Reactions to Arthropods

WHEN TO REFER

- Patients with rigid abdomen and severe pain should be evaluated in the nearest Emergency Department.
- Refer to the appropriate local Emergency Department for antivenin administration.

cramping or severe pain with numbness spreads from the bite to involve the entire torso. The most common complaints are generalized abdominal, back, and leg pain that progress to severe abdominal pain and spasm similar to acute surgical abdomen. Spasm of the abdominal wall leading to boardlike rigidity of the musculature is a sign of latrodectism.

Hyperactive deep tendon reflexes may be seen. Associated symptoms include headache, sweating, nausea, vomiting, and dizziness. Reactions to the bite generally increase in severity up to 24 hours and then subside in the next 2 to 3 days. Weakness, tingling, and transient muscle spasm may persist for months after recovery from acute latrodectism. Recovery from serious reaction usually offers systemic immunity to subsequent bites.

Diagnosis

Differential diagnosis. Acute surgical abdomen, bites from insects or other arthropods.

Diagnostic methods. The appearance of small, red fang marks and clinical history are suggestive. Biopsies may be performed at the site of inoculation for spider mouth parts.

Therapy

Immediate care: ice should be applied to the bite site to restrict spread of venom. The area should be elevated.

Within 90 hours, black widow spider-specific antivenin alone or in combination with IV opioids, benzodiazepines, aspirin, or muscle relaxants (calcium gluconate, 10%, 10 mL IV) can relieve pain and muscle spasms.

Course and Complications

Most cases recover with conservative therapy as outlined above. Convulsions, paralysis, shock, and death occur in 5% of cases, usually in children or the elderly.

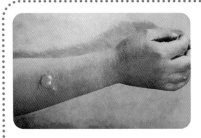

A 45-year-old man is removing old flattened moving boxes from his basement. He will soon be moving from North Carolina. As he is moving a pile of boxes, a large brown spider falls from the boxes onto his bare arm and bites. The bite site is shown 24 hours later (Fig. 8-5). What is the most likely spider? What consequences of this bite are worrisome?

BROWN RECLUSE SPIDER

Background

The brown recluse (*Loxoscelidae reclusus*) spider grows to 1.5 cm in length and has a characteristic dark violin-shaped marking on its back. It is found most commonly in the southern half of the United States. These spiders avoid light and are most commonly found under radiators, in woodpiles, and in barns and basements.

Pathogenesis

Sphingomyelinase D and hyaluronidase present in the spider venom allows for the digestion of skin and deeper tissues, leading to eschar formation. Large-vessel vasculitis and neutrophilic infiltration of the lesion may lead to extensive necrosis seen in severe cases.

Clinical Presentation

Bites are generally located on the extremities and cause mild localized swelling, erythema, and sharp pain. Bites in more fatty areas of the body, such

KEY FEATURES

- The brown recluse spider is prevalent in southern half of the United States. It is recognized by dark "fiddle-shaped" area on its back.

- It generally lives in dark places such as in woodpiles, closets, basements.

- Reactions to bite are generally mild, but can lead to dermonecrosis, eschar formation, and disseminated intravascular coagulation (DIC).

as the buttocks and thighs, can lead to more serious reactions. If the bite is in the neck, airway patency may be compromised. A severe reaction can lead to dermonecrosis within 4 hours (Fig. 8-5). The necrotic changes that can take place due to loxoscelism begin with a rapidly expanding bluish macular ring around the site of the bite. The center of the ring eventually sinks below the normal skin surface and sloughs off dead tissue, leading to a dry, necrotic eschar or ulceration. The lesion may take months to heal and lead to significant scarring.

Diagnosis

In an ideal situation, the spider that envenomated the patient is caught and saved for identification. In general, these spiders are not subtle and will be noticed at the time of biting, though it is rare that the spider is caught. Some patients will present with the chief complaint of "spider bite." In general, unless a spider was seen, other diagnoses in addition to a bite reaction should be entertained.

Differential diagnosis
- Cutaneous bacterial and viral infections
- Arterial insufficiency ulceration
- Venous ulcerations
- Pyoderma gangrenosum
- Cutaneous and systemic vasculitis

Diagnostic Methods

- Enzyme immunoassay to detect spider venom in a skin biopsy or plucked hair (up to 4 days after bite)
- Passive hemagglutination inhibition test (up to 3 days after bite)

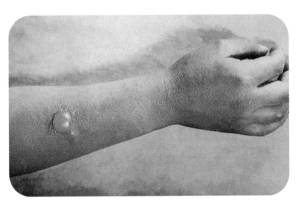

Figure 8-5 Bullous reaction 24 hours following a Chilean brown recluse spider bite. Courtesy of CDC/Harold G. Scott.

Therapy

Most bites can be treated with ice and local elevation. Moderate to severe skin necrosis requires antibiotics as prophylaxis for the ulcerations and analgesics for pain. Antivenin and dapsone are given in moderate to severe cases, though use of dapsone has not been clearly shown to decrease the size of necrosis or shorten time to healing. A glucose-6-phosphodiesterase level should be checked to assess for deficiency when prescribing dapsone. Severe systemic reactions to the bite may be treated additionally with prednisone and aspirin and a serial complete blood count (CBC) should be obtained. Surgical excision of necrotic areas is not recommended.

Complications

Rarely, a severe systemic reaction will occur. Usually seen in children, within 12 to 24 hours of a bite, the victims will have fever, chills, nausea, vomiting, arthralgias, and hives. Thrombocytopenia or hemolytic anemia leading to DIC, renal failure, or even death may occur.

WHEN TO REFER

Refer to Emergency Department if signs of systemic reaction are observed. Skin ulcerations may be managed by a skilled wound care expert such as a dermatologist or, if available, a wound care nurse.

NOT TO BE MISSED

- Administration of antivenin must be done in a timely manner if desired (within 90 hours).

ICD9 Codes	
910.4	*Insect bite, nonvenomous of face, neck, and scalp except eye, without mention of infection*
910.5	*Insect bite, nonvenomous of face, neck, and scalp except eye, infected*

911.4	Insect bite, nonvenomous of trunk, without mention of infection
911.5	Insect bite, nonvenomous of trunk, infected
912.4	Insect bite, nonvenomous of shoulder and upper arm, without mention of infection
912.5	Insect bite, nonvenomous of shoulder and upper arm, infected
913.4	Insect bite, nonvenomous of elbow, forearm, and wrist, without mention of infection
913.5	Insect bite, nonvenomous, of elbow, forearm, and wrist, infected
914.4	Insect bite, nonvenomous, of hand(s) except finger(s) alone, without mention of infection
914.5	Insect bite, nonvenomous, of hand(s) except finger(s) alone, infected
915.4	Insect bite, nonvenomous, of fingers, without mention of infection
915.5	Insect bite, nonvenomous of fingers, infected
916.4	Insect bite, nonvenomous, of hip, thigh, leg, and ankle, without mention of infection
916.5	Insect bite, nonvenomous of hip, thigh, leg, and ankle, infected
917.4	Insect bite, nonvenomous, of foot and toe(s), without mention of infection
917.5	Insect bite, nonvenomous, of foot and toe(s), infected
918.0	Superficial injury of eyelids and periocular area
919.4	Insect bite, nonvenomous, of other, multiple, and unspecified sites, without mention of infection
919.5	Insect bite, nonvenomous, of other, multiple, and unspecified sites, infected
989.5	Toxic effect of venom
707.00	Pressure ulcer, unspecified site
707.01	Pressure ulcer, elbow
707.02	Pressure ulcer, upper back
707.03	Pressure ulcer, lower back
707.04	Pressure ulcer, hip
707.05	Pressure ulcer, buttock
707.06	Pressure ulcer, ankle
707.07	Pressure ulcer, heel
707.09	Pressure ulcer, other site
707.10	Unspecified ulcer of lower limb
707.11	Ulcer of thigh
707.12	Ulcer of calf
707.13	Ulcer of ankle
707.14	Ulcer of heel and midfoot
707.15	Ulcer of other part of foot
707.19	Ulcer of other part of lower limb
707.20	Pressure ulcer, unspecified stage
707.21	Pressure ulcer stage I
707.22	Pressure ulcer stage II
707.23	Pressure ulcer stage III
707.24	Pressure ulcer stage IV
707.25	Pressure ulcer, unstageable
707.8	Chronic ulcer of other specified sites
707.9	Chronic ulcer of unspecified site

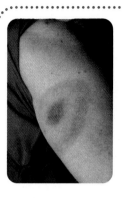

A 40-year-old man from Connecticut presents with muscle pain, joint pain, and a slight fever in late August, 2 weeks after a hiking trip. The patient does not recall having been stung or bitten by any bugs during the hike and had consistently applied bug repellent on his arms and legs. Physical exam was normal except for an area of expanding rash with a central clearing on the patient's central abdomen (Fig. 8-6). What is the most likely diagnosis? What should the treatment be?

KEY FEATURES

- Ticks are blood-sucking ectoparasites that attach onto their human hosts tightly from a few hours to 10 days.

- May be characterized as a "new mole" by patients or may be hidden in patient's hair.

- Tick bites elicit pruritus and rash after the tick is done feeding or is removed.

- Important vectors for disease transmission.

(Continued)

Ticks

BACKGROUND

Ticks are blood-sucking ectoparasites that serve as vectors for numerous bacterial, viral, and parasitic infections. There are two primary categories of ticks: hard-bodied and soft-bodied. Hard-bodied ticks are most frequently the vector for serious illnesses and are difficult to remove compared to soft-bodied ticks. Ticks attach to their hosts by waiting at the tips of grass or bushes and latching onto prey that happen to brush by. Hard ticks can attach to their hosts for up to 10 days. Diverse tick species are differentially distributed around the United States and affect the regional concentration of vector-borne illnesses. These species are outlined in Table 8-3. Identification of the specific species of tick in a patient who has been bitten is important for diagnosis of these illnesses.

CLINICAL PRESENTATION

Oftentimes, patients will present to the physician with the tick still attached to their bodies, mistaking the tick for a "new mole" (Fig. 8-7). The most common areas for tick attachment include the head, neck, and upper trunk. Hypersensitivity reactions to tick bites often develop after the tick is done feeding or is removed. Development of erythematous plaques; pruritus; or papular, nodular, or vesiculobullous reactions at the site of tick bites are common. Erythema migrans (Fig. 8-6), a skin manifestation of cutaneous infection with *Borrelia*, may occur soon after a tick bite. It presents initially as an erythematous macule or papule at the site of tick attachment. Erythema enlarges a few centimeters per day over many days, often with

CHAPTER 8 Derm Reactions to Arthropods

Table 8-3 Major Tick-borne Illnesses in the United States

DISEASE	TICK VECTOR	AGENT	REGION	CLASSIC SIGNS/ SYMPTOMS
Lyme disease	*Ixodes*	*Borrelia burgdorferi*	Northeast, Great Lakes	Erythema chronicum migrans, arthralgia, myalgia
Babesiosis	*Ixodes*	*Babesia microti*	Northeast	Mild fever, anemia
Ehrlichiosis	*Ixodes, Amblyomma*	*Ehrlichia chaffeensis*	South, Southeast	Fever, headache, myalgias
Rocky Mountain spotted fever	*Dermacentor*	*Rickettsia rickettsii*	South Atlantic, Pacific, Southwest	Fever, headache, myalgias, rash spreading from distal to proximal
Colorado tick fever	*Dermacentor*	*Coltivirus*	West	Fever, chills, headaches, pain behind eyes, rash
Tularemia	*Dermacentor, Amblyomma*	*Francisella tularensis*	Arkansas, Missouri, Oklahoma	Fever, headache, fatigue, lymphadenopathy
Tick paralysis	*Dermacentor, Amblyomma*	Toxin	Northwest, South	Ascending paralysis

KEY FEATURES (Continued)

- Treatment of reaction to tick bite must be accompanied by assessment of associated symptoms and possible serological tests.

- Suspicion of Rocky Mountain spotted fever or Lyme disease should lead to prescription of prophylactic antibiotics.

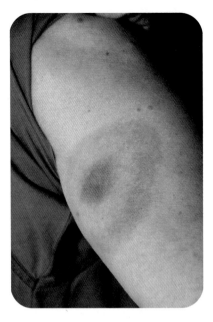

Figure 8-6 Erythema chronicum migrans on the outer upper arm. Courtesy of James Gathany/CDC.

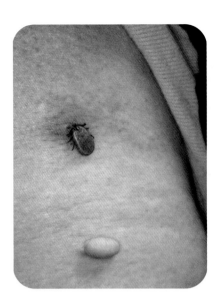

Figure 8-7 An engorged tick on the outer thigh. This man presented with the chief complaint of "new black spot."

central clearing thus giving a target-shaped appearance. Lesions are rarely persistent for more than a few months. A Borrelial lymphocytoma (a B-cell pseudolymphoma) may present in a current or prior area of erythema migrans. Acrodermatitis chronica atrophicans is a longer-duration, progressive cutaneous finding in disseminated *Borrelia* infection (Lyme disease). It begins as symmetric edema and erythema on the distal extensor extremities most commonly. It slowly begins to clear centrally, over years becoming cigarette-paper–like and atrophic. These later findings may be associated with peripheral neuropathy.

It is important to identify the type of tick and to monitor the patient carefully for signs of vector-borne illnesses.

DIAGNOSIS

Tick bites are often misdiagnosed as insect bites. The bite of a tick will sometimes exhibit unusually intense pruritus and pain. A recent history of camping and spending time outdoors should raise suspicion of tick bites. It is crucial to thoroughly examine all areas of the body for possible ticks that are still attached to the patient, including the scalp. Assess for signs and symptoms of vector-borne illnesses and obtain serology. For diseases such as Rocky Mountain spotted fever, immediate empiric treatment is essential to prevent significant morbidity and mortality. Lyme disease can be diagnosed with ELISA titers or enzyme immunoassay tests. False negatives may occur early in the disease course. The Centers for Disease Control (CDC) recommends following up initial positive tests with a confirmatory Western blot test.

THERAPY

- Steroids: mild tick bite reactions respond to topical corticosteroids such as triamcinolone 0.1% bid. However, more severe reactions may require corticosteroid injections into the affected area. Surgical removal of site may be necessary in some cases to relieve nonresolving pain and pruritus.

- Tick removal: if tick is present, it will need to be correctly extracted from the patient's skin. There are inexpensive plastic devices that can be used to correctly remove the tick, but it can also be done with a plastic spoon, credit card, or forceps. During the procedure, be sure not to squeeze the abdomen of the tick or use a twisting motion while pulling out the tick, as this will lead to retention of the tick mouth part in the skin. Make sure to wear gloves and do not touch the tick with bare hands.
  - Use a set of tweezers or forceps and grasp the tick as close to the skin as possible
  - Pull upward with constant pressure and speed
- Antibiotic prophylaxis: in cases where the tick identified has high risk of carrying tick-borne diseases and the tick is heavily engorged, antibiotic prophylaxis (i.e., doxycycline 100 BID × 10 days) is recommended. Rocky Mountain spotted fever must be treated empirically as soon as possible to prevent significant morbidity and mortality.
- Disseminated disease: erythema migrans and disseminated *Borrelia*, when treated early, generally respond to doxycycline 100 mg PO BID × 21 days. Acrodermatitis atrophicans should be treated for 28 days. An alternate therapy for children under 9 is amoxicillin 250 to 500 mg PO TID; not to exceed 3 g/d.
- Tick control: Permethrin-treated clothing and DEET application on the skin are effective ways to prevent future tick bites.

WHEN TO REFER

Refer to Emergency Room if emergent signs of Rocky Mountain spotted fever are present.

NOT TO BE MISSED

- Treat cases of suspected Rocky Mountain spotted fever empirically with doxycycline.
- Antibiotic prophylaxis following a tick bite.

"AT A GLANCE" THERAPY

- Steroids: mild tick bite reactions respond to topical corticosteroids such as triamcinolone 0.1% BID topically or intralesionally.
- Tick removal: if tick is present, it will need to be correctly extracted from the patient's skin.
- Antibiotic prophylaxis: doxycycline 100 BID × 10 days is recommended.
- Disseminated disease: erythema migrans and disseminated *Borrelia*, when treated early, generally respond to doxycycline 100 mg PO BID × 21 days. Acrodermatitis atrophicans should be treated for 28 days. An alternate therapy for children under 9 is amoxicillin 250 to 500 mg PO TID; not to exceed 3 g/d.

ICD9 Codes	
088.81	*Lyme disease*
529.1	*Geographic tongue*

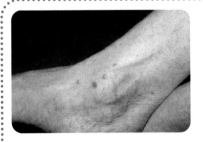

A 51-year-old man presents with multiple pruritic erythematous papules on his lower legs (Fig. 8-8). The family has recently acquired a cat, which is allowed to be both inside the house as well as outside. The house has wall-to-wall carpets. What is the most likely cause of this insect bite?

Fleas

BACKGROUND

Fleas are ubiquitous pests with laterally flattened bodies and large hind legs, which they use to jump as high as 18 cm from host to host. *Pulex irritans* is the human flea, but since most fleas show little host specificity, any mammalian flea can generally bite humans as well. Unfortunately, fleas are also important vectors of disease and are responsible for the transmission of clinically significant diseases such as endemic typhus and bubonic plague, especially in the southwestern United States.

KEY FEATURES

- Fleas are ubiquitous pests with a laterally flattened body and large hind legs used to jump from host to host.

- Fleas show little host specificity (any type of flea may bite humans).

- Bites are intensely pruritic and usually occur on lower limbs.

- Treatment of fleas require thorough evaluation of source of infestation.

- Fleas are vectors for endemic typhus and bubonic plague in the American Southwest.

PATHOGENESIS

The distinct papules and pruritus are caused by a type IV delayed type hypersensitivity reaction to the flea saliva injected into the skin while feeding.

CLINICAL PRESENTATION

Flea bites are intensely pruritic. Papulovesicular or purpuric lesions usually appear on the lower legs, to which fleas have easier access, but may also occur on any part of the body (Fig. 8-8). Allergic reactions are also common in previously sensitized individuals. Look for systemic signs of microbial infection that may accompany flea infestations because fleas are common carriers for bacteria responsible for endemic typhus and bubonic plague.

DIAGNOSIS

Patients will present with intensely pruritic papulovesicular or purpuric lesions, usually on the lower extremities. Diagnosis is most often clinical. Biopsy is rarely indicated. Patients may also have pets that are likely infested with fleas.

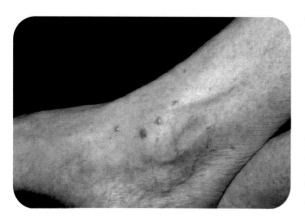

Figure 8-8 Flea bites on the ankles. From Goodheart HP. *Goodheart's Photoguide to Common Skin Disorders,* 3rd ed. Philadelphia: Lippincott Williams & Wilkins, 2009.

THERAPY

Eradicating fleas is a difficult task and may require professional extermination services. Fleas may survive on mice, rats, house pets, and even carpets. Therefore, extermination of fleas requires elimination of rodents and a thorough evaluation of the potential source of fleas. House pets should be taken to veterinarians if flea infestation is suspected. Lufenuron can be used as an oral formulation for cats and dogs to prevent fleas from reproducing. Fipronil is a topical agent to prevent flea infestations on pets. Flea bites are self-limited and do not require any therapy. Symptomatic relief from pruritus may be obtained by topical corticosteroids or intralesional injections (triamcinolone 3 mg/cc ~0.3 cc per lesion) for severely pruritic lesions.

COURSE AND COMPLICATIONS

Fleas are vectors for disease in the American Southwest. The most common diseases transmitted by fleas are endemic typhus and bubonic plague. The features of these infections are outlined in Table 8-4. Serology should be obtained if signs and symptoms indicate transmission of infection.

Table 8-4 Common Flea-borne Diseases in the United States

DISEASE	RESERVOIRS	ORGANISM	SIGNS/SYMPTOMS	GEOGRAPHY	TREATMENT
Endemic typhus	Rats	*Rickettsia typhi*	Fever, headache, rash	Southwestern United States	Doxycycline
Bubonic plague	City rats, squirrels, prairie dogs	*Yersinia pestis*	Hot, tender, red lymphadenopathy; high fever, conjunctivitis	Southwestern United States	Streptomycin, gentamicin, doxycycline

WHEN TO REFER

In general, flea bites do not need referral. For patients in whom the lesions are questionable, referral to a dermatologist may be useful.

NOT TO BE MISSED

- Flea-borne infections such as endemic typhus and bubonic plague.
- The fleas and flea eggs must be eradicated from the patient's environment if resolution is desired.

ICD9 Codes

910.4	Insect bite, nonvenomous of face, neck, and scalp except eye, without mention of infection
910.5	Insect bite, nonvenomous of face, neck, and scalp except eye, infected
911.4	Insect bite, nonvenomous of trunk, without mention of infection
911.5	Insect bite, nonvenomous of trunk, infected
912.4	Insect bite, nonvenomous of shoulder and upper arm, without mention of infection
912.5	Insect bite, nonvenomous of shoulder and upper arm, infected
913.4	Insect bite, nonvenomous of elbow, forearm, and wrist, without mention of infection
913.5	Insect bite, nonvenomous, of elbow, forearm, and wrist, infected
914.4	Insect bite, nonvenomous, of hand(s) except finger(s) alone, without mention of infection
914.5	Insect bite, nonvenomous, of hand(s) except finger(s) alone, infected
915.4	Insect bite, nonvenomous, of fingers, without mention of infection
915.5	Insect bite, nonvenomous of fingers, infected
916.4	Insect bite, nonvenomous, of hip, thigh, leg, and ankle, without mention of infection
916.5	Insect bite, nonvenomous of hip, thigh, leg, and ankle, infected
917.4	Insect bite, nonvenomous, of foot and toe(s), without mention of infection
917.5	Insect bite, nonvenomous, of foot and toe(s), infected
918.0	Superficial injury of eyelids and periocular area
919.4	Insect bite, nonvenomous, of other, multiple, and unspecified sites, without mention of infection
919.5	Insect bite, nonvenomous, of other, multiple, and unspecified sites, infected

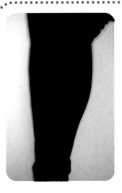

A 34-year-old immigrant presents with multiple pruritic nodules, primarily on his lower legs (Fig. 8-9). He has a few similar lesions on his arms and trunk. Another dermatologist gave him the diagnosis of lichen planus. He continues to get new lesions and is concerned. A skin biopsy is consistent with a hypersensitivity reaction, not a lichenoid dermatitis. He is treated with topical clobetasol and counselled about bedbugs. On follow-up, he has no new lesions and the old lesions are resolving. He relates that he moved to a new apartment and got a new mattress, as he found bedbugs in the old bedding. He has complete resolution.

Bedbugs

BACKGROUND

Bedbugs are blood-sucking ectoparasitic insects that belong to various genera, including *Cimex*, *Leptocimex*, *Oeciacus*, and *Hematasiphon*. They have flat oval bodies and can grow up to 8 mm long. During the day, bedbugs hide in cracks and dark places, but at night, they come out to feed on birds and mammals.

CLINICAL PRESENTATION

Bedbug bites manifest as linear bites, often in groups of three (Figs. 8-9, 8-10). The bites themselves can lead to a range of reactions, from small purpuric macules to generalized allergic reactions. Bedbugs are generally not vectors for diseases, but may have a role in the transmission of hepatitis B.

KEY FEATURES

- Nocturnal blood-sucking insects.

- Hide in cracks and crevices during the day and come out to feed on mammals or birds at night.

- Bites in linear pattern, often in groups of three.

- Insecticides, insect repellants, and elimination of cracks and crevices can help eradicate bedbugs.

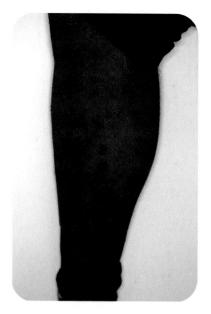

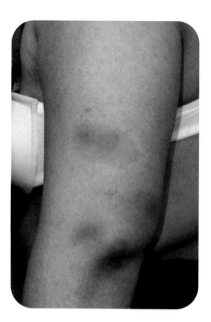

Figure 8-9 Chronic prurigo nodularis, hyperpigmentation, and active new bedbug bites on the lower leg.

Figure 8-10 Multiple acute bedbug bites on the arm.

DIAGNOSIS

Linear purpuric macules, oftentimes in groups of three, may be visualized.

THERAPY

Insecticides such as dichlorvos can be used to eradicate bedbugs. Elimination of cracks and crevices in the walls of the patient's living quarters and roosting areas for bats or birds can help to destroy areas where bedbugs normally dwell in the daytime. Although insect repellants have some efficacy, it has been noticed that bedbugs will often take smaller bites on an individual, but will draw blood from many more individuals, increasing the likelihood of disease transmission. These bites are self-limited and do not require any therapy. Symptomatic relief from pruritus may be obtained by topical corticosteroids or intralesional injections (triamcinolone 3 mg/cc ~0.3 cc per lesion) for severely pruritic lesions.

COURSE AND COMPLICATIONS

Fecal matter from bedbugs may contribute to asthmatic reactions. Once the environmental infestation is resolved, new lesions will cease to appear.

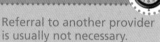

WHEN TO REFER

Referral to another provider is usually not necessary.

NOT TO BE MISSED

- Recommend professional exterminator services for home consultation in all cases of suspected bedbugs.

ICD9 Codes	
910.4	Insect bite, nonvenomous of face, neck, and scalp except eye, without mention of infection
910.5	Insect bite, nonvenomous of face, neck, and scalp except eye, infected
911.4	Insect bite, nonvenomous of trunk, without mention of infection
911.5	Insect bite, nonvenomous of trunk, infected
912.4	Insect bite, nonvenomous of shoulder and upper arm, without mention of infection
912.5	Insect bite, nonvenomous of shoulder and upper arm, infected
913.4	Insect bite, nonvenomous of elbow, forearm, and wrist, without mention of infection

913.5	*Insect bite, nonvenomous, of elbow, forearm, and wrist, infected*
914.4	*Insect bite, nonvenomous, of hand(s) except finger(s) alone, without mention of infection*
914.5	*Insect bite, nonvenomous, of hand(s) except finger(s) alone, infected*
915.4	*Insect bite, nonvenomous, of fingers, without mention of infection*
915.5	*Insect bite, nonvenomous of fingers, infected*
916.4	*Insect bite, nonvenomous, of hip, thigh, leg, and ankle, without mention of infection*
916.5	*Insect bite, nonvenomous of hip, thigh, leg, and ankle, infected*
917.4	*Insect bite, nonvenomous, of foot and toe(s), without mention of infection*
917.5	*Insect bite, nonvenomous, of foot and toe(s), infected*
918.0	*Superficial injury of eyelids and periocular area*
919.4	*Insect bite, nonvenomous, of other, multiple, and unspecified sites, without mention of infection*
919.5	*Insect bite, nonvenomous, of other, multiple, and unspecified sites, infected*
989.5	*Toxic effect of venom*

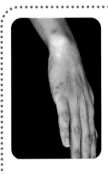

A 32-year-old woman presents to the clinic with new itchy bumps on her right outer hand and lower arm (Fig. 8-11). She had recently moved from Boston to New Hampshire and a friend took her mushroom hunting for the first time. She thinks these might be mosquito bites, but is not sure. What is your diagnosis?

KEY FEATURES

- Mosquitoes are blood-sucking insects present in temperate and tropical climates.

- They are significant disease vector around the world.

- Bites are generally round, pruritic erythematous papules.

- Prevention of bites requires applying insect repellant on skin (DEET) and clothing (Permethrin) as well as using netting around bedding at night.

- Systemic signs following mosquito bites should increase suspicion of encephalitic viruses.

Mosquitoes

BACKGROUND

Mosquitoes are disease vectors in tropical and temperate zones across the world. The most common genus of mosquito to be found in the continental United States belongs to the genus *Aedes*. Mosquitoes in the United States can carry some encephalitic viruses and symptoms should be noted. Bites from female *Anopheles* mosquitos are the vector in many parts of the tropical and subtropical world for malarial infection caused by *Plasmodium spp.* (*P. ovale*, *P. vivax*, *P. malaria*, and *P. falciparum*). Malaria is not endemic to the United States, Western Europe, or Russia at this time, but awareness of its symptoms is essential in this age of world travel. Over a million new infections are acquired each year, with hundreds being first seen in the United States following travel.

PATHOGENESIS

The bite of the mosquito itself causes an urticarial and pruritic reaction at the site where the mosquito has inserted its blood tube into the skin. This reaction is an allergic response to irritants and anticoagulants present in the saliva of the mosquito. Arthus-type hypersensitivity reactions can develop. Anaphylaxis is rare.

CLINICAL PRESENTATION

Mosquito bites will manifest as intensely pruritic and erythematous papules (Fig. 8-11). Generally, in children, the reaction to mosquito bites is more pronounced than in adults. Mosquitoes tend to prefer warmer areas on the body of young and strongly scented individuals. Bright colors and areas of higher carbon dioxide concentrations will also attract mosquitoes.

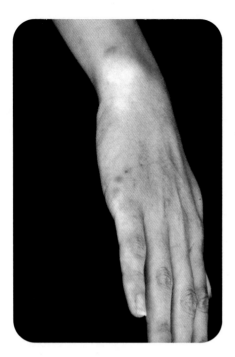

Figure 8-11 Mosquito bites on the lower arm and hand.

DIAGNOSIS

Patients will present with pruritic papular lesions, especially after having been outside. These lesions can occur anywhere on the body, but are most often located in areas of exposed skin on the legs, arms, and neck.

THERAPY

Because mosquitoes are attracted to body odor, the best way to prevent mosquito bites is for the patient to apply insect repellant on the skin before participating in outdoor activities. The most effective insect repellant is DEET and can be co-applied with Permethrin on clothing. The combination can prevent most mosquito bites. Reapplication of repellant is necessary when mosquitoes begin to land on the skin. Thiamine hydrochloride (vitamin B1) can be taken orally during the summer as a way of preventing mosquito bites, although the effectiveness is controversial. Once bitten, an individual can apply hydrocortisone, antihistamines, or general antipruritic medications to treat the symptoms of the bite.

COURSE AND COMPLICATIONS

Mosquito bites fully resolve in 1 to 2 weeks, but it is important that signs and symptoms of vector-borne diseases be assessed. Mosquito-borne encephalitic diseases must be addressed as soon as possible since the mortality rate is extremely high. This group of diseases manifest as headache, fever, lethargy, lymphadenopathy, and stupor and require immediate supportive care. The viruses responsible in the United States include West Nile virus, St. Louis encephalitis virus, California encephalitis virus, and equine encephalitis viruses.

WHEN TO REFER

Any patient with nonhealing lesions should be evaluated by a dermatologist. If recurrent fevers occur in an individual with recent travel to malarial areas, evaluation for malaria should be considered. Those with signs of encephalitic disease should be carefully evaluated.

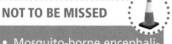

NOT TO BE MISSED

- Mosquito-borne encephalitis diseases such as West Nile virus.

ICD9 Codes	
910.4	Insect bite, nonvenomous of face, neck, and scalp except eye, without mention of infection
910.5	Insect bite, nonvenomous of face, neck, and scalp except eye, infected
911.4	Insect bite, nonvenomous of trunk, without mention of infection
911.5	Insect bite, nonvenomous of trunk, infected
912.4	Insect bite, nonvenomous of shoulder and upper arm, without mention of infection
912.5	Insect bite, nonvenomous of shoulder and upper arm, infected
913.4	Insect bite, nonvenomous of elbow, forearm, and wrist, without mention of infection
913.5	Insect bite, nonvenomous, of elbow, forearm, and wrist, infected
914.4	Insect bite, nonvenomous, of hand(s) except finger(s) alone, without mention of infection
914.5	Insect bite, nonvenomous, of hand(s) except finger(s) alone, infected
915.4	Insect bite, nonvenomous, of fingers, without mention of infection
915.5	Insect bite, nonvenomous of fingers, infected
916.4	Insect bite, nonvenomous, of hip, thigh, leg, and ankle, without mention of infection

916.5	Insect bite, nonvenomous of hip, thigh, leg, and ankle, infected
917.4	Insect bite, nonvenomous, of foot and toe(s), without mention of infection
917.5	Insect bite, nonvenomous, of foot and toe(s), infected
918.0	Superficial injury of eyelids and periocular area
919.4	Insect bite, nonvenomous, of other, multiple, and unspecified sites, without mention of infection
919.5	Insect bite, nonvenomous, of other, multiple, and unspecified sites, infected
989.5	Toxic effect of venom

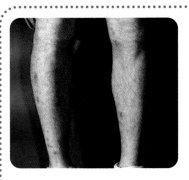

A 45-year-old man from Alabama is brought to the clinic in moderate distress by his spouse after he began to experience burning pain on his right leg followed by trouble breathing. He had knelt down to take a photograph while in the nearby woods when he noticed ants on his lower legs. The bites were painful and burning. Upon examination, multiple red tender papules were noted on the right leg above the ankle (Fig. 8-12) and wheezing was heard upon auscultation of the lungs. What is the most likely diagnosis? What is the cause of the breathing difficulty?

Fire Ants

BACKGROUND

Fire ants, originally from South America, are now endemic in Arizona, California, and New Mexico in the southwestern United States. They are small insects that can range from yellow and red to black and have a set of large pincers on their head and a stinger at the tip of their abdomen. Fire ants thrive in sandy environments, where they like to build their mounds. Their preferred environment often overlaps with areas where people reside, leading to a high incidence of stings. It is estimated that 30% to 60% of people who live in areas endemic for fire ants are stung each year. Particularly vulnerable are children, who get bitten when playing in sand boxes and playgrounds.

CHAPTER 8 Derm Reactions to Arthropods

PATHOGENESIS

The sting of a fire ant is painful, but transient. The venom is made primarily of piperidine alkaloids. The protein induces an IgE response in the victim and leads to the formation of a pustule or in severe cases anaphylaxis. When provoked, fire ants attack en masse, and each ant is capable of holding onto the victim with its jaws and inflicting up to 20 stings in a circular pattern.

KEY FEATURES

- Fire ants are small insects with a large jaw and a stinger on the tail that are endemic in southwestern United States.

- They often attack in groups when provoked.

- Often, these ants build mounds in sandy areas, including playgrounds.

- Bite manifestations range from clustered pustules on the skin to anaphylaxis.

- Pustules and local reactions to bites can be treated by application of ice, oral antihistamines, and/or topical steroids.

CLINICAL PRESENTATION

Fire ant stings are initially extremely painful, but the pain subsides in a matter of minutes. Urticaria follows and resolves within an hour. Eight to 24 hours later, umbilicated pustules form at the site of the stings (Figs. 8-12, 8-13), usually in a circular pattern. In the middle of the pustules may be two red dots where the jaw of the fire ant attached. Some patients have a late-phase reaction where an erythematous indurated pruritic plaque forms around the sting area a few days after the sting. Some individuals will manifest severe anaphylaxis.

DIAGNOSIS

Depending on the amount of time since the sting, one could expect to see multiple pustules in clusters, often on the legs of children. In a patient presenting

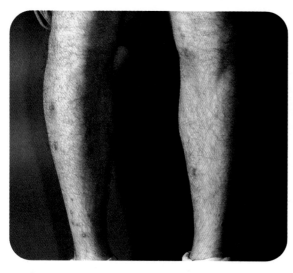

Figure 8-12 Fire ant bites on the legs of an adult man. Courtesy of CDC/ Dr. Harold G. Scott.

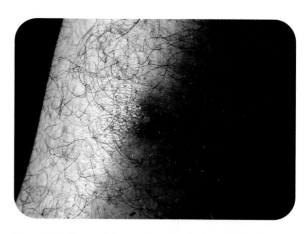

Figure 8-13 The pustular reaction after the fire ant bite. Courtesy of CDC/ Dr. Harold G. Scott.

with signs of anaphylaxis in an area endemic for fire ants, check between his/her toes for indications of bites.

THERAPY

External treatments include hydrocortisone cream and application of ice. Antihistamines can also be taken orally to alleviate some of the swelling and prednisone should be prescribed for more severe local reactions. Some individuals with known severe allergic reaction to fire ant stings can undergo immunotherapy with fire ant whole body extract. Anaphylaxis should be treated immediately with epinephrine.

COURSE AND COMPLICATIONS

Anaphylactic reactions occur in some individuals and are life-threatening. Thirty-two deaths from fire ant stings were reported in a 1-year period in the Southern United States in 1989.

WHEN TO REFER

Any signs of anaphylaxis should be treated emergently.

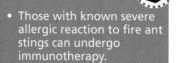

NOT TO BE MISSED

- Those with known severe allergic reaction to fire ant stings can undergo immunotherapy.
- Anaphylaxis should be treated immediately with epinephrine.

ICD9 Codes

910.4	Insect bite, nonvenomous of face, neck, and scalp except eye, without mention of infection
910.5	Insect bite, nonvenomous of face, neck, and scalp except eye, infected
911.4	Insect bite, nonvenomous of trunk, without mention of infection
911.5	Insect bite, nonvenomous of trunk, infected
912.4	Insect bite, nonvenomous of shoulder and upper arm, without mention of infection
912.5	Insect bite, nonvenomous of shoulder and upper arm, infected
913.4	Insect bite, nonvenomous of elbow, forearm, and wrist, without mention of infection
913.5	Insect bite, nonvenomous, of elbow, forearm, and wrist, infected
914.4	Insect bite, nonvenomous, of hand(s) except finger(s) alone, without mention of infection
914.5	Insect bite, nonvenomous, of hand(s) except finger(s) alone, infected

915.4	Insect bite, nonvenomous, of fingers, without mention of infection
915.5	Insect bite, nonvenomous of fingers, infected
916.4	Insect bite, nonvenomous, of hip, thigh, leg, and ankle, without mention of infection
916.5	Insect bite, nonvenomous of hip, thigh, leg, and ankle, infected
917.4	Insect bite, nonvenomous, of foot and toe(s), without mention of infection
917.5	Insect bite, nonvenomous, of foot and toe(s), infected
918.0	Superficial injury of eyelids and periocular area
919.4	Insect bite, nonvenomous, of other, multiple, and unspecified sites, without mention of infection
919.5	Insect bite, nonvenomous, of other, multiple, and unspecified sites, infected
989.5	Toxic effect of venom

STINGS AND REACTIONS
Bees, Wasps, and Hornets
BACKGROUND

Bees, wasps, and hornets belong to the *Hymenoptera* order of insects that sting when threatened. Although the method and pattern of stings may vary between members of this group, reactions to the stings are generally similar. Honeybees, for example, die after inflicting a sting because their hooked stingers are left in the victim. Wasps and hornets do not shed their stingers during the attack and are able to sting repeatedly. However, reactions to the stings are similar, ranging from mild toxic reactions to life-threatening anaphylaxis.

PATHOGENESIS

Reactions are histamine-related type I IgE-mediated immediate reactions. Immediate urticaria, respiratory distress, and anaphylaxis may occur from *Hymenoptera* stings. There are many components in the venom, that cause reactions including mast cell degranulating peptide, mastoparan, phospholipase, histamine, bradykinin, acetylcholine, dopamine, and serotonin.

CLINICAL PRESENTATION

The stinger may still be lodged in the sting site if the culprit is a honeybee and should be removed by a flicking motion of the fingernail. Grabbing the stinger and pulling out may exacerbate the toxicity of the sting by pumping additional venom into the site. Toxic reactions to stings manifest as a sharp pain and limited induration at the site of the sting in most individuals. A burning sensation will be present that will subside after a few hours.

Allergic reactions can be localized or systemic. Localized reactions include an urticarial response to the sting that can expand to greater than 10 cm and last longer than 5 days. Generalized reactions are rare (0.4%), but can be very serious. Although some may develop hives and urticaria all over their bodies, specific causes for concern are signs of shortness of breath, wheezing, nausea, and abdominal cramping.

DIAGNOSIS

Recent stings will manifest as erythematous indurated wheals around the site of the sting. History will be significant for intense, sharp pain during the sting

KEY FEATURES

- Bees, wasps, and hornets sting when provoked.

- Stings result in immediate sharp pain followed by a burning sensation that lasts a few hours.

- Localized reactions can usually be cleared by applying ice or taking oral antihistamines.

- In some individuals, severe systemic allergic reaction may occur and requires the administration of epinephrine and antihistamines.

WHEN TO REFER

Acute referral is not necessary unless the patient has a systemic anaphylactic reaction. Consultation with an allergist may be helpful in cases in which desensitization is desired.

NOT TO BE MISSED

- Treat generalized allergic reactions with antihistamines and epinephrine.

followed by burning and pruritus over the next few hours. A nonallergic reaction to the sting will not have urticaria or systemic systems unless significant numbers of stings are found. In individuals with severe or systemic allergic reaction to the sting, skin tests should be done 3 or more weeks after the sting to determine sensitivity to various species.

THERAPY

Localized toxic reactions can be treated with ice and localized allergic reactions can be treated using antihistamines. Generalized allergic reactions should be immediately treated with epinephrine, followed by administration of antihistamines. Anaphylaxis has a high mortality rate, so it is not advisable to wait until systemic symptoms appear in patients with known allergies before administration of epinephrine. Patients with a history of severe systemic reactions should have epinephrine (Epi-Pen) available to carry with them. Desensitization immunotherapy can also be considered for these individuals to help prevent reactions if stung again.

COURSE AND COMPLICATIONS

Anaphylactic reactions occur in some individuals and are life-threatening. Wasp envenomation and following anaphylaxis is the most common bite-related cause of death in the United States.

ICD9 Codes

989.5   Toxic effect of venom

Suggested Reading

American Academy of Pediatrics. Committee on Infectious Diseases. Prevention of Lyme disease. *Pediatrics.* 2000;105(1 Pt 1):142–147.

Azad AF, Radulovic S, Higgins JA, et al. Flea-borne rickettsioses: ecologic considerations. *Emerg Infect Dis.* 1997;3(3):319–327.

Bilo BM, Rueff F, Mosbech H, et al. Diagnosis of *Hymenoptera* venom allergy. *Allergy.* 2005;60(11):1339–1349.

Bonifazi F, Jutel M, Bilo B, et al. Prevention and treatment of *Hymenoptera* venom allergy: guidelines for clinical practice. *Allergy.* 2005;60(12):1459–1470.

Chosidow O. Clinical practices. Scabies. *N Engl J Med.* 2006;354(16):1718–1727.

Davidovici BB, Pavel D, Cagnano E, et al. Acute generalized exanthematous pustulosis following a spider bite: report of 3 cases. *J Am Acad Dermatol.* 2006;55(3):525–529.

Diaz JH, Leblanc KE. Common spider bites. *Am Fam Physician.* 2007;75(6):869–873.

Fizgerald KT, Flood AA. *Hymenoptera* stings. *Clin Tech Small Anim Pract.* 2006;21(4):194–204.

Fradin MS, Day JF. Comparative efficacy of insect repellents against mosquito bites. *N Engl J Med.* 2002; 347(1):13–18.

Frankowski BL. American Academy of Pediatrics guidelines for the prevention and treatment of head lice infestation. *Am J Manag Care.* 2004;10(9 Suppl):S269–S272.

Heukelbach J, Walton SF, Feldmeier H. Ectoparasitic infestations. *Curr Infect Dis Rep.* 2005;7(5):373–380.

Heukelbach J, Feldmeier H. Scabies. *Lancet.* 2006;367(9524):1767–1774.

Jacobson CC, Abel EA. Parasitic infestations. *J Am Acad Dermatol.* 2007;56(6):1026–1043.

Jones KN, English JC 3rd. Review of common therapeutic options in the United States for the treatment of pediculosis capitis. *Clin Infect Dis.* 2003;36(11):1355–1361.

Karthikeyan K. Treatment of scabies: newer perspectives. *Postgrad Med J.* 2005;81(951):7–11.

Ko CJ, Elston DM. Pediculosis. *J Am Acad Dermatol.* 2004;50(1):1–12; quiz 13–14.

Lebwohl M, Clark L, Levitt J. Therapy for head lice based on life cycle, resistance, and safety considerations. *Pediatrics.* 2007;119(5):965–974.

McGinley-Smith DE, Tsao SS. Dermatoses from ticks. *J Am Acad Dermatol.* 2003;49(3):363–392.

Pasaoglu G, Sin BA, Misirligil Z. Rush hymenoptera venom immunotherapy is efficacious and safe. *J Investig Allergol Clin Immunol.* 2006;16(4):232–238.

Romero A, Potter MF, Potter DA, et al. Insecticide resistance in the bed bug: a factor in the pest's sudden resurgence? *J Med Entomol.* 2007;44(2):175–178.

Russell FE, Gertsch WJ. For those who treat spider or suspected spider bites. *Toxicon.* 1983;21(3):337–339.

Spach DH, Liles C, Campbell GL, et al. Tick-borne diseases in the United States. *N Engl J Med.* 1993;329(13): 936–947.

Vankawala HH, Park R. *Hymenoptera* Stings. Available at: http://emedicine.medscape.com/article/768764-overview. Accessed April 17, 2009.

Zhu YI, Stiller MJ. Arthropods and skin diseases. *Int J Dermatol.* 2002;41(9):533–549.

CHAPTER 9 Fungal Infections

Fátima Akrouh, Sam Rodriguez, and Peter C. Schalock

This chapter reviews the common cutaneous fungal infections likely to be encountered in a primary care setting. Superficial fungal infections primarily invade keratinized tissues, hair, and nails. These are some of the most common skin diseases worldwide and are particularly significant in immunocompromised hosts. Dermatophytes are fungi that digest and live on keratin. Common species include *Trichophyton*, *Epidermophyton*, and *Microsporum* species. Dermatophyte infection is common, with a 10% to 20% lifetime risk of developing a cutaneous fungal infection. Therefore, rapid and accurate diagnosis of such infections reduces morbidity and likelihood of spread. Dermatophytes possess enzymes that enable them to digest keratin, resulting in scaling, erythema, and injury of the involved structures. Tinea infection typically presents as "ringworm," a lesion with central clearing and an elevated erythematous round border. Individuals with allergies and other immune deficiencies typically present with more pronounced and more numerous lesions. Bacterial superinfection and topical steroid use may also affect the presenting lesion and associated findings.

In diagnosing a fungal infection, it is important to note that many fungi are dimorphic and exist as both spores and hyphae. Spores are the reproducing form of yeast and are seldom observed on skin scrapings. The gold standard for diagnosis of fungal infection of the skin is the potassium hydroxide (KOH) preparation, which often demonstrates hyphae, which are branching filamentous forms of fungi (Fig. 9-1).

Cutaneous fungal infections (Tinea) are generally classified by the area of the body they affect. Below, the different locations will be discussed. Tinea can present in multiple locations. When atypical or disseminated infection is observed, this should suggest the possibility of an underlying systemic deficiency or immune problem such as human immunodeficiency virus (HIV) or diabetes mellitus.

General Treatment Principles

When selecting a treatment regimen for superficial fungal infections important factors to consider are efficacy, method of delivery, and cost. Topical treatment is first line for most superficial fungal infections but success rates vary highly on infection type, location, and patient compliance. Delivery methods include sprays, lotions, creams, powders, and gels (Table 9-1). Patients who do not respond to topical treatments or present with severe infections may be treated with oral antifungal agents.

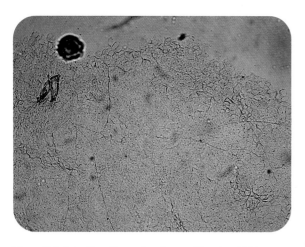

Figure 9-1 Branching filamentous forms of fungi on KOH exam.

While most skin dermatophyte infections are treated topically, tinea unguium (onychomycosis) and tinea capitis are primarily treated with oral agents. Oral antifungals have the ability to target areas where topical treatment is not practical or adequate such as the hair and nails, but carry the risk of greater systemic side effects such as hepatitis and gastrointestinal issues, potential drug interactions, Stevens-Johnson syndrome/toxic epidermal necrolysis, and cytochrome P450 inhibition. The most commonly used oral agents are terbinafine and itraconazole. Treatment regimens are summarized in their specific sections.

Consider obtaining a fungal culture for identification or confirming the presence of a dermatophyte from a nail clipping before starting any systemic medication. There are various methods for obtaining cultures or clippings, which are summarized in Table 9-2. Treating nails that are dystrophic from psoriasis or lichen planus with antifungal is ineffective, and exposes the patient to unnecessary risks from side effects.

Table 9-1 Topical Antifungals

	AVAILABLE FORMS	FREQUENCY OF APPLICATION
Terbinafine (Lamisil)	Cream 1%: 15 g, 30 g Gel 1%: 5 g, 15 g, 30 g	Twice daily
Clotrimazole (Lotrimin)	Cream 1%: 15 g, 30 g, 45 g, 90 g Lotion 1%: 30 mL Solution 1%: 10 mL, 30 mL	Twice daily

Tolnaftate (Tinactin)*	Cream 1%: 15 g, 30 g
	Gel 1%: 15 g
	Powder 1%: 45 g, 90 g
	Topical aerosol:
	   liquid (1%): 59.2 mL, 90 mL,
	     120 mL
	   powder (1%): 56.7 g, 100 g,
	     105 g, 150 g
	Solution 1%: 10 mL
		Twice daily

Miconazole (Monistat-Derm)	Cream 2%: 15 g, 30 g, 56.7 g, 85 g	Twice daily
Ketoconazole (Nizoral)	Cream 2%: 15 g, 30 g, 60 g	Twice daily
Ciclopirox (Loprox)	Cream 1%: 15 g, 30 g, 90 g Lotion 1%: 30 mL, 60 mL Topical suspension 0.77%: 30 mL, 60 mL	Twice daily
Naftifine (Naftin)	Cream 1%: 15 g, 30 g, 60 g Gel 1%: 20 g, 40 g, 60 g	Twice daily
Oxiconazole (Oxistat)	Cream 1%: 15 g, 30 g, 60 g Lotion 1%: 30 mL	Twice daily
Sulconazole (Exelderm)	Cream 1%: 15 g, 30 g, 60 g Solution 1%: 30 mL	Twice daily
Econazole (Spectazole)	Cream 1%: 15 g, 30 g, 85 g	Twice daily
Sertaconazole (Ertaczo)	Cream 2%: 30 g	Twice daily

Table 9-2 How to Collect a Fungal Specimen

SKIN

Clean skin with alcohol, allowing it to dry completely. Scrapings are traditionally taken with a sterile scalpel blade or the edge of a glass slide. When collecting specimens from children, a toothbrush or moist gauze may be used to minimize irritation.

HAIR

Remove several hairs from affected area with tweezers, sending any hairs that fluoresce under Wood's lamp examination. Scrape scalp lesion with scalpel blade or glass slide. If no hair sample is required a cotton swab, toothbrush, or moist gauze may be used.

NAIL

Clean nail with soap and water or alcohol, allowing it to dry completely. Clip the nail as proximally as possible, collecting subungual specimen with 1 to 2 mm serrated curette or scalpel blade. If only small fragments of nail are easily obtainable, send these as-is for fungal culture. If a larger specimen is obtained, this also can be sent for culture or alternately it may be sent for histopathologic examination. Periodic acid-Schiff (PAS) staining under light microscopy will frequently show dermatophyte infection.

PREPARING A SPECIMEN

- Examine hair and skin samples with KOH.
- Nail samples may be KOH-positive but are often challenging to interpret immediately. Ideally, the specimen would be examined 2 to 3 hours after placing in KOH to allow for digestion of the keratin and easier identification of hyphae.
- Consider sending nail clippings for PAS staining.
- Samples for culture should be collected in sterile container and/or placed on culture media.

Adapted from Bolognia JL: Fungal Diseases. *Dermatology.* Mosby:1171–1198, 2003; Trovato MJ, Schwartz RA, Janniger CK: Tinea capitis: current concepts in clinical practice. *Cutis.* 2006;77:93–99(1,5).

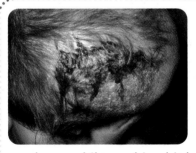

A 2-year-old boy is brought to his primary care doctor by his mother for a flaky plaque with raised borders on his scalp (Fig. 9-2). She first noticed the round, 3-cm area on his left occiput 1 week ago while combing his hair. The hair over the plaque is slightly shorter than the rest of his hair. His mother wants to know if this is "just dandruff." She also noted enlarged lymph nodes on the back of his neck.

KEY FEATURES

- Tinea capitis is the most frequent dermatophyte infection in children under 10 years of age.
- Most commonly caused by dermatophytes from the *Trichophyton* and *Microsporum* genus.

(*Continued*)

Tinea Capitis

BACKGROUND/EPIDEMIOLOGY

Tinea capitis (TC) is a common fungal infection, especially in young, school-aged children. The actual incidence is unknown, but the most commonly infected patient are African American boys under age 10 years. TC is by far the most common dermatophyte infection for children under 10 years of age (92.5%).

PATHOGENESIS

Tinea capitis is most commonly caused by dermatophytes from the *Trichophyton* and *Microsporum* genus. The infections are broken down into ectothrix and endothrix, defined by the location of the arthroconidia of the dermatophyte. Ectothrix infections have external arthroconidia and will fluoresce under Wood's lamp exam with a green-yellow color. Endothrix infections have internal arthroconidia and do not fluoresce. The most common causes of each type of infection are listed in Table 9-3. In the United States, the most prevalent type is commonly referred to as the "black dot" form and is caused by *Trichophyton tonsurans*.

CLINICAL PRESENTATION

This infection typically causes scaling and alopecia in a circumferential pattern on the scalp with a raised border. The alopecia is often incomplete and

KEY FEATURES (*Continued*)

- Scaling and alopecia in a circumferential pattern on the scalp with a raised border.
- Lymphadenopathy of the neck is common.
- Oral antifungal therapy is treatment of choice.

Table 9-3 Causes of Tinea Capitis

ECTOTHRIX	ENDOTHRIX
M. canis	*T. tonsurans*
M. gypseum	*T. violaceum*
T. equinum	
T. verrucosum	

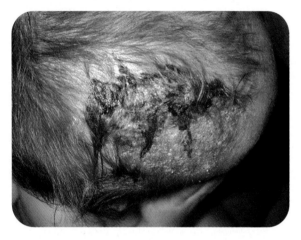

Figure 9-2 Tinea capitis before oral antifungal therapy.

commonly affects the scalp, although it may also be found on eyelashes, eyebrows, facial hair, and pubic hair. Many patients are asymptomatic although some will complain of pruritus. In some cases the infection can cause marked alopecia, lichenification, or a severe inflammatory reaction known as a kerion (Fig. 9-2). Kerions are inflamed, granulomatous nodules that are often extremely painful and may be associated with sinus drainage, scarring, and alopecia. Complications of tinea capitis include secondary infection, often by *Staphylococcus aureus*, or kerion formation. Transmission may occur from person to person or via animals, soil, or fomites.

DIAGNOSIS

Assessment should include careful examination of the scalp, face, and skin. Particular attention should be paid to the eyebrows, eyelashes, and facial hair. Wood's lamp examination has been used to identify some tinea capitis types, though it has limited utility in North America as *T. tonsuran* does not fluoresce. Patients may also present with lymphadenopathy, particularly in the occipital nodes. Other diagnoses to consider when presented with a scaling plaque on the scalp are presented in Table 9-4.

Scrapings of the rash can be prepared using 10% KOH and examined on a glass slide. See Chapter 3 for a detailed description of this technique. When collecting specimens from children for culture or KOH, a toothbrush or moist gauze may be used to minimize irritation. Fungal cultures may also be obtained with either a blade or sterile swab and inoculated onto Sabouraud agar or Mycosel. Fungal colony growth requires approximately 6 weeks (Table 9-1).

TREATMENT

The first-line therapy for tinea capitis is systemic antifungal treatment. Topical therapies are not effective for the treatment of tinea capitis, as they do not penetrate the hair shaft, which may harbor organisms. The most common medication is griseofulvin dosing at 15 to 25 mg/kg daily micronized form and

Table 9-4 Differential Diagnosis for Tinea Capitis

Seborrheic dermatitis	Chronic cutaneous lupus erythematosus
Alopecia areata	Psoriasis
Cellulitis	Traction alopecia
Dissecting folliculitis	Trichotillomania
Impetigo/Bacterial pyoderma	

WHEN TO REFER

Patients should be referred if tinea capitis persists despite 6 to 8 weeks of oral treatment, or if there is significant spread, suspected kerion formation, or secondary bacterial infection despite adequate oral treatment.

NOT TO BE MISSED

- Treat all cases of tinea capitis with oral therapy; topicals are not enough.
- Consider treatment of all family members with an antifungal shampoo.

10 mg/kg in the ultramicronized form for 6 to 8 weeks although treatment may take upward of 3 months. If treatment lasts less than 3 months in a healthy individual, blood counts and liver function tests (LFTs) are usually not indicated. The newer oral antifungal agents are equally effective in treating TC in most studies, but are significantly more expensive.

Some practitioners will concurrently start topical shampoos to reduce contagion, but they should not be used as monotherapy. Special attention should be paid to potential asymptomatic carriers. The infection may spread within those in close contact by fomite spread. Scalp cultures may be obtained to identify possible carriers who are often treated with selenium sulfide shampoo.

"AT A GLANCE" TREATMENT

- Systemic antifungal therapy is necessary for tinea capitis
  - Griseofulvin dosing at 15 to 25 mg/kg daily micronized form or 10 mg/kg in the ultramicronized form for 6 to 8 weeks
  - Also consider antifungal shampoo (ketoconazole 2% or selenium sulfide OTC)

COURSE AND COMPLICATIONS

Systemic treatment usually results in complete resolution, although treatment duration is often variable. The clinical course is highly individual as some patients may simply be asymptomatic carriers while others can have significant spread, inflammation, and permanent scarring alopecia.

ICD9 Codes

110.0	*Dermatophytosis of scalp and beard*

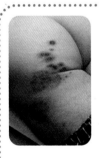

A 16-year-old male athlete comes in with a 10-day history of a scaly, itchy rash on his trunk (Fig. 9-3). He thought it was dry skin, but it did not resolve with topical moisturizers. It has been enlarging in size. He is worried that it might be ringworm, as some other members of his wrestling team are also currently being treated.

KEY FEATURES

- Tinea corporis presents as a scaling plaque on the trunk or extremities.
- It spreads centrifugally with central clearing within 2 to 3 weeks of infection.
- The most common pathogens are *T. rubrum* and *T. tonsurans*.

(Continued)

Tinea Corporis

BACKGROUND/EPIDEMIOLOGY

Tinea corporis is a dermatophyte fungal infection of the skin of the body, primarily the trunk. It begins as a round erythematous scaly patch or plaque, which spreads centrifugally with central clearing. Tinea corporis affects all age groups, though those most commonly affected are adolescents and women of childbearing age. Children are more likely to have infections acquired from animals (zoonotic infection).

PATHOGENESIS

The infection can be caused by any dermatophyte but most pathogens are *T. rubrum* (47%), *T. tonsurans*, and *Microsporum canis* (13%). Transmission can occur from contact with human or animal carriers and from the soil. Autoinoculation may occur secondary to a prior or concurrent infection with tinea capitis or pedis. Risk factors include immunosuppression and exposure to skin-to-skin contact during athletics (e.g., wrestling, locker rooms).

CLINICAL PRESENTATION

Initial clinical presentation typically occurs between 1 and 3 weeks after exposure. The lesion is typically annular with raised borders although shape and

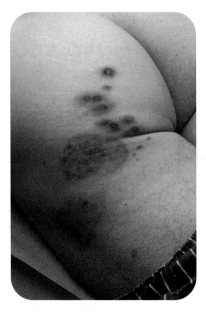

Figure 9-3 Inflammatory tinea corporis on the buttock.

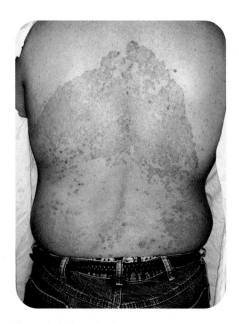

Figure 9-4 Extensive tinea corporis.

size may be highly variable. The lesion is usually scaly but vesicular, granulomatous, and verrucous variants have also been reported (Figs. 9-3, 9-4). The degree of inflammation will vary depending on causative organism and can be excessive in the clinical variant, tinea profunda,which results from an intense inflammatory response to the organism.

Prior treatment with corticosteroids can result in atypical presentations that may lack scaling and exacerbation of the infection when steroids are discontinued. This "tinea incognito" is important to consider in skin lesions that were presumed to be dermatitis but are not responding to therapy and often worsening. In many cases, the lesion(s) may have subtle scale and are copiously KOH positive on exam.

DIAGNOSIS

Clinical exam of the affected site(s) with KOH exam of all scaling plaques as described in Chapter 3 is necessary for any lesions thought to be tinea corporis. Fungal culture may be useful in cases recalcitrant to topical therapy. Rarely is a skin biopsy indicated.

It is important to distinguish tinea corporis from psoriasis. As shown in Figure 9-4, the distribution may be similar to psoriatic plaques. A KOH exam in this situation would easily differentiate between psoriasis and a dermatophyte infection.

TREATMENT

Treatment with a topical antifungal is usually sufficient. A typical starting regimen for an adult would include topical ketoconazole, econazole, or terbinafine applied once daily to the affected area. Treatment duration varies based on severity of infection and typically requires 2 to 3 weeks of therapy. Patients who fail to respond to topical treatment may be candidates for oral therapy agents such as terbinafine, itraconazole, fluconazole, and ketoconazole.

Corticosteroids should, in most cases, be avoided as they may suppress physical signs and worsen the infection. Rarely, cases of inflammatory tinea will respond to both antifungal and corticosteroid therapy. A moderate-potency steroid such as triamcinolone acetonide and a separate antifungal such as econazole nitrate cream is recommended. For inflammatory, pruritic cases, if an anti-inflammatory is necessary, treat with triamcinolone twice daily for 1 week and continue the antifungal for a total of 3 weeks.

"AT A GLANCE" TREATMENT

- First-line therapy: topicals such as clotrimazole, miconazole, ketoconazole, econazole, or terbinafine applied once daily to the affected area
- Patients who fail to respond to topical treatment may be candidates for oral therapy. Terbinafine 250 mg PO QD × 2 weeks often is successful
  - Alternate oral therapy: itraconazole, fluconazole, ketoconazole, or griseofulvin
- Avoid topical corticosteroids other than in cases of inflammatory tinea

COURSE AND COMPLICATIONS

Tinea corporis infections may resolve without therapy. As the infections are bothersome, therapy is often desired. TC responds well to topical therapy.

ICD9 Codes	
110.5	Dermatophytosis of the body
696.1	Other psoriasis and similar disorders

WHEN TO REFER ?

Patients with recurrent or recalcitrant infections despite multiple topical and/or oral treatments as well as preventative measures should be referred for further workup. Special consideration should be given to patients who are immunocompromised, as they may have atypical presentations and may be subject to more complications.

NOT TO BE MISSED

- Differentiate between psoriasis and tinea corporis in extensive cases.
- Avoid usage of topical corticosteroids if possible.

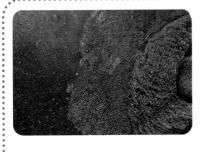

A 67–year-old man with a history of well-controlled type II diabetes comes to your office complaining of 2 weeks of itching "down there" (Fig. 9-5). He says that he noticed a raised, reddish patch on his upper inner thigh extending into the inguinal fold. He has been using baby powder and a "medicated powder" for the itching, but they have not provided relief. The itching is driving him crazy and he wants to know what treatment options are available.

KEY FEATURES

- Tinea cruris is a dermatophyte infection of the inguinal folds and inner thighs/buttocks/abdomen.
- The scrotum/vulva are nearly always spared.
- Treatment is with topical antifungals. Recalcitrant cases may require oral therapy.

Tinea Cruris

BACKGROUND/EPIDEMIOLOGY

Tinea cruris is a common dermatophyte infection of the inguinal folds, but may extend to the inner thighs, buttocks, and abdomen. It is rarely seen in children and is three times more likely to be seen in males.

PATHOGENESIS

Tinea cruris is a dermatophyte infection most often caused by E. floccosum, T. rubrum, and T. mentagrophytes. Risk factors include obesity, abrasive garments, and excessive perspiration.

CLINICAL PRESENTATION

Tinea cruris typically presents as an erythematous, pruritic plaque in the inguinal folds, inner thigh, or between the scrotum/labia majora and inner thigh. Like other dermatophyte infections, the lesion often has a raised border that can have vesicles or pustules in active edges. The scrotum is often spared and scrotal involvement should prompt suspicion of a candidal infection. Several examples of tinea cruris are shown in Figures 9-5 and 9-6. Secondary lesions may result from bacterial superinfections. Chronic cases may progress to include lichen simplex chronicus or prurigo nodules.

DIAGNOSIS

A KOH exam is important for confirming the diagnosis of a dermatophyte infection. The areas of highest yield to scrape organisms from are active border

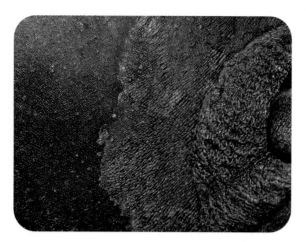

Figure 9-5 Tinea cruris on the thighs of an African male.

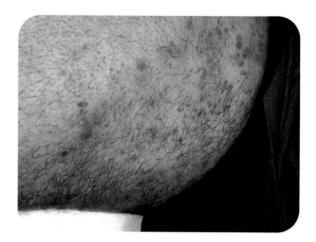

Figure 9-6 Tinea cruris on the thigh of a white male.

regions. Equivocal specimens should be sent for culture. Assessment should include careful examination of the scalp, face, skin, fingernails, and groin. Diagnoses also to be considered include: candidiasis, cellulitis, intertrigo, psoriasis, or contact dermatitis (allergic or irritant) (Table 9-5).

TREATMENT

Similar to tinea corporis, first-line treatment for tinea cruris infections consists of topical antifungals. Patients who are refractory to topical treatment may be candidates for systemic antifungal therapy. As this condition may recur in many patients, prevention is an important part of treatment. Patients should be instructed to wear loose-fitting clothing, wash contaminated clothing, dry completely after bathing, and lose weight. Use of topical drying powders is often helpful. Additionally, patients should be advised to avoid touching the groin area after contact with the feet because tinea cruris is often caused by hyphae carried from fungal-infected feet and/or nails.

"AT A GLANCE" TREATMENT

- Initial therapy is with topical agents. Refractory cases may be treated systemically.
- Patients should be instructed to wear loose-fitting clothing, wash contaminated clothing, dry completely after bathing, and lose weight. Use of topical drying powders is often helpful (Zeasorb AF powder OTC).

ICD9 Codes

110.3   *Dermatophytosis of groin and perianal area*

WHEN TO REFER

Patients with recurrent or recalcitrant infections despite multiple topical and/or oral treatments as well as preventative measures should be referred for further workup. Special consideration should be given to patients who are immunocompromised, as they may have atypical presentations and may be subject to more complications.

NOT TO BE MISSED

- Recommend lifestyle changes, such as thorough drying of the inguinal area.

Table 9-5 Differential Diagnosis for Tinea Cruris

Candidiasis	Psoriasis
Contact dermatitis (irritant or allergic)—often from the topical agents used to treat tinea	Intertrigo
	Lichen simplex chronicus
Miliaria	Impetigo
Lichen simplex chronicus	

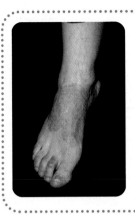

A 30-year-old man comes into your primary care office with a complaint of extreme itchiness and blistering on his plantar feet for 5 days (Fig. 9-7). He is athletic and attends a gym every other day where he swims in the indoor pool. He has had "athlete's foot" for years but this eruption is different. He is worried.

Tinea Pedis

BACKGROUND/EPIDEMIOLOGY

Dermatophyte fungi are present in the environment and acquisition most likely occurs from walking barefoot in moist areas, although there is a high degree of variation in susceptibility despite similar levels of exposure.

PATHOGENESIS

This infection, like many other types, is caused by dermatophytes, most commonly of the *Trichophyton*, *Epidermophyton*, and *Microsporum* genera.

CLINICAL PRESENTATION

Tinea pedis is the most common dermatophyte infection and occurs on the feet and toes. The four major types include interdigital, inflammatory, moccasin, and ulcerative. The differences in these subtypes are summarized in Table 9-6. Typical cases of tinea pedis are shown in Figures 9-7 and 9-8.

There are several variants of tinea pedis. These present differently from the typical "athlete's foot" with scaling, erythema, and itching. Inflammatory tinea pedis presents with multiloculated bullae (Fig. 9-9) in addition to scaling KOH-positive plaques. In some cases, only the bullae are present. To obtain a positive

KEY FEATURES

- Tinea pedis infection is most commonly of the plantar surface and inter-digital spaces.
- Variants include inflammatory, multiloculated bullae, or darkly pigmented tinea nigra.
- Topical antifungal agents are the primary therapy.

CHAPTER 9 Fungal Infections

Table 9-6 Major Types of Tinea Pedis

TYPE	CAUSATIVE ORGANISM	CLINICAL PRESENTATION	TREATMENT
Interdigital	*T. Mentagrophytes* *T. rubrum* *E. floccosum* *S. hyalinum* *S. dimidiatum* *Candida* spp.	Most common subtype Commonly presents within the inter-digital spaces with erythema, scaling, and cracking Subject to secondary bacterial infection	Topical antifungals Antibiotics for secondary bacterial infection
Inflammatory	*T. mentagrophytes*	Presents on medial surface of foot, often with vesicles and bullae	Topical antifungals Antibiotics for secondary bacterial infection
Moccasin	*T. Rubrum* *E. floccosum* *S. hyalinum* *S. dimidiatium*	Presents with erythema, scaling, cracking, and hyperkeratosis on plantar surfaces	Topical antifungals Additional product with urea or lactic acid; often requires oral antifungals
Ulcerative	*T. rubrum* *T. mentagrophytes* *E. floccosum*	Often an exacerbation of interdigital form Seen in diabetics and immuno-compromised	Topical antifungals Often requires oral and/or topical antibiotics for secondary bacterial infection

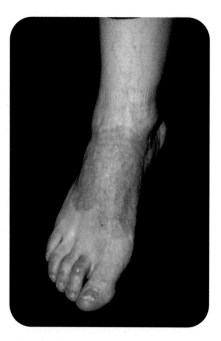

Figure 9-7 Tinea pedis.

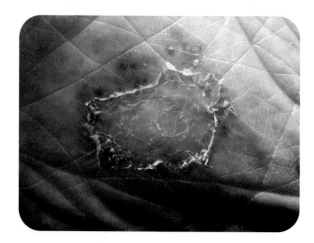

Figure 9-8 Pustular variant of tinea pedis.

KOH, the bullae should be unroofed and the inner surface of the bulla scraped and examined. Alternately, the blister roof may be sent for culture or histopathologic examination.

A rare variant of tinea pedis is dark, irregular scaling plaques on the plantar surface or web spaces. A typical example is shown in Figure 9-10. This condition is known as tinea nigra and is due to an infection by pigment producing *Hortaea werneckii*. It is important to recognize that this condition, though rare, is possible, and consider performing a KOH before performing a biopsy for what usually is a changing, irregular pigmented lesion. A positive KOH will rule out the possibility of an evolving acral lentiginous melanoma.

DIAGNOSIS

Examination should include thorough assessment of feet, toes, and toenails, as well as examination for other concurrent dermatophyte infections of the hands, fingernails, and crural areas. Other diagnoses to consider include contact dermatitis or cellulitis. KOH can be used to differentiate dermatophyte infection from other conditions that may have a similar presentation (Table 9-7).

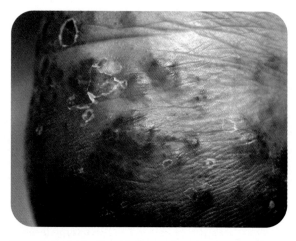

Figure 9-9 Multiloculated bullae in inflammatory tinea pedis.

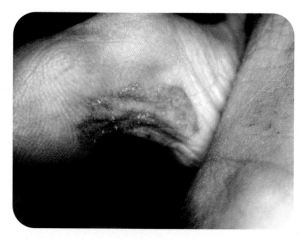

Figure 9-10 Tinea nigra caused by dematiaceous fungi.

Table 9-7 Differential Diagnosis for Tinea Pedis

Contact dermatitis

Psoriasis

Secondary syphilis

Erythrasma

Bacterial infection

Pitted keratolysis

Acral lentiginous melanoma (tinea nigra)

TREATMENT

Infections tend to be chronic and recurrent, thus prevention is an important part of any treatment strategy. Patients should be instructed to wear nonocclusive shoes, absorbent cotton socks, and alternate footwear every few days. Topical antifungals may be used for minor infections, but more extensive infections may require an oral antifungal. Tinea pedis is also prone to secondary bacterial infections, and oral antibiotics should be considered if there is a high degree of inflammation or bacterial infection is suspected. In such cases a bacterial culture should be sent. Oral antifungals should be given strong consideration in the immunocompromised, diabetics, and those with the moccasin form.

"AT A GLANCE" TREATMENT

- First-line mild infection: topical antifungals may be used for minor infections
- Extensive infection: oral antifungals such as terbinafine.
- Consider secondary bacterial infections. Treat with oral antibiotics if there is a high degree of inflammation or bacterial infection is suspected. Send a bacterial culture.
- Wear nonocclusive shoes and alternate footwear every few days

ICD9 Codes

110.4   Dermatophytosis of foot

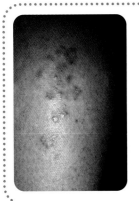

A 35-year-old woman comes to your office with an itchy "rash" on her left shin for the last two months. The rash is a well-circumscribed oval plaque with overlying pustules surrounding the hair follicles (Fig. 9-11). She reports daily shaving of her legs. She has been applying a strong topical steroid cream for 6 weeks, but the rash has only worsened.

Majocchi Granuloma

BACKGROUND/EPIDEMIOLOGY

The incidence of Majocchi granuloma is highest in childhood and has been associated with the use of potent topical steroids for dermatophyte infections. A second common form is seen in young women who shave their legs. Often, coexisting tinea pedis or corporis will be present near these lesions, suggesting this diagnosis.

PATHOGENESIS

Majocchi granuloma is a deep folliculitis due to dermatophyte infection. It is typically produced by *T. rubrum*. *Epidermophyton floccosum* and *T. mentagrophytes* have also been observed but less frequently.

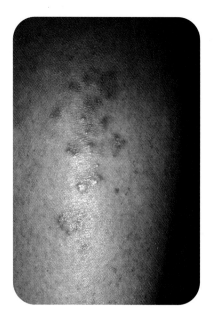

Figure 9-11 Majocchi granulomas on the shin of a young woman.

CLINICAL PRESENTATION

Majocchi granuloma presents as grouped or isolated papules or nodules near the border of a plaque and may evolve to perifollicular nodules. Lesions often appear in the scalp, face, forearms, hands, or legs and may become suppurative if superinfection occurs. The two forms of Majocchi granuloma are a superficial small perifollicular form common in women who frequently shave their legs (Fig. 9-11) and those who use topical steroids for a pre-existing dermatophyte infection, and a deeper subcutaneous form, which typically occurs in chronically immunosuppressed patients.

DIAGNOSIS

KOH exam may be positive from tinea on the surface adjacent to Majocchi papules and plaques. In some cases, a skin biopsy is necessary to define the etiology of the folliculitis.

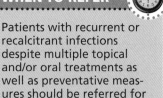

TREATMENT

Topical antifungals are often ineffective as they do not penetrate into the follicle. Oral griseofulvin, itraconazole, or terbinafine are often effective. For patients declining oral therapy, consider treating with a topical azole antifungal agent such as econazole nitrate 2% BID for a minimum of 3 months. Occlusion with plastic wrap may help increase penetration into the hair follicle.

"AT A GLANCE" TREATMENT

- Topical therapy is rarely effective. If necessary, try a generic azole antifungal such as econazole nitrate 2% BID for a minimum of 3 months
- Oral therapy: terbinafine 250 mg PO × 4 to 6 weeks. Other options include griseofulvin or itraconazole

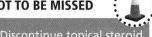

COURSE AND COMPLICATIONS

Full clinical resolution is expected with appropriate systemic antifungal therapy. Scarring and alopecia are rare complications. In immunocompromised patients, more widespread cutaneous or fungal septicemia is possible.

ICD9 Codes
110.5   *Dermatophytosis of the body*

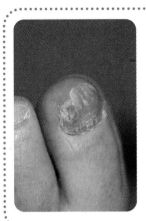

A 73-year-old retired university professor presents for yellow, brittle nails that are painful with walking (Fig. 9-12). He plays tennis 3 to 4 times weekly and the pain from his nails is affecting his game. He would like his nails fixed before a tournament next week. What is the most likely diagnosis? Is treatment within a week possible?

Tinea Unguium (Onychomycosis)

Chao Li, Fátima Akrouh, Sam Rodriguez, Peter C. Schalock

BACKGROUND/EPIDEMIOLOGY

Onychomycosis (OM) is a very common form of dermatophyte infection. It is found worldwide, with incidences of 2% to 13% in North America and 3% to 8% of the population in the United Kingdom. The infections are caused by typical dermatophyte fungi, yeasts such as *Candida*, and molds. Incidence increases with age. Very few children have nail infections, while many elderly individuals may have tinea unguium. Children under 18 years old have approximately 3% rate of OM while elderly individuals have up to a 90% chance of having nail infections.

KEY FEATURES

- Onychomycosis presents with dystrophic, discolored nails on hands and/or feet.
- Incidence increases with increasing age.
- Treatment is indicated for pain with walking or problems with dexterity. In some cases, treatment for cosmetic reasons may be indicated.
- Successful treatment is only seen with the use of oral antifungals.

PATHOGENESIS

Primary onychomycosis is the invasion of a healthy nail, and often occurs when there is a defect in the blood supply, innervation, or after trauma of the extremities. Secondary onychomycosis usually occurs in an abnormal nail, such as one that is affected by psoriasis or trauma; toenail infection can also occur secondarily to tinea pedis, while fingernail infection can occur secondarily to tinea manuum or by scratching of other areas affected by tinea.

CLINICAL PRESENTATION

Dystrophy, brittleness, and separation of the nail plate from the nail bed are all common signs of onychomycosis (Figs. 9-12, 9-13). In many cases, the nail is

CHAPTER 9 Fungal Infections

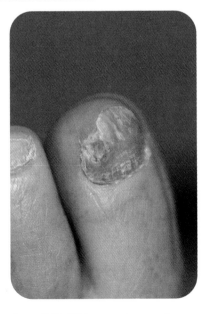

Figure 9-12 DLS type onychomycosis.

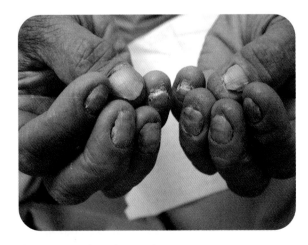

Figure 9-13 Nail onychomycosis.

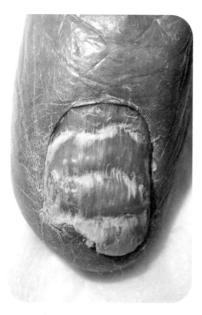

Figure 9-14 Superficial white type onychomycosis.

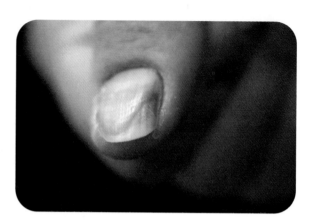

Figure 9-15 Nail infection with *Pseudomonas aeruginosa.*

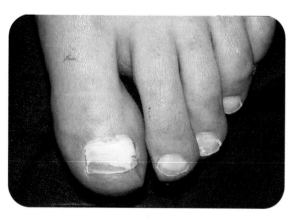

Figure 9-16 White proximal subungual onychomycosis. From Goodheart HP. *Goodheart's Photoguide to Common Skin Disorders,* 3rd ed. Philadelphia: Lippincott Williams & Wilkins, 2009.

discolored, often yellowish. Other subtypes present with white changes in the surface of the nail (Fig. 9-14). In some cases, a green-black pigmentation may be present, which would suggest an infection not with a fungus, but from the pyocyanin producing *Pseudomonas aeruginosa* (Fig. 9-15). There are multiple subtypes of OM, which are summarized in Table 9-8.

Many patients want OM treated for cosmetic reasons, but there are also important medical indications for treatment. A common presentation is pain during walking or other activities secondary to nail dystrophy. OM may allow secondary bacterial infections to develop, especially in diabetic or immunosuppressed individuals (Figs. 9-12 to 9-14, 9-16).

DIAGNOSIS

There are many causes of dystrophic nails that can be confused with a dermatophyte or candidal infection. It is essential that these other conditions be diagnosed, or at least suspected before prescribing for OM. See Tables 9-9 and 9-10 for other diagnoses to be considered when evaluating a dystrophic nail. Also, a detailed discussion of nail infections is found in Chapter 25.

Diagnostic Methods

Laboratory testing is important for confirming onychomycosis before initiating oral antifungal treatment.

- KOH examination: larger sample sizes and repeating collections reduce false-negative results.
- Nail biopsy: there is minimal dermal inflammatory response but fungal hyphae can be observed in the ventral nail and nail bed stratum corneum layer. Periodic acid-Schiff (PAS) staining of nail clippings is the most sensitive test.
- Fungal culture: isolation of pathogens in culture is the most specific test, and helps identify the organism.

Table 9-8 Types of Onychomycosis

TYPE	PHYSICAL FINDINGS	NOTES
Distal lateral subungual	Hyperkeratotic/opacified nail plate, subungual hyperkeratosis, onycholysis. Discoloration of nail varies (Fig. 9-12)	Most common type Caused by invasion of fungus from distal skin or through hyponychium
Superficial white	White discoloration on dorsal surface of nail (Fig. 9-14)	Caused by dermatophyte directly invading surface of nail
White proximal subungual	White discoloration of the proximal nail fold. May invade through nail. The nail stays normal distally (Fig. 9-16)	Rare; often seen in HIV infection
Endonyx	White discoloration of nail plate. No subungual hyperkeratosis or onycholysis	Variant of distal lateral subungual type
Candidal	3 Types: • *Onycholysis* • *Paronychia* • *Chronic mucocutaneous (CM)*	CM type—significant subungual hyper-keratosis/inflammation observed. Affected digits may become bulbous/drumstick-like; entire nail thickness may be involved
Total dystrophic	See Figure 9-13	End stage of any of the above types

Adapted from Blumberg M, Kantor GR. Onychomycosis. Available at: http://emedicine.medscape.com/article/1105828-overview. Accessed April 25, 2009.

Table 9-9 Differential Diagnosis of Nail Dystrophy

COMMON

Psoriasis

Lichen planus

Irritant dermatitis

POSTTRAUMATIC

Onychomycosis

INFREQUENT

Bacterial paronychia (including pseudomonal infection)

Darier disease

Pachyonychia congenita

Drug reaction (e.g., tetracyclines, quinolones, psoralens)

Periodic nail shedding

Thyroid disease

Yellow nail syndrome

Systemic illness

Table 9-10 Differential Diagnosis of Nail Pigmentation

Malignant melanoma

Melanonychia (caused by malignant melanoma)

Pseudomonas infection

Longitudinal melanonychia

Nail matrix nevus

Heme under nail secondary to trauma

Drug deposition (i.e., minocycline)

THERAPY

Oral antifungal therapy is the primary treatment of OM. There are multiple choices for medications, which are summarized in Table 9-11. The most commonly used medications at this time are terbinafine and pulsed dosed itraconazole. These medications should be used with caution, being aware of the multiple potential problems and interactions. The side effects and interactions that should be taken into account before therapy are summarized in Table 9-12.

Topical therapy may be successful in some mild cases. In the United States, the only approved topical antifungal for OM is ciclopirox. Amorolfine can also be effective and is available over the counter (OTC) in the United Kingdom, but is not available in the United States. Combination therapy has been shown to be more effective than topical or oral treatments alone. In one study of 80 patients, oral terbinafine given along with ciclopirox nail lacquer improved cure rates from 65% with oral agent alone to 88% with combined therapy. In a similar study of 147 patients, oral terbinafine with amorolfine nail lacquer improved cure rates from 37% with oral agent alone to 72% with combined therapy.

Table 9-11 Therapy of Onychomycosis

MEDICATION	DOSE	TREATMENT REGIMEN	
Oral		**Toenails**	**Fingernails**
Terbinafine	250 mg PO QD	12–16 weeks	6 weeks
Itraconazole	200 PO BID	1 week on 3 weeks off = 1 pulse. 3 pulses	2 pulses
Fluconazole	150–300 mg PO Q week	9–15 months	4–9 months
Ketoconazole		Not recommended due to risk of hepatotoxicity	
Griseofulvin Microfine	500 mg PO QD	6–12 mo	6–12 mo
Topical			
Amorolfine	5% lacquer	6–12 mo (not available in United States)	6–12 mo
Ciclopirox	8% lacquer	QD × 48 weeks	Same

Adapted from Gupta AK, Cooper EA. Update in antifungal therapy of dermatophytosis. *Mycopathologia.* 2008;166:353–367.

CHAPTER 9 Fungal Infections

Table 9-12 Overview of Important Facts about Terbinafine and Itraconazole

	TERBINAFINE	ITRACONAZOLE
Metabolism	CYP2D6—Liver metabolism	CYP3A4—Liver metabolism
Contraindications and cautions	• Active liver disease/cirrhosis/elevated liver function tests (LFT) • Renal disease (CCr <50 mL/min) • Cutaneous or systemic lupus • Patients on warfarin (increase risk of agranulocytosis)	• Congestive heart failure or h/o CHF • Active liver disease, cirrhosis, elevated liver function tests • Discontinue if neuropathy develops • Oral hypoglycemic: may require dosage adjustment, monitor for hypoglycemia

Common S/E	• Headache: 12.9%
	• GI disturbances: 2.2%–5.6%
	• Liver function abnormalities – 3.3%
	• Pruritus: 2.8%
	• Taste disturbance (can last > 1y): 2.8%
	• Urticaria: 1.1%
		• GI:
		  • Diarrhea, dyspepsia, flatulence, abdominal pain (4%)
		  • Others: nausea, appetite increase, constipation, gastritis, gastroenteritis
		• Rash (4%)
		• CNS: headache (10%), dizziness, abnormal dreaming
		• Hepatic/Renal: liver function/enzyme abnormality (3%–4%), urinary tract infection (3%)

Lab testing	• Baseline: LFT, CBC, BUN, Cr • At 6 weeks: Repeat above	No monitoring recommended for pulse therapy For cautious providers, consider: • Baseline: LFT, CBC, BUN, Cr, basic metabolic panel (including K) • Repeat above after 3 cycles

Adapted from Gupta AK, Cooper EA. Update in antifungal therapy of dermatophytosis. Mycopathologia. 2008;166:353–367 and Lamisil package insert. Available at: http://www.pharma.us.novartis.com/product/pi/pdf/Lamisil_tablets.pdf Accessed April 26, 2009.

WHEN TO REFER

Patients with recurrent or recalcitrant infections despite first-line oral treatments as well as preventative measures should be referred for further workup. Special consideration should be given to patients who are immunocompromised, as they may have atypical presentations and may be subject to more complications. Consider consultation with podiatry for patients with comorbidities.

"AT A GLANCE" TREATMENT

• Oral therapy is the mainstay of treatment. See Table 9-11 for suggested topical and oral therapies for OM.

COURSE AND COMPLICATIONS

Most uncomplicated cases of OM treated with oral agents respond to therapy. It is important to explain to the patient that it takes time before clinical response is apparent as clearing is usually from the proximal nail fold, growing distally. For fingernails, a nail grows out in 3 to 6 months and a toenail will take 6 to 12 months to grow out completely. With this in mind, counseling the patient that it may take 2 to 3 months before any signs of clearing may help prevent concerns of treatment failure. While most (60% to 70%) individuals do show signs of treatment success, recurrence rate within 2 years is very high.

NOT TO BE MISSED

- OM may allow for secondary bacterial infections to develop, especially in diabetic or immunosuppressed individuals.

Onychomycosis can be complicated by comorbidities such as diabetes and HIV/AIDS. Candida onychomycosis can invade the entire nail plate in immunosuppressed populations and cause onycholysis in diabetics. Furthermore, onychomycosis has also been identified as a risk factor for development of diabetic foot. With these comorbidities, good foot care including treatment of OM is necessary.

ICD9 Codes

110.1   Dermatophytosis of nail

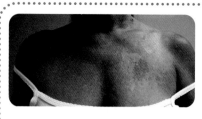

A 44-year-old woman comes to your office complaining of white splotches on her upper chest after a 2-week trip in Puerto Rico (Fig. 9-17). She was there on vacation, surfing and residing in youth hostels. The skin changes appeared three days before she returned to the United States. Her boyfriend told her that it was probably just a reaction to "too much sun." He recently noticed similar "blotches" on his upper arms.

CUTANEOUS YEAST INFECTIONS

Tinea Versicolor

BACKGROUND/EPIDEMIOLOGY

Tinea versicolor (alternatively pityrosporum versicolor or pityriasis versicolor) is a common cause of mild hypo- and hyperpigmentation with fine scaling on the trunk and upper extremities, most often of young individuals. It is rare in children, but once sebaceous gland activity increases the rate of infection goes up. No race or gender is predominantly affected, but the 15- to 24-year-old age group is most commonly infected.

PATHOGENESIS

Tinea versicolor (TV) is caused by *Malassezia furfur*, a dimorphic lipophilic yeast found in 90% to 100% of adults as normal flora. The infection is in the stratum corneum of the epidermis, but a tyrosinase produced by the organism can inhibit melanocytes production of pigment, thus leading to hypopigmented patches. It is also capable of causing inhibition of melanosome breakdown, thus leading to hyperpigmentation.

CLINICAL PRESENTATION

There are three forms of TV. Tinea versicolor most commonly presents as hypo- or hyperpigmented patches on the trunk, back, and upper arms. Characteristic lesions are oval or round macules and papules which may eventually become confluent (Fig. 9-17). These findings are generally noted more often in summer as areas that do not tan with sunlight exposure. The second form of TV is an inverse pattern, with similar types of plaques appearing on the face, body folds, and extremities. This type is more often associated with immunosuppressed individuals. A third, distinctive type of TV is called pityrosporum folliculitis. This is caused by infection of the hair follicle on skin with prominent sebaceous glands (face/chest/axilla), most often the chest with *M. furfur*. Deep-seated follicular pustules without scaling or pigmentary changes are often present, which may be challenging to differentiate from a bacterial folliculitis. Patients working in humid environments, with diabetes mellitus, or those being treated with steroids, antibiotics or immunosuppressive agents are all more susceptible.

Patients may be asymptomatic, presenting only due to the pigmentary complaints, while others may complain of pruritus. Tinea versicolor has a

KEY FEATURES

- Tinea versicolor is a superficial infection of the epidermis by the yeast, *Malassezia furfur*.

- It most commonly presents as hypo- or hyperpigmented patches on the trunk, back, and upper arms.

- There is a distinctive pattern on KOH exam ("spaghetti and meatballs").

- Treatment with topical therapy is usually successful.

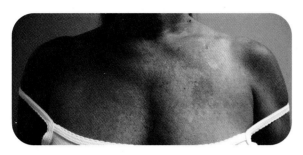

Figure 9-17 Tinea versicolor on the chest of a woman.

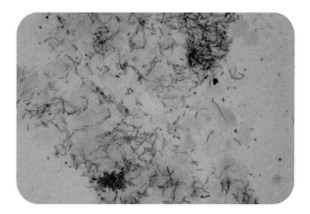

Figure 9-18 Positive KOH exam for *M. furfur*.

predilection for oily skin of the trunk and upper extremities. It typically presents in teenagers and young adults when skin sebum production is at its highest. This condition is rarely seen in very young children or older adults.

DIAGNOSIS

Diagnosis by Wood's lamp demonstrates a yellow or gold color in one-third of cases. Because of the lack of sensitivity of this test, a scraping for light microscopy is the diagnostic tool of choice. Specimens should be collected from the border of a lesion. Microscopy reveals typical "spaghetti and meatballs" (Fig. 9-18) of yeast clusters and short curved septated hyphae. Skin biopsy is rarely indicated unless the suspicion of other dermatoses is high. Other diagnoses to consider are discussed in Table 9-13.

TREATMENT

Tinea versicolor is responsive to topical and oral antifungals. Oral therapy is indicated in cases resistant to topical therapy. Oral treatments usually have better patient compliance rates while topical agents are safer, especially for children. Prophylactic oral treatments with ketoconazole have been shown to prevent relapse in particularly susceptible patients.

"AT A GLANCE" TREATMENT

- Initial therapy is with topical agents. Recalcitrant case may benefit from systemic therapy. Treatment options are summarized in Table 9-14.

COURSE AND COMPLICATIONS

Ninety-seven percent of patients are cured with oral agents. Tinea versicolor recurs after treatment at a rate of 60% by the first year and 80% by the second year. For patients with recurrent disease, prophylactic topical or oral therapy may be indicated.

WHEN TO REFER

Patients with recurrent or recalcitrant infections despite multiple topical and/or oral treatments as well as preventative measures should be referred for further workup. Special consideration should be given to patients who are immunocompromised as they may have atypical presentations and may be subject to more complications.

NOT TO BE MISSED

- Secondary syphilis has similar morphology to TV. Due to the serious long-term sequelae, this diagnosis must be considered in cases of "tinea versicolor" that are widespread and treatment resistant.

Table 9-13 Differential Diagnosis for Tinea Versicolor

Vitiligo	Seborrheic dermatitis
Guttate psoriasis	Pityriasis alba
Erythrasma	Pinta
Tinea corporis	Secondary syphilis

Table 9-14 Treatment Options for Tinea Versicolor

TOPICAL	DOSING	ORAL	DOSING
Selenium sulfide	QD with 10 minute application (for shampoo), overnight for lotion. Treat for 2 weeks	Ketoconazole	400 mg PO × 1 dose
Sodium sulfacetamide	QHS × 2 weeks		200 mg PO QD × 10 days
Ciclopiroxamine	QHS × 2 weeks, then once weekly for 2 months to prevent recurrence	Fluconazole	150–300 mg PO every week × 2–4 weeks
Azoles (i.e., ketoconazole)	QHS × 2 weeks, then once weekly for 2 months to prevent recurrence. Shampoo application for 10 minutes followed by showering off may be effective	Itraconazole	200 mg PO QD × 7 days
Allylamines (i.e., terbinafine)	QHS × 2 weeks, then once weekly for 2 months to prevent recurrence. *M. furfur* may be resistant to allylamines		

ICD9 Codes

| 111.0 | *Pityriasis versicolor* |
| 097.9 | *Syphilis, unspecified* |

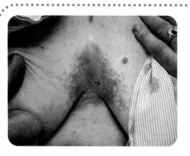

A 47-year-old woman presents complaining of a rash in her central chest, between and under her breasts (Fig. 9-19). She describes eroded patches that are mildly tender and quite itchy. The whole area is slightly red and there are small pustules surrounding the eroded patches. This summer has been particularly hot and she says that she is sweating more than usual.

KEY FEATURES

- *Candida* species colonize the mucous membranes of 50% of normal hosts.

- *C. albicans* species is responsible for the majority of infections and may present as intertrigo, paronychia, or oral thrush.

(Continued)

Candidiasis

BACKGROUND/EPIDEMIOLOGY

Candida species colonize mucous membranes of 50% of normal hosts. It is often found as a commensal organism in the vaginal mucosa of some healthy women. In elderly and diabetic patients, it is the cause of up to 50% of intertrigo.

PATHOGENESIS

While many *Candida* species may cause cutaneous infection, *C. albicans* species is responsible for the majority of infections. Yeasts that are capable of infecting the skin have virulence factors including proteases. Yeasts weakly expressing virulence factors have minimal virulence, strongly expressing yeasts cause more infection. Epidermal adhesion is essential for eventual penetration and hyphae formation. Immune modulation of infection is important in controlling infection. Immunosuppressed patients, especially those with HIV/AIDS, may progress from mucocutaneous infection with *C. albicans* to invasive systemic infections.

CLINICAL PRESENTATION

Cutaneous candidal infections can present in a variety of ways: intertrigo, nail paronychia, diaper rashes in infants, or mucosal infections/thrush. Intertrigo is

KEY FEATURES *(Continued)*

- Treatment is usually successful with topical therapies such as azoles, terbinafine cream, or nystatin. Oral fluconazole is another option for recalcitrant cases.

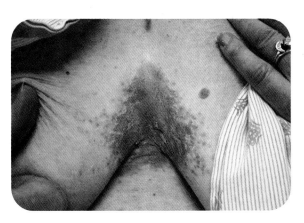

Figure 9-19 Inflammatory candidal infection of the central chest.

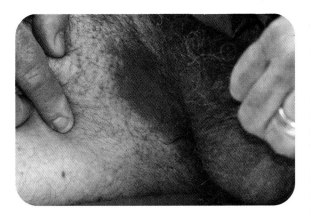

Figure 9-20 Candidal intertrigo.

WHEN TO REFER

Patients with recurrence or recalcitrant infections despite multiple topical and/or oral treatments as well as preventative measures should be referred for further workup. Special consideration should be given to patients who are immunocompromised, as they may have atypical presentations and may be subject to more complications.

characterized by erythematous, "beefy-red," eroded patches with satellite pustules and scale (Fig. 9-19). These lesions are particularly common in warm, moist, macerated folds of glabrous skin such as axillary, gluteal, inframammary, scrotum (Fig. 9-20), and interdigital. Obesity, diabetes mellitus, systemic antibiotics, and chafing clothing are common risk factors. Diaper rashes in infants can result from *C. albicans* infection. Mucosal candidiasis may present in a variety of manners. Candida paronychia is characterized as painful, erythematous swellings of the skin around the nail plate. This is often seen in patients whose occupation involves frequent immersion of the hands in water.

Candida may also be found in chronic paronychia, but is not always causative. Anticandidal therapy therefore may not always be successful.

Oral candidiasis can present as thrush (nonadherent white material on the buccal mucosa) or glossitis. Risk factors include oral contraceptive use, long-term use of antibiotics, malnutrition, or immunosuppression. Candida vulvovaginitis is defined by an oozing, infection with "cottage cheese-like" exudates, often seen in pregnant women, diabetics, and with chronic antibiotic use.

DIAGNOSIS

Assessment should include careful examination of the scalp, face, skin, fingernails, and groin. KOH exam shows thin-walled budding yeast with pseudohyphae. *Candida* can be cultured on Sabourad's media in 4 to 5 days.

TREATMENT

Candida infections including mucocutaneous sites respond to topical therapies such as azoles, terbinafine cream, or nystatin. Oral antifungals are only necessary with extensive or disseminated disease. In candidal paronychia infections, minimizing water contact is very important. The patient should minimize handwashing and use gloves for other wet work (dishes, housework, etc.). The use of an antifungal solution such as nystatin solution is often helpful. Candidal intertrigo infections should be treated with frequent bathing followed by thorough drying. For patients with large intertriginous areas (pendulous breasts or pannus) with frequent or chronic intertrigo, drying the area following bathing with a hair dryer on low heat setting may be very helpful. Follow drying with application of a topical antiyeast agent in a lotion form. Avoid ointment usage as it may cause further maceration. To keep the area dry following self-care, a thin cotton cloth material (such as a t-shirt cut to appropriate size) may be placed between the two opposing layers of skin (under a large breast for example). Avoid use of paper-based products (i.e., paper towels) as they are often adherent and removal causes further inflammation/irritation. Use of a drying powder such as Zeasorb AF may also be useful. If the skin is inflamed, a mild-potency topical steroid such as hydrocortisone cream may give relief from pruritus. Rarely is the use of a combination agent with a superpotent steroid such as betamethasone dipropionate indicated.

Diaper-area skin infections with *Candida* in diaper-aged children occur due to maceration of the occluded skin, allowing for yeast colonization. Up to 75% of diaper rashes lasting longer than 3 days are candidal infections. The yeast is fecal in origin and is not part of normal flora. Treatment with oral antibiotics may worsen this condition.

NOT TO BE MISSED

- Consider immunocompromised state for patients with recalcitrant or with multiple recurrent infections.

"AT A GLANCE" TREATMENT

- Treatment is usually successful with topical therapies such as ketoconazole 2% cream BID × 1 to 2 weeks or other over-the-counter azoles, terbinafine cream, or nystatin.
- Oral fluconazole is another option for recalcitrant cases.

CLINICAL COURSE

Mucocutaneous candidiasis has an excellent prognosis and usually resolves with topical antifungals. However, repeated infections could be harbingers of an immunocompromised host.

ICD9 Codes

| 112.3 | Candidiasis of skin and nails |
| 112.0 | Candidiasis of mouth |

Suggested Reading

Alvarez MS, Silverberg NB. Tinea capitis. Cutis.2006;78:189–196.

Blumberg M, Kantor GR. Onychomycosis. Available at: http://emedicine.medscape.com/article/1105828-overview. Accessed April 25, 2009.

Bolognia JL. Fungal diseases. Dermatology. 2003:1171–1198.

Burkhart CG, Gottwald L, Burkhart CN. Tinea versicolor. Available at: http://emedicine.medscape.com/article/1091575-overview. April 27, 2009.

Chang SE, Lee DK, Choi JH, et al. Majocchi's granuloma of the vulva caused by Trichophyton mentagrophytes. Mycoses. 2005;48:382–384.

Gonzalez U, Seaton T, Bergus G, et al. Systemic antifungal therapy for tinea capitis in children. Cochrane Database Syst Rev. 2007; CD004685.

Gupta AK, Chaudhry M, Elewski B. Tinea corporis, tinea cruris, tinea nigra, and piedra. Dermatol Clin. 2003;21:395–400.

Gupta AK, Cooper EA, Ryder JE, et al. Optimal management of fungal infections of the skin, hair, and nails. Am J Clin Dermatol. 2004;5:225–237.

Gupta AK, Cooper EA. Update in antifungal therapy of dermatophytosis. Mycopathologia. 2008;166:353–367.

Hall JC. Sauer's Manual of Skin Diseases. Philadelphia: Lippincott Williams & Wilkins; 2006:244–266.

Hay RJ. The management of superficial candidiasis. J Am Acad Dermatol. 1999;40: S36–42.

Janniger CK. Majocchi's granuloma. Cutis. 1992;50:267–268.

Lamisil package insert. Available at: http://www.pharma.us.novartis.com/product/pi/pdf/Lamisil_tablets.pdf Accessed April 26, 2009.

Loo DS. Cutaneous fungal infections in the elderly. Dermatol Clin. 2004;22:33–50.

Lott MER, Zember G. Tinea corporis. Available at: http://emedicine.medscape.com/article/1091473-overview. Accessed April 26, 2009.

Noble SL, Forbes RC, Stamm PL. Diagnosis and management of common tinea infections. Am Fam Physician. 1998;58:163–174.

Schwartz RA. Superficial fungal infections. Lancet. 2004;364:1173–1182.

Trovato MJ, Schwartz RA, Janniger CK. Tinea capitis: current concepts in clinical practice. Cutis. 2006; 77:93–99.

CHAPTER 10 Viral Infections of the Skin

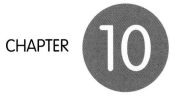

Jennifer K. Tan-Billet and Andrew A. Nelson

Viruses cause a myriad of skin conditions, ranging from benign nonspecific morbilliform eruptions to potentially life-threatening disseminated disease. With several hundred viruses in existence, it is not possible to comprehensively discuss all viral-mediated cutaneous eruptions in this chapter. Rather, this section will focus on the most common and important cutaneous manifestations of viral disease, with emphasis on presentation to primary care providers and initial management. The development of vaccines for diseases such as measles, mumps, rubella, and varicella has greatly diminished the frequency of these previously common diseases; as a result, not all of these entities will be discussed. We hope that this chapter will serve as an overview and introduction to the cutaneous manifestations of viral infections.

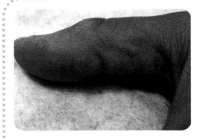

A 12-year-old boy is brought into the clinic by his mother. She complains of "warts" on his hands, which are embarrassing to him (Fig. 10-1A). They have tried numerous over-the-counter wart therapies, but none have worked. Several of his classmates have similar lesions. What is the most likely diagnosis? What is the best treatment option?

KEY FEATURES

- Verruca vulgaris is an extremely common condition, affecting nearly 20% of schoolchildren.

- They are associated with human papilloma virus (HPV) infections, specifically HPV types 1, 2, and 4.

(Continued)

Verruca Vulgaris (Common Warts)

BACKGROUND

Verruca vulgaris (VV) lesions represent infection by the human papilloma virus (HPV), a type of DNA virus. While the term *verruca vulgaris* is used to describe common warts, *verruca plantaris* refers to plantar warts and *verruca plana* refers specifically to flat warts. To date, more than 100 different HPV types have been identified; common warts are most associated with infections of HPV types 1, 2, and 4. While the majority of verruca vulgaris lesions are benign and self-resolve, they can be cosmetically unappealing and occasionally painful to patients. Treatment of these lesions is quite challenging for they are often refractory to repeated exposures to many therapeutic modalities.

PATHOGENESIS

Human papilloma viruses are a type of DNA virus. HPV can only complete its full life cycle when infecting squamous epithelial cells, particularly proliferating basal epithelial cells. Once the virus infects these proliferating basal epithelial cells, cell proliferation is upregulated. The epidermis then becomes thickened and hyperkeratotic through increased cellular division.

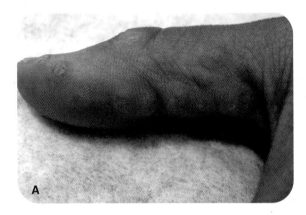
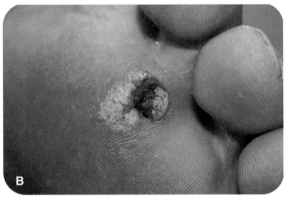

Figure 10-1 A Multiple verruca vulgaris on the thumb. **B** Verruca plantaris. Note the black dots (capillary thromboses).

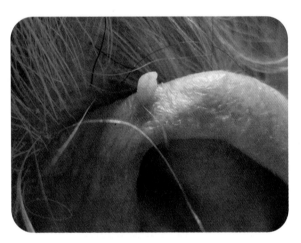

Figure 10-2 Verruca vulgaris on the helix of the ear.

CLINICAL PRESENTATION

Verruca vulgaris typically present as hyperkeratotic, rough, exophytic, round papules (Fig. 10-1A). These papules often have pinpoint black dots, which result from thrombosed capillary loops (Fig. 10-1B). The most common locations include the fingers, dorsum of the hands, and other sites exposed to trauma. Verruca vulgaris can be spread by autoinoculation; there may therefore be a linear arrangement of lesions as a result of this phenomenon. The majority of lesions are asymptomatic, although the lesions can be quite painful, particularly when located on the soles of the feet. HPV infects fully differentiated squamous epithelium, resulting in the massively thickened epidermis and stratum corneum that characterizes the cutaneous lesions. In some cases, VV can form a cutaneous horn which may be indistinguishable from an actinic keratosis, such as that shown in Figure 10-2.

DIAGNOSIS

Differential Diagnosis

The differential diagnosis includes plantar clavi (corns), seborrheic keratoses, actinic keratoses, and squamous cell carcinoma. Rarely, a type of skin cancer called a verrucous carcinoma may be mistaken for a common wart; verrucous carcinoma tends to develop on the feet and is resistant to treatment (see Treatment section). When the lesion is adjacent to a nail, particular concern should be paid to possible amelanotic melanoma and invasive squamous cell carcinoma (see Chapter 25).

Diagnostic Methods

Most often the lesions can be diagnosed clinically. If the lesions do not respond to therapy, or there is any question regarding the diagnosis, a shave biopsy can be performed for confirmation.

THERAPY

There is no current medication to "cure" HPV. Rather, current therapies focus on destroying the verrucous lesions or inducing an immune response against those cells infected with HPV. Because about 40% to 65% of warts resolve spontaneously in 2 years, providing no initial treatment is both reasonable and cost-effective. If warts are symptomatic, enlarging, spreading, or persistent, there are several treatment modalities to consider.

KEY FEATURES (*Continued*)

- The majority of lesions self-resolve in 1 to 2 years.
- Therapeutic options consist of either destructive or immunomodulatory therapies; treatment can be challenging, typically multiple treatments over several months are necessary.

- **Destructive therapies** (local anesthesia should be used for several of these therapies):
  - **Salicylic acid peels:** Available over-the-counter in products such as Mediplast, Compound W, Wart Off, Duofilm, or Dr. Scholls Clearaway. Of the current topical treatment modalities, there is sufficient evidence based on controlled trials available to support the use of this therapy. Patients should be instructed to apply 1 to 2 times daily and warned that effects are slow to achieve. This treatment is often used in combination with a pumice stone to pare down the lesion.
  - **Cryotherapy (liquid nitrogen):** Often applied using an open-spray or cotton-tipped applicator for approximately 10 to 30 seconds to generate a 2 to 3 mm iceball around the wart (with cooling duration of approximately 20 to 60 seconds). Thin, filiform warts (Fig. 10-2) require freezing only of the lesion itself with little to no involvement of surrounding normal skin. For warts on the hand, a double freeze-thaw cycle likely confers little benefit over a single cycle and may result in increased discomfort and blister formation. For plantar warts, two freeze-thaw cycles appear to be more effective. Cryotherapy may be used in combination with paring of warts or salicylic acid application, though there is currently inconclusive evidence available to support the use of cryotherapy over salicylic acid as initial therapy for warts.
  - **Cantharidin:** This therapy, derived from the blister beetle, is painted on warts in a physician's office. Application is painless but may cause subsequent blister formation in the next several hours. Cantharidin 0.7% is painted on to the wart and 1 mm of surrounding skin; the patient should not touch or remove the cantharidin initially. The cantharidin is then washed off 2 to 4 hours later.
  - **Electrocautery:** Care should be taken, as HPV has been reported to be aerosolized following electrocautery.
  - **Laser therapy:** Treatment with pulsed dye laser or ablative therapy with CO_2 laser is typically employed. HPV can be aerosolized with this treatment.
  - **Surgical excision:** Though useful for stubborn lesions, surgical excision often results in increased scarring and the wart may recur following excision.
- **Immunomodulators:**
  - **Imiquimod:** Stimulates toll-like receptors 7 and 8, increasing the production of inflammatory cytokines to kill the HPV-infected cells. Patients may apply 5% cream 3 to 5 times weekly for up to 16 weeks.
  - **Cimetidine:** An oral H2 blocker that has been reported to treat verruca through an unclear immunomodulatory effect. This may be a useful option for young patients that cannot tolerate destructive therapies. Doses of 25 to 40 mg/kg/day divided QID are typically prescribed, though results are generally varied and a double-blinded, placebo-controlled trial demonstrated no benefit.
  - **Interferon and bleomycin:** Intralesional forms of these agents are sometimes used as second-line agents for recalcitrant warts. However, these injections can be painful for patients.
- **Alternative therapies:**
  - **Duct tape application:** Apply to warts daily. Alternatively, patients may apply the duct tape and leave in place for up to 6 days. Duct tape requires up to 1 month or longer of treatment to be effective.
  - **Hypnosis:** Reported success in up to 25% to 50% of patients.
  - **Hot water immersion:** The affected area is soaked in hot water 2 to 3 times weekly for 30 to 45 minutes.

"AT A GLANCE" TREATMENT

- There are many suggested second-line therapies for warts that are summarized in the text.

- First-line therapy includes:
  - **Destructive therapies:**
  - **Salicylic acid peels:** Available over-the-counter in products such as Mediplast, Compound W, Wart Off, Duofilm, or Dr. Scholls Clearaway. Patients should apply 1 to 2 times daily. If using with imiquimod, apply one in the morning and one at night. This treatment is often used in combination with a pumice stone to pare down the lesion. This may take months to achieve success.
  - **Cryotherapy (liquid nitrogen):** Cryotherapy may be used in combination with paring of warts or salicylic acid application
- **Imiquimod:** Apply 5% cream 3 to 5 times weekly for up to 16 weeks QD. Use in conjunction with monthly liquid nitrogen and salicylic acid.

COURSE AND COMPLICATIONS

Verruca vulgaris lesions can be quite refractory to therapy. The HPV infects keratinocytes at the base of the lesions. Thus, interventions are often unsuccessful, as they treat the lesions from the outside-in. Patients should be counseled that it will take many treatments spread over several months (usually one visit per 3 to 4 weeks) to treat these lesions and that there is no "cure" for warts. Additionally, patients should be instructed that warts can be passed from one person to another by direct physical contact and sometimes by sharing an object that has been touched by someone infected with HPV (such as gym mats and floors of showering facilities). Trauma, excess hand moisture, nail biting, and swimming pools can all increase the transmission of warts.

KEY FEATURES

- Condyloma acuminata is a common, highly prevalent sexually transmitted infection in young adults spread via intimate contact. It can be a manifestation of sexual abuse in young children.

- Typically presents as soft exophytic growths in the groin and anogenital region.

- Condyloma acuminata are caused by HPV infections. HPV types 16, 18, 31, and 33 are "high-risk," and are associated with an increased risk of cervical cancer. HPV types 6 and 11 are "low-risk" and are not associated with an increased risk of cervical cancer.

- Treatment consists of topical destructive therapy or immunomodulatory therapies. Lesions can be quite refractory to therapy.

- A vaccine has been developed that helps to protect against HPV types 6, 11, 16, and 18 in HPV naïve patients.

> **ICD9 Codes**
>
> 078.10   *Viral warts, unspecified*

Condyloma Acuminata (Genital Warts)

Condyloma acuminata (Figs. 10-3A,B) are associated with infections by the human papilloma virus (HPV). In contrast to common warts, condyloma lesions are caused by infections with HPV types 6, 11, 16, 18, and others. In the

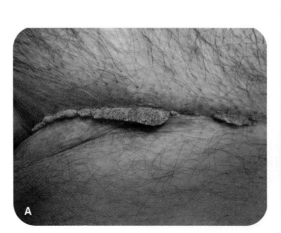
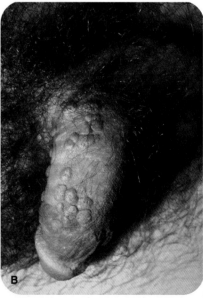

Figure 10-3 A Perianal and gluteal cleft condyloma acuminate. **B** Penile condyloma acuminate. Image from Rubin E, Farber JL. *Pathology*, 3rd ed. Philadelphia: Lippincott Williams & Wilkins, 1999.

1970s, the association between HPV infections and cervical cancer was first recognized. However, more recently, it has become apparent that certain specific "high-risk" HPV types are more closely associated with the development of cervical cancer. Condyloma acuminata are discussed in detail in Chapter 13.

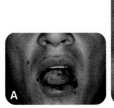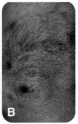

A 18-year-old male with a longstanding history of severe atopic dermatitis presents to your clinic with a recurrence of a cold sore that he has had on and off for several years as well as a new rash. He says that he had a similar rash with the flare of his last cold sore, but this time it is much worse. He reports that he has ulcerations on his tongue and buccal mucosa as well as lesions on his arms, legs, and body, which "look kind of like targets." He is feeling a bit more tired than normal and feels like he is "getting a cold" but he declines fevers or chills. The flare seemed to have started with a few painful "sores" around the mouth. He has cutaneous lesions as described above (Figs. 10-4A,B). What is the best diagnosis? What treatment is necessary at this time?

Human Herpes Viruses

BACKGROUND

Herpes simplex virus is a common, ubiquitous infection. In fact, nearly 90% of the world's population between the ages of 20 and 40 are thought to have been exposed to HSV-1, as measured by positive antibodies. HSV-1 infections are most common on the lips and mouth; however, HSV-1 can also be the cause of genital herpes in approximately 10% to 20% of cases. HSV-1 infections can be primary, latent, and/or recurrent. The majority of affected patients are in the latent phase. Thus, while the majority of the population may have been previously exposed to HSV-1, a much smaller proportion has a clinical outbreak of HSV-1 at any given time.

PATHOGENESIS

Transmission of HSV-1 can occur during symptomatic outbreaks or during asymptomatic latent periods. HSV-1 is most commonly spread through contaminated saliva or other secretions. The HSV-1 virus infects localized keratinocytes, and replicates locally. It can then spread up the nerve to the dorsal root ganglion, where it becomes latent. The virus can then be reactivated by multiple stimuli and result in recurrent infections.

CLINICAL PRESENTATION

Primary HSV-1 infections typically develop a few days after exposure to the virus. These initial outbreaks are usually symptomatic, with systemic symptoms such as fever, malaise, and lymphadenopathy developing 2 to 3 days before any cutaneous lesions. Primary HSV-1 infections commonly manifest as gingivostomatitis or pharyngitis with mononucleosis-like symptoms. The outbreak consists of multiple grouped "herpetiform" vesicles on an erythematous base (Fig. 10-4A). The lesions then crust and resolve over several weeks. In contrast to recurrent aphthous stomatitis ("canker sores"), HSV infections typically affect keratinized surfaces of the mouth such as the gingivae and hard palate; aphthous stomatitis tends to occur on the buccal mucosa and underside of the tongue.

Following the primary infection, HSV-1 infections can become latent. During this latent phase, the virus is localized to the dorsal root ganglion, where it is dormant. No clinical lesions or symptoms are present during this phase. The virus is then reactivated and spreads down the nerve to cause a clinical eruption. Reactivation can be caused by stress, sunlight, fever, sickness, or may occur spontaneously.

KEY FEATURES

- Common, ubiquitous infection with nearly 90% of patients between ages of 20 and 40; infection is with herpes simplex virus (HSV)-1 (positive antibodies).

- Most commonly appears as grouped vesicles on an erythematous base on lips/mouth; however, can be a cause of genital herpes as well.

- Clinically manifests as primary infections, latent infections, or recurrent infections.

- Diagnosed via Tzanck prep, direct fluorescent antibody (DFA) testing, viral culture.

- Treated with topical or oral antiviral agents such as acyclovir, famciclovir, and valacyclovir.

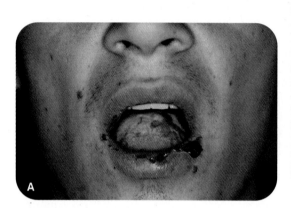
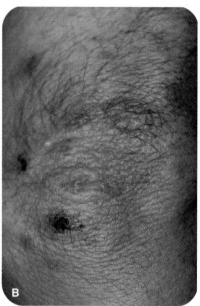

Figure 10-4 A Crusted plaque at the lateral oral commissure consistent with herpes simplex type I infection. **B** Erythema multiforme with typical target lesions on the knee in a man with recurrent HSV type I oral infections.

Recurrent outbreaks are often preceded by symptoms of burning and tingling in the lips, which may begin 1 to 2 days before the cutaneous outbreak. These symptoms are presumably related to the virus spreading down the nerve. Cutaneous lesions associated with recurrent HSV-1 are typically localized to the vermillion border of the lips and are characterized by small grouped vesicles on an erythematous base. The majority of these recurrent outbreaks are not associated with systemic symptoms, although lymphadenopathy and fatigue may occur. Recurrent outbreaks are typically milder and resolve quicker than primary infections, with the outbreak lasting approximately 1 week.

Recurrent flares of erythema multiforme (EM) are nearly always associated with flares of herpes simplex. As described in the case, patients' EM will flare in conjunction with reactivation of HSV (Figs. 10-4A,B). Appropriate oral therapy for HSV will also suppress the EM flare.

DIAGNOSIS

Differential Diagnosis

Aphthous ulcers or "canker sores," which are typically located on the buccal mucosa or undersurface of the tongue; erythema multiforme, a mucocutaneous condition which may be triggered by HSV; Stevens-Johnson syndrome, which usually has cutaneous target lesions in addition to oral lesions; pharyngitis associated with mononucleosis (EBV infections)

Diagnostic Methods

- Historically, HSV infections were diagnosed by a Tzanck smear. This procedure involves unroofing a vesicle, scraping the base of the lesion, and applying cells to a microscope slide. Giemsa stain is then used to fix the specimen, followed by a brief rinse with water. A positive Tzanck is characterized by the presence of multinucleated giant cells, which represent infected keratinocytes. Although this technique allows for the rapid diagnosis of a human herpes virus (HHV) infection, it does not distinguish between HSV-1, HSV-2, and VZV infections.
- Direct fluorescent antibody (DFA) testing utilizes antibodies specific to the different HHV types. This test is performed similarly to a Tzanck to obtain

basal keratinocytes and apply them to a microscope slide to be sent for DFA testing. Fluorescent antibodies to HSV-1, HSV-2, and VZV are then applied to the slide; a rinse is then performed. If HSV or VZV infection is present, the specific antibody will bind to infected keratinocytes and will not be washed away with the rinse. The slides are then examined under a fluorescent microscope. If an HSV infection is present, the fluorescent antibodies will be seen. The DFA is a rapid test, but the true benefit is in the differentiation of HSV-1, HSV-2, and VZV.

- Viral culture is performed by sampling the fluid beneath a vesicle. HSV-1 and −2 grow rapidly in culture, but a diagnosis still requires a few days. Viral culture can help differentiate HSV-1, HSV-2, and VZV. However, it is important to note that VZV grows poorly in culture, and a negative culture does not necessarily exclude the diagnosis.
- Antibody testing for HSV can also be performed. IgM antibodies can establish the diagnosis of a primary HSV infection. IgG antibodies only establish whether a patient has been previously exposed; they do not necessarily establish a diagnosis of recurrent HSV infection.

TREATMENT

Primary HSV infections are often severe and symptomatic and most patients are treated with antiviral therapy. A systematic review of acyclovir for treating primary herpetic gingivostomatitis found only weak evidence that acyclovir effectively reduces the number of oral lesions and prevents the development of new extraoral lesions. Patients with recurrent HSV may be treated with topical agents, such as 1% penciclovir or 5% acyclovir ointment, with limited expectations of useful effects. Oral therapy with acyclovir (dosed 5 times per day) or valacyclovir (dosed twice daily) is also an option for severe cases. Currently, no oral agents are Food and Drug Administration (FDA) approved for the treatment of primary oral HSV, though several dosing regimens have been reported in the literature. Mild, asymptomatic HSV-1 outbreaks require no therapy. However, topical agents and oral therapy can potentially abort or shorten an outbreak if given at the first sign of an infection, such as tingling in the lips. Therapy regimens are summarized in Table 10-1.

Finally, for patients with significant, frequent, recurrent outbreaks (including recurrent EM), suppressive therapy with either oral acyclovir or valacyclovir given on a low-dose daily basis is a therapeutic option. The dosing schedules for suppressive and episodic outbreaks are FDA-approved.

"AT A GLANCE" TREATMENT

- HSV type I therapy is summarized in Table 10-1.

Table 10-1 HSV Therapy

	ACYCLOVIR	FAMCICLOVIR	VALACYCLOVIR
Treatment for primary oral HSV*	15 mg/kg 5 times daily × 7 days	500 mg BID × 7 days	1 g BID × 7 days
Episodic treatment for recurrent oral HSV	200 mg 5 times daily × 5 days	1.5 g × 1 dose	2 g BID × 1 day
Suppressive treatment	400 mg BID	250 mg BID	500 mg once daily

*This dosing schedule is not FDA approved.

WHEN TO REFER

Cases refractory to treatment should be referred.

NOT TO BE MISSED

• For patients with recurrent erythema multiforme, consider suppressive antiviral therapy if they have more than several episodes per year.

COURSE AND COMPLICATIONS

Primary HSV-1 infections can be quite painful and severe. They are self-limited infections, with symptoms resolving over 4 to 6 weeks. Unfortunately, the virus travels retrograde up the nerves and becomes latent, with the potential to reactivate.

Recurrent HSV-1 infections tend to be less severe and shorter than primary infections. However, they can be painful and occasionally associated with systemic symptoms such as lymphadenopathy. These outbreaks typically last 1 week, but can be potentially shortened or aborted with early antiviral therapy.

ICD9 Codes

054.9	Herpes simplex without mention of complication
695.10	Erythema multiforme, unspecified
695.11	Erythema multiforme minor
695.12	Erythema multiforme major
695.13	Stevens-Johnson syndrome
695.14	Stevens-Johnson syndrome-toxic epidermal necrolysis overlap syndrome
695.15	Toxic epidermal necrolysis
695.19	Other erythema multiforme

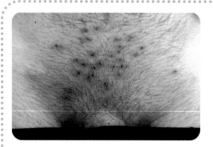

A 21-year-old college student presents to the student health service with an 8-day history of painful suprapubic, penile, and scrotal ulcerations (Fig. 10-5A). He noticed a few lesions on his lower pubis and decided to shave his pubic hair to get a better view. He is feeling poorly, reporting a fever, and has noticed some tender lymph nodes in his groin area. He recently had unprotected sexual intercourse and oral sex with his girlfriend, who came to his college for a short visit from her school in another state. He has done some Internet research and is confused because he thinks the skin lesions and his symptoms are consistent with "herpes" but does believe he could have gotten the infection as his girlfriend "only sleeps with me." What is his diagnosis? What tests could be done to prove to him that this is a primary HSV infection?

Herpes Simplex Virus Type II

BACKGROUND

Genital herpes is most commonly caused by infection with the herpes simplex virus type 2 (HSV-2). While HSV-2 infections preferentially affect the genitalia, approximately 10% to 20% of genital herpes outbreaks are caused by HSV-1. In some cases HSV-2 may be the cause of oral herpes as HSV-2 infection is spread via sexual contact. As a result, HSV-2 infections before adolescence are rare.

PATHOGENESIS

HSV-2 infections are spread through close intimate contact. The virus then integrates into keratinocytes and spreads in a retrograde fashion to a dorsal root ganglion where it becomes eventually becomes latent.

CLINICAL PRESENTATION

HSV-2 infections, similar to HSV-1, are grouped into primary, latent, and recurrent. Primary HSV-2 infections are often severe and extremely painful. In men, the primary outbreak is characterized by painful, erosive, grouped vesicles on an erythematous base, usually located on the shaft of the penis or glans penis. It can be spread by shaving or trauma to adjacent skin/hair follicles (Fig. 10-5A). In women, the primary outbreak is characterized by painful, erosive, grouped

KEY FEATURES

- Herpes simplex virus type 2 is a common sexually transmitted infection, principally affecting young, sexually active patients.

- HSV-2 is the most common cause of genital herpes.

- Clinically it manifests as grouped vesicles and erosions on an erythematous base. Eruptions are divided into primary, latent, and recurrent.

- It is diagnosed with Tzanck prep, DFA testing, viral culture.

- Treatment is with oral antiviral agents. Patients must be educated that they can spread HSV-2 even in the absence of a clinical eruption (asymptomatic viral shedding).

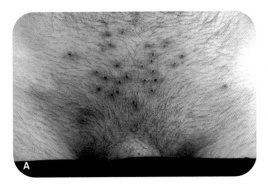
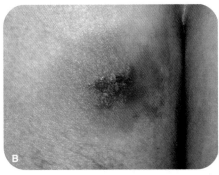

Figure 10-5 A HSV-2 outbreak on the penis and suprapubic skin. **B** Recurrent HSV-2 outbreak on the buttock.

vesicles on an erythematous base located on the vulva or vagina; however, lesions can also be found on the perineum, perianally, and the cervix. Another common location for recurrence is on the buttocks (Fig. 10-5B). Systemic symptoms such as lymphadenopathy, fever, dysuria, and rarely aseptic meningitis may occur.

In the latent phase, the HSV-2 virus is localized to a dorsal root ganglion, and no clinically active lesions are present. Triggers such as stress, immunosuppression, and acute medical illness may lead to reactivation. Recurrent HSV-2 infections clinically manifest as grouped vesicles on an erythematous base on the buttocks, perineum, vulva, or shaft of the penis. Again, these outbreaks are often heralded by a sense of tingling or pain in the region. There is a wide variety in the number of outbreaks per year. Outbreaks typically last approximately 1 week.

It is also important to note that many patients demonstrated to have serologic evidence of infection are asymptomatic and/or report no history of genital disease. Subclinical shedding of the herpes virus has been shown to occur in such patients.

DIAGNOSIS

Differential Diagnosis

Syphilis, chancroid, and lymphogranuloma venereum should be considered.

Diagnostic Methods

Similar to HSV-1 infection, a Tzanck smear can be performed on the vesicles to identify a herpes infection. However, DFA or viral culture should be performed to differentiate between HSV-1, HSV-2, and VZV infections.

In a case such as that presented above, proving the infection through culture and DFA is helpful. HSV-2 IgM and IgG antibodies can also be helpful in diagnosing primary infection.

TREATMENT

Treatment regimens are summarized in Table 10-2. Oral antiviral agents such as acyclovir, valacyclovir, and famciclovir have been shown to reduce the intensity and duration of both primary and recurrent HSV-2 outbreaks. For recurrent outbreaks, the medication should be taken as soon as the first signs of an outbreak are noted as an abortive medication.

Patients with severe recurrent outbreaks can be treated with suppressive therapy with these antiviral agents. Suppressive therapy not only decreases the frequency of outbreaks, it also reduces asymptomatic viral shedding thereby reducing the likelihood of transmitting HSV-2 to seronegative partners.

WHEN TO REFER

Treatment refractory cases may benefit from a dermatology and/or infectious disease consultation.

NOT TO BE MISSED

- Treat HSV-2 patients with a seronegative partner with daily suppressive therapy to prevent transmission.

Table 10-2 Treatment Regimens for Genital HSV

	ACYCLOVIR	FAMCICLOVIR	VALACYCLOVIR
Primary genital herpes infection	200 mg 5 times daily × 10 days	Not FDA approved	1 g BID × 10 days
Recurrent genital herpes outbreak	200 mg 5 times daily × 5 days	1 g BID × 1 day	500 mg BID × 3 days
Suppressive dose (healthy patients)	400 mg BID	250 mg BID	1 g or 500 mg once daily
Suppressive dose (immunocompromised patients)	Not established	Not established	500 mg BID

"AT A GLANCE" TREATMENT

- HSV type 2 therapy is summarized in Table 10-2.

COURSE AND COMPLICATIONS

HSV-2 infections can be challenging to treat as a result of their latent infection in the dorsal root ganglion. Primary infections and recurrent outbreaks can be managed with oral antiviral agents. However, even between outbreaks, patients can spread HSV-2. Asymptomatic viral shedding occurs in a high number of patients, and may be responsible for high rates of transmission. As a result, patients with partner who is seronegative for HSV-2 should be treated with daily suppressive therapy.

ICD9 Codes
054.9	*Herpes simplex without mention of complication*

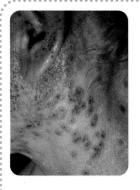

A 25-year-old male with a longstanding history of severe atopic dermatitis presents to your clinic with flaring atopic dermatitis over the last few days, and is not responding to the usual topical steroids. The flare seemed to have started with a few painful "sores" around the mouth, which then seemed to spread in the areas on his face and neck in which he has active eczema. He has cutaneous lesions as shown (Fig. 10-6). What is the best diagnosis? What treatment is necessary at this time?

Eczema Herpeticum

BACKGROUND

Eczema herpeticum, also known as Kaposi's varicelliform eruption, represents a widespread infection of HSV. It occurs in patients with a history of atopic dermatitis (eczema) or another dermatologic disease that impairs the barrier function of the epidermis, such as burns, ichthyosis vulgaris, Darier disease, pemphigus, or cutaneous T-cell lymphoma. These patients then develop an HSV outbreak that spreads rapidly across the skin due to epidermal impairment.

PATHOGENESIS

The impaired barrier function of the epidermis in certain dermatologic conditions allows for widespread dissemination of HSV. It is unclear exactly which molecular defects in these diseases allow for the dissemination to occur.

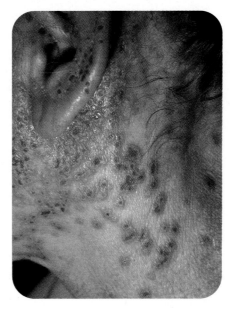

Figure 10-6 Eczema herpeticum in a patient with underlying atopic dermatitis.

CLINICAL PRESENTATION

Eczema herpeticum is most commonly seen in young children with a history of eczema. They are usually brought to the physician or emergency room for a severe eczema flare that is not responding to topical steroids. The preceding dermatologic disease is readily observed. Superimposed on this disease are monotonous vesicles, which transform into punched-out, grouped erosions and ulcers (Fig. 10-6). Oftentimes, the erosions become so closely grouped together that they overlap, forming larger erosions with a characteristic scalloped borders.

DIAGNOSIS

A high index of suspicion is necessary, as eczema herpeticum can become so widespread that the classic grouped vesicles on an erythematous base are not clinically apparent.

Similar to HSV infections, diagnosis is made via Tzanck smear, DFA, or viral culture. However, if there is a clinically high likelihood of eczema herpeticum, treatment should be initiated before the diagnostic laboratory results are available.

TREATMENT

Patients with eczema herpeticum require intravenous (IV) therapy with acyclovir. IV acyclovir at a dose of 10 mg/kg IV TID should be continued until all lesions have crusted over. The patient should then complete a 7 to 10 day course of treatment with oral agents, at doses appropriate for HSV as previously described. Patients may also benefit from long-term suppressive therapy with oral acyclovir or valacyclovir to prevent future recurrences, again at doses appropriate for HSV infections.

"AT A GLANCE" TREATMENT

• These patients require intravenous therapy with acyclovir 10 mg/kg IV TID until all lesions are crusted.
• The patient should then complete a 7- to 10-day course of treatment with oral agents, at doses appropriate for HSV as previously described in Table 10-2.

COURSE AND COMPLICATIONS

Patients with severe eczema herpeticum require close observation. If the eruption involves the face, an ophthalmologist should be consulted to evaluate for HSV keratitis, which may lead to blindness. If treated early, there are no long-term sequelae from eczema herpeticum. Bacterial superinfection may also occur; bacterial cultures should also be considered.

NOT TO BE MISSED

- Ophthalmologic evaluation is important in any patient with facial involvement.
- Treatment should initially be intravenous for all eczema herpeticum patients.

ICD9 Codes	
691.8	Other atopic dermatitis and related conditions
054.9	Herpes simplex without mention of complication
054.0	Eczema herpeticum

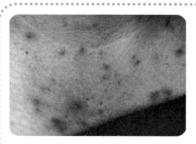

A 32-year-old woman presents with the chief complaint of, "I've got chicken pox!" She has three children at home, one of which has active "chicken pox" acquired at the day care center. The patient has never had a vaccination for varicella, and she did not have the primary infection as a child. On skin exam, she presents with pruritic, erythematous papules and vesicles on her face, trunk, and extremities (Fig. 10-7). Some lesions are crusted. How would you proceed with diagnosis and treatment?

Varicella Zoster Virus

BACKGROUND

Varicella zoster virus (VZV) is the cause of varicella (chicken pox) in children and zoster (shingles) in adults. While chickenpox and smallpox were differentiated in 1767, it was not until 1888 that physicians recognized the association between varicella and zoster.

PATHOGENESIS

Varicella is very contagious and is typically spread by respiratory droplets. VZV replicates and spreads throughout the body for approximately 2 weeks before the development of the cutaneous eruption. The patient is infectious until all skin lesions have crusted. During the cutaneous eruption, VZV invades nerves and spreads retrograde to involve the dorsal root ganglion where it becomes latent.

Zoster occurs from reactivation and replication of VZV in the dorsal root ganglion. Reactivation may be due to stress, illness, and immunosuppression or may occur spontaneously. The virus then spreads down the sensory nerve causing prodromal symptoms and the characteristic dermatomal cutaneous eruption.

CLINICAL PRESENTATION

Varicella typically begins with a viral prodrome of fevers, muscle pains, and fatigue for 1 to 2 days before the cutaneous eruption. Initial cutaneous lesions consist of extremely pruritic, erythematous macules and papules that begin on the face and spread downward. These papules then evolve quickly into small vesicles surrounded by an erythematous halo, known as "dew drops on a rose petal" (Fig. 10-7). As these vesicles mature, they crust over. Lesions in multiple stages of evolution are characteristic of varicella.

Zoster typically manifests with intense pain and pruritus for several days prior to developing the characteristic cutaneous eruption of grouped vesicles on an erythematous base (Fig. 10-8). Involvement of the 5th cranial nerve (Fig. 10-9) may lead to corneal involvement (Fig. 10-10).

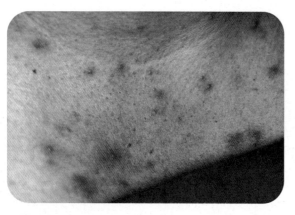

Figure 10-7 Primary varicella infection in a woman.

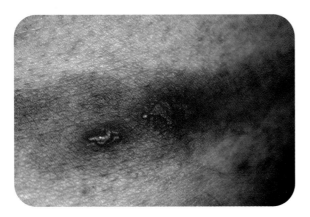

Figure 10-8 Dermatomal distribution of herpes zoster.

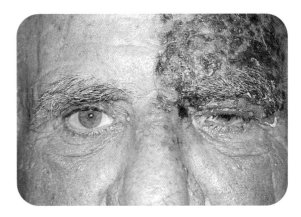

Figure 10-9 Herpes zoster in the fifth cranial nerve. From Tasman W, Jaeger E. *The Wills Eye Hospital Atlas of Clinical Ophthalmology*, 2nd ed. Lippincott Williams & Wilkins, 2001.

These patients should be evaluated by ophthalmology. Another variant is zoster involving the ear or conchal bowl—Ramsay-Hunt syndrome (Fig. 10-11). This syndrome should be considered in patients with facial nerve palsies, loss of taste, and dry mouth in addition to zosteriform lesions in the ear. Classically, the eruption is localized to a single dermatome; however, involvement of adjacent dermatomes can occur, as can widespread lesions in cases of "disseminated zoster." Bilateral zoster is rare, and should raise suspicion for immunodeficiency states such as HIV/AIDS.

DIAGNOSIS

Differential Diagnosis

Varicella: HSV, viral exanthems, drug eruption, pityriasis lichenoides et varioliformis acuta (PLEVA), and smallpox (characterized by monomorphic lesions, all at a single stage of development)

   Zoster: HSV, localized contact dermatitis, arthropod bites

KEY FEATURES

- Varicella zoster virus is the cause of varicella in children, and when reactivated, zoster in adults.

- Varicella presents clinically with pruritic, erythematous papules and vesicles classically described as "dew drops on a rose petal".

- Lesions of primary varicella are in multiple stages of development.

- Zoster presents clinically with a prodrome of burning, stinging, and itching for several days prior to developing the characteristic vesicles in a dermatomal distribution.

- Treatment for varicella consists of supportive therapy and possible early oral antiviral therapy.

- Treatment for zoster consists of oral antiviral therapy to reduce the severity of the infection and the likelihood of developing posterpetic neuralgia.

- Vaccines are currently available for both varicella and zoster.

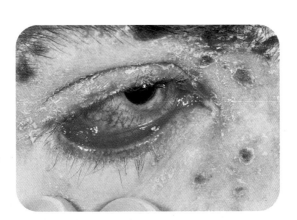

Figure 10-10 Herpes zoster ophthalmicus. From Gold DH, MD, and Weingeist TA. *Color Atlas of the Eye in Systemic Disease*. Baltimore: Lippincott Williams & Wilkins, 2001.

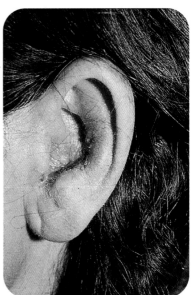

Figure 10-11 Herpes zoster in the 7th cranial nerve distribution (Ramsay-Hunt syndrome). Courtesy of Steven D. Handler, MD, MBE.

Diagnostic Methods

- Tzanck smear: performed as for HSV-1. However, does not differentiate HSV from VZV.
- Direct fluorescent antibody: again, performed as for HSV-1. DFA is a rapid test to differentiate HSV-1, HSV-2, and VZV.
- Viral culture: a very specific test, but not sensitive. VZV is difficult to culture and grows slowly, requiring at least 1 week.

TREATMENT

- Treatment regimens are summarized in Table 10-3.
- Primary varicella: supportive therapy consisting of antipyretics and antihistamines in healthy children. For children older than 2 years old and adults, oral acyclovir is FDA approved; it has been shown to decrease the severity and duration of VZV infection. Varicella zoster immunoglobulin (VZIG) can be administered within 96 hours of exposure to prevent primary varicella. VZIG is utilized in immunocompromised patients to prevent severe disease and in pregnant patients to prevent neonatal varicella.
- Zoster: acyclovir, valacyclovir, and famciclovir are all FDA approved for the treatment of zoster, and should ideally be initiated within 72 hours of onset. If the lesions are outside of a single dermatome (disseminated zoster), IV acyclovir therapy should be initiated.
- Postherpetic neuralgia: early initiation of antiviral therapy in zoster has been shown to reduce the incidence of postherpetic neuralgia. Topical therapies such as EMLA cream, lidocaine patches, and capsaicin cream can be used. However, severe cases should be treated with oral gabapentin (300 to 600 mg PO TID, to discontinue, taper over 7 days) and tricyclic antidepressants (nortriptyline 25 mg PO TID/QID; not to exceed 150 mg/d or amitriptyline 30 to 100 mg PO QHS)
- Vaccines:
  - Varivax®: a live, attenuated strain of VZV. The vaccine is administered in two doses (age 12 months, and 4 to 6 years). It has been shown to be 70% to 90% effective in preventing all cases of varicella, and more than 95% effective in preventing severe varicella infections. This vaccine is also available in a quadrivalent formulation (ProQuad®) with measles, mumps, and rubella vaccines.
  - Zostavax®: related to Varivax®, but approximately 14 times more concentrated. FDA approved for patients more than 60 years old with no history of previous zoster. Zostavax® has been shown to reduce the rates of zoster and postherpetic neuralgia.

Table 10-3 Treatment Regimens for Varicella/Herpes Zoster

	ACYCLOVIR	FAMCICLOVIR	VALACYCLOVIR
Varicella (pediatric dose)	20 mg/kg 4 times daily × 5 days	Not established	20 mg/kg TID × 5 days
Varicella (adult dose)	800 mg 4 times daily × 5 days	Not established	1 g TID × 5 days
Zoster	800 mg 5 times daily × 7–10 days	500 mg TID × 7 days	1 g TID × 7 days
Disseminated zoster (pediatric dose)	20 mg/kg IV q 8 hours × 7 days	Not established	Not established
Disseminated zoster (adult dose)	10 mg/kg IV q 8 hours × 7 days	Not established	Not established

WHEN TO REFER

- Primary varicella: adults and teenagers with systemic symptoms.

- Zoster: if lesions are disseminated or the patient develops severe postherpetic neuralgia.

- All patients with V1 (fifth cranial nerve) involvement should be evaluated by ophthalmology.

NOT TO BE MISSED

- Fifth cranial nerve involvement (V1) may cause herpes zoster ophthalmicus and untreated, blindness.

- Early antiviral therapy is helpful in preventing postherpetic neuralgia.

"AT A GLANCE" TREATMENT

- Treatment regimens for varicella/herpes zoster are summarized in Table 10-3.
- Postherpetic neuralgia:
  - Initiate antiviral therapy early.
  - Topical therapies such as EMLA cream, lidocaine patches, and capsaicin cream can be used.
  - Severe cases should be treated systemically:
    - oral gabapentin (300 to 600 mg PO TID, to discontinue, taper over 7 days)
    - nortriptyline 25 mg PO TID/QID; not to exceed 150 mg/d or amitriptyline 30 to 100 mg PO QHS
- Vaccines:
  - Varivax®: a live, attenuated strain of VZV. The vaccine is administered in two doses (age 12 months, and 4 to 6 years). This vaccine is also available in a quadrivalent formulation (ProQuad®) with measles, mumps, and rubella vaccines.
  - Zostavax®: FDA approved for patients older than 60 years with no history of previous zoster.

COURSE AND COMPLICATIONS

Primary varicella is typically a benign, self-limited infection and requires no intervention for healthy children. Rare, serious side effects such as Reye syndrome and cerebellar ataxia can occur. Adults developing primary varicella typically have a much more significant disease, with increased risk of VZV pneumonia, hepatitis, glomerulonephritis, optic neuritis, and vasculitis.

Zoster is also typically benign and self-limited. However, if it involves specific nerves, there may be serious side effects. Zoster involving the tip of the nose indicates involvement of the nasociliary nerve, and possible involvement of the optic nerve; ophthalmology should be consulted to evaluate. Also, if there are lesions on the ear or conchal bowl, Ramsay-Hunt syndrome should be considered and the patient evaluated for facial nerve palsies, loss of taste, and dry mouth. Finally, regardless of the affected region, patients may develop postherpetic neuralgia, characterized by severe pain persisting after the cutaneous eruption resolves. The risk of postherpetic neuralgia increases with age and immunosuppression.

ICD9 Codes	
052.9	Varicella without mention of complication
053.9	Herpes zoster without mention of complication
053.20	Herpes zoster dermatitis of eyelid

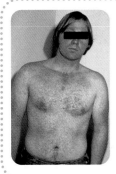

A 32-year-old man presents with a 2-day history of fevers and fatigue, and the development of a cutaneous eruption characterized by bright red erythema of his bilateral cheeks (Fig. 10-12). What is the most likely diagnosis? What systemic manifestations should be considered?

Viral Exanthems

BACKGROUND

Exanthems are defined as cutaneous manifestations of a general disease; enanthems are an eruption of the mucous membranes as a sign of a general disease. Viruses are the most common cause of exanthems in young children. While some viruses may result in characteristic eruptions, many viruses manifest with a nonspecific appearance.

PATHOGENESIS

Nonspecific viral exanthems are thought to be related to an immune reaction to the underlying viral infection. Following the initial infection and incubation period, a transient viremia occurs. Patients then mount an immune response to this viremia, which is thought to cause the cutaneous exanthem.

CLINICAL PRESENTATION

Nonspecific viral exanthems are characterized clinically by erythematous, blanchable macules and papules on the body (Fig. 10-12). These lesions typically begin on the trunk and spread to the extremities; sparing of the face is often observed. This eruption is also referred to as "maculopapular" or "morbilliform" for its resemblance to the cutaneous eruption of measles. Nonspecific viral exanthems may be associated with systemic symptoms such as fever, myalgias, fatigue, headaches, and gastrointestinal (GI) discomfort.

DIAGNOSIS

Differential Diagnosis

Nonspecific viral exanthems: enteroviruses and respiratory viruses (adenovirus, para-influenza virus, respiratory syncytial virus [RSV] and influenza virus); adverse cutaneous drug reactions (drug rashes)

   Specific viral exanthems: A full discussion is beyond the scope of this chapter, but includes such diseases as measles, rubella, roseola, Epstein-Barr virus (EBV), and parvovirus.

TREATMENT

No treatment is necessary for the majority of these exanthems. They are asymptomatic and self-limited. However, supportive care with antipyretics, oral antihistamines, and topical steroids may help the patient to be more comfortable.

KEY FEATURES

- Exanthems are manifestations of an underlying general disease.

- Viral exanthems can be very specific for an underlying disease or may be nonspecific manifestations.

- Clinically exanthems appear as blanchable, erythematous macules and papules. In some cases they may be associated with systemic symptoms.

- Majority of viral exanthems are benign, self-limited, and require no therapeutic intervention.

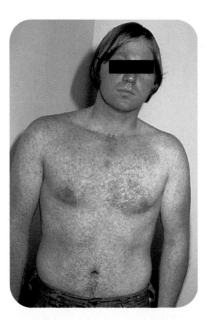

Figure 10-12 Viral exanthem. From Goodheart HP. *Goodheart's Photoguide to Common Skin Disorders,* 3rd ed. Philadelphia: Lippincott Williams & Wilkins, 2009.

CHAPTER 10 Viral Infections of the Skin

WHEN TO REFER

Patients should be referred when the exanthema does not resolve on its own in 1 to 2 weeks or when severe systemic symptoms develop.

NOT TO BE MISSED

- Exanthems associated with a clear viral infection should clear within 1 to 2 weeks. Quickly progressive or blistering rashes should be evaluated immediately.

- Exanthems with associated mucositis should be immediately evaluated by dermatology for progressive Stevens-Johnson syndrome.

"AT A GLANCE" TREATMENT

- Most exanthems do not require therapy as they are asymptomatic and self-limited
- Supportive care:
  - antipyretics (i.e., appropriate doses of acetaminophen or ibuprofen)
  - oral antihistamines (OTC diphenhydramine in appropriate dosage for age)
  - topical steroids (triamcinolone acetonide 0.1% BID as needed)

COURSE AND COMPLICATIONS

Nonspecific viral exanthems are considered benign and self-limited with the majority spontaneously self-resolving in 1 to 2 weeks. They are not typically associated with any severe systemic effects, although transient mild fatigue, fever, headaches, abdominal pain, and hepatic transaminitis may occur.

ICD9 Codes

057.9   Viral exanthem, unspecified

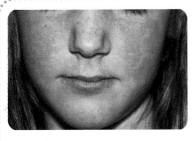

A 7-year-old girl presents with red cheeks (Fig. 10-13). Her mother reports she has had a low-grade fever and increased fatigue for about 3 days before the rash developed. She is otherwise feeling well. Mom would like to know if this is "slapped cheek disease."

Parvovirus B19 ("Erythema Infectiosum," "Fifth Disease")

BACKGROUND

Erythema infectiosum was first described clinically in 1889; it is also known as fifth disease in the numerical classification of childhood exanthems. While it was long considered to be related to a viral infection, it was not until 1975 that parvovirus B19 was isolated. Furthermore, it was not until 1983 that the causal association between parvovirus B19 and erythema infectiosum was identified.

KEY FEATURES

- Erythema infectiosum is caused by infection with Parvovirus B19.

- Clinically it manifests in two stages. First stage shows classic "slapped cheeks" appearance. Second stage manifests as erythematous macules of reticular appearance on extremities.

- Most cases are benign and self-limited with no treatment necessary.

(Continued)

PATHOGENESIS

Parvovirus B19 has a strong predisposition toward infecting erythroid progenitor cells. There is actually a specific cellular receptor on erythrocytes to which the virus binds. Following an incubation period of approximately 2 to 3 weeks, a transient viremia occurs. During this viremic period, anemia and reticulocytopenia may occur. Finally, as the patient develops IgG antibodies to parvovirus B19, the characteristic clinical appearance develops.

CLINICAL PRESENTATION

Erythema infectiosum occurs most commonly in children between the ages of 6 and 10. They often present with several days of prodromal symptoms such as fever and fatigue before developing an exanthem.

The initial clinical appearance consists of bright red erythematous macules on the bilateral cheeks with sparing of the midline face, nose, and perioral

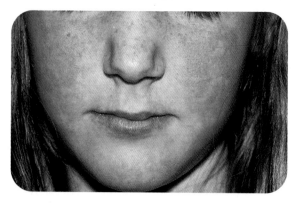

Figure 10-13 Erythema infectiosum secondary to parvovirus B19 infection. From Goodheart HP. *Goodheart's Photoguide to Common Skin Disorders*, 3rd ed. Philadelphia: Lippincott Williams & Wilkins, 2009.

areas (Fig. 10-13). Erythema infectiosum is also known as "slapped cheeks" disease for this characteristic clinical appearance during the first stage of the disease. A second stage develops 1 to 3 days later, consisting of erythematous macules in a reticular, lacy configuration on the extremities. The clinical eruption may also be accompanied by diffuse arthralgias.

A separate clinical entity associated with parvovirus B19 infection has been described in young adults. Patients develop typical edema and erythema of the palms and soles, as well as associated petechiae and purpura. This eruption is known as papular-purpuric gloves-and-socks syndrome and is also benign, requiring only supportive therapy.

DIAGNOSIS

Differential Diagnosis

Scarlet fever, rubella, measles, and nonspecific viral exanthem associated with enteroviral infection

Diagnostic Methods

The majority of cases can be diagnosed clinically when the classic eruption is present. However, in challenging cases, IgM antibodies to parvovirus B19 can be used to demonstrate an acute infection. Polymerase chain reaction (PCR) testing is also available.

TREATMENT

As erythema infectiosum is generally a benign, self-limited eruption, healthy children require only supportive therapy. There is no specific antiviral therapy or vaccine available for parvovirus B19 infections.

Transient aplastic crisis, a rare severe effect seen following parvovirus B19 infections, may require packed red blood cell transfusions. Fetuses of patients infected during the first or second trimester may also develop fetal anemia or hydrops fetalis; these patients require close, periodic ultrasound monitoring and possible in utero blood transfusions.

"AT A GLANCE" TREATMENT

- Erythema infectiosum is generally benign and self-limited. No cutaneous therapy is necessary
- Transient aplastic crisis rarely occurs. This requires inpatient management.
- Maternal infection with parvovirus B19:
  - Fetuses of patients infected during the first or second trimester may also develop fetal anemia or hydrops fetalis; these patients require close, periodic ultrasound monitoring and possible in utero blood transfusions.

COURSE AND COMPLICATIONS

The majority of cases of erythema infectiosum are benign and self-limited. However, in some cases, symptomatic and severe transient aplastic crisis can develop, particularly in those patients with pre-existing anemia or blood dyscrasias. Finally, pregnant patients developing acute parvovirus B19 infections are at risk of transmitting the infection transplacentally, causing fetal anemia or hydrops fetalis. As a result, patients with parvovirus B19 infections should be counseled to avoid pregnant women.

ICD9 Codes

057.0	Erythema infectiosum (fifth disease)
778.0	Hydrops fetalis not due to isoimmunization
284.01	Constitutional red blood cell aplasia
284.09	Other constitutional aplastic anemia
284.81	Red cell aplasia (acquired) (adult) (with thymoma)
284.89	Other specified aplastic anemias
284.9	Aplastic anemia, unspecified

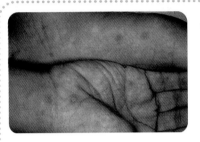

A 4-year-old boy presents with his mother due to his not feeling well. Mom noticed bumps on his hands and feet. He has had several days of fever and fatigue before the development of cutaneous lesions. Skin exam reveals small vesicles on an erythematous base on the palms and soles (Fig. 10-14) and about 10 yellow shallow ulcers on the tongue, buccal mucosa, palate, and tonsillar pillars.

Coxsackie Virus ("Hand-Foot-and-Mouth Disease")

BACKGROUND

Hand-foot-and-mouth disease (HFMD) was initially reported in 1958 following an outbreak of Coxsackie A16 virus in Toronto. A second outbreak occurred several years later in England. The eruptions were characterized by fever, oral lesions, and an acral vesicular eruption.

PATHOGENESIS

HFMD is most commonly associated with infections of coxsackie virus A16, a member of the enterovirus family. Enteroviruses are usually spread via respiratory or fecal-oral routes. They then infect epithelial cells in the pharynx or digestive tract, and initially replicate in lymphoid tissues. A viremia then results, producing an exanthem.

CLINICAL PRESENTATION

HFMD typically presents with a mild viral prodrome characterized by several days of fever and fatigue prior to the development of cutaneous lesions. The cutaneous manifestations of HFMD include small vesicles on an erythematous base on the palms and soles; similar lesions may be seen on the dorsum of the hands and feet (Fig. 10-14). Oral lesions manifest as erosive stomatitis, with

KEY FEATURES

- Hand-foot-and-mouth disease is associated most commonly with Coxsackie virus A19 infection, and more rarely, enterovirus-71 infection.

- Clinically it manifests as small vesicles on erythematous base on the palms and soles, as well as yellow shallow ulcers in the mouth.

- Typically it is a benign condition that requires no intervention.

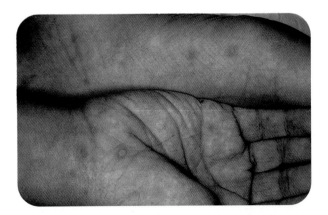

Figure 10-14 Hand-foot-and-mouth disease: vesicular papules on the palms secondary to Coxsackie A16 virus infection. From Fleisher GR, MD, Ludwig W, MD, Baskin MN, MD. *Atlas of Pediatric Emergency Medicine*. Philadelphia: Lippincott Williams & Wilkins, 2004.

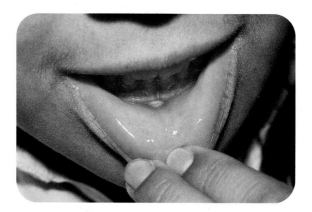

Figure 10-15 Hand-foot-and-mouth disease: shallow oval ulceration on the oral mucosa. From Goodheart HP. *Goodheart's Photoguide to Common Skin Disorders*, 3rd ed. Philadelphia: Lippincott Williams & Wilkins, 2009.

yellow shallow ulcers typically located on the tongue, buccal mucosa, palate, and tonsillar pillars (Fig. 10-15).

DIAGNOSIS

Differential Diagnosis

Aphthous ulcers/stomatitis or "canker sores," HSV infection, herpangina (similar oral ulcers, but no cutaneous exanthem, usually associated with Coxsackie virus infection), erythema multiforme, drug reaction, Kawasaki disease are in the differential.

Diagnostic Methods

This eruption is typically diagnosed clinically. A Tzanck smear, DFA, and/or viral culture can exclude HSV infection.

TREATMENT

No treatment is necessary, as the eruption is benign and self-limited. Lidocaine solution or gel may be used on painful erosive stomatitis either as a swish-and-spit (solution) or application of a thin layer of the gel 1 to 3 times daily as necessary.

"AT A GLANCE" TREATMENT

- No therapy is necessary.
- Symptomatic therapy for oral pain—lidocaine solution or gel—swish and spit 1 to 3 times daily as needed for pain

COURSE AND COMPLICATIONS

The majority of cases are mild, benign, and self-limited, particularly when associated with coxsackie A16 infections. Recently, however, there was an epidemic of severe HFMD associated with enterovirus-71 in Taiwan; these cases were associated with severe pulmonary and neurologic complications, as well as rare deaths associated with HFMD.

WHEN TO REFER

Patients should be referred if lesions do not self-resolve over several weeks. Additionally, patients with severe systemic symptoms should be referred for evaluation of pulmonary and neurologic manifestations.

NOT TO BE MISSED

- This infection is an enterovirus and may be quite infectious. Counsel patients to avoid close contact and to practice good hygiene while skin lesions are active.

ICD9 Codes

074.3   *Hand, foot, and mouth disease*

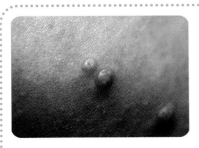

A 7-year-old girl presents with her mother due to "spreading bumps" on her face and neck. The girl participates in beauty pageants and her mother wants these lesions gone immediately. They have already tried a topical cream, which did not work, and they are frustrated. On exam, she has four discrete flesh colored 2- to 3-mm papules with a central umbilication on her right cheek and neck (Fig. 10-16). What is the most likely diagnosis? What therapy would be the next logical step?

Molluscum Contagiosum

BACKGROUND

Molluscum contagiosum is a relatively common and benign disease. It is present in two main age groups: (a) children who develop these lesions on the face, extremities, and hands through transmission by close play contact; and (b) young adults who develop these lesions on the genitalia through sexual contact.

PATHOGENESIS

Molluscum contagiosum is caused by a pox virus. There are actually two different molecular subtypes of the virus, molluscum contagiosum virus (MCV) I and II. These two different subtypes cause clinically and pathologically indistinguishable lesions.

KEY FEATURES

- Molluscum contagiosum is a common, benign viral infection caused by the poxvirus.

- Clinically lesions manifest as small white, shiny, umbilicated papules.

- In children, lesions often develop on face and extremities due to play.

- In young adults, lesions often develop in the groin due to sexual contact.

- Most lesions self-resolve in 1 to 2 years. If patients would like treatment, destructive therapies are necessary.

CLINICAL PRESENTATION

Molluscum lesions are firm white to waxy papules, typically 2 to 4 mm in size (Fig. 10-16). The classic description of a molluscum lesion includes a central umbilication. Depending on the age of the patient, lesions either occur on the face/extremities or in the groin. Disseminated, large lesions of molluscum can be a sign of immune dysfunction, particularly in the setting of HIV infection.

DIAGNOSIS

Differential Diagnosis

Condyloma acuminata, particularly when located in the groin. In severely immunosuppressed patients, infections such as cutaneous cryptococcus and histoplasmosis may appear very similar to molluscum.

Diagnostic Methods

Classic molluscum lesions can be diagnosed by visual inspection, particularly when the central umbilication is present. If there is any doubt, a small skin biopsy can be performed to demonstrate the characteristic molluscum bodies (Henderson-Patterson bodies), which are large intracytoplasmic inclusion bodies in the keratinocytes.

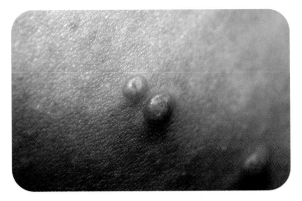

Figure 10-16 Molluscum contagiosum. Note the central umbilication on these discrete papules.

TREATMENT

The majority of molluscum lesions spontaneously self-resolve, although new spots may erupt as older ones disappear. For many children, treatment of the lesions may be more traumatic to the child than the actual molluscum lesion. If lesions are large, symptomatic, unsightly, embarrassing, or if parents are very concerned it is then reasonable to move forward with therapy. Most adult patients prefer to have their lesions treated.

WHEN TO REFER

Patients with numerous, large lesions should be evaluated for immune dysfunction and may require referral.

Treatment consists primarily of locally destructive options:

- Cryotherapy with liquid nitrogen: often applied using an open-spray or cotton-tipped applicator for approximately 10 to 30 seconds to generate a 2- to 3-mm iceball around the lesion (with cooling duration of approximately 20 to 60 seconds).
- Topical salicylic acid: available as monotherapy in over-the-counter products such as Mediplast, Compound W, Wart Off, Duofilm, or Dr. Scholls Clearaway. Additionally, topical salicylic acid administered in conjunction with other topical therapies may result in a synergistic effect. In a randomized study, combining 50% salicylic acid plaster products with topical 10% povidone-iodine solutions resulted in greater cure rates than salicylic acid alone. Topical salicylic acid 5% under occlusion administered with 5% sodium nitrite once daily was also more effective than salicylic acid alone.
- Topical imiquimod: a small amount of imiquimod (Aldara®) is applied to each lesion of molluscum three times a week. If there is no response, patients may need to increase application frequency to five times a week or even daily. Often requires 12 to 16 weeks of continuous therapy to observe a therapeutic effect.
- Curettage: manual scraping away of the molluscum lesion. In clinical trials, 80% of patient's molluscum lesions resolved after one treatment with curettage. However, this modality may be painful for young children and often requires the application of a topical anesthetic such as EMLA (Eutectic mixture of local anesthetics) in order for children to tolerate the procedure.
- Oral cimetidine: cimetidine is given at a dose of 35 mg/kg/day for at least 4 months. Approximately 50% of patients responded in a clinical trial, but this improvement was not statistically significant when compared to placebo.

"AT A GLANCE" TREATMENT

- Treatment is primarily destructive:
  - Liquid nitrogen
  - Curettage
  - Topical salicylic acid such as Compound W (salicylic acid 18% solution)
- Imiquimod 5% cream applied daily, up to 16 weeks may be successful in clearing lesions.

COURSE AND COMPLICATIONS

As mentioned, the majority of molluscum lesions spontaneously self-resolve. If treatment is offered, multiple visits and treatments may be necessary. There are no major complications associated with molluscum infections.

NOT TO BE MISSED

- Counsel adult patients with lesions confined to the genitalia that their sexual partner may have similar lesions. Both partners should have treatment to prevent passing the infection back and forth between partners.

ICD9 Codes

078.0   *Molluscum contagiosum*

Suggested Reading

Bacelieri R, Johnson SM. Cutaneous warts: an evidence-based approach to therapy. *Am Fam Physician.* 2005;72(4):647–652.

Berth-Jones J, Bourke J, Eglitis H, et al. Value of a second freeze-thaw cycle in cryotherapy of common warts. *Br J Dermatol.* 1994;131(6):883–886.

Cernik C, Gallina K, Brodell R. The treatment of herpes simplex infections: An evidence-based review. *Arch Intern Med.* 2008;168(11):1137–1144.

Cook K, Brownell I. Treatments for genital warts. *J Drugs Dermatol.* 2008;7(8):801–807.

Garland SM, Hernandez-Avila M, Wheeler CM, et al. Quadrivalent vaccine against human papillomavirus to prevent anogenital diseases. *N Engl J Med.* 2007;356(19):1928–1943.

Gibbs S, Harvey I. Topical treatments for cutaneous warts. *Cochrane Database Syst Rev* 2006;3:CD001781. DOI: 10.1002/14651858.CD001781.pub2.

Hengge UR, Esser S, Schultewolter T, et al. Self administered topical 5% imiquimod for the treatment of common warts and molluscum contagiosum. *Br J Dermatol.* 2000;143(5):1026–1031.

Lebrun-Vignes B, Bouzamondo A, Dupuy A, et al. A meta-analysis to assess the efficacy of oral antiviral treatment to prevent genital herpes outbreaks. *J Am Acad Dermatol.* 2007;57(2):238–246.

Nasser M, Fedorowicz Z, Khoshnevisan MH, et al. Acyclovir for treating primary herpetic gingivostomatitis. *Cochrane Database Syst Rev.* 2008;4: CD006700. DOI: 10.1002/14651858.CD006700.pub2.

Oxman MN, Levin MJ, Johnson GR, et al. A vaccine to prevent herpes zoster and postherpetic neuralgia in older adults. *N Engl J Med.* 2005;352:2271–2284.

Scott LA, Stone MS. Viral exanthems. *Dermatol Online J.* 2003;9:4.

van der Wouden JC, et al. Interventions for cutaneous molluscum contagiosum. *Cochrane Database Syst Rev.* 2006;2: CD004767. DOI: 10.1002/14651858.CD004767.pub2.

von Krogh G. Management of anogenital warts (condylomata acuminata). *Eur J Dermatol.* 2001;11(6):598–603.

Wald A, Zeh J, Selke S, et al. Reactivation of genital herpes simplex virus type 2 infection is asymptomatic seropositive persons. *N Eng J Med.* 2000;342:844–850.

Weibel RE, Neff BJ, Kuter BJ, et al. Live attenuated varicella virus vaccine. Efficacy trial in healthy children. *N Engl J Med.* 1984;310:1409–1415.

Yilmaz E, Alpsoy E, Basaran E. Cimetidine therapy for warts: a placebo-controlled, double-blinded study. *J Am Acad Dermatol.* 1996;34(6):1005–1007.

CHAPTER 11 Benign Neoplasms

Juliana L. Basko-Plluska

Neoplasms of the skin are derived from proliferation of the different types of cells residing in the epidermis, dermis, or subcutaneous tissue. Epidermal growths are due to the proliferation of basal cells and keratinocytes and are characterized clinically by excessive accumulation of keratin or scale. Pigmented growths are due to the proliferation of pigment-forming cells and melanocytes, and they have a characteristic light to dark brown color. Finally, dermal growths are derived from the proliferation of the various types of cells residing in the dermis (e.g., fibroblasts, neurons, endothelial cells) and present clinically as firm, indurated papules or nodules. This chapter will provide a general overview of the most commonly encountered benign neoplasms of the skin.

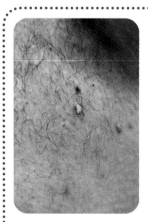

A 55-year-old diabetic woman complains of an old skin growth on her axilla (Fig. 11-1). She first noted a tiny, nonpainful "soft bump" last year, but over time, the lesion grew larger. The patient denies any symptoms but is concerned about the few times when the lesion got irritated by rubbing on jewelry. Upon examination, a 2-mm skin-colored, pedunculated papilloma is present on the right side of the neck. It is nontender and easily moveable with manipulation. What is the most likely diagnosis?

Skin Tags

BACKGROUND/EPIDEMIOLOGY

A skin tag, also known as an acrochordon, is a very common, benign epidermal growth in middle-aged individuals and the elderly. The overall prevalence in the adult population is approximately 25%; the prevalence reaches 60% at the age of 70. Skin tags are more common in females than males and typically affect the intertriginous areas (axilla, groin, and inframammary regions) as well as the neck and the eyelids. Patients usually complain of slow-growing fleshy bumps, which are cosmetically unappealing.

PATHOGENESIS

The pathogenesis of acrochordons remains unknown. They are an obligatory lesion in acanthosis nigricans (Fig. 11-2), and are commonly associated with acromegaly and pregnancy, suggesting that high levels of circulating growth hormone may play a role. Recent studies have shown that patients with multiple skin tags have a higher frequency of diabetes (23% versus 8.51%). It is likely that multiple skin tags may serve as a cutaneous marker for impaired insulin sensitivity in patients with no previously known impaired glucose metabolism.

KEY FEATURES

- Skin tags are benign epidermal growths, common in middle-aged individuals and the elderly.

- Typically they present as an asymptomatic, skin-colored, pedunculated papilloma.

- Typical sites of distribution are the intertriginous areas, neck, and eyelids.

- Diagnosis is made by visual inspection.

- Treatment is indicated for cosmetic purposes unless the lesion is frankly inflamed or has questionable morphology for a skin cancer.

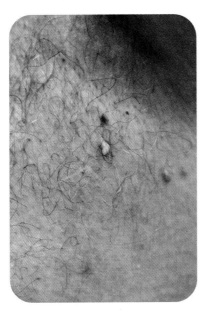

Figure 11-1 Small, 1- to 2-mm furrowed papules, commonly found in the neck and the axilla.

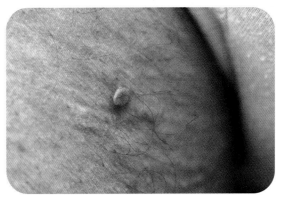

Figure 11-2 Large, pedunculated papillomas on the lower parts of the body.

Occasionally, multiple acrochordons and multiple flesh-colored facial papules (fibrofolliculoma/trichodiscoma) are seen. These patients should be evaluated for Birt-Hogg-Dube (BHD) syndrome, although it remains to be determined whether skin tags can be used as markers for these two conditions. In patients with other skin findings of BHD syndrome, consider gene analysis for definite diagnosis. Patients with BHD have an increased risk for pulmonary cysts/spontaneous pneumothoraces and renal cell carcinoma; therefore, screening abdominal ultrasounds are suggested for the patient and first-degree family members.

Unlike adult skin tags, childhood skin tags deserve special attention, as they may be the first manifestation of nevoid basal cell carcinoma syndrome, a rare autosomal dominant syndrome characterized by multiple basal cell carcinomas and multiple systemic anomalies.

CLINICAL PRESENTATION

Three types of acrochordon have been classically described:

- Small, 1- to 2-mm furrowed papules, commonly found in the neck and the axilla (often called "skin tags") (Fig. 11-1)
- Single or thread-like, 2- to 5-mm papules on areas other than the neck and the axilla
- Large, pedunculated papillomas on the lower parts of the body, often called "fibroepithelial polyps" (Fig. 11-2)

Wiggling of the pedunculated lesions back and forth does not ordinarily elicit any tenderness, unless there is irritation or torsion of the skin tag.

DIAGNOSIS

Differential Diagnosis

Skin tags can be confused with pedunculated seborrheic keratosis (SK), compound melanocytic nevus, solitary neurofibroma, viral warts, or molluscum contagiosum (Table 11-1).

Diagnostic Methods

Diagnosis is made by visual inspection.

WHEN TO REFER

Referral to a dermatologist for simple acrochordon(s) is not necessary. If nevoid basal cell carcinoma syndrome is suspected, referral to a pediatric dermatologist is indicated. If a history or a question of Birt-Hogg-Dube syndrome arises, consider a renal ultrasound and referral to dermatology for a full skin exam and appropriate biopsies. Also, gene analysis may be obtained for more definitive diagnosis.

Table 11-1 Differential Diagnosis of Skin Tags

DIAGNOSIS	KEY FEATURES
Pedunculated seborrheic keratosis	Tan to dark-brown papules or plaques with stuck-on appearance and greasy surface. Mainly on the sun-exposed areas, sparing the palms and soles. Often asymptomatic, but may itch or bleed.
Compound melanocytic nevus	Tan to brown, up to 6 mm dome-shaped nevus with symmetric borders and uniform pigmentation. May be congenital or acquired.
Solitary neurofibroma	Asymptomatic hyperpigmented nodules measuring few mm to 4–5 cm. Occasional positive Tinel sign.
Viral warts	Firm papules with verrucous surface, mainly on the fingers and soles. Often asymptomatic, except plantar warts. Transmission by autoinoculation, direct skin contact, or sexual contact.
Molluscum contagiosum	Dome-shaped papule with central umbilication and pearly appearance. Tends to spare the palms and soles. Children and immunosuppressed patients are mostly affected.

TREATMENT

Asymptomatic skin tags are removed if indicated for cosmetic purposes.

- Cryotherapy: liquid nitrogen is used to freeze the lesion at the base. Side effect: temporary posttreatment hypopigmentation.
- Snipping with scissors at the base: no local anesthesia is required
- Excision with sharp blade: no local anesthesia is required
- Ligation with suture tied around the base: no local anesthesia is required, but it hurts
- Electrodessication: an electric current is used to destroy the skin tag; cauterization can be used to stop the bleeding. Side effects: temporary posttreatment hypopigmentation

"AT A GLANCE" THERAPY

- First-line therapy:
  - Liquid nitrogen: quick and easy. Downside is that LN2 hurts more and it takes about a week for the lesion to fall off.
  - Scissors (sharp Gradle scissors work best): snip at base of lesion
- Second-line therapy:
  - Sharp blade excision (#15 blade)
  - Ligation at base with a tied suture
  - Electrodessication

NOT TO BE MISSED

- Skin tags in children should elevate suspicion for nevoid basal cell carcinoma syndrome.
- Patients with multiple fleshy facial papules and multiple neck and axillary skin tags should be evaluated for Birt-Hogg-Dube syndrome.

COURSE AND COMPLICATIONS

Skin tags are permanent growths with no potential for malignant transformation. They tend to recur after surgical removal.

ICD9 Code

701.9   *Unspecified hypertrophic and atrophic conditions of skin*

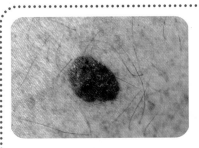

A 50-year-old woman with a history of chronic sunburns complains of several skin lesions on her back and chest area, which have recently started to itch (Fig. 11-3). The patient denies any other symptoms but is worried about skin cancer. Upon examination, a few scattered warty-like lesions with a "stuck-on" appearance are noted. What is the most likely diagnosis?

Seborrheic Keratosis

BACKGROUND/EPIDEMIOLOGY

Seborrheic keratosis (SK) is a common benign epidermal tumor, which results from the clonal proliferation of immature keratinocytes. It is found with increasing numbers and increasing age. In one study, individuals older than age 64 years were examined and 88% had at least one SK lesion. These lesions are less common on darker-skinned individuals and there is no gender predominance.

KEY FEATURES

- Seborrheic keratosis (SK) is a common benign epidermal tumor, possibly related to chronic sun exposure.

- Typically they present as a verrucous, warty-like papule with a "stuck-on" appearance.

- Typical locations are the trunk and extremities, starting in middle-aged individuals; it tends to spare the palms, soles, and mucosal surfaces.

- Diagnosis is made by visual inspection.

- Therapy is not needed, but when necessary or desired it consists of cryotherapy or curettage.

PATHOGENESIS

The precise etiology of SK is not well understood. Higher incidence on the sun-exposed areas suggests that chronic sun exposure may play a role. Some studies suggest SK may be inherited in an autosomal dominant fashion; a clear genetic locus has not yet been determined. Mutations in fibroblast growth factor receptor 3, which regulates cell growth, have been noted in 40% to 85% of examined SK lesions. The deeply pigmented variant of SK often has a mutation in endothelin-1. The exact cause of the growth due to these mutations is not yet known.

CLINICAL PRESENTATION

Seborrheic keratosis starts as a sharply defined, light-brown macule, which later develops into a verrucous, warty-like papule with a "stuck-on" appearance. It affects mainly middle-aged to elderly individuals; almost everyone over the age of 50 has at least one SK. The lesions are usually asymptomatic, but can occasionally itch or bleed upon irritation. The trunk is most often affected; the palms, soles, and the mucosal surfaces are often spared. Dark-skinned individuals tend to develop a variant of SK, called *dermatosis papulosa nigra*, which presents as smaller, heavily pigmented lesions in younger individuals, often presenting on the face (Fig. 11-4).

Seborrheic keratoses are totally benign. Collision tumors of SK and other skin malignancies have been reported, mainly squamous cell carcinoma and rarely melanoma. In cases of a typical-appearing SK, a biopsy is not necessary for confirmation. When a typical SK changes or the appearance is atypical, a biopsy is indicated.

An association between the sudden, explosive appearance of multiple seborrheic keratoses and internal malignancies, most often adenocarcinoma of the gastrointestinal tract, has also been reported, known as "the sign of Leser-Trélat." This type of sudden explosive growth of SK may also accompany severe sunburn, eczema flare, or other severe inflammatory dermatosis. Finally, eruptive seborrheic keratoses may also occur in association with leukemia, lymphoma, or human immunodeficiency virus (HIV).

DIAGNOSIS

Upon examination, well-circumscribed, light- to dark-brown papules or plaques with an adherent greasy scale and tiny keratotic dots studding the surface are noted. They may vary in size from 1 mm to 5 cm or greater and are often uniformly pigmented. Close inspection with a hand lens demonstrates the presence of pseudohorn cysts and dark keratin plugs. Typical examples of

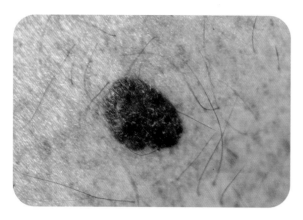

Figure 11-3 Seborrheic keratosis: this is an atypical-appearing lesion with clearly visible pseudohorn cysts.

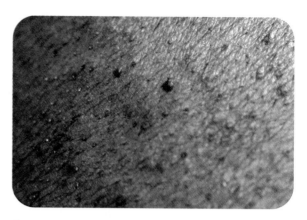

Figure 11-4 Dermatosis papulosis nigra on the cheek of an African-American woman.

benign SK are shown in Figures 11-3 to 11-7. An irritated and subsequently necrotic SK is shown in Figure 11-7.

Differential Diagnosis

SK can oftentimes be confused with malignant melanoma, squamous cell carcinoma, actinic keratosis, viral warts, and solar lentigo (Table 11-2).

Diagnostic Methods

Diagnosis is made by visual inspection. A biopsy is indicated for questionable or changing lesions.

THERAPY

Benign-appearing seborrheic keratoses are treated, if indicated, for cosmetic purposes. The following treatment modalities exist:

- Cryotherapy: the standard treatment for thin seborrheic keratoses, which produces cosmetically acceptable results to patients. The downside is the risk for post-treatment hypopigmentation and recurrence.

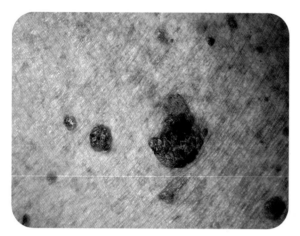

Figure 11-5 Multiple seborrheic keratoses on the back.

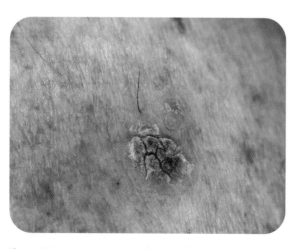

Figure 11-6 Waxy-appearing seborrheic keratosis.

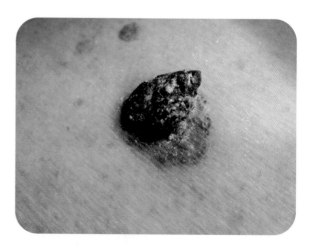

Figure 11-7 Necrotic and irritated seborrheic keratosis.

Table 11-2 Differential Diagnosis of Seborrheic Keratosis

DIAGNOSIS	KEY FEATURES
Malignant melanoma	Dark brown to black, nonhomogenous melanocytic lesions measuring >6 mm in diameter, which may itch or bleed. Lesions have a tendency for rapid growth. Risk factors: light skin, prolonged sun exposure, dysplastic nevi, family history of melanoma
Squamous cell carcinoma	Sharply defined, scaly, erythematous patch, papule, or nodule, which may ulcerate. Risk factors: light skin, chronic sun exposure/phototherapy, exposure to industrial carcinogens, organ transplantation/ immunosuppression
Actinic keratosis	Discrete, yellow-brown to slightly erythematous papules with adherent scale and a rough/ sandpaper-like consistency on the habitually sun-exposed areas
Viral wart	Firm papules with verrucous surface affecting mainly the fingers and soles
Solar lentigo	Asymptomatic, evenly pigmented light brown patch on the sun-exposed areas. It may not be possible to differentiate lentigo from flat SK.

- Electrocautery: less effective than cryotherapy for thin lesions. The downside risk is for posttreatment skin hypopigmentation.
- Shave excision: horizontal slicing of the affected skin extending to the level of mid-dermis. Well-suited for epidermal growths. There is postoperative scarring and occasionally pigmentary change.
- Curettage: lesions are very superficial and "stuck-on." They can be removed with a curette or edge of a #15 scalpel blade.

"AT A GLANCE" THERAPY

- First-line therapy:
  - Cryotherapy: the standard treatment for thin seborrheic keratoses
- Second-line therapy:
  - Electrocautery: carefully done, this method is very effective for thin SK; not appropriate for thick lesions.
  - Shave excision: horizontal slicing of the affected skin extending to the level of mid-dermis. Well-suited for thicker epidermal growths. There is postoperative scarring and occasionally pigmentary change. Best option for thick SK.

WHEN TO REFER

Referral to a dermatologist is recommended when the lesions appear suspicious for skin cancer or when inflammation, bleeding, and/or ulceration occur. Dermatologists may also perform cosmetic removals of SK lesions.

COURSE AND COMPLICATIONS

Seborrheic keratoses are permanent growths that may enlarge and become thicker over time, but have no potential for malignant transformation.

NOT TO BE MISSED

- Changing lesions with atypical features should be biopsied to evaluate for malignant melanoma.

ICD9 Codes

702.11   *Inflamed seborrheic keratosis*
702.19   *Other seborrheic keratosis*

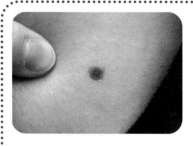

A 24-year-old white woman presents for an evaluation of a nonpainful brown "mark" on her left breast, which she first noticed a month ago. The patient denies any family history of melanoma or other skin cancers. On exam, you find a hyperpigmented macule with well-defined borders and uniform coloration, measuring 4 × 5 mm (Fig. 11-8). What is the most likely diagnosis?

Nevi

BACKGROUND/EPIDEMIOLOGY

A nevus, commonly referred to as a mole, is a benign overgrowth (hamartoma) of melanocytes, the pigment-producing cells. During the early developmental stages of a nevus, melanocytes migrate from the neural crest and aggregate at the dermoepidermal junction and give rise to a junctional nevus. Melanocytic aggregates may grow into the underlying dermis forming a compound nevus. As melanocytic aggregates migrate further down into the dermis (leaving the epidermis entirely), a dermal nevus is formed. This histologic progression of nevus cells correlates with the physical appearance of the nevus. Normally, junctional nevi appear flat whereas compound and dermal nevi are raised.

KEY FEATURES

- Nevi are benign hamartomas of melanocytes within the epidermis and/or dermis.

- Physical findings vary on the specific type of the nevus; symmetry, regular borders, uniform pigmentation, and diameter <6 mm are characteristic of a benign nevus.

- Diagnosis is made by visual inspection.

- The majority of benign nevi require no treatment.

- Lesions with atypical features and/or with changing features should be biopsied to evaluate for evolving malignant melanoma.

PATHOGENESIS

The number of nevi in an individual is determined by a combination of genetic factors and the degree of sun exposure. Some benign nevi are present at birth, which likely represent errors in embryologic migration. Most nevi are acquired during childhood, reaching a peak in adulthood (4th to 5th decades). Late-acquired nevi have a higher risk of transforming into a melanoma.

CLINICAL PRESENTATION

Benign nevi are classified into several major types and are defined in Table 11-3 (Figs. 11-8 to 11-12).

DIAGNOSIS

Differential Diagnosis

Malignant melanoma, seborrheic keratosis, dermatofibroma are in the differential.

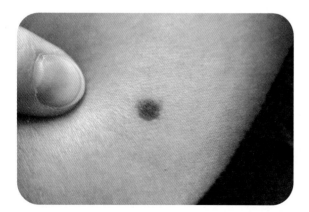

Figure 11-8 Compound nevus on the outer breast of a woman.

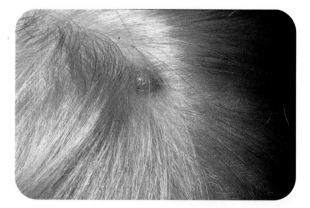

Figure 11-9 Spindle and epithelioid cell nevus (Spitz) on the scalp of a child. From Elder AD, Elenitsas R, Johnson BL, et al. *Synopsis and Atlas of Lever's Histopathology of the Skin*. Lippincott Williams & Wilkins, Philadelphia, 1999:2, 163, 167.

Table 11-3 Characteristics of Nevi

TYPE OF NEVUS	TYPICAL FEATURES
Congenital/ Acquired nevus Fig. 11-8	*Epidemiology:* appear at birth (congenital); childhood (early-acquired); or into middle age *Pathogenesis:* proliferation of normal melanocytes at the dermoepidermal junction. *History:* undergo morphologic changes until body growth completed. Minimal risk of malignant transformation. The types are indistinguishable later in life. *Physical exam:* well-circumscribed, evenly pigmented light to dark-brown nevus measuring <6 mm in diameter. Larger congenital nevi can measure up to 20 mm and often have a pebbled and hairy surface. No preferential body site
Spindle and epithelioid cell (Spitz) nevus Fig. 11-9	*Epidemiology:* found exclusively in fair-skinned individuals, usually as a solitary lesion. ~50% appear by age 10. Rarely seen in patients older than age 40 *Pathogenesis:* unknown *History:* characterized by a rapid initial growth phase; lesions develop abruptly within months but may regress with time *Physical exam:* hairless, well-circumscribed papule or nodule. Color may vary from pink to red to brown or black. Most commonly distributed on the head and neck region
Blue nevus Fig. 11-10	*Epidemiology:* appears in childhood or late adolescence and is more common in the Asian populations *Pathogenesis:* dermal melanocytes producing heavy pigmentation *History:* asymptomatic *Physical exam:* blue or blue-black papules to nodules, usually <10 mm in diameter Most commonly on the dorsa of the hands or feet (50%)
Halo nevus Fig. 11-11	*Epidemiology:* overall prevalence 1%. Onset usually during the first three decades. Seen in association with vitiligo (18%–26%) or in patients with metastatic melanoma. *Pathogenesis:* immune reaction against self-melanocytes, resulting in a decrease of melanin production or disappearance of melanocytes at the dermoepidermal junction *History:* most often undergo spontaneous involution, with regression of the centrally located pigmented nevus *Physical exam:* <5 mm papules with a peripheral rim of hypopigmentation and a centrally located pigmented nevus
Dysplastic nevus Fig. 11-12	*Epidemiology:* most common in fair-skinned individuals. May develop at any age and may be associated with heritable melanoma syndrome or dysplastic nevus syndrome *Pathogenesis:* de novo vs. transformation of a pre-existing nevus *History:* high risk of malignant transformation *Physical exam:* a light to dark brown papule or nodule exhibiting one of the ABCDEs of melanoma (asymmetry, irregular borders, irregular color, diameter >6 mm, evolution)

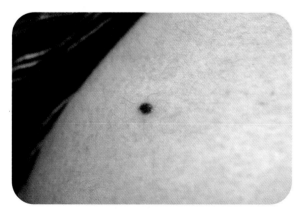

Figure 11-10 Blue nevus on the inner thigh.

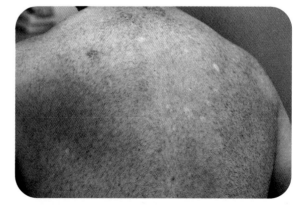

Figure 11-11 Multiple depigmented patches on the back of a man with vitiligo. These lesions are halo nevi, though most of the nevi within are gone.

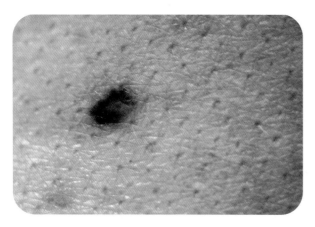

Figure 11-12 Atypical nevus. On biopsy, this lesion was graded as severely atypical.

Diagnostic Methods

Diagnosis is made by visual inspection. Biopsy may be indicated for histologic confirmation of the following types of nevi if they appear clinically suspicious: Spitz, blue, halo, and dysplastic nevi.

THERAPY

Most congenital nevi do not require any treatment and are followed clinically or with routine photographs to document changes.

- Congenital/early-acquired nevi: surgical excision, or dermabrasion can be used if indicated for cosmetic purposes. Laser therapy is not indicated for removal of nevi.
- Spitz nevi: treatment remains controversial. Some dermatologists believe that no treatment is necessary, whereas others recommend a subtotal excision with clinical follow-up when pathology is unequivocal. Yet other dermatologists recommend complete excision with re-excision if positive margins. Recently, a treatment algorithm was proposed, according to which all Spitz nevi should be biopsied. Those with typical pathology should be followed clinically, whereas those with atypical pathology can be either followed clinically or completely excised; this is left to the discretion of the dermatologist.
- Blue nevi: do not need to be excised if stable and less than 10 mm in diameter. Atypical morphologic changes should be followed with excision and histologic evaluation to rule out melanoma.
- Halo nevi: treatment remains controversial. Halo nevi with banal features are usually not treated; an atypical halo nevus with color variation and irregular borders must be excised.
- Dysplastic nevi: all suspicious atypical nevi with multiple concerning features should undergo biopsy. All patients with multiple dysplastic nevi should be followed by a dermatologist at regular intervals.

COURSE AND COMPLICATIONS

Almost all nevi remain unchanged through life and risk of malignant transformation is low. Dysplastic nevi have a higher rate of malignant transformation than the other types and must be followed periodically.

It is important to recognize that not all melanomas develop in pre-existing nevi. In patients with many dysplastic nevi, even removal of every nevus would not prevent a melanoma from occurring. Fifty to sixty percent of melanomas arise from previously normal skin and not from a "precursor" lesion such as a dysplastic nevus. Therefore, removal of only suspicious atypical or changing lesions is recommended.

WHEN TO REFER

- Referral to a dermatologist is warranted if the nevus displays any of the ABCDEs of melanoma. Consider referring patients with many questionable or atypical lesions and/or a family history of melanoma in a primary relative (i.e., mother/father/brother/sister) for a minimum of a yearly skin exam.

- If biopsies are done in a primary care situation, it is important to be aware of the standards of care for re-excision of atypical lesions. A conservative rule of thumb is to re-excise with a reasonable margin of normal tissue (3 to 5 mm) any nevus with at least any moderate atypia and involved margins. All severely atypical nevi, whether pathologic margins are clear or involved, should be re-excised with an elliptical excision with a margin of 5 mm. Refer any questionable lesions to a dermatologist for consultation.

- A good rule for deciding whether to biopsy: if the patient is worried about the lesion and it is changing, consider biopsy or referral for complete removal.

ICD9 Codes	
216.X	*Nevus*
216.0	*Benign neoplasm of skin of lip*
216.1	*Benign neoplasm of eyelid, including canthus*
216.2	*Benign neoplasm of ear and external auditory canal*
216.3	*Benign neoplasm of skin of other and unspecified parts of face*
216.4	*Benign neoplasm of scalp and skin of neck*
216.5	*Benign neoplasm of skin of trunk, except scrotum*

NOT TO BE MISSED

- Dysplastic nevi with changing features.

- Atypical halo nevi.

- Partial biopsies of nevi are not sufficient to rule out melanoma in a suspicious lesion. Sampling of the entire lesion is necessary, especially if histopathology does not match clinical suspicion.

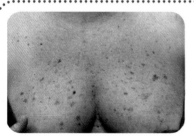

A 55-year-old white woman complains of brown "marks" on her chest for years (Fig. 11-13). She denies any changes in morphology or any symptoms associated with these lesions. Upon examination, multiple 2- to 10-mm uniformly brown macules are on sun-exposed areas of the previously sun-exposed chest, neck, and on the face. The lesions are nontender and nonkeratotic on palpation. What is the differential diagnosis?

Solar Lentigines

BACKGROUND/EPIDEMIOLOGY

Solar lentigo (plural: lentigines), also commonly referred to as a "liver spot" or "old-age" spot. Fair-skinned individuals are at higher risk; dark-skinned individuals who have more melanin at baseline are rarely affected. Solar lentigines typically first appear during the fourth decade of life and subsequently increase in number with age. More than 90% of people at the age of 60 have developed solar lentigines.

CHAPTER 11 Benign Neoplasms

KEY FEATURES

- Solar lentigines are a benign proliferation of normal melanocytes secondary to chronic solar damage.

- Typically they appear as an asymptomatic light brown macules.

- They appear primarily on sun-exposed areas sites.

- Diagnosis is made by visual inspection.

- Treatment options, if indicated for cosmetic purposes, include laser surgery, cryosurgery, topical retinoids, and chemical peel.

PATHOGENESIS

A solar lentigo is a benign proliferation of normal melanocytes secondary to chronic solar damage. On histology, an increased number of melanocytes are seen at the dermoepidermal junction with subsequent increased melanin production. Solar lentigines occur mainly on the sun-exposed areas.

CLINICAL PRESENTATION

Upon examination, sharply demarcated, evenly pigmented light to dark brown macules ranging in size from 1 to 5 cm (Fig. 11-13) are noted on the sun-exposed areas (the face, dorsa of the hands, arms, and the back). Occasionally, several macules may coalesce into larger lesions in the areas that have undergone severe solar damage.

DIAGNOSIS

In general, a solar lentigo is uniform in pigmentation, both at a distance and on close examination. Solar lentigo can be confused with superficial spreading malignant melanoma; lentigo maligna (in situ melanoma); lentigo maligna melanoma (invasive); SK; and freckles (ephilid).

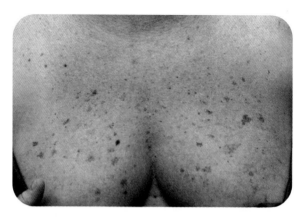

Figure 11-13 Solar lentigines on the chest of a woman.

Diagnostic Methods

Diagnosis is made by visual inspection.

THERAPY

Solar lentigines are treated if indicated for cosmetic purposes. Effective treatment options include:

- Cryosurgery: cycles of liquid nitrogen spraying for a total of 3 to 5 seconds to the affected areas × 1. Melanocytes, which are more sensitive to liquid nitrogen than other types of skin cells, are selectively destroyed. If liquid nitrogen is applied for more than 10 sec/cycle, skin depigmentation can occur.
- Topical retinoids (tretinoin alone or in combination with mequinol) may help.
- Chemical peeling with trichloroacetic acid
- Laser surgery: currently the treatment of choice. Specific lasers, which selectively destroy the pigment within the lesion, can eliminate up to 80% of lesions in one single treatment, with few side effects.

COURSE AND COMPLICATIONS

Solar lentigines are completely benign lesions.

WHEN TO REFER

There is no need for referral when the diagnosis is certain. For irregular or changing lesions, consider referral to a dermatologist for biopsy.

NOT TO BE MISSED

- Any changing lesion should be biopsied to evaluate for lentigo maligna-type melanoma.

ICD9 Codes

709.09	Other dyschromia
172.0	Malignant melanoma of skin of lip
172.1	Malignant melanoma of skin of eyelid, including canthus
172.2	Malignant melanoma of skin of ear and external auditory canal
172.3	Malignant melanoma of skin of other and unspecified parts of face
172.4	Malignant melanoma of skin of scalp and neck
172.5	Malignant melanoma of skin of trunk, except scrotum
172.6	Malignant melanoma of skin of upper limb, including shoulder
172.7	Malignant melanoma of skin of lower limb, including hip
172.8	Malignant melanoma of other specified sites of skin
172.9	Melanoma of skin, site unspecified
702.19	Other seborrheic keratosis

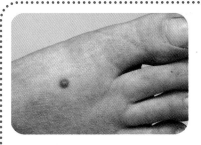

A 35-year-old woman complains of a slightly painful, firm nodule on her dorsal right foot (Fig. 11-14). She first noted it a few months ago at the site where she had sustained a prior black fly bite. Upon examination, a firm, light brown nodule measuring 1 cm in diameter is noted on the right dorsal foot. The nodule is slightly tender to palpation and dimples inward with lateral compression. What is the most likely diagnosis?

Dermatofibroma

BACKGROUND/EPIDEMIOLOGY

Solitary dermatofibroma, also known as benign fibrous histiocytoma, is a common lesion which affects mainly young to middle-aged females (female-to-male, 4:1). A dermatofibroma typically occurs on the lower extremities, and is hardly ever found on the head, palms, and soles. It is usually asymptomatic but can occasionally become slightly tender and pruritic.

PATHOGENESIS

The exact pathophysiology of a dermatofibroma is not well understood. Whether a dermatofibroma is a reactive inflammatory process or a true neoplasm is still debated. Often, the development of a dermatofibroma is preceded by injury (e.g., an insect bite or ruptured folliculitis), suggesting the possibility of an abnormal response to injury and inflammation, analogous to the formation of a hypertrophic scar or keloid. Occasionally, multiple lesions (>15) may appear over a period of about 4 months, known as multiple eruptive dermatofibromas (MEDF). Eruption of multiple dermatofibromas has been associated with immune-mediated processes, mainly systemic lupus erythematosus (SLE), HIV infection, and immunosuppression therapy. These observations suggest that immune mechanisms may play a role in the development of MEDF and possibly solitary dermatofibroma.

KEY FEATURES

- Dermatofibromas are benign hyperproliferation of normal dermal fibroblasts within a dense matrix of collagen.

- Typically these lesions present as an asymptomatic, light to dark brown, firm papule or nodule which exhibits the "dimple sign".

- Typically occurs on the lower extremities of young to middle-aged females.

- Diagnosis is made by visual inspection.

- Treatment consists of cryosurgery if indicated for cosmetic purposes.

CLINICAL PRESENTATION

Upon examination, firm papules or nodules with smooth surface, measuring 3–10 mm in diameter may be noted (Fig. 11-14). The lesions have a light pink to brown pigmentation, which fades out, toward the periphery. They characteristically dimple with lateral compression (i.e., the dimple sign) (Fig. 11-15).

CHAPTER 11 Benign Neoplasms

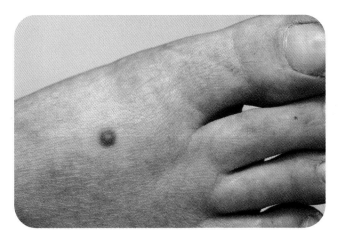

Figure 11-14 Dermatofibroma.

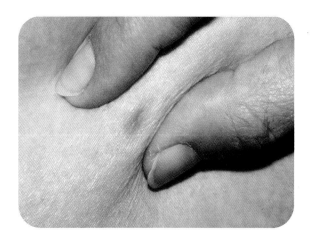

Figure 11-15 Dermatofibroma with a positive dimple sign. From Goodheart HP. *Goodheart's Photoguide to Common Skin Disorders*, 3rd ed. Philadelphia: Lippincott Williams & Wilkins, 2009.

WHEN TO REFER

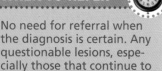

No need for referral when the diagnosis is certain. Any questionable lesions, especially those that continue to enlarge, should be biopsied.

NOT TO BE MISSED

- Any quickly evolving or questionable lesion should be biopsied to rule out melanoma.

DIAGNOSIS

Differential Diagnosis

Dermatofibroma can be confused with melanocytic lesions (benign nevus or melanoma), insect bite reaction, and angiomas.

Diagnostic Methods

Diagnosis is made by visual inspection and the presence of the "dimple sign." The "dimple sign" is positive when the lesion buckles and depresses with lateral pressure.

THERAPY

Dermatofibromas are treated in the setting of repeated trauma or if indicated for cosmetic purposes.

- The most effective treatment is cryotherapy: tissue freezing by liquid nitrogen cycles for a total of 3 to 5 seconds to the affected areas. The main side effect of cryosurgery is skin depigmentation if liquid nitrogen is applied for more than 10 sec/cycle. This may decrease symptoms and thin the lesion, but it is rarely effective in improving the cosmetic appearance.
- Surgical removal often leaves a scar worse than the original lesion.
- Strong topical or intralesional steroids are injected to treat pruritic lesions.

COURSE AND COMPLICATIONS

Dermatofibromas have an indolent course. A few lesions may actively grow up to 2 cm in diameter. Lesions tend to recur following treatment.

ICD9 Code	
210.0	Benign neoplasm of lip
216.0	Benign neoplasm of skin of lip
216.1	Benign neoplasm of eyelid, including canthus
216.2	Benign neoplasm of ear and external auditory canal
216.3	Benign neoplasm of skin of other and unspecified parts of face
216.4	Benign neoplasm of scalp and skin of neck
216.5	Benign neoplasm of skin of trunk, except scrotum
216.6	Benign neoplasm of skin of upper limb, including shoulder
216.7	Benign neoplasm of skin of lower limb, including hip
216.8	Benign neoplasm of other specified sites of skin
216.9	Benign neoplasm of skin, site unspecified
221.2	Benign neoplasm of vulva

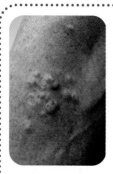

A 25-year-old healthy man complains of a group of "bumps" in his right arm arising in the last year (Fig. 11-16). They have recently grown in size and now feel slightly painful to touch. The patient denies any other symptoms. Upon examination, a solitary, flesh-colored nodule is noted on the left arm, which is tender to palpation. What is the most likely diagnosis?

Neurofibroma

BACKGROUND/EPIDEMIOLOGY

Neurofibroma is a benign dermal tumor that originates from neural tissue, mainly from the superficial cutaneous nerves, although it can arise from any nerve in the body. Frequently, the tumor grows on spinal nerve roots producing minimal symptoms. Occasionally, it may compress the spinal cord, resulting in motor and sensory issues.

PATHOGENESIS

There are two types of neurofibromas: *the sporadic type*, which is more common, and *the inherited type*, which is associated with neurofibromatosis type 1 (NF1; an autosomal-dominant inherited disorder characterized by neurofibromas, acoustic nerve schwannomas, café-au-lait spots, and pigmented nodules of the iris).

The exact pathophysiology of neurofibromas is not well-understood. The *sporadic-type neurofibromas* present as solitary lesions that have an extremely small risk for malignant transformation. They occur in young adults and are usually asymptomatic. Occasionally, they produce pain or motor weakness depending on the location and size of the tumor. The *inherited-type neurofibromas* may be single or part of multiple neurofibromas, as is the case in NF1. The lesions rarely develop before puberty and are usually larger and more painful than the sporadic-type neurofibromas. Patients with NF1-associated neurofibromas also complain of multiple organ system dysfunction (e.g., gastrointestinal, cardiovascular, neurologic, and musculoskeletal symptoms).

CLINICAL PRESENTATION

The physical findings vary according to the type of neurofibroma.

- Sporadic-type:
  - Skin-colored, pink to brown single papules or nodules varying from a few mm to 1 cm (Fig. 11-16)
  - Lesions may be tender if there is involvement of the nerve
- Inherited-type:
  - 1 to 100 skin-colored, tender nodules measuring up to 4 to 5 cm and distributed throughout the body
  - Café-au-lait spots or pigmented nodules of the iris may also be observed
  - Positive Tinel sign (electric-like shooting pain by tapping on a lesion) suggests nerve involvement

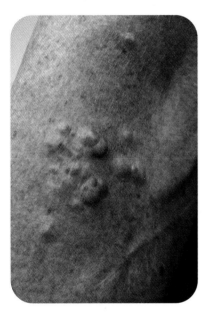

Figure 11-16 Multiple neurofibromas on the arm of a young man.

DIAGNOSIS

Differential Diagnosis

Neurofibromas can sometimes be confused with nevi, amelanotic melanoma, malignant melanoma, and dermatofibroma.

Diagnostic Methods

- The "buttonhole sign" is pathognomonic for neurofibroma.
- Biopsy is indicated to distinguish it from amelanotic melanoma or malignant melanoma.

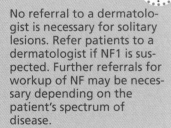

THERAPY

Symptomatic neurofibromas may be surgically removed; asymptomatic neurofibromas of either type are removed only if indicated for cosmetic purposes.

COURSE AND COMPLICATIONS

Sporadic neurofibromas have a very small risk of malignant transformation over time and they do not tend to recur after excision. NF1-associated neurofibromas, on the other hand, have a significant rate of malignant transformation and must be followed closely. For this reason, patients with NF1 have a higher mortality rate than those with sporadic neurofibromas.

NOT TO BE MISSED

- Multiple neurofibromas may suggest a diagnosis of neurofibromatosis.

ICD9 Code

215.0	*Other benign neoplasm of connective and other soft tissue of head, face, and neck*
215.2	*Other benign neoplasm of connective and other soft tissue of upper limb, including shoulder*
215.3	*Other benign neoplasm of connective and other soft tissue of lower limb, including hip*
215.4	*Other benign neoplasm of connective and other soft tissue of thorax*
215.5	*Other benign neoplasm of connective and other soft tissue of abdomen*
215.6	*Other benign neoplasm of connective and other soft tissue of pelvis*
215.7	*Other benign neoplasm of connective and other soft tissue of trunk, unspecified*
215.8	*Other benign neoplasm of connective and other soft tissue of other specified sites*
215.9	*Other benign neoplasm of connective and other soft tissue, site unspecified*

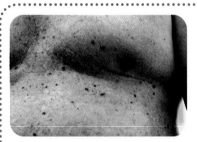

A 75-year-old man complains of a few "red spots" on his abdomen and chest that have increased in number since the last year (Fig. 11-17). He denies any symptoms, but finds the spots cosmetically unappealing. Upon examination, he has multiple scattered 2- to 3-mm bright red papules on the chest, abdomen, and back. There is no associated tenderness to palpation. What is the most likely diagnosis?

Cherry Angioma

BACKGROUND/EPIDEMIOLOGY

Cherry angioma is an exceedingly common vascular lesion, the pathophysiology of which is not well understood. On histology, dilated capillaries with flattened endothelial cells are surrounded by an edematous stroma. Cherry angiomas first appear around the age of 30 to 40 and slowly increase in number and size over the years. More than 70% of people at the age of 70 have several such lesions. There is no racial or gender predisposition.

PATHOGENESIS

The pathogenesis of cherry angiomas is not known.

CLINICAL PRESENTATION

Cherry angiomas mostly affect the trunk and upper extremities, although they can develop anywhere in the body, except the mucous membranes. They are largely asymptomatic, unless irritated.

PHYSICAL FINDINGS

Upon examination, symmetric bright-to-violaceous papules or nodules usually measuring 3 to 5 mm are noted (Fig. 11-17). If hemorrhagic, the lesions may appear dark brown to almost black. They are nontender and blanch upon palpation.

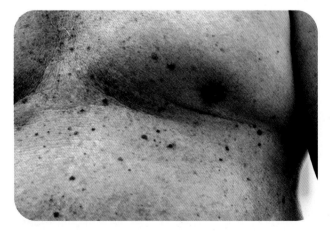

Figure 11-17 Cherry angiomas on the chest.

KEY FEATURES

- Cherry angiomas are exceedingly common benign lesions which first appear during the third or fourth decade of life; the number of lesions increases over the years.

- Typically they present as an asymptomatic, bright to red violaceous, dome-shaped papule.

- Typical sites of distribution are the trunk; the mucous membranes are spared.

- Diagnosis is made by visual inspection.

- Treatment consists of electro- or laser coagulation for cosmetic purposes.

Table 11-4 Differential Diagnosis of Cherry Angiomas

DIAGNOSIS	KEY FEATURES
Amelanotic melanoma	Asymmetric, nonpigmented nodular lesion. Oftentimes, can itch or bleed. +/− family history of melanoma
Pyogenic granuloma	Red, friable, solitary or grouped nodules, mainly on the facial and acral areas. Very common in children and during pregnancy. Can bleed easily
Solitary glomus tumor	A solitary blue to red vascular papule or nodule that occurs mainly under the nail and is tender to palpation
Angiokeratoma	Red papules, some with hyperkeratosis. Most commonly found on the scrotum, shaft of penis, labia majora, inner thigh, or lower abdomen

DIAGNOSIS

Differential Diagnosis

Cherry angioma is most commonly considered in the differential for amelanotic melanoma, pyogenic granuloma, angiokeratoma, and solitary glomus tumor (Table 11-4). Small lesions may be confused with petechiae.

Diagnostic Methods

Diagnosis is made by visual inspection.

THERAPY

Asymptomatic cherry angiomas are treated if indicated for cosmetic purposes. Effective treatment options include:

- Electrocoagulation: destruction of dilated blood vessels by radio waves
- Laser coagulation: destruction of dilated blood vessels through a laser
- Cryosurgery (tissue freezing with liquid nitrogen) is not as effective.

COURSE AND COMPLICATIONS

Cherry angiomas are permanent growths with excellent prognosis given their benign nature. They grow in size and number over the years and may bleed due to frequent irritation by clothes.

WHEN TO REFER

No need for referral when the diagnosis is certain.

NOT TO BE MISSED

- Changing, suspicious, or atypical lesions should be biopsied.

ICD9 Code

448.1   Nevus, nonneoplastic

Suggested Reading

Argenziano G, Zalaudek I, Ferrara G, et al. Proposal of a new classification system for melanocytic naevi. Br J Dermatol. 2007;157:217–227.

Goldstein BG, Goldstein AO. Benign neoplasms of the skin. UpToDate. 2008.

Heaphy MR Jr, Millns JL, Schroeter AL. The sign of Leser-Trélat in a case of adenocarcinoma of the lung. J Am Acad Dermatol. 2000;43(2 Pt 2):386–390.

Hui P, Glusac EJ, Sinard JH, et al. Clonal analysis of cutaneous fibrous histiocytoma (dermatofibroma). J Cutan Pathol. 2002;29:385–389.

Lindelöf B, Sigurgeirsson B, Melander S. Seborrheic keratoses and cancer. J Am Acad Dermatol. 1992; 26(6):947–950.

Kameya S, Noda A, Isobe E, et al. The sign of Leser-Trélat associated with carcinoma of the stomach. Am J Gastroenterol. 1988;83(6):664–666.

Luba MC, Bangs SA, Mohler AM, et al. Common benign skin tumors. *Am Fam Physician.* 2003;67:729–738.

Marghoob AA, Borrego JP, Halpern AC. Congenital melanocytic nevi: treatment modalities and management options. *Semin Cutan Med Surg.* 2007;26:231–240.

Murphy ME, Boyer JD, Stashower ME, et al. The surgical management of spitz nevi. *Dermatol Surg.* 2002;28:1065–1069.

Naeyaert JM, Brochez L. Clinical practice. Dysplastic nevi. *N Engl J Med.* 2003;349:2233.

Niemi KM. The benign fibrohistiocytic tumors of the skin. *Acta Derm Venereol.* 1970; 50 (Suppl. 63): 1–66.

Ortonne J-P, Pandya AG, Lui H, et al. Treatment of solar lentigines. *J Am Acad Dermatol.* 2006;54(5):S262–271.

Ortonne J-P. Pigmentary changes of the aging skin. *Br J Dermatol.* 1990;122 (Suppl 35):21–28.

Rasi A, Soltani-Arabshahi R, Shahbazi N. Skin tag as a cutaneous impaired carbohydrate metabolism: a case-control study. *Int J Dermatol.* 2007;46:1155–1159.

Requena L, Sangüeza OP. Benign neoplasms with neural differentiation: a review. *Am J Dermatopathol.* 1995;17:75.

Savar A, Cestari DM. Neurofibromatosis type I: genetics and clinical manifestations. *Semin Ophthalmol.* 2008;23(1):45–51.

Vun Y, De'Ambrosis B, Spelman L, et al. Seborrheic keratosis and malignancy: collision tumor or malignant tranformation. *Austral J Dermatol.* 2006;47:106–108.

Wolff K, Johnson RA, Suurmond D. Benign neoplasms and hyperplasias: Skin tag. In *Fitzpatrick's Color Atlas & Synopsis of Clinical Dermatology.* 5th ed. New York: McGraw-Hill 2005;9:224.

Wolff K, Johnson RA, Suurmond D. Benign neoplasms and hyperplasias: Cherry angioma. In *Fitzpatrick's Color Atlas & Synopsis of Clinical Dermatology.* 5th ed. New York: McGraw-Hill 2005;9:192–193.

Wolff K, Johnson RA, Suurmond D. Benign neoplasms and hyperplasias: Seborrheic keratosis. In *Fitzpatrick's Color Atlas & Synopsis of Clinical Dermatology.* 5th ed. New York: McGraw-Hill 2005;9:204–207.

Wolff K, Johnson RA, Suurmond D. Benign neoplasms and hyperplasias. In *Fitzpatrick's Color Atlas & Synopsis of Clinical Dermatology.* 5th ed. New York: McGraw-Hill 2005;9:166–175.

Wolff K, Johnson RA, Suurmond D. Benign neoplasms and hyperplasias. In *Fitzpatrick's Color Atlas & Synopsis of Clinical Dermatology.* 5th ed. New York: McGraw-Hill 2005;10:260–262.

Wolff K, Johnson RA, Suurmond D. Benign neoplasms and hyperplasias. In *Fitzpatrick's Color Atlas & Synopsis of Clinical Dermatology.* 5th ed. New York: McGraw-Hill 2005;9:218–219.

Wolff K, Johnson RA, Suurmond D. Benign neoplasms and hyperplasias. In *Fitzpatrick's Color Atlas & Synopsis of Clinical Dermatology.* 5th ed. New York: McGraw-Hill 2005;15:463–466.

CHAPTER 12 Papulosquamous Diseases

Susan J. Huang and Arturo Saavedra-Lauzon

Papulosquamous disorders are a varied group of conditions, all sharing the common morphologic feature of scaling papules and plaques. Psoriasis is one of the most common papulosquamous disorders, seen in almost 2% of the general population. Seborrheic dermatitis, pityriasis rosea, and keratosis pilaris are dissimilar but common conditions, which are frequently seen in primary care. Lichen planus is an uncommon condition that can be idiopathic, caused by common oral medications or even by systemic viral infections such as hepatitis B and C. Lastly, pityriasis rubra pilaris is very rare, idiopathic condition that is challenging to treat. All of these conditions will be reviewed in detail in this section.

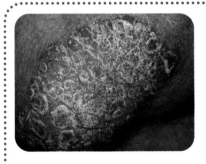

Ms. K is a 25-year-old white student who complains of a 2-month history of an itchy rash. She states that the rash first started as raised bumps, which then coalesced into plaques. She also states that her mother is being treated for a longstanding skin condition. On examination, well-demarcated papules and plaques with overlying thick, white scale (Fig. 12-1) over an erythematous base involve her elbows, knees, and her lower back. The patient also shows you areas where the lesions have appeared after scratching. When gently curetting the scale off a lesion, the scale lifts off in intact sheets. Removal of the scale reveals pinpoint bleeding, consistent with the Auspitz sign.

Psoriasis

BACKGROUND/EPIDEMIOLOGY

Psoriasis is a fairly common skin condition in the United States, affecting up to 2% of individuals. In its common form, it is marked by thick white or silvery lamellated scale (often called micaceous) with or without accompanying pruritus, often in visible areas. Such visibility, accompanying symptoms, and chronic nature can severely decrease quality of life. Individuals with psoriasis have a higher incidence of depression. Furthermore, patients with psoriasis are at increased risk of having lymphoma, metabolic syndrome, and cardiovascular disease. Psoriasis primarily affects adults with bimodal age peaks in the second and fifth decades of life, though any age may be affected.

PATHOGENESIS

A positive family history predisposes an individual to psoriasis. Studies have shown that between 36% and 91% of patients with psoriasis have positive family histories. Furthermore, certain HLA types including HLA-B13, B17, B37, Bw16, and DR7 are more common among those with psoriasis. Clinically, there

KEY FEATURES

- Psoriasis affects ~2% of individuals.

(Continued)

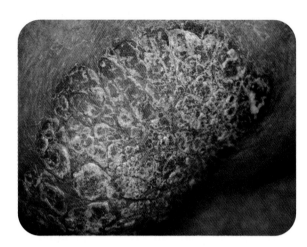

Figure 12-1 Micaceous scale overlying an erythematous plaque consistent with psoriasis on the elbow.

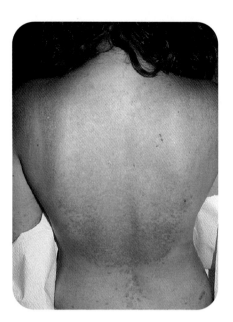

Figure 12-2 The Koebner phenomenon is localized to the area of sunburn. The region that had been covered by the patient's bathing suit is almost free of lesions. From Goodheart HP. *Goodheart's Photoguide of Common Skin Disorders*, 3rd ed. Philadelphia: Lippincott Williams & Wilkins, 2009.

are several triggers and exacerbating factors. Streptococcal infection often leads to guttate psoriasis, and viral exanthems are known to trigger episodes. Life stressors; direct cutaneous trauma; medications such as lithium, beta blockers, nonsteroidal anti-inflammatory drugs (NSAIDs); and steroid tapers have all been reported to trigger psoriasis. Human immunodeficiency virus (HIV) infection does not increase the incidence of psoriasis but is linked to more aggressive psoriasis.

CLINICAL PRESENTATION

The most frequent type of psoriasis accounting for 90% of cases is plaque psoriasis. Other variants include pustular, guttate, erythrodermic, inverse, and nail psoriasis.

The most common form of psoriasis is plaque psoriasis. Lesions are well-demarcated circular, oval, or polycyclic papules or plaques marked by erythema and overlying silvery micaceous scale (Fig. 12-1). They are generally distributed symmetrically and often affect the scalp, elbows, knees, trunk, presacral region, hands, and feet. On hands and feet, painful fissuring can occur. Genitals are affected in 30% of cases. Lesions may be accompanied by pruritus or pain. In developing lesions, the active edge appears more erythematous and small papules may surround the lesion. Arrangement of lesions may be linear, perhaps reflecting the Koebner phenomenon, where lesions develop in sites of cutaneous trauma such as scratching (Fig. 12-2). The scales of psoriatic lesions can be lifted in coherent sheets. Upon removing the scales and then the overlying membrane, pinpoint bleeding can be observed. This is known as the Auspitz sign. In some cases, an inverse pattern of psoriasis may be observed. In these cases, thin erythematous plaques without scale are present in intertriginous or flexural areas such as the axilla, groin, inguinal crease, or under breasts.

Pustular psoriasis is a less common form of cutaneous psoriasis and can manifest as localized or generalized sterile pustules (Fig. 12-3). In many cases,

KEY FEATURES (Continued)

- The most common presentation is with thick white or silvery lamellated scale on typical areas: elbows, knees, scalp, umbilicus.

- It primarily affects adults, with bimodal age peaks in the second and fifth decades of life, though any age may be affected.

- Psoriasis patients are at increased risk of having lymphoma, metabolic syndrome, and cardiovascular disease.

- Treatment of psoriasis is complicated, and individualized regimens are needed depending on the extent and severity of disease. No cure exists, so treatment is aimed at controlling the disease.

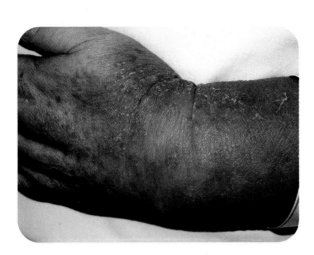

Figure 12-3 Pustular psoriasis on the lower arm and hand.

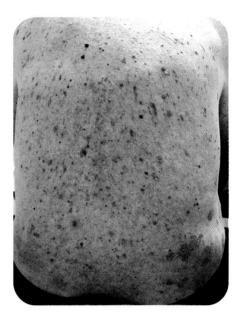

Figure 12-4 Guttate psoriasis on the trunk.

these patients are systemically ill, requiring hospitalization. It is a diagnosis of exclusion and as such, other causes of pustules such as infection must be ruled out.

Guttate psoriasis presents as hundreds of small ~1- to 10-mm plaques of psoriasis on the trunk and extremities (Fig. 12-4), often in an explosive manner. This is the most common type of psoriasis outbreak in those under the age of 30 years. In many cases, group A beta-hemolytic streptococcal infections (S. *pyogenes*), often pharyngitis, precede outbreak and are the cause of this type of psoriasis. This may be the first presentation of psoriasis. Treatment with appropriate oral antibiotics will often lead to completely clearance, though not all cases are infection-related. In some, this will be the only eruption of psoriasis, though many eventually develop plaque type psoriasis.

Erythrodermic psoriasis is another form of cutaneous psoriasis and is a medical emergency. Often it is in the setting of worsening or uncontrolled psoriasis, although it is sometimes the first presentation of psoriasis. Erythema and exfoliation affect large areas of skin. The condition can lead to infection and significant fluid, electrolyte, and protein imbalances, which can be fatal. Of note, hypocalcemia is a complication of erythrodermic psoriasis. These patients should be managed as inpatients.

Psoriasis affecting the nails occurs in almost 80% of psoriasis patients. Nails may exhibit pitting, keratotic collections, "oil spots" (yellow-brown discoloration), and onycholysis (Fig. 12-5) (lifting of the distal nail).

Psoriatic arthritis occurs in about 10% of psoriasis cases. The majority of cases present as asymmetric arthritis of finger and toe joints, which in time can lead to a "sausage digit." In patients with joint disease, tendons may also be affected. For patients with psoriatic arthritis, consider referring to dermatology or rheumatology for consideration of a systemic therapy, which will not only treat the psoriasis but also reduce joint inflammation and destruction.

DIAGNOSIS

Diagnosis of cutaneous lesions is usually clinical but a biopsy may aid in diagnosis in questionable cases. To evaluate the

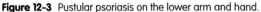

Figure 12-5 Nail psoriasis.

differential diagnosis of fungal infection, a potassium hydroxide (KOH) test of a skin scraping can be performed. This test has high sensitivity and low specificity, so a fungal culture should be obtained if you suspect a false negative KOH test (see Chapter 9).

Joint disease typically coincides or follows cutaneous lesions, but could also precede cutaneous lesions. To evaluate joint disease, erythrocyte sedimentation rate (ESR), rheumatoid factor (RF), and radiologic studies may help determine the cause of disease. Contrary to rheumatoid arthritis, psoriatic arthritis is a seronegative arthritis. ESR is usually normal, serologies are negative, and radiographic erosive changes are present.

Differential diagnoses for psoriasis includes atopic dermatitis, lichen simplex chronicus, seborrheic dermatitis, pityriasis rosea, fungal infection, and syphilis. Psoriatic lesions may be secondarily infected. Consider the possibility of allergic contact dermatitis for psoriasis that is worsening despite adequate topical therapy. There are many preservatives that are potential causes of allergy and will worsen psoriasis if the patient becomes allergic.

TREATMENTS

Treatment of psoriasis is complicated, and individualized regimens are needed depending on the extent and severity of disease. No cure exists so treatment is aimed at controlling the disease. Patients should be referred to a dermatologist and/or rheumatologist for long-term care. However, it is appropriate to start initial therapy for plaque psoriasis.

For involvement of less than 5% of the body surface area (BSA), topical medication should first be used. Topical steroids, coal tar, vitamin D analogs (e.g., calcipotriol, calcipotriene), or a topical retinoid (e.g., tazarotene) may be useful. Potent steroids should be avoided for the face and genital areas. For lesions of the palms and soles, topical therapy may be insufficient. Patients may benefit from local phototherapy and/or systemic treatment such as oral methotrexate, acitretin, or cyclosporine.

A typical regimen for a newly diagnosed patient with plaque psoriasis on elbows, knees, and scalp (<5% BSA) could consist of the following topicals: a vitamin D analog (calcipotriene) twice daily to affected areas on weekdays and a superpotent topical steroid (clobetasol propionate) ointment twice daily on weekends. For scalp involvement, a topical solution or foam such as fluocinonide 0.05% is usually helpful. An over-the-counter coal tar shampoo used 3 to 4 times weekly is helpful for many patients. It is important that the patient leave the shampoo in for 5 to 10 minutes before rinsing to receive full benefit. If palms and/or soles are involved, consider narrow-band UVB therapy (if available), a super-potent topical steroid, and a keratolytic such as salicylic acid 6% cream.

If lesions involve a larger percentage of the body surface area, systemic therapy, phototherapy with or without topical therapy should be considered. Oral methotrexate, acitretin, or cyclosporine can be used. If treatment is refractory, consider the use of biologics. These biologics include alefacept, efalizumab, adalimumab, etanercept, infliximab, and ustekinumab. Patients needing these medications should be referred to a dermatologist.

"AT A GLANCE" TREATMENT

- Treatment of psoriasis is complicated and individualized regimens are needed depending on the extent and severity of disease. No cure exists.
- Less than 5% BSA:
  - Primary: topical medications: vitamin D analog (calcipotriene) BID to affected areas on weekdays and a superpotent topical steroid (clobetasol propionate) ointment twice daily on weekends.
  - Scalp: a topical solution/foam such as fluocinonide 0.05%. An over-the-counter coal tar shampoo used 3 to 4 times weekly. Leave in for 5 minutes.

- Palmoplantar psoriasis:
  - Primary: super-potent topical steroid and a keratolytic such as salicylic acid 6% cream
  - Secondary: may require local phototherapy and/or systemic treatment such as oral methotrexate, acitretin, or cyclosporine
- More than 5% BSA:
  - Topical therapy as appropriate as above
  - Systemic therapy, phototherapy with or without topical therapy should be considered. Oral methotrexate, acitretin or cyclosporine can be used.
  - If treatment is refractory, consider the use of biologics including alefacept, adalimumab, etanercept, infliximab, and ustekinumab. Patients needing these medications should be referred to a dermatologist.

WHEN TO REFER

- Psoriasis is a chronic condition requiring follow-up and tailored treatment regimens. As such, the patient should be referred to a dermatologist and/or rheumatologist for advanced or recalcitrant disease.
- Erythrodermic or pustular psoriasis patients should receive emergent care.

NOT TO BE MISSED

- Erythrodermic psoriasis requires emergent treatment.

COURSE AND COMPLICATIONS

In plaque psoriasis, individual lesions start as papules, which may then coalesce into plaques with variable amount of scaling. Lesions may last months to years in the same location. With treatment, lesions first clear centrally and clearance then proceeds outward. Upon resolution, postinflammatory hypo- or hyperpigmentation may be present. Improvement with therapy may be evaluated based on the Psoriasis Area and Severity Index (PASI) score or on quality-of-life scores. The PASI score considers the surface area affected, redness, thickness, and amount of scaling.

Psoriatic arthritis develops in about 10% of patients with cutaneous psoriasis. Usually joint disease coincides with or follows cutaneous disease, although this is not always the case. Psoriatic arthritis is usually progressive and may lead to long-term destruction of affected joints.

ICD9 Code

696.1   *Other psoriasis and similar disorders*

CHAPTER 12 Papulosquamous Diseases

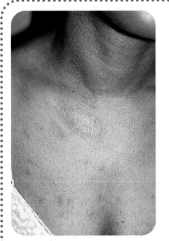

Ms. K is a 26-year-old waitress who complains of pruritic pink patches on her chest, back, and upper arms (Fig. 12-6). One week prior, she noticed a solitary pink ovoid patch on her abdomen, which then enlarged over the next few days. Starting 2 days ago, she noticed similar patches developing on her trunk. Ms. K recently had an upper respiratory infection before the onset of her rash, but otherwise has had no other medical issues. She is particularly concerned about the appearance of her lesions and wants to know if her lesions are contagious and when they will subside.

Pityriasis Rosea

BACKGROUND/EPIDEMIOLOGY

Pityriasis rosea (PR) is a common mild and self-resolving skin condition which most often affects healthy children and young adults between the ages of 10 and 35. In the typical scenario, a single salmon-colored patch called a "herald patch" appears first, frequently on the trunk. Multiple other similar lesions then appear, often on the trunk and proximal extremities and following skin cleavage lines, although other patterns may occur. Thus, on the back, these lesions may create the classical "Christmas tree" distribution. Patients often complain of pruritus, which can be severe. Variants of PR exist and include localized and inverse pityriasis rosea, and papular, urticarial erythema multiforme-like, vesicular, pustular, and purpuric variants.

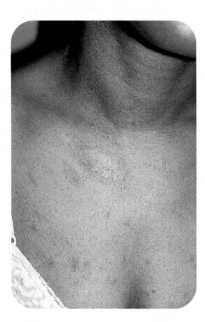

Figure 12-6 Pityriasis rosea. From Goodheart HP. *Goodheart's Photoguide of Common Skin Disorders*, 3rd ed. Philadelphia: Lippincott Williams & Wilkins, 2009.

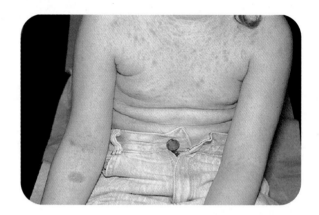

Figure 12-7 Pityriasis rosea. The herald patch is on the flexor forearm. From Goodheart HP. *Goodheart's Photoguide of Common Skin Disorders*, 3rd ed. Philadelphia: Lippincott Williams & Wilkins, 2009.

PATHOGENESIS

An exact etiology is unknown, although viral etiologies—specifically, HHV-6 or HHV-7 infection—have been implicated. Some cases are preceded by a viral prodrome marked by headache, fever, malaise, abdominal discomfort, and/or arthralgias. PR has also been reported to occur more frequently in the spring and fall seasons. Infectivity is low to none.

CLINICAL PRESENTATION

The herald patch in 80% of the cases precedes the wave of lesions and is frequently located on the trunk or neck. This patch is a single discrete pink or salmon-colored ovoid patch or plaque, which enlarges over the course of a few days. It is marked by a collarette of scale as well as fine central scale which may clear with time. After days or weeks, crops of other lesions in different phases arise, most often on the trunk and proximal extremities and neck, although other distributions are also possible. For instance, the palms, soles, and face are usually spared but may be affected in variant forms of PR. The lesions are similar to the herald patch in morphology but are often smaller in size (Figs. 12-6, 12-7). They are often arranged with their long axis along skin cleavage lines, thus resulting in the classic "Christmas tree" distribution on the back. Most of patients report either no symptoms or mild pruritus. In individuals with dark skin, lesions are more often hyperpigmented and papular and more widespread.

DIAGNOSIS

Several other conditions can mimic PR (Table 12-1). Of primary importance, secondary syphilis should be ruled out (Fig. 12-8). Clinical suspicion increases with the presence of condyloma lata, a chancre, split papules (fissured papules seen at the angle of the mouth), and/or peripheral lymphadenopathy. It is important to be aware that, while unlikely to spread with minimal contact, the skin lesions of secondary syphilis may be infectious. Mucosal involvement is

KEY FEATURES

- Pityriasis rosea is a self-limited condition presenting initially as a single salmon-colored, thin scaling plaque on the trunk, then many smaller scaling plaques develop.

- It is likely caused by a viral infection, though pathogenesis has not been proven.

- Be aware that secondary syphilis is a mimic; screen appropriate cases.

- Treatment is symptomatic: topical corticosteroids and antipruritics.

Table 12-1 Differential Diagnosis for Pityriasis Rosacea	
Tinea corporis	Pityriasis lichenoides
Viral exanthem	Secondary syphilis
Nummular eczema	

also more common in secondary syphilis. A rapid plasma reagin (RPR), Venereal Disease Research Laboratory (VDRL) and fluorescent treponemal antibody-absorption (FTA-ABS) along with a biopsy can help distinguish between pityriasis rosea and secondary syphilis.

Drug eruptions may mimic PR (Table 12-2). In these cases, lesions tend to be fewer in number and larger in size and often lack the preliminary herald patch. Tinea corporis can also resemble pityriasis rosea and can be ruled out by a KOH preparation of a scraping. Viral exanthems can mimic pityriasis rosea although lesions are usually nonscaling. Nummular eczema and pityriasis lichenoides should also be excluded. In acquired immunodeficiency syndrome (AIDS) patients, a more chronic pityriasis rosea-like condition has been described.

STUDIES

Additional studies are unnecessary in straightforward cases, but should be performed to rule out other conditions such as secondary syphilis (see Table 12-1).

TREATMENT

Lesions and symptoms typically resolve without therapy, but acyclovir (800 mg QID × 1 week) may shorten the duration of lesions and reduce the severity of the itch. For more severe cases, narrow-band ultraviolet B (UVB) therapy may help. Pruritus can be symptomatically treated with a moderate-potency topical steroid such as triamcinolone 0.1% cream twice daily and emollients. If pruritus is severe, oral antihistamines, oral steroids, and UVB or sunlight therapy can be used. Patients should be reassured that the lesions will resolve over time and that infectivity is low to none.

"AT A GLANCE" TREATMENT

- No therapy necessary in most cases
- Acyclovir 800 mg PO QID × 1 week may shorten the course
- Symptomatic therapy of pruritus may be beneficial
  - Triamcinolone 0.1% cream BID
  - Emollients
  - In severe cases: oral antihistamines, oral steroids, and UVB or sunlight therapy

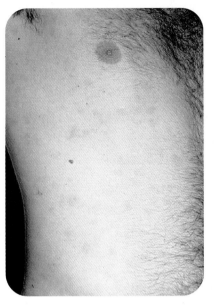

Figure 12-8 Secondary syphilis: body. From Goodheart HP. *Goodheart's Photoguide of Common Skin Disorders*, 3rd ed. Philadelphia: Lippincott Williams & Wilkins, 2009.

Table 12-2 Causes of Pityriasis Rosacea-like Drug Reactions	
ACE inhibitors	Clonidine
Arsenic	Gold
Barbiturates	Isotretinoin
Beta-blockers	Metronidazole
Bismuth	Sulfa drugs

WHEN TO REFER

For severe cases of PR, phototherapy with UVB may be helpful and referral is warranted.

NOT TO BE MISSED

- HIV-associated PR mimics.
- Consider secondary syphilis in all PR patients with appropriate history.

COURSE AND COMPLICATIONS

PR is most often acute, asymptomatic, and self-limited to 4 to 8 weeks, although it can last for months. Postinflammatory hyperpigmentation may occur, especially in those with dark skin. Recurrence is unusual. A viral etiology is suspected and individuals may gain immunity after an episode of pityriasis rosea.

ICD9 Codes	
696.3	Pityriasis rosea
091.3	Secondary syphilis of skin or mucous membranes
091.4	Adenopathy due to secondary syphilis
091.50	Syphilitic uveitis, unspecified
091.51	Syphilitic chorioretinitis (secondary)
091.52	Syphilitic iridocyclitis (secondary)
091.61	Secondary syphilitic periostitis
091.62	Secondary syphilitic hepatitis
091.69	Secondary syphilis of other viscera
091.7	Secondary syphilis, relapse
091.81	Acute syphilitic meningitis (secondary)
091.82	Syphilitic alopecia
091.89	Other forms of secondary syphilis
091.9	Unspecified secondary syphilis
995.27	Other drug allergy

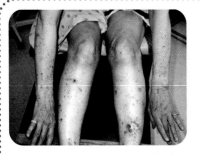

Ms. S is a 35-year-old woman who presents with a 2-month history of an itchy purple rash. She states that the rash first started as flat purple spots, which then became raised. Examination reveals flat-topped polygonal purple papules of her lower back, inner wrists, legs, and inner ankles (Fig. 12-9). The buccal mucosa reveals patches with overlying fine white lines. The patient tells you that she does not feel discomfort or pain in her mouth. You tell the patient that she has lichen planus affecting the skin and mouth. You prescribe oral antihistamines and topical steroids for symptomatic and therapeutic treatment.

Lichen Planus

BACKGROUND/EPIDEMIOLOGY

Lichen planus (LP) is a relatively rare disease. In its cutaneous form, lichen planus affects less than 1% of the population. The oral form affects 1% to 2% of adults, and accounts for 60% to 70% of lichen planus cases. Nails are involved in 10% of lichen planus patients. Although lichen planus can affect individuals of any age it most commonly affects adults between 30 and 60 years of age.

PATHOGENESIS

The cause of LP is unknown, but it is likely immune-mediated. Possible etiologies include viral infection, genetic influence, and contact allergens. Hepatitis C (HCV) infection is more common in LP patients and could serve as an antigen for the inflammatory infiltrate. Hepatitis B (HBV), HIV, and *Helicobacter pylori* infection have also been implicated as possible etiologies. However, LP itself is neither infectious nor contagious. Certain contact allergens such as dental amalgams have also been implicated in oral LP. Removal of the offending agents often leads to resolution of the lesions.

CLINICAL PRESENTATION

The cutaneous form of LP starts as macules and then develops into lesions characterized by the "P's": purple pruritic polygonal papules which are often shiny

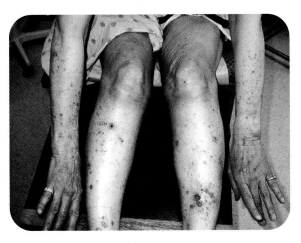

Figure 12-9 Lichen planus. Flat-topped polygonal purple papules of her lower back, inner wrists, legs, and inner ankles.

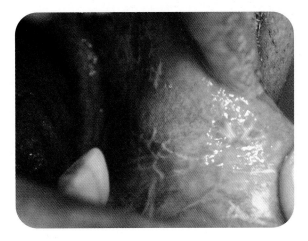

Figure 12-10 Wickham's striae on the buccal mucosa.

KEY FEATURES

- Lichen planus is an uncommon skin disease presenting characteristically as purple, polygonal papules on skin and mucous membranes.

- It most commonly affects adults between 30 and 60 years.

- Lichen planus is seen more often in patients with hepatitis B and C.

- The disease may be limited to one body site (i.e., nails, mucosa, skin).

and flat-topped (Fig. 12-9). These papules can then further spread and may be discrete or grouped. Distribution is often symmetric, favoring flexor surfaces such as the wrist. Involvement of the face, palms, and soles is unusual but possible. Lesions often exhibit overlying Wickham striae, fine lacy white or gray lines (Fig. 12-10). Lesions may erode or ulcerate and may exhibit Koebnerization, where lesions arise in sites of trauma. In addition to the classic presentation of cutaneous LP, several variants exist. In hypertrophic LP, thick hyperkeratotic plaques are common. Involvement of the shins (Fig. 12-11) and legs are common (Fig. 12-12). Vesicles and bullae may be present in vesiculobullous LP.

Oral LP affects a large proportion of patients. In the most common form, the reticular form, asymptomatic lesions of the buccal mucosa with or without involvement of the gums are present. Lesions are characterized by Wickham striae. In the erosive form, uncomfortable or painful erosions and ulcers of the buccal mucosa and tongue are present. These lesions may be aggravated by acidic, rough, or spicy foods and by caffeinated beverages. Of note, a fraction of erosive LP can degenerate to oral squamous cell carcinoma.

LP of the scalp is known as lichen planopilaris. Lesions present as keratotic follicular papules, which may be surrounded by a violaceous rim. These papules may coalesce into patches. Over time and without treatment, lichen

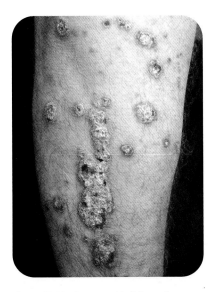

Figure 12-11 Hypertrophic lichen planus on the shins.

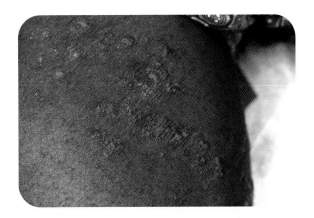

Figure 12-12 Hypertrophic lichen planus on the thighs of a man with type V skin.

CHAPTER 12 Papulosquamous Diseases

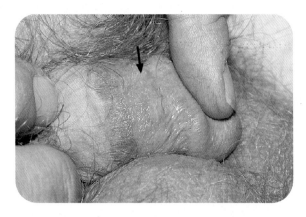

Figure 12-13 Penile lichen planus. From Goodheart HP. *Goodheart's Photoguide of Common Skin Disorders,* 3rd ed. Philadelphia: Lippincott Williams & Wilkins, 2009.

planopilaris can lead to scarring alopecia and permanent hair loss.

In women, LP can involve the vulva and vagina. These cases may manifest as patches of leukoplakia or erythroplakia. Erosions or ulcers may also be present. Lesions may be asymptomatic, or they may lead to burning, pruritus, or dyspareunia. Often there is a thin vaginal discharge. Over time, lesions may lead to vaginal adhesions, so timely treatment is necessary.

LP can also involve the penis, where it primarily affects the glans (Fig. 12-13). Lesions may be annular or vesicular. If lesions are vesicular, then a differential diagnosis of herpes should be raised.

When LP involves the nails, it may manifest with longitudinal grooves or ridges, thinning of the nail plate, and/or distal splitting (Fig. 12-14). Rarely, lesions may scar and then lead to nail loss.

DIAGNOSIS

Differential diagnoses for cutaneous LP include lichenoid drug eruptions (LDE), psoriasis, lichen simplex chronicus (thickening of the skin caused by repeated trauma to the skin), secondary syphilis, chronic graft-versus-host disease (GVHD), and pityriasis rubra pilaris (PRP). A short list of medications that can lead to LDE is shown in Table 12-3. LDE lesions are more eczematous in nature and often occur in photodistributed areas. In secondary syphilis, lesions lack Wickham striae, and palms and soles may be affected. Serologic studies can help distinguish the different entities.

If oral lesions are present, it is important to rule out immunobullous disease such as pemphigus vulgaris and cicatricial pemphigoid. Vesicular penile lesions may mimic HSV infection.

Diagnostic Methods

LP is usually diagnosed clinically. A punch biopsy is often helpful in aiding diagnosis. If the patient has LP, it is important to rule out underlying hepatitis C virus (HCV) or hepatitis B virus (HBV). Liver function tests and serologies should be obtained.

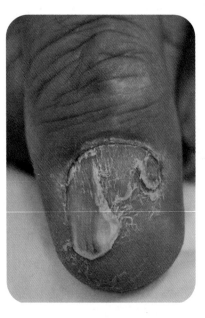

Figure 12-14 Nail pterygium of lichen planus. From Goodheart HP. *Goodheart's Photoguide of Common Skin Disorders,* 3rd ed. Philadelphia: Lippincott Williams & Wilkins, 2009.

TREATMENT

For cutaneous lesions, oral antihistamines may help control pruritus. Topical or intralesional steroids remain the first-line therapies for localized cutaneous lesions. Systemic steroids remain the mainstay of therapy for generalized cutaneous lesions. Note that lesions may recur with steroid

Table 12-3 Common Medications Causing Lichenoid Drug Reactions	
ACE inhibitors	Ketoconazole
Antimalarials	Methyldopa
Calcium channel blockers	Naproxen
Diuretics	Penicillamines
Gold	Quinidine
Ibuprofen	Sulfonylureas

CHAPTER 12   Papulosquamous Diseases

Table 12-4 Summary of Lichen Planus Treatment by Affected Site

SITE		TREATMENT
Cutaneous	First-line	Pruritus: oral antihistamines, topical pramoxine, menthol Localized skin lesions: topical steroids, intralesional steroids Generalized lesions: oral steroids
	Second-line	Oral steroids, oral metronidazole, oral retinoids (isotretinoin, acitretin), narrowband UVB, PUVA
	Third-line	Other antimicrobials (trimethoprim-sulfamethoxazole, griseofulvin, itraconazole), cyclosporine, hydroxychloroquine, topical immunomodulators (e.g., tacrolimus)
Oral	First-line	Topical lidocaine (for pain), topical steroids, intralesional steroids, topical tacrolimus ointment, oral retinoid, oral immunomodulators, miconazole/chlorhexidine (for oral candida if necessary)
	Second-line	Oral steroids
	Third-line	Cyclosporine, griseofulvin, hydroxychloroquine
Scalp	First-line	Topical steroids, intralesional steroids
	Second-line	Oral steroids, hydroxychloroquine
	Third-line	Cyclosporine, tetracycline, oral retinoids, griseofulvin, topical immunomodulators
Vulvar and penile		Topical corticosteroids
Nail		Oral retinoid

taper. In such rebound cases, consider alternative forms of therapy, as listed in Table 12-4.

"AT A GLANCE" TREATMENT

- Therapy of LP is often complicated and dependent on body site. See Table 12-4 for a summary based on site and a graduated approach.

COURSE AND COMPLICATIONS

Individual lesions progress from macules to papules that may disseminate, ulcerate, erode, or atrophy. Lesions may resolve with postinflammatory hyperpigmentation, especially in darker-skinned patients. Over half of papules and plaque lesions resolve spontaneously within 6 months to a year. About 85% subside within 18 months. However, over half relapse within 1 to 2 years. Most cases of oral LP are chronic, with an average duration of 5 years. It is also often the hardest to treat and has a small risk of progression to oral squamous cell carcinoma. For this reason, patients should avoid tobacco and alcohol intake and should be screened yearly for potential progression of oral lesions.

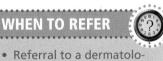

WHEN TO REFER

- Referral to a dermatologist is warranted if the LP is severe, if it is unresponsive to treatment, or if phototherapy is needed.
- Oral LP patients may benefit from consultation with an oral medicine specialist.

NOT TO BE MISSED

- HCV or HBV infection.
- Differential diagnosis of penile lesions: HSV, psoriasis.
- Oral squamous cell carcinoma.

ICD9 Code

697.0	*Lichen planus*

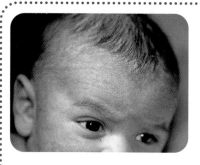

A mother brings in her 2-month-old infant for a rash on his scalp (Fig. 12-15). She states that the infant does not appear to be bothered by the rash and is otherwise well. Examination reveals thick yellow greasy scales of the scalp. In addition to reassuring the mother about this benign self-resolving condition, you recommend shampooing and using mineral oil to loosen the scale.

Seborrheic Dermatitis

BACKGROUND/EPIDEMIOLOGY

Seborrheic dermatitis is a common skin condition that affects 1% to 3% of adults. The condition is also common in infants, where it is often referred to as "cradle cap." In these cases, seborrheic dermatitis is rarely pruritic and infants are not usually bothered by the condition. An infant with generalized seborrheic dermatitis is rare and may represent a sign of immunodeficiency.

Although an aggravating factor is often not identified, known factors include exposure to sun, heat, fever, topical agents, or having a mustache or beard. Some patients may experience pruritus. Most cases of seborrheic dermatitis are not associated with other conditions, but in some cases, seborrheic dermatitis may be associated with Parkinson disease, other debilitating neurologic disease, or steroid taper. Extensive and therapy-resistant cases of seborrheic dermatitis can occur in HIV-infected patients.

PATHOGENESIS

While the cause of seborrheic dermatitis is controversial, suspected etiologies include the normal commensal yeast M. *furfur* as well as sebum overproduction, both of which are often coincident with the condition. A hormonal link has also been suspected.

CLINICAL PRESENTATION

Examination reveals well-demarcated yellow or reddish patches or plaques with flaky, greasy scales in areas with many sebaceous glands including, the scalp, face, ears, presternal region, and intertriginous areas. In infants, seborrheic dermatitis often presents as thick white or yellow greasy scales of the scalp (Fig. 12-15). On the face, the lateral nose, nasolabial folds, eyebrows, and

KEY FEATURES

- Seborrheic dermatitis is a common nonemergent skin condition which affects 1% to 3% of adults.

- It is most likely caused by *Malassezia furfur* and sebum overproduction.

- Presentation is with well-demarcated yellow or reddish patches or plaques with flaky, greasy scales in areas with sebaceous glands.

- The first-line treatment is with topical antifungals and/or low-potency topical corticosteroid.

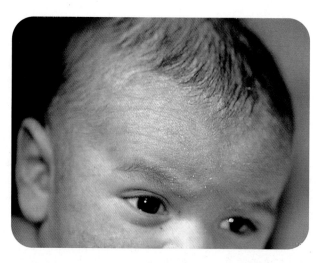

Figure 12-15 Seborrheic dermatitis (cradle cap) on the scalp and face. From Fleisher GR, Ludwig S, Baskin MN. *Atlas of Pediatric Emergency Medicine.* Philadelphia: Lippincott Williams & Wilkins, 2004.

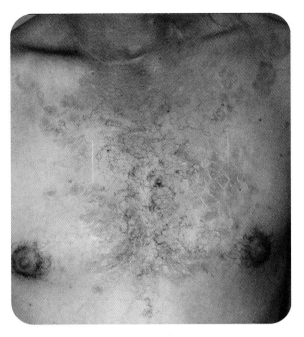

Figure 12-16 Seborrheic dermatitis on the trunk. From Berg D, Worzala K. *Atlas of Adult Physical Diagnosis*. Philadelphia: Lippincott Williams & Wilkins, 2006.

glabella are commonly affected. Rarely, vesicles and crusting are present. On the chest, lesions tend to be small reddish brown follicular or perifollicular papules, which can coalesce into plaques (Fig. 12–16). As lesions may be pruritic, patients may scratch lesions, leading to erosions and possibly secondary infections. The condition, known as dandruff (pityriasis simplex capillitii), is also a form of seborrheic dermatitis and presents as diffuse, fine white or greasy scales with minimal inflammation.

Differential diagnoses to consider include atopic dermatitis, candidiasis, dermatophytosis, psoriasis, and rosacea.

Diagnostic Methods

In typical cases of seborrheic dermatitis, the diagnosis is clear and additional studies are unnecessary. If the condition is generalized further evaluation for HIV is warranted. A fungal culture can distinguish tinea infection from seborrheic dermatitis.

TREATMENT

For seborrheic dermatitis affecting the scalp, shampoos containing azoles, salicylic acid, tar, selenium, sulfur, zinc, or ciclopirox can be used. For nonscalp lesions, topical azoles, topical ciclopirox, oral terbinafine, short-term low-potency topical steroids, and metronidazole gel, in addition to shampoos may be used.

For cradle cap, if treatment is desired, daily shampooing with unmedicated shampoo is recommended. The application of mineral oil before shampooing to soften scales can first be attempted. Antidandruff shampoos with zinc pyrithione, selenium sulfide, or ketoconazole can also be used. In more resistant cases, 1% hydrocortisone cream can be used although cases of adrenocortical suppression have been reported in children.

"AT A GLANCE" TREATMENT

- Scalp: shampoos containing azoles, salicylic acid, tar, selenium, sulfur, zinc, or ciclopirox.
- For nonscalp lesions, topical azoles (ketoconazole 2% cream), topical ciclopirox, oral terbinafine, short-term low-potency topical steroids, and metronidazole gel

WHEN TO REFER

For severe treatment-resistant seborrheic dermatitis, consider referral to a dermatologist for alternative therapies.

NOT TO BE MISSED

- HIV infection.
- Generalized infantile seborrheic dermatitis linked to immunodeficiency.

COURSE AND COMPLICATIONS

Seborrheic dermatitis is a chronic relapsing condition so ongoing therapy is needed. Cradle cap often self-resolves by 8 months of age.

ICD9 Code	
690.10	Seborrheic dermatitis, unspecified
690.11	Seborrhea capitis
690.12	Seborrheic infantile dermatitis
690.18	Other seborrheic dermatitis

CHAPTER 12 Papulosquamous Diseases

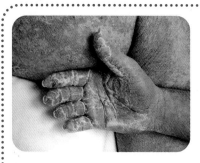

Mr. H is a 40-year-old man who complains of a rough orange rash that has spread from his head downward over the course of a few weeks (Fig. 12-17). He states that his rash began on his face and then moved toward his trunk and extremities. On examination, he has rough red-orange patches on his face, neck, upper torso, elbows, knees, and dorsal hands, with interspersed islands of sparing. His palms and soles appear thickened, orange, and waxy with prominent cracks. You suspect pityriasis rubra pilaris and direct Mr. H to use emollients to relieve the cracking and prescribe acitretin, an oral retinoid.

Pityriasis Rubra Pilaris

BACKGROUND/EPIDEMIOLOGY

PRP is a papulosquamous disease of the skin with a bimodal distribution. It most commonly affects those in their first, second, or sixth decades of life. There are no race or gender predilections.

PATHOGENESIS

The etiology of PRP remains unknown. Most cases are acquired although a minority of cases may be autosomal dominant. Inducing factors include light exposure, infection, and trauma of the skin. Reported associated diseases include myasthenia gravis, celiac sprue, myositis, inflammatory arthritis, hypothyroidism, and HIV.

CLINICAL PRESENTATION

It commonly progresses in a cephalocaudal direction and may progress to generalized erythroderma with characteristic islands of sparing. Under the Griffiths categorization, there are six types of pityriasis rubra pilaris, with three being juvenile forms (Table 12-1). Type II, the classic juvenile type, occurs in roughly 10% of cases and presents in a similar fashion as the classic type but occurs between 1 and 2 years of age. The classic type (Type I) of pityriasis rubra pilaris accounts for roughly 55% of cases. Presentation is with small, rough follicular papules on an erythematous base. The papules can coalesce into plaques and may be accompanied by erythroderma or exfoliation with areas of unaffected skin, referred to as "islands of sparing." Affected skin appears orange or red. One-fifth of patients will report pruritus or a burning sensation. Lesions begin on the head and neck and proceed caudally. The dorsal fingers, trunk, and extremities are frequently affected. On the palms and soles, orange or red keratoderma likened to wax and possibly accompanied by cracks and pain may be present. Figure 12-17 shows the characteristic islands of sparing and the palmar keratoderma occasionally referred to as "carnauba wax"

KEY FEATURES

- Pityriasis rubra pilaris (PRP) is a rare disorder of either sporadic or familial etiology.

- It presents characteristically with small rough follicular papules on an erythematous base that coalesce into plaques. Characteristic "islands of sparing" of unaffected skin. Affected skin appears orange or red.

- Primary therapy is with oral retinoids (acitretin).

- HIV-related PRP is recalcitrant to therapy and chronic in duration.

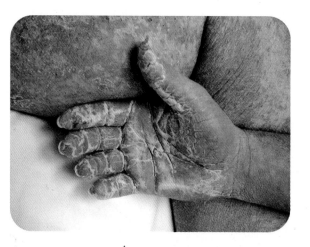

Figure 12-17 Pityriasis rubra pilaris on the hands/trunk.

Table 12-5 Clinical Presentation Summary of Pityriasis Rubra Pilaris by Griffiths Categorization

TYPE		FREQUENCY (%)*	DESCRIPTION	COURSE
I	Classic adult	>50	Follicular papules coalescing into plaques with "islands of sparing," palmoplantar keratoderma	80% clear within 3 years
II	Atypical adult	5	Ichthyosiform eczematous patches especially of the elbows and knees	Chronic
III	Classic juvenile	10	As in Type I	Most clear within 3 years
IV	Circumscribed juvenile	25	Localized areas of follicular keratosis and erythema, especially of the elbows and knees	Uncertain
V	Atypical juvenile	5	Follicular hyperkeratosis	Chronic
VI	HIV associated	—		

*Clayton BD, Jorizzo JL, Hitchcock MG, et al. Adult pityriasis rubra pilaris: A 10-year case series. *JAAD*. 1997;36:959–964. Type VI was not studied.

changes. If the nails are affected, they may have a thick plate and have yellow-brown, subungual debris. On the scalp, erythroderma or fine scale may be present. Adult-onset PRP should be distinguished from psoriasis. The lack of the Auspitz sign where lifting of scales reveals pinpoint bleeding and the presence of islands of sparing, palmoplantar keratoderma, and follicular papules point to PRP. Pitting of the nails and nail dystrophy is also uncommon in PRP. PRP may also mimic dermatomyositis and seborrheic dermatitis. Other types of PRP are reviewed in Table 12-5.

Diagnostic Methods

PRP may be difficult to diagnose in the early stages. Continued follow-up to examine progression of lesions as well as skin biopsy can aid diagnosis.

TREATMENTS

Treating PRP can be difficult and patients often require several different treatments. Thus far, there are no comprehensive studies regarding the treatment of PRP, though one small case series suggests that 80% of classic type PRP patient improve in 4 to 6 months with oral retinoid therapy. A reasonable first-line treatment includes oral retinoids such as acitretin. Methotrexate therapy, with or without oral retinoids, can also be used depending on the severity of lesions. Treatments that have varied efficacy include topical vitamin D analog, azathioprine, corticosteroids, cyclosporine, anabolic steroids, and narrowband UVB/UVA or PUVA treatment. Pediatric patients should receive mild treatment. HIV-associated (type VI) PRP is less responsive to the above treatments but is responsive to highly active antiretroviral treatment (HAART), even if the CD4 count is not low enough to otherwise necessitate HAART. Emollients, keratolytics, and antihistamines can be used for symptomatic treatment.

WHEN TO REFER

Referral to a dermatologist is helpful for refractory cases of PRP or cases requiring phototherapy.

NOT TO BE MISSED

- HIV-associated PRP (type VI).

"AT A GLANCE" TREATMENT

- Therapy is challenging, with many patients not improving quickly.
- First-line therapy: oral retinoids such as acitretin
- Second-line: methotrexate therapy, with or without oral retinoids
- Other treatments: topical vitamin D analog, azathioprine, corticosteroids, cyclosporine, anabolic steroids, and narrowband UVB/UVA or PUVA treatment
- HIV-related PRP should be treated with HAART.

COURSE AND COMPLICATIONS

In the classic type, 80% of the adult cases and the majority of the juvenile cases clear within 3 years and usually do not relapse. HIV-associated PRP, type VI, carries a worse prognosis.

ICD9 Code	
696.4	*Pityriasis rubra pilaris*

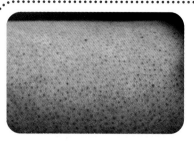

A 20-year-old woman presents to your office complaining of chronic "chicken bumps" on her outer upper arms and thighs (Fig. 12-18). She first noticed these bumps as a teenager, but postponed seeking medical attention, as the lesions were asymptomatic. She reports that her mother has similar skin findings. On examination, the patient has numerous small rough pink folliculocentric papules of her upper arms and thighs with a sandpaper-like texture and xerosis of her upper and lower extremities.

Keratosis Pilaris

BACKGROUND/EPIDEMIOLOGY

Keratosis pilaris (KP) is a common skin condition, affecting up to 40% of adults worldwide. Lesions are most frequently asymptomatic, although accompanying pruritus is possible.

PATHOGENESIS

KP is a variant of normal and is associated with the hyperkeratinization of hair follicles. The etiology may be inherited in an autosomal dominant pattern with variable penetrance.

CLINICAL PRESENTATION

Examination of the skin reveals small, rough flesh-colored, pink or erythematous folliculocentric papules especially located on the upper arms, thighs, buttocks, and cheeks (Fig. 12-18). Pruritus is generally absent. The skin is sometimes described as resembling "goose bumps" or "chicken skin."

Associated conditions include xerosis (acquired dry skin), ichthyosis (a genetic disorder of dry skin), atopic dermatitis, phrynoderma (vitamin A deficiency), and type 1 diabetes mellitus. Differential diagnoses include folliculitis and follicular eczema. Folliculocentric pustules may be present in folliculitis and should be treated with antibiotics. Follicular eczema is an atopic condition treated with topical steroids and emollients.

DIAGNOSIS

The diagnosis of KP is made clinically. Additional laboratory studies and biopsies are generally unnecessary.

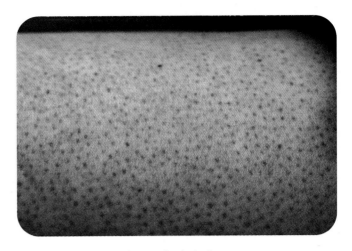

Figure 12-18 Keratosis pilaris on the thigh of a young woman.

TREATMENT

The mainstay of therapy for KP is the prevention of dry skin. In addition to emollients, lactic acid, other alpha-hydroxy acid, salicylic acid, or urea-containing emollients or keratolytics, and topical retinoids such as tretinoin or tazarotene may be helpful. The use of a loofah sponge or microdermabrasion can help remove excess keratin. Topical steroids or topical immunomodulators may be used as second-line treatment. Retinoids should be avoided in young children and pregnant women.

"AT A GLANCE" TREATMENT

- Prevention of xerosis is primary therapy.
- Emollients may help but are not curative.
  - Lactic acid, tretinoin, tazarotene, alpha-hydroxy acid, urea, or salicylic acid
- In general, KP may improve with time and is treatment resistant.

COURSE AND COMPLICATIONS

Keratosis pilaris is a variant of normal and is chronic, with flares and remissions. Thus, ongoing therapy is needed if treatment is desired. The condition often resolves with age.

ICD9 Code	
757.39	*Other specified congenital anomalies of skin*
701.1	*Keratoderma, acquired*

Suggested Reading

Allison DS, el-Azhary RA, Calobrisis SD, et al. Pityriasis rubra pilaris in children. *JAAD.* 2002;47:386–389.

Chuh A, Lee A, Zawar V, et al. Pityriasis rosea – An update. *Int J Dermatol Venereol Leprol.* 2005;71(5):311–315.

Chuh AA, Dofitas BL, Comisel GG, et al. Interventions for pityriasis rosea. *Cochrane Database Syst Rev.* 2007;(2):CD005068.

Clayton BD, Jorizzo JL, Hitchcock MG, et al. Adult pityriasis rubra pilaris: A 10-year case series. *JAAD.* 1997;36:959–964.

Gerbig AW. Treating keratosis pilaris. *JAAD.* 2002;47(3):457.

Gonzalez LM, Allen R, Janniger CK, et al. Pityriasis rosea: An important papulosquamous disorder. *Int J Dermatol.* 2005;44:757–764.

Gottlieb A, Korman NJ, Gorman KB, et al. Guidelines of care for the management of psoriasis and psoriatic arthritis: Section 2. Psoriatic arthritis: overview and guidelines of care for treatment with an emphasis on the biologics. *J Am Acad Dermatol.* 2008;58(5):851–864.

Gottlieb AB, Chao C, Dann F. Psoriasis comorbidities. *J Derm Treat.* 2008;19(1):5–21.

Gupta AK, Bluhm R. Seborrheic dermatitis. JEADV. 2004;18: 13–26.

Kang H, Alzolibani AA, Otberg N, et al. Lichen planopilaris. *Dermatologic Therapy.* 2008;21(4):249–256.

Katta R. Lichen planus. *Amer Fam Phys.* 2000;61:3319–24,3327–3328.

Kourosh AS, Miner A, Menter A. Psoriasis as the marker of underlying systemic disease. *Skin Therapy Lett.* 2008;13(1):1–5.

Lateef A, Schwartz RA. Keratosis pilaris. *Cutis.* 1999;63(4):205–207.

Lebwohl MG, van de Kerkhof P. Psoriasis. Treatment in skin: Comprehensive Therapeutic Strategies. 550–559.

Menter A, Gottlieb A, Feldman SR, et al. Guidelines of care for the management of psoriasis and psoriatic arthritis: Section 1. Overview of psoriasis and guidelines of care for the treatment of psoriasis with biologics. *J Am Acad Dermatol.* 2008;58(5):826–850.

Rasi A, Tajziehchi L, Savabi-Nasab S. Oral erythromycin is ineffective in the treatment of pityriasis rosea. *J Drugs Dermatol.* 2008;7(1):35–38.

Schwartz RA, Janusz CA, Janniger CK. Seborrheic dermatitis: An overview. *Am Fam Physician.* 2006; 74(1):125–130.

Sehgal VN, Srivastava G. (Juvenile) Pityriasis rubra pilaris. *Int J of Derm.* 2006;45(4):438–446.

Sheffield RC, Crawford P, Wright ST, et al. What's the best treatment for cradle cap? *J Fam Pract.* 2207; 56(3):232–233.

Tosti A, Piraccini BM, Cambiaghi S, et al. Nail lichen planus in children. *Arch Dermatol.* 2001;137(8):1027–1032.

White KL. Pityriasis rubra pilaris. *Derm Online Journal.* 9(4).

CHAPTER 12   Papulosquamous Diseases

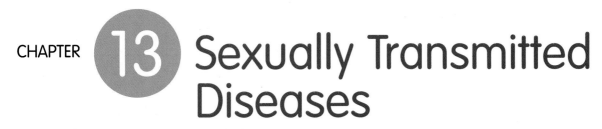

CHAPTER 13 Sexually Transmitted Diseases

Pranav Pancholi, Mahendra Pancholi, and Ellen K. Roh

With over 19 million annual cases of sexually transmitted diseases (STDs) in the United States, it is important for the primary care provider to have a good understanding of the field of STDs. STDs have for a long time been a component of dermatology but with the advent of the era of human immunodeficiency virus (HIV) are often managed by infectious disease specialists. The subsequent sections will emphasize mainly dermatologic STDs but references will be made to other STDs as well for a comprehensive review.

The following diseases are classified as STDs:

- Chancroid
- Chlamydia
- Donovanosis (granuloma inguinale)
- Genital herpes
- Genital human papilloma virus (HPV) infection (condyloma acuminatum)
- Gonorrhea
- Hepatitis B/C
- HIV
- Lymphogranuloma venereum
- Molluscum contagiosum (in some cases)
- Mycoplasma and ureaplasma urethral infections (not pneumonia)
- Pubic lice and scabies
- Syphilis
- Trichomoniasis

The above list tries to cover most of the important causes of STDs. In many instances patients may present with signs and symptoms of just one STD, but a careful history and examination should be done to search for other STDs. Up to 23% of patients presenting for the evaluation of an STD have been found to have multiple infection types.

A general template for the workup in males and females is discussed below. The workup for an STD may vary depending on the history and physical examination—for example, in males practicing sex with males (MSM), tests for Hepatitis A and B antibodies should be included, so that the vaccines can be offered to patients with negative serologies. As with any STD the importance of patient education and subsequent testing of sexual partners cannot be overstated. Every effort must be made to reach out to these individuals to discuss abstinence, monogamy, and protective techniques. Baseline studies are summarized in Table 13-1.

Table 13-1 Baseline Evaluation for Suspected Sexually Transmitted Diseases

Urethral smear	• Gonococci culture • Gram stain • PCR for *Chlamydia* • pH
Cervical smear	• Gonococci culture • Gram stain • PCR for *Chlamydia* • Wet mount for Trichomonads

HIV serology
Hepatitis B and C serology
Syphilis VDRL or RPR or FTA-ABS

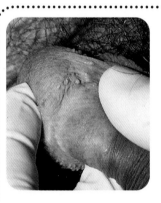

Thomas is a 16-year-old boy who comes to see you with a complaint of an "STD." He says that he noticed some warts on his penis. On further probing he denies any sexual intercourse but confesses that he saw them after he masturbated for the first time. He reports that they don't seem to change in size or disappear. On examination, you notice circumferentially arranged, skin-colored papules on the corona and sulcus of the penis (Fig. 13-1).

NONVENEREAL SKIN DISEASE

Normal Anatomic Variants

Pranav Pancholi, Mahendra Pancholi, and Ellen K. Roh

BACKGROUND

Genital lesions can be a cause of great alarm and anxiety in patients, especially when noticed after sexual intercourse for the first time or after sexual intercourse with a new partner. A good number of young men are obsessed with their genitals during puberty and will inspect their genitalia frequently. This can be a source of anxiety for the young adolescent who may be under the impression that he has been plagued by an STD.

Familiarity with normal genital anatomy and physiology is essential to be able to recognize normal anatomic variants and processes. Patients often present with worries about their own genitals, such as size, shape, retractibility of the prepuce and the distribution of pubic hair, as well as questions about vaginal/penile discharge. The normal variants of genital morphology are listed in Table 13-2 (Figs. 13-1 to 13-5).

Table 13-2 Normal Variants on Genital Skin

SIZE AND SHAPE VARIATIONS

Pubic hair distribution	Dependent on Tanner staging (Figs. 13-2A,B)
Pigmentation	Melanocytic nevi, melanotic macules/lentigines
Fordyce spots	Prominent sebaceous glands on the labia, glans, or penile shaft
Smegma	Natural white secretion by the glands of Tyson on either side of the frenulum
Pearly penile papules	Asymptomatic circumferentially arranged skin-colored papules on the corona and sulcus of the penis (Fig. 13-1). A similar variant called "vestibular papules" can be found in women on the inner labia minora
Circumcision	May be for cultural, religious, or medical reasons (Fig. 13-3)
Angiokeratoma	Discrete red papules on the scrotum or labia (Figs. 13-4, 5)

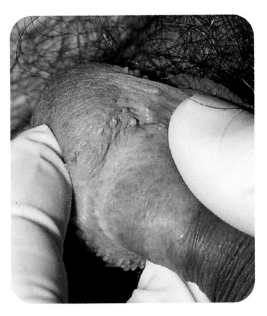

Figure 13-1 Pearly penile papules. From Goodheart HP. *Goodheart's Photoguide to Common Skin Disorders,* 3rd ed. Philadelphia: Lippincott Williams & Wilkins, 2009.

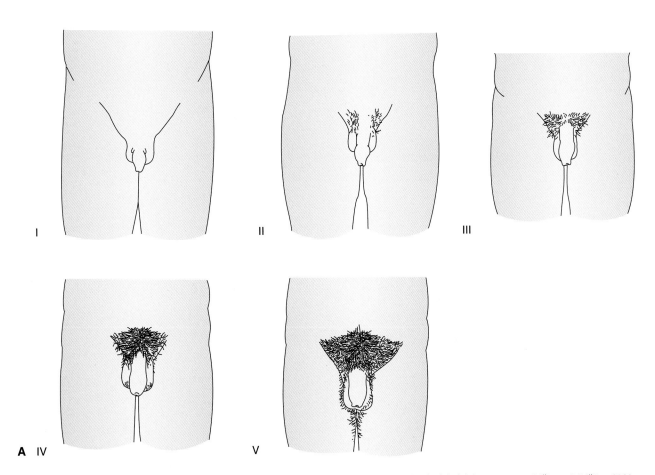

Figure 13-2 A. Tanner stages I–V in males. From Pillitteri A. *Maternal and Child Nursing,* 4th ed. Philadelphia: Lippincott Williams & Wilkins, 2003.

CHAPTER 13 Sexually Transmitted Diseases

CHAPTER 13 Sexually Transmitted Diseases

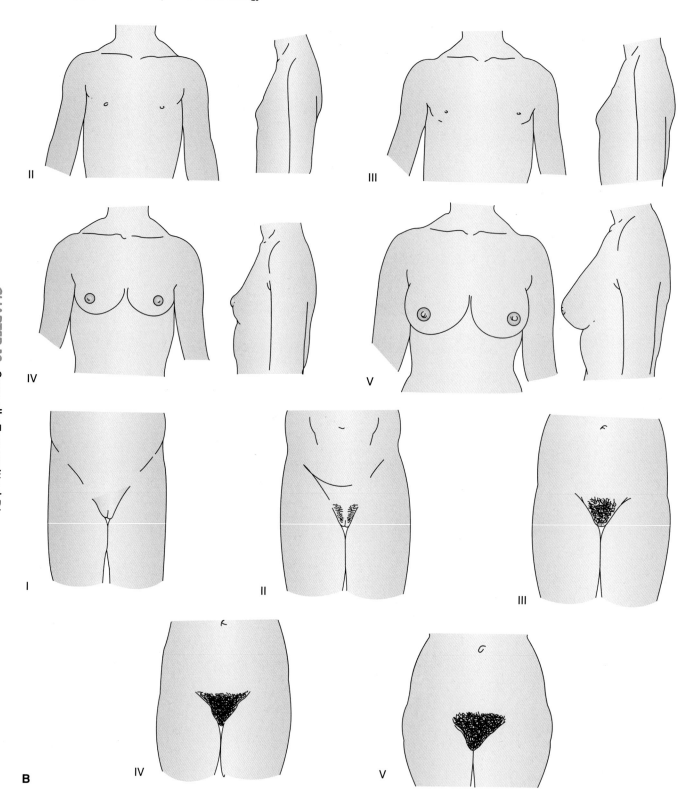

Figure 13-2 B. Tanner stages I–V in females. From Pillitteri A. *Maternal and Child Nursing,* 4th ed. Philadelphia: Lippincott Williams & Wilkins, 2003.

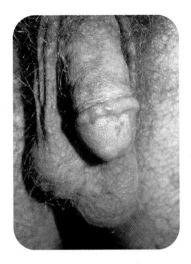

Figure 13-3 A circumcised penis. The papules present are secondary to scabies infection. From Goodheart HP. *Goodheart's Photoguide to Common Skin Disorders*, 3rd ed. Philadelphia: Lippincott Williams & Wilkins, 2009.

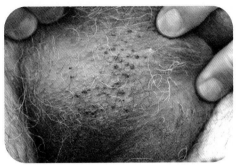

Figure 13- 4 Angiokeratoma of the scrotum.

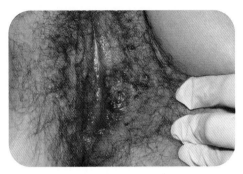

Figure 13-5 Angiokeratoma of the vulva. From Goodheart HP. *Goodheart's Photoguide to Common Skin Disorders*, 3rd ed. Philadelphia: Lippincott Williams & Wilkins, 2009.

Nonvenereal Genital Lesions

Pranav Pancholi, Mahendra Pancholi, and Ellen K. Roh

Some individuals may harbor a myth that every genital lesion is a sexually transmitted disease. Most skin conditions may present themselves in the anogenital region, and it is important to be aware of their presentations so that a false diagnosis of an STD is not made. Many of the conditions that are found on the genitals are common dermatoses also found on other body sites. Three conditions should be highlighted in this section: lichen sclerosus, lichen planus, and psoriasis. All of these conditions are inflammatory in nature, commonly present on the genitalia, and are not sexually transmitted.

Lichen planus and psoriasis are discussed in detail in Chapter 12. Psoriasis on the genitalia presents in similar fashion to other body sites, with erythematous scaling plaques (Fig. 13-6). It may involve the penis/scrotum or vulva, perianal skin, and gluteal cleft. In many cases, it is challenging to treat and is a significant cause of discomfort for the patient. Lichen planus presents with purple papules and plaques as well as whitish surface changes (Fig. 13-7) called Wickham's

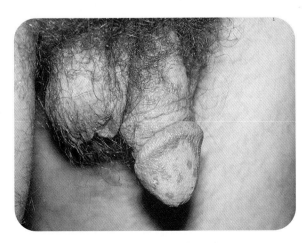

Figure 13-6 Penile psoriasis. From Goodheart HP. *Goodheart's Photoguide to Common Skin Disorders*, 3rd ed. Philadelphia: Lippincott Williams & Wilkins, 2009.

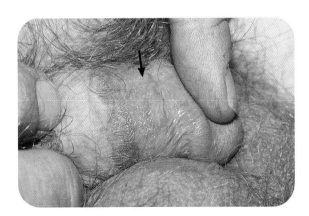

Figure 13-7 Penile lichen planus. Note the Wickham's striae at the arrow. From Goodheart HP. *Goodheart's Photoguide to Common Skin Disorders*, 3rd ed. Philadelphia: Lippincott Williams & Wilkins, 2009.

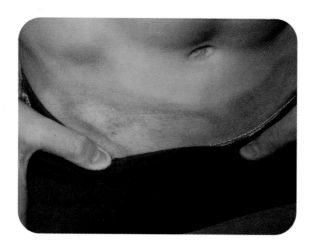

Figure 13-8 Cutaneous lichen sclerosus. Courtesy of Artesia Assets.

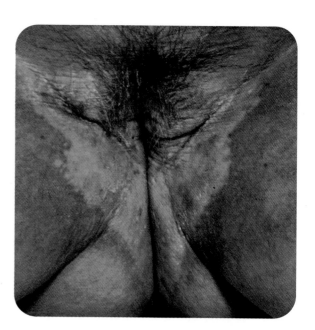

Figure 13-9 Vulvar lichen sclerosus. Image from Rubin E, Farber JL. *Pathology*, 3rd ed. Philadelphia: Lippincott Williams & Wilkins, 1999.

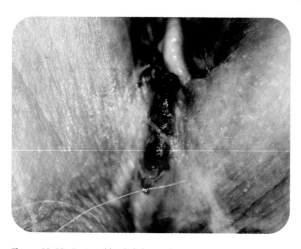

Figure 13-10 Perineal body lichen sclerosus.

striae. In women, the vaginal mucosa may be involved, leading to a thin vaginal discharge. All women with suspected or confirmed lichen planus should have regular vaginal exams and intravaginal treatment for their lichen planus.

Lichen sclerosus is an inflammatory condition of the penis or vulva of unknown etiology. It presents in middle age or older individuals, characteristically with atrophic hypopigmented patches/plaques on the genitalia most commonly. Other body sites may also be involved (Fig. 13-8). Symptoms generally are burning and itching, but the long-term scarring causes significant morbidity in some. In males, balanitis xerotica obliterans may cause both phimosis and paraphimosis in the male. In females, gradual scarring may lead to obliteration of the external anatomy (clitoris, labia minora) (Fig. 13-9), stenosis of the introitus, and involves the perineal body/perianal skin (Fig. 13-10). Chronic treatment with a potent corticosteroid is necessary.

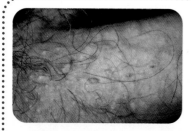

Jose is a 24-year-old who presents with a "swelling" on his penis that he noticed 2 weeks ago. He says that it does not bother him but his partner told him to get it checked. On further questioning he admits to having had multiple partners with whom he occasionally uses protection. On examination, you find a few unevenly distributed papular lesions that have a "cauliflower-like" appearance (Fig. 13-11). On application of 5% acetic acid, the lesions become whitish.

Human Papillomavirus Infection

Jennifer K. Tan-Billet, Andrew A. Nelson, Pranav Pancholi, Mahendra Pancholi, and Ellen K. Roh

BACKGROUND/EPIDEMIOLOGY

Condyloma acuminatum (CA) derives its origin from the Greek word "kondylos" meaning knob or knuckle. It is the most common STD with a 1% incidence in sexually active adults. The CDC reports that at least 50% of sexually active adults are affected at some point in their lives. The risk of disease increases with the number of lifetime sexual partners. CA is associated with infections by the human papilloma virus (HPV). In the 1970s, the association between HPV infections and cervical cancer was first recognized. However, more recently, it has become apparent that certain specific "high-risk" HPV types are more closely associated with the development of cervical cancer.

KEY FEATURES

- Condyloma acuminatum (genital warts) (CA) are wart-like lesions in the genital region caused by human papillomavirus (HPV) infection.

- Typically CA presents as soft exophytic growths in the groin and anogenital region.

- CAs are caused by HPV infections. HPV types 16, 18, 31, and 33 are "high-risk," and are associated with an increased risk of cervical cancer. HPV types 6 and 11 are "low-risk" and are not associated with an increased risk of cervical cancer.

- Common, highly prevalent sexually transmitted infection in young adults spread via intimate contact. It can be a manifestation of sexual abuse in young children.

- Treatment consists of topical destructive therapy or immunomodulatory therapies. Lesions can be quite refractory to therapy.

- A vaccine has been developed which helps to protect against HPV types 6, 11, 16, and 18 in HPV-naïve patients.

PATHOGENESIS

Similar to verruca vulgaris, CA is caused by infection with HPV. HPV infects the proliferating basal keratinocytes, causing upregulation of the cell cycle and dysregulated cellular proliferation. This results in the characteristic hyperkeratotic, exophytic lesions.

As mentioned, HPV types 16, 18, 31, 33, and 45 are "high-risk" HPV types, associated with an increased risk of cervical cancer. Of these types, HPV 16 and 18 are the most common cause of cervical cancer. It is not clear why these particular HPV types are oncogenic, although it is thought that when this HPV type DNA integrates into host DNA, it inhibits specific cellular proteins (E6 and E7 proteins). The E6 and E7 proteins normally regulate p53 and pRb genes; their inhibition results in dysregulated cell division and oncogenic potential.

CLINICAL PRESENTATION

CA are typically soft, papillated exophytic growths located in the anogenital region (perineum and perianally); the external genitalia (labia, shaft of the penis, scrotum) (Fig. 13-11); or the adjacent areas (inguinal fold, mons pubis). They are usually skin-colored or pink and lack the thick hyperkeratotic surface of common warts. Early small lesions may be easily missed during a routine examination; larger lesions can be easily recognized. Many patients have subclinical infection and may be unaware that they can spread HPV. Patients with a pre-existing sexually transmitted infection are at increased risk for disease. Although nonsexual transmission is possible (such as during the passage through an infected vaginal canal during birth), when found in children it is imperative to look for signs of sexual abuse.

Soft, moist, pink- or flesh-colored papular eruptions with normal surrounding skin are typically present. However larger nodular growths or plaques may also be seen. In males, the shaft of the penis and the prepuce are the most commonly affected sites. The labia and the posterior fornix are the most commonly affected sites in women. Individuals participating in anal intercourse may have warts around the anal region.

DIAGNOSIS

The diagnosis is based on clinical findings. However, if in doubt, 3% to 5% acetic acid can be applied with a cotton swab to look for whitening of the lesion. Aceto-whitening can also help to identify affected areas not easily apparent to the naked eye. If still uncertain, a biopsy can be performed for a more definitive diagnosis. A biopsy may also be indicated if there is any suspicion of malignant change. In women, a Papanicolaou smear should be performed. Anoscopy is recommended for patients with anal lesions. A workup for other STDs may be warranted depending on the clinical history and physical findings.

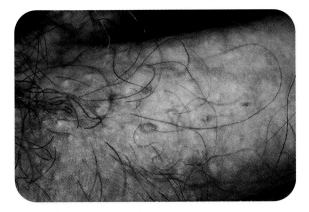

Figure 13-11 Condyloma acuminata on the penis.

Differential Diagnosis

Condyloma lata, associated with secondary syphilis can be a diagnostic consideration. Serologic testing for syphilis is recommended in high-risk patients. When only a single lesion is present, a squamous cell carcinoma should be considered.

Molluscum contagiosum (MC) in the genital area is also in the differential diagnosis with CA. While these lesions are spread by close contact they are not considered a STD in all cases. Lesions in the genital area of children are not necessarily transmitted sexually as MCs are easily spread by the patient's own genital contact. If appropriate, abuse should be considered. In adults, lesions confined to the genitals are often spread by close physical contact. See Chapter 10 for a complete discussion of MC.

Diagnostic Methods

- Many lesions can be recognized clinically. However, early lesions can be difficult to detect, particularly when they are located in the vagina
- 5% acetic acid can be applied to possible condylomatous lesions; if these lesions whiten with acetic acid, this supports the diagnosis of CA
- Colposcopy can help visualize and identify the lesions in the vagina
- A skin biopsy may be necessary to definitively identify the lesions. This is particularly true in young children, where the diagnosis of condyloma may be an indicator of sexual abuse
- HPV testing via polymerase chain reaction (PCR) can be performed to differentiate high-risk versus low-risk HPV, which can be of critical importance for female patients and their possible risk of cervical cancer.

THERAPY/TREATMENT

Many cases of CA are subclinical, with significant multifocal infection with HPV. As a result, high rates of recurrence are noted regardless of which therapeutic modality is utilized. Therapeutic options are broadly divided into locally destructive and immunomodulators.

- Destructive therapies (local anesthesia should be used for several of these therapies)
  - Podophyllin/Podophyllotoxin: Podophyllin is a root extract that acts as a local cytotoxic agent. It is physician-applied weekly to bi-weekly and requires rinsing 4 hours following application to prevent systemic toxicity. Podophyllotoxin (podofilox) is a preferred, less toxic agent that is applied by patients. It is used BID for 3 days, which is then followed by a 4-day medication-free period prior to repeating the cycle 2 to 3 times. No rinse is required between each application of podophyllotoxin.
  - Cryotherapy (liquid nitrogen): Often applied using an open-spray or cotton-tipped applicator for approximately 10 to 30 seconds to generate a 2- to 3-mm iceball around the lesion (with cooling duration of approximately 20 to 60 seconds). No clinical trials have compared cryotherapy with placebo for the treatment of genital HPV infection.
  - Trichloroacetic acid: 80% to 90% solution is used, resulting in keratinocyte necrosis. Repeated weekly application is performed. Severe burning and pain may result from therapy.
  - Electrocautery: Care should be taken, as HPV has been reported to be aerosolized following electrocautery.
  - Surgical excision: Particularly useful for large, disfiguring lesions or those lesions that impair bowel function. This is often a debulking procedure and may require adjuvant treatment with another destructive/immunomodulatory agent.
- Immunomodulators
  - Imiquimod: Stimulates toll-like receptors 7 and 8, stimulating production of inflammatory cytokines to kill HPV-infected cells. Patients may apply 5%

cream three times weekly until there is clearance or for a maximum of 16 weeks. Patients with HIV/AIDS may require up to 20 weeks of treatment,
- Interferon and bleomycin: Intralesional forms of these agents are sometimes used as second-line agents for recalcitrant lesions. However, these injections can be painful for patients.

PREVENTION

Safe sexual practice is key in preventing CA, as skin-to-skin transmission is the main route of transmission. Male latex condoms confer some protection, but skin-to-skin transmission may still be possible. In 2006, a vaccine (Gardasil®) was approved for use in female patients between the ages of 9 and 26. The vaccine protects against HPV types 6, 11, 16, and 18 and is most effective if administered prior to initial engagement in sexual activity. HPV 6 and 11 have been shown to cause approximately 90% of all cases of benign CA. HPV 16 and 18 are associated with approximately 70% of all cervical cancers. Thus, this vaccine not only protects against the high-risk HPV types, but also the most common low-risk HPV types. The vaccine requires three injections over a 6-month period. Common side effects include injection site pain, bruising, fever, vomiting, and syncope. While the vaccine can help prevent primary infection in HPV naïve patients, it does not have a role in the treatment of patients previously infected with HPV.

"AT A GLANCE" TREATMENT

- Cryotherapy with liquid nitrogen: the wart is frozen for 5 to 10 seconds with a 2- to 3-mm margin, left to thaw and then the procedure is repeated a second time.
- 5% imiquimod (Aldara) cream used three times weekly for up to 16 weeks.
- Podofilox 0.5% gel is a treatment option that can be applied by the patient at home. It is to be used twice daily for 3 days, with a break for 4 days and the repeated. Four such cycles may be carried out.
- Podophyllin resin 25% in a tincture of iodine is applied by the physician in the office, and then washed off by the patient 1 to 4 hours later. The procedure is repeated weekly until clearance. It is an FDA pregnancy category × drug.
- Trichloroacetic acid (TCA) can be used in concentrations of up to 90% to destroy genital warts. It is applied by the physician in the office, and is most effective when used for small, moist lesions. Uninvolved skin must be carefully avoided to prevent any unnecessary damage.
- Other treatment options include electrodessication, ablative carbon dioxide laser treatment, and intralesional injections of 5-fluorouracil, bleomycin, or interferon.

COURSE AND COMPLICATIONS

CA can be difficult to treat, often recurs, and as a result, has significant psychological effects on patients. Beyond the difficulty in treating lesions, there is a well-defined association between certain HPV types and an increased risk of cervical cancer. HPV types 16, 18, 31, 33, and 45 are considered "high-risk" HPV types, and are well associated with increased risk of cervical cancer. On the other hand, HPV types 6 and 11 are "low-risk" HPV types in CA and are not associated with an increased risk of cervical cancer. Female patients with CA should undergo HPV testing to determine their potential risk of cervical cancer. Due to the highly contagious nature of HPV, all patients should be counseled regarding disease transmission and the importance of engaging in protected sexual intercourse.

WHEN TO REFER

- Patients with potential lesions inside the vagina should be referred to a specialist for colposcopy.
- Patients with refractory lesions should also be referred for treatment.
- For young children affected with CA, it may be necessary to involve child protective services to evaluate for possible sexual abuse.
- Lack of response to at least two different modalities.
- If a wart is rapidly growing, pigmented, or ulcerated, the patient should have a dermatological consult to rule out a possible malignancy.

CHAPTER 13 Sexually Transmitted Diseases

NOT TO BE MISSED

- Malignant transformation of genital warts.

More than two-thirds of people who have sexual contact with an infected person will develop genital warts, followed by an incubation period of weeks to months. Lesions can increase in size and number and often persist, though they can occasionally spontaneously regress (as many as 30% over 4 months). Recurrence is common, occurring within 3 months in 25% to 67% of cases. Immunosuppressed patients are more likely to have resistance to treatment, recurrence, and malignant transformation.

ICD9 Codes

078.11	*Condyloma acuminatum*
078.10	*Viral warts, unspecified*

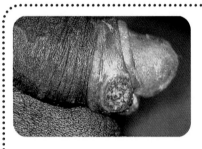

Joe, a 29-year-old long-distance truck driver, presents to the clinic with a "condition" on his penis. On further probing he admits to having had unprotected sexual intercourse with a commercial sex worker about a month ago on one of his journeys. He states that the lesion started off as a small pimple that has now changed into its present state. On examination you notice an oval 2x1 cm ulcer with indurated edges (Fig. 13-12). On palpation the ulcer is painless and inguinal lymphadenopathy is noted.

KEY FEATURES

- A single painless ulcer on the external genitalia most commonly (or other site of primary infection).

- Syphilis is caused by the spirochete *Treponema pallidum*.

- The incubation period of syphilis is 9–90 days, however most lesions appear within 3 weeks of contact.

- Primary syphilis typically begins as a small red papule that rapidly progresses into a single, shallow, painless ulcer.

(Continued)

Genital Ulcer Disease Syphilis

Pranav Pancholi, Mahendra Pancholi, and Ellen K. Roh

BACKGROUND/EPIDEMIOLOGY

The name of the condition is derived from a poem written by Girolamo Francastoro of Verona in 1530 known as *syphilis sive morbus gallicus* in which a mythical swineherd Syphilis is afflicted by *morbus gallicus* as a punishment for insulting Apollo, the Greek god of the sun. Syphilis is also known as the great impostor because of its variety of presentations and its ability to mimic other infections and immune-mediated processes. After a steady decline in its incidence over five decades, the number of syphilis cases to the U.S. Centers for Disease Control and Prevention has been increasing again yearly since 2000. Most of these cases have been in men, particularly in men who have sex with men.

PATHOGENESIS

Syphilis is a multisystem chronic infectious disease caused by the spirochete *Treponema pallidum*. The organism enters the body through mucous membranes or breaks in the skin, and rapidly spreads via blood vessels and lymphatics. The main route of transmission is unprotected sexual intercourse. Other routes of transmission include in utero transfer and rarely blood transfusions or needle-stick injuries.

CLINICAL PRESENTATION

Primary Syphilis

The incubation period of syphilis is 9 to 90 days, however most lesions appear within 3 weeks of contact. Primary syphilis typically begins as a small red papule that rapidly progresses into a single, shallow painless ulcer (Fig. 13-12). The ulcer is round or oval and well-defined with indurated edges and a clean base that can produce a serous exudate. Inguinal lymph nodes are enlarged, rubbery, painless, and discrete.

This primary ulcer, or chancre, heals spontaneously in 4 to 8 weeks, so may go unnoticed, especially in females. And though the classic chancre is painless,

KEY FEATURES (*Continued*)

- Secondary syphilis: When primary syphilis goes untreated, it is followed by generalized widespread manifestations mainly on the skin and mucus membranes (*Syphilides*).
  - Generalized, symmetrical, and nonitchy, pink, macular lesions involving the trunk, limbs, palms, and soles. The macular lesions may then progress to coppery-red papular or papulosquamous lesions.
  - At mucocutaneous junctions and other areas with excessive moisture and friction the lesions become confluent and flattened and are termed condyloma lata.

- Tertiary syphilis manifests itself after 3 to 20 years. Skin lesions are known as gummas, which form as a result of focal granulomatous tissue destruction. Clinically, they usually appear as an isolated ulcerated nodule on the lower leg.

- Treatment is with benzathine penicillin intramuscular injections.

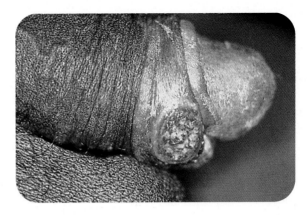

Figure 13-12 Primary syphilis. From Goodheart HP. *Goodheart's Photoguide to Common Skin Disorders*, 3rd ed. Philadelphia: Lippincott Williams & Wilkins, 2009.

patients can occasionally present with pain if there is a secondary bacterial infection or co-infection with herpes or chancroid.

Secondary Syphilis

When primary syphilis goes untreated, it is followed by generalized widespread manifestations mainly on the skin and mucous membranes termed as secondary syphilis. These appear around 4 to 10 weeks after the initial chancre. During the secondary stage, the patient may also have constitutional symptoms such as fever, malaise, headache, myalgia, and anorexia. The skin lesions also known as syphilides occur in 75% to 80% of patients. They are generalized, symmetrical and nonitchy, pink, macular lesions (Fig. 13-13). These usually involve the trunk, limbs, palms, and soles. The macular lesions may then progress to coppery-red papular or papulosquamous lesions. At mucocutaneous junctions and other areas with excessive moisture and friction the lesions become confluent and flattened and are termed condyloma lata (Fig. 13-14). In the mucous membranes eroded papules may coalesce to

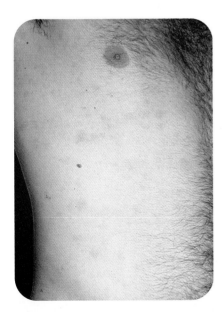

Figure 13-13 Secondary syphilis: papulosquamous lesions on the body, similar to pityriasis rosea. From Goodheart HP. *Goodheart's Photoguide to Common Skin Disorders*, 3rd ed. Philadelphia: Lippincott Williams & Wilkins, 2009.

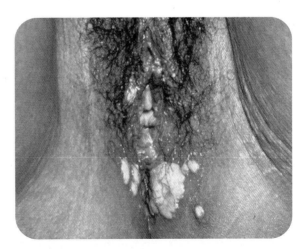

Figure 13-14 Condyloma lata on the vulva. From Goodheart HP. *Goodheart's Photoguide to Common Skin Disorders*, 3rd ed. Philadelphia: Lippincott Williams & Wilkins, 2009.

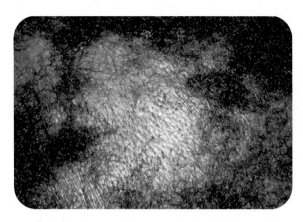

Figure 13-15 "Moth-eaten" appearance of the alopecia of secondary syphilis. From Goodheart HP. *Goodheart's Photoguide to Common Skin Disorders*, 3rd ed. Philadelphia: Lippincott Williams & Wilkins, 2009.

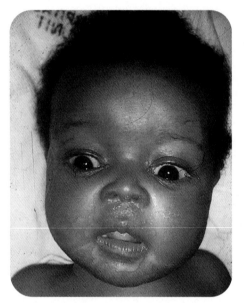

Figure 13-16 Saddle-nose deformity of congenital syphilis. From Bickley LS, Szilagyi P. *Bates' Guide to Physical Examination and History Taking*, 8th ed. Philadelphia: Lippincott Williams & Wilkins, 2003.

form "snail-track" ulcers. Syphilitic alopecia may result in patchy hair loss on the sides and back of the head, giving it a "moth eaten" appearance (Fig. 13-15). Syphilis can also involve the nails, resulting in paronychia.

Fifty percent of patients with secondary syphilis may have generalized lymphadenopathy. The lymph nodes are painless, discrete, rubbery, mobile, and vary in size from 0.5 to 2 cm. Other manifestations of secondary syphilis include arthritis, periostitis, tenosynovitis, iritis, choroidoretinitis, hepatitis, glomerulonephritis, and neurologic disease.

Tertiary Syphilis

Tertiary syphilis manifests itself after 3 to 20 years. Skin lesions are known as gummas, which form as a result of focal granulomatous tissue destruction. Clinically, they usually appear as an isolated ulcerated nodule on the lower leg. Gummas may also form on the mucous membranes, sub-mucus tissue, and bone. Other manifestations of tertiary syphilis include cardiovascular syphilis (may cause aortic aneurysm) and neurosyphilis (Argyll Robertson pupils, tabes dorsalis, positive Romberg sign).

Congenital Syphilis

T. pallidum is able to cross the placenta after the fourth month of gestation and may cause fetal infections. Infants born with syphilis infections are often normal at birth but develop signs of infection within the first 2 years of life. The most frequent and often first finding is "snuffles" due to a perforated septum. In some cases, the child may have a saddle nose deformity (Fig. 13-16). Cutaneous lesions most resemble secondary syphilis. Other less common findings include syphilitic pemphigus (bullous eruption), rhagades, condyloma lata, Parrot pseudoparalysis (epiphysitis causing pain leading to infant's refusing to move). These children may also have neurosyphilis.

DIAGNOSIS

Dark ground microscopy is the only definitive means of establishing the diagnosis, however a negative result does not rule out syphilis. Dark ground microscopy should be repeated for 2 consecutive days if negative. It should be avoided on oral lesions due to the presence of oral commensal treponemes that may obscure the diagnosis.

Serologic Tests

The following tests are used in the diagnosis of syphilis:

- VDRL (Venereal Disease Research Laboratory)
- RPR (Rapid plasma reagent)
- FTA-ABS (fluorescent treponemal antibody)
- MHA-TP (microhemagglutination assay for *Treponema pallidum*)

RPR and VDRL are also known as nonspecific tests. A positive nonspecific test should always be confirmed with specific tests such as the FTA-ABS or MHA-TP.

The following points should be noted when performing serologic tests on patients:

- Serologic tests become positive 3 to 5 weeks after the infection or 1 to 2 weeks after appearance of the chancre. Hence a negative test does not rule out syphilis and repeat testing is recommended. An initially negative test that becomes positive later is highly diagnostic.

- A single nonspecific positive test result (VDRL or RPR) does not mean that the lesion is due to syphilis, as there may be other conditions such as autoimmune disease, e.g., lupus, vaccination, or pregnancy that may give a false-positive result.
- A single positive test should be confirmed with another test as false positives can occur.
- Watch out for false negatives due to the prozone phenomenon inherent in the RPR and VDRL tests. This is rare.

TREATMENT

Primary Syphilis, Secondary Syphilis, and Early Latent Syphilis (Less than 1 Year)

A single dose of intramuscular, benzathine penicillin G 2.4 million units is adequate. A 2-week course of doxycycline 100 mg BID may be used as an alternative for penicillin-sensitive patients. Penicillin desensitization is recommended for pregnant allergic patients.

Syphilis of Undetermined Duration and Late Syphilis

Three consecutive weeks of intramuscular, benzathine penicillin G, 2.4 million units is adequate. For penicillin allergic patients a 4-week doxycycline regime may be used. Patients with primary and secondary syphilis should be informed of the Jarisch-Herxheimer reaction before initiation of penicillin therapy. This is a transient phase that lasts for about 24 hours after penicillin initiation. Symptoms include transient enlargement the chancre and skin lesions and a flu-like syndrome consisting of headache, fever, malaise, chills, and arthralgias.

"AT A GLANCE" TREATMENT

- The treatment of choice of syphilis remains intramuscular benzathine penicillin G, 2.4 million units in a single dose
- For penicillin allergic patients: doxycycline 100 mg PO BID × 2 weeks

WHEN TO REFER

- Individuals co-infected with HIV should be managed by infectious disease specialists.
- If there is any suspicion of internal organ involvement.
- Pregnant patients with syphilis should be evaluated by a high-risk obstetrician.

NOT TO BE MISSED

- Systemic complications, especially cardiovascular and neurologic.

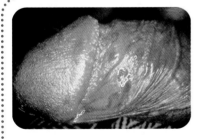

John is a 20-year-old college student who presents with recurring painful genital sores. They tend to occur when he is stressed (he is currently studying for finals) and last for about 1 week.

He can sometimes predict an outbreak, as he will have a tingling sensation the day before. He is worried because he is in a new relationship and does not want his partner to find out. On exam, there are several grouped erosions and vesicles on the penis that are tender to palpation (Fig. 13-17).

Other Conditions Causing Genital Ulcers

Pranav Pancholi, Mahendra Pancholi, and Ellen K. Roh

BACKGROUND/EPIDEMIOLOGY

The variety of conditions that fall under the category of genital ulcer disease can usually be differentiated based on the history and physical examination and a few simple lab tests. It is important to note that even though most causes of genital ulcer disease are sexually transmitted agents, others causes should be sought for when the history does not suggest sexual transmission.

The cause of the above case report, herpes simplex, is the most common of the genital ulcer diseases. In 2008, the CDC found that at least 45 million people ages 12 and older have had a genital HSV infection. HSV 1 and 2 are discussed in detail in Chapter 10. This section will include brief discussion on

HSV-related disease, though the overarching purpose is to review the many causes of genital ulcerations. Other less common causes of genital ulcerations are chancroid, lymphogranuloma venereum, and granuloma inguinale.

Chancroid is a rare STD in the United States that is most common in sexually active heterosexual men. Uncircumcised men are more at risk for developing the infection than circumcised men.

Lymphogranuloma venereum (LGV) is a primarily cutaneous STD that is also rare in the United States, though is endemic is some developing countries (India and Africa). It occurs in all races, and is the most common in young adults (Andrews).

Granuloma inguinale (or donovanosis) is very rarely reported in the United States, and most cases are thought to be acquired during foreign travel. It is endemic in tropical and subtropical climates, such as Papua New Guinea, Brazil, parts of South Africa, India, and Indonesia, and among the aborigines of Australia (Velho).

PATHOGENESIS

All venereal genital ulcer diseases have an infectious etiology. HSV-2 is the responsible for most cases of genital herpes, though HSV-1 has been increasing identified as the infectious agent in up to 40% cases of genital herpes. It is spread by skin-to-skin contact. Active lesions contain live virus, but patients can also have asymptomatic shedding between outbreaks. Chancroid is caused by the bacteria *Haemophilus ducreyi*. The unique serotypes L1, L2, and L3 of the bacteria *Chlamydia trachomatis* is the causative organism for lymphogranuloma venereum. Granuloma inguinale is a result of infection with *Klebsiella granulomatis* (formerly known as *Calymmatobacterium granulomatis* or *Donovania granulomatis*).

CLINICAL PRESENTATION

The most important clues to making the diagnosis are:

- Single lesion or multiple lesions
- Painful or painless
- Incubation period (determined from sexual history)

DIAGNOSIS/THERAPY

For details on diagnosis and therapy of genital ulcerative disease, see the discussion in Table 13-3 (Figs. 13-17 to 13-20). Table 13-3 lists the five main causes of genital ulcer disease caused by sexually transmitted diseases. Other nonvenereal causes that should also be in the differential diagnosis include balanitis/vulvitis, erythema multiforme, Stevens-Johnson syndrome, folliculitis, scabies, Crohn disease, tuberculosis, and squamous cell carcinoma need to be considered.

"AT A GLANCE" TREATMENT

- See Table 13-3 for a primary and secondary treatment recommendations

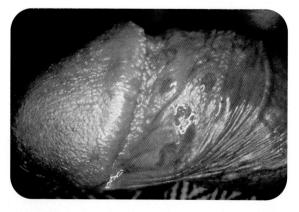

Figure 13-17 Herpes simplex type II infection on the penis. From Goodheart HP. *Goodheart's Photoguide to Common Skin Disorders,* 3rd ed. Philadelphia: Lippincott Williams & Wilkins, 2009.

COURSE AND COMPLICATIONS

All of the genital ulcer diseases described above can have a recurring course if left untreated. Rupture of buboes and fistula development have been reported with chancroid.

Table 13-3 Genital Ulcerations (LAD)

CONDITION	CAUSE	ULCER	LAD	NOTES	PRIMARY TREATMENT	SECONDARY TREATMENT
Chancroid Fig. 13-18	*Haemophilus ducreyi*	Painful	Painful	Soft/nonindurated shallow ulcer with undermined ragged edges and a sloughing base. Painful, tender lympha-denopathy (+ buboes)	• Azithromycin 1 g PO in a single dose	• Ceftriaxone 250 mg IM in a single dose • Ciprofloxacin 500 mg PO BID for 3 days • Erythromycin base 500 mg TID for 7 days
Granuloma inguinale Fig. 13-20	*Calymmatobac-terium granulomatis*	Painless	None	Nodule that often ulcerates with beefy red granulomatous tissue that bulges out, above the level of surrounding skin	• Trimethoprim/sulfamethoxazole One DS tab (800 mg/160 mg) PO BID • Doxycycline 100 mg PO BID Therapy for at least 3-week course, until full resolution	• Ciprofloxacin 750 mg PO BID • Erythromycin 500 mg PO QID • Azithromycin 1 g PO q wk
Herpes simplex Fig. 13-17	Herpesvirus	Painful	Painful	Primary infection is often accompanied by systemic "flu-like" symptoms	• See Chapter 10, Table 10-2	
Lymphogran uloma venereum Fig. 13-19	*Chlamydia trachomatis* L1–L3	Painless	Painful	Ulcer, vesicle, papule or pustule (~5 mm), heals spontaneously. Followed by exquisitely tender, matted lymphadenopathy that ulcerates through the overlying skin+ buboes and groove sign	• Doxycycline 100 mg PO BID × 21 days	• Erythromycin 500 mg PO QID for 21 days
Primary syphilis Fig. 13-12	*Treponoma pallidum*	Painless	Painless	Ulcer is round, well-defined with indurated edges and a clean base that produces a serous exudate	• **Adult Primary/secondary:** Benzathine penicillin G 2.4 million U IM in a single dose **Latent/unknown duration/tertiary** Benzathine penicillin G 2.4 million U IM qwk for 3 wk • **Pediatric Primary/secondary:** Benzathine penicillin G 50,000 U/kg IM single dose; not to exceed 2.4 million U **Latent/unknown duration/tertiary** Benzathine penicillin G 50,000 U/kg IM qwk for 3 wk • **Adult Neurosyphilis** Penicillin G procaine (Crysticillin) 2.4 million U IM qd for 17–21 d + probenecid 500 mg PO QID for 17–21d • **Pediatric Neurosyphilis:** Crystalline penicillin G 50,000 U/kg IM (up to 2.4 million U); give 3 doses at 1-wk intervals	Penicillin-allergic patients should undergo penicillin allergy skin testing and penicillin desensitization, if necessary (U.S. CDC) Alternate: Doxycycline • Primary/secondary/early latent: 100 mg PO BID × 2 wk • Late latent: 100 mg PO BID × 1 mo • Neurosyphilis: 200 mg PO QID × 1 mo

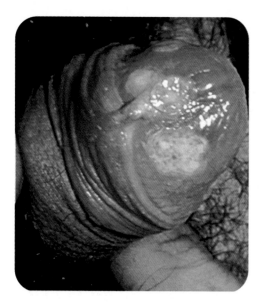

Figure 13-18 Chancroid. From Goodheart HP. *Goodheart's Photoguide to Common Skin Disorders*, 3rd ed. Philadelphia: Lippincott Williams & Wilkins, 2009.

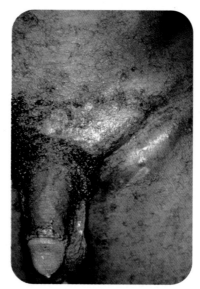

Figure 13-19 Lymphogranuloma venereum. Regional lymphadenitis ("the groove sign") is present. From Goodheart HP. *Goodheart's Photoguide to Common Skin Disorders*, 3rd ed. Philadelphia: Lippincott Williams & Wilkins, 2009.

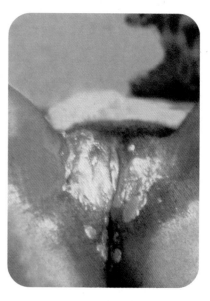

Figure 13-20 Granuloma inguinale. From Sweet RL, Gibbs RS. *Atlas of Infectious Diseases of the Female Genital Tract.* Philadelphia: Lippincott Williams & Wilkins, 2005.

WHEN TO REFER

- If patients have co-infection with HIV.
- If disease is not responsive to standard treatment.

NOT TO BE MISSED

- Cases of syphilis, gonorrhea, and chlamydia must all be reported to the local health department.

Scarring can also occur with lymphogranuloma venereum, as well as rare systemic complications. Chronic lesions of granuloma inguinale can heal with a deforming scarring and rarely become malignant (basal cell carcinoma and squamous cell carcinoma). Patients who have co-infection with HIV can have a more recalcitrant disease course.

ICD9 Codes

097.9	*Syphilis, unspecified*
098.0	*Gonococcal infection (acute) of lower genitourinary tract*
054.9	*Herpes simplex without mention of complication*

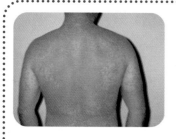

A 32-year-old man presents with a new rash on his trunk and extremities. He is feeling poorly with many symptoms. He reports fever, general malaise, headache, myalgia, nausea, vomiting, diarrhea, and a generalized morbilliform skin rash (Fig. 13-21) that involves the palms and soles. He reports having a new partner with whom he has been having unprotected intercourse. An HIV screening is positive.

External Markers of HIV

Pranav Pancholi, Mahendra Pancholi, and Ellen K. Roh

BACKGROUND/EPIDEMIOLOGY

In 1985, the human immunodeficiency virus (HIV) was identified as the causative agent for acquired immunodeficiency syndrome (AIDS). It was initially thought to be a disease of homosexual men, but today it is present in every country and affects homosexual and heterosexual men and women. In 2000, the CDC estimated that 50 million people were infected worldwide. It is most commonly spread through sexual intercourse, but can also be spread by contaminated needles, during pregnancy, contact with contaminated fluids, and blood transfusion.

PATHOPHYSIOLOGY

HIV is a retrovirus that mainly infects CD4 T cells, resulting in their depletion and an impaired cell-mediated immunity. Once the CD4 T cell count is 200 or less, the patient is defined as having AIDS and becomes susceptible to opportunistic pathogens.

CLINICAL PRESENTATION

The cutaneous manifestations of HIV are often the initial signs of infection, and recognition of these markers can help the provider make an earlier diagnosis. The first manifestation of HIV on the skin occurs during the seroconversion period. This consists of a flu-like syndrome with fever, general malaise, headache, myalgia, nausea, vomiting, diarrhea, and a generalized morbilliform skin rash that involves the palms and soles (Fig. 13-21). This rash lasts 12 to 15 days, after which it disappears spontaneously. The presentation of cutaneous manifestations can be divided into early (prior to immunosuppression); intermediate (immunosuppressed but prior to diagnosis of AIDS); and late manifestations (AIDS-associated), as discussed in Table 13-4 (Figs. 13-22 to 13-26). Most of the listed conditions worsen/increase in intensity with increasing immunosuppression.

HIV infection is associated with multiple cutaneous malignancies:

- AIDS-related B-cell non-Hodgkin lymphoma with cutaneous nodules
- Anal carcinoma/cervical intraepithelial neoplasia; progressive and recalcitrant
- Intraoral, multiple squamous cell carcinoma, Bowen disease metastatic basal cell carcinoma
- Kaposi sarcoma may present at any point in the course of HIV/AIDS.
- Malignant melanoma is more aggressive in HIV.
- Pediatric AIDS patients may develop leiomyosarcoma.
- Squamous cell carcinoma of anal mucosa

DIAGNOSIS

There are two subtypes of the HIV virus, type 1 and type 2. Type 1 is more common in the United States. ELISA is used to check for both subtypes and then this is confirmed by Western blotting.

It is important to note that there is a window period of at least 6 weeks following exposure to HIV during which time the virus will be undetectable. Hence it

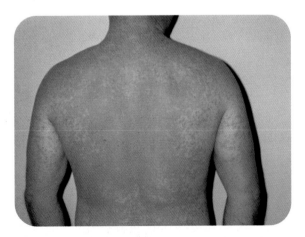

Figure 13-21 Morbilliform dermatitis of acute HIV infection. From Goodheart HP. *Goodheart's Photoguide to Common Skin Disorders*, 3rd ed. Philadelphia: Lippincott Williams & Wilkins, 2009.

Table 13-4 Cutaneous Manifestations of HIV Infection

Early

Condyloma and verruca	Extensive genital warts may be treatment resistant. Increase in number in early stage. No increase in later stages
Generalized wasting	Greater than 10% weight loss with general skin laxity
Kaposi sarcoma (KS)	Reddish purple papulonodular lesions secondary to human herpesvirus-8 infection (Fig. 13-22). May present early, intermediate or late
Morbilliform dermatitis	During the seroconversion period lasting 2–3 weeks. Clears spontaneously
Papulosquamous eruption of HIV	Generalized xerosis and pruritus. 4.5% of HIV patients report itch
Seborrheic dermatitis	Treatment resistant and often extensive

Intermediate

Aphthous ulcers	Multiple, tiny reddish ulcers with a yellow center
Dermatophyte infection	Tinea corporis, tinea cruris, tinea pedis, pityriasis versicolor
Disseminated scabies	Crusted, scaling plaques, discreet or generalized. Extremely contagious due to the thousands of *Sarcoptes* mites present
Ecthyma and abscesses	More common in IV drug abusers
Eosinophilic folliculitis	Papular, pruritic eruption with pustules
Herpes infections	Multiple, tiny, painful ulcers. May be extensive and recalcitrant
Molluscum contagiosum	Shiny, dome-shaped, umbilicated papules. Differentiate from cutaneous cryptococcal infections
Onychomycosis	Fungal nail infection mainly in the proximal nail plate
Oral/vaginal candidiasis	White crusted lesions in the mouth easily removable by scraping. Oral hairy leukoplakia will not scrape off (Fig. 13-26). Increases in severity/prevalence with increasing immunosuppression
Papular pruritic eruption	Itchy red papules on the head/neck/upper trunk (Fig. 13-25)
Pigmentary changes	Hyperpigmentation, sometimes drug related

Late Complications

Bacillary angiomatosis	Differentiated from KS by biopsy (Fig. 13-23)
Drug reactions	Due to the numerous drugs used in therapy various drug reactions ranging from mild pruritus to Stevens-Johnson syndrome may occur
Erythema multiforme	Target-like papulovesicular lesions with a red center
Herpes zoster	Painful papulovesicular lesions on an erythematous base, usually involving one dermatome but in HIV recurrent multidermatomal attacks are not uncommon
Lipodystrophy	Facial wasting with collection of fat in the abdominal region
Mycobacterium avium complex	Disseminated disease. Skin findings are nonspecific, but including scaling plaques, ulcerations, panniculitis and draining sinuses
Oral hairy leukoplakia	Whitish crusty lesions on the side of the tongue that are not easily removable by scraping (Fig. 13-24)
Photosensitivity	UVB>UVA sensitivity. Increased risk for photo-induced lichenoid drug reactions

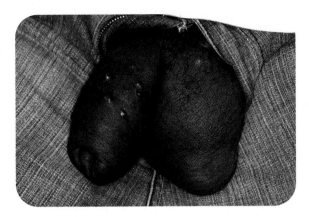

Figure 13-22 HIV infection-associated Kaposi sarcoma.

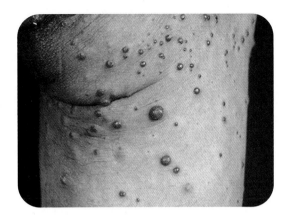

Figure 13-23 Bacillary angiomatosis in HIV infection. From Goodheart HP. *Goodheart's Photoguide to Common Skin Disorders*, 3rd ed. Philadelphia: Lippincott Williams & Wilkins, 2009.

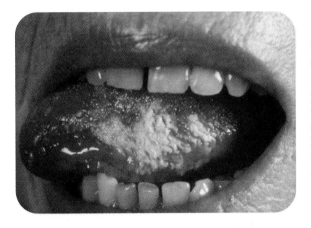

Figure 13-24 Oral hairy leukoplakia in HIV, secondary to Epstein-Barr virus infection. From Goodheart HP. *Goodheart's Photoguide to Common Skin Disorders*, 3rd ed. Philadelphia: Lippincott Williams & Wilkins, 2009.

is advisable to check for HIV at 6 weeks, 3 months, and finally at 6 months before ruling out the possibility of infection.

A comprehensive baseline assessment of an HIV-positive patient will include but not be limited to the following tests: STD screening, hepatitis screening, Papanicolaou smear in women, complete blood count, blood chemistry, liver function tests, lipid profile, CD4+ count, viral load, viral resistance assay, *Toxoplasma* screen, tuberculin skin test, and a chest X-ray. Other tests may be performed as deemed necessary.

TREATMENT

The mainstay of therapy is the HAART regime (Highly Active Anti-Retroviral Treatment). This consists of a combination

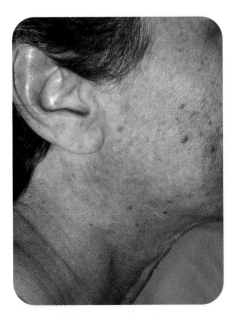

Figure 13-25 Papular pruritic eruption. Erythematous papules, plaques in a woman with AIDS (CD4 count of 80).

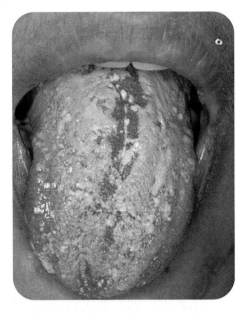

Figure 13-26 Oral candidiasis in HIV. From Goodheart HP. *Goodheart's Photoguide to Common Skin Disorders*, 3rd ed. Philadelphia: Lippincott Williams & Wilkins, 2009.

CHAPTER 13 Sexually Transmitted Diseases

Table 13-5 Therapy Suggestions for Conditions Prevalent in HIV/AIDS

Nonspecific pruritus	• Antihistamines: cetirizine, loratadine, hydroxyzine, doxepin. See Chapter 17 for details.
Xerosis	• Moisturizing creams such as Cerave
Seborrheic dermatitis	• Mild potency steroids (i.e., hydrocortisone 1%) • Coal tar preparations • Topical antifungals (i.e., ketoconazole 2% cream BID)
Aphthous ulcers	• Local anesthetic mouthwash (lidocaine) PRN • Clobetasol gel BID • Aphthae major: thalidomide
Oral candidiasis	• Nystatin or ketoconazole mouth wash
Vaginal candidiasis	• Nystatin or ketoconazole
Dermatophyte infection including onychomycosis	• Ketoconazole, griseofulvin, terbinafine (see Chapter 7 for treatment details based on infection type/location)
Eosinophilic folliculitis	• Mild to moderate potency steroids
Molluscum contagiosum	• Cryotherapy, surgical removal
Warts (genital or common)	• Cryotherapy, imiquimod
Herpes infections	• Valacyclovir 500 mg PO BID is only FDA-approved agent for suppression
Ecthyma and abscesses	• Oral antibiotics (base on culture and site) • Incise and drain abscesses
Kaposi sarcoma (KS)	• Cryotherapy, IV chemotherapeutic agents
Bacillary angiomatosis	• Erythromycin 1 g BID for 4 weeks. • Serious infection: consider adding a third-generation cephalosporin or an aminoglycoside
Lipodystrophy	• Change of antiviral regime, injectable poly-L-lactic acid (Sculptura), autologous fat transplants

therapy using drugs from the three categories; nucleoside reverse transcriptase inhibitors (NRTIs); nonnucleoside reverse transcriptase inhibitors (NNRTIs); and protease inhibitors (PIs). Treatment success is monitored by regular CD4+ counts and viral load measurements and is aimed at a CD4+ count above 500 and an undetectable viral load. With appropriate antiretroviral treatment, most of the cutaneous manifestations will also improve. Table 13-5 lists a few conditions and their treatments.

WHEN TO REFER

• HIV therapy should be managed by an infectious disease specialist.

• The cutaneous manifestations can be referred if unresponsive to standard treatments.

"AT A GLANCE" TREATMENT

• The mainstay of HIV therapy is a combination therapy using drugs from the three categories; nucleoside reverse transcriptase inhibitors (NRTIs), non-nucleoside reverse transcriptase inhibitors (NNRTIs), and protease inhibitors (PIs).
    • This is most often managed by infectious disease specialists
• Therapy suggestions for conditions prevalent in HIV/AIDS are summarized in Table 13-5.

NOT TO BE MISSED

• Opportunistic infections.

ICD9 Codes

042	*Human immunodeficiency virus (hiv) disease*
690.10	*Seborrheic dermatitis, unspecified*
690.11	*Seborrhea capitis*

690.12	*Seborrheic infantile dermatitis*
690.18	*Other seborrheic dermatitis*
698.9	*Unspecified pruritic disorder*
078.0	*Molluscum contagiosum*
078.10	*Viral warts, unspecified*
078.11	*Condyloma acuminatum*

Suggested Reading

CDC. Primary and secondary syphilis—United States, 2003–2004. *MMWR Morb Mortal Wkly Rep.* 2006; 55(10):269–273.

Erdal E, Zalewska A, Schwartz RA. Cutaneous Manifestations of HIV Disease. http://emedicine.medscape.com/article/1133746-overview. Accessed January 25,2010.

Kurgis B. Skin manifestations of human immunodeficiency virus (HIV): Part 1. Infectious manifestations. *J Am Osteopath Assoc.* 1993;93:106.

Kurgis B. Skin manifestations of human immunodeficiency virus (HIV): Part 2. Noninfectious skin manifestations. *J Am Osteopath Assoc.* 1993;93:223.

O'Rourke E, Schweon S. Syphilis. Still a public health danger. *RN.* 2007;70(7):26–31.

Pabst KM, Reichart CA, Knud-Hansen CR, et al. Disease prevalence among women attending a sexually transmitted disease clinic varies with reason for visit. *Sexually Transmitted Diseases.* 1992;19:88–91.

Panagiotis C, Efthimios D, Konstantinos P, et al. Human papilloma virus: Diagnostic, treatment and preventive issues. *Akush Ginekol (Sofiia).* 2008;47(1):35–38.

Rigopoulos D, Paparizos V, Katsambas A. Cutaneous markers of HIV infection. *Clin Dermatol.* 2004;22(6): 487–498.

Scheinfeld N, Lehman DS. An evidence-based review of medical and surgical treatments of genital warts. *Dermatol Online J.* 2006;12(3):5.

Velho PE, Souza EM, Belda JW. Donovanosis. *Braz J Infect Dis.* 2008;12(6):521–525.

Wang KL. Human papillomavirus and vaccination in cervical cancer. *Taiwan J Obstet Gynecol.* 2007;46(4): 352–362.

CHAPTER 14 Pigmentary Disorders

Vinod E. Nambudiri

Much like the height and weight of individuals, the spectrum of skin pigmentation is a continuous, fluid distribution of hues. The pigment-containing cells of the skin, the melanocytes, are thought to be present in roughly equal number across all skin types. However, the distribution of melanosomes, subcellular organelles rich in the primary skin pigment melanin contained within melanocytes, varies in concentration. Greater melanosome density results in darker baseline pigmentation. This chapter examines disorders in pigmentation, with consideration given to the common specific pigmentary aberrations of melasma and vitiligo, as well as generalized disease processes such as postinflammatory hyperpigmentation.

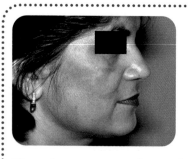

A 39-year-old primigravid Indian woman presents to her physician at 30 weeks gestation concerned about the appearance of several new dark-colored patches of skin on her cheeks and forehead. These have appeared over the last few weeks. On physical exam, you note that she has a baseline brown complexion. There are multiple darker brown, nonelevated, blotchy patches of skin on her face, primarily involving the forehead, cheeks, and nose (Fig. 14-1). On further history taking, she reveals that she spends a considerable time outdoors enjoying the sunny weather. She also recalls her mother and sister mentioning similar episodes during their respective pregnancies. What is the most likely diagnosis? What if any treatments are you able to offer her?

Melasma

BACKGROUND/EPIDEMIOLOGY

The term "melasma" derives from the Greek words describing a "black spot" and was originally used in medical literature to refer to the increased skin pigmentation arising in the lower extremities due to venous stasis. In modern clinical dermatology, the term has been used to refer to conditions resulting in patchy or generalized hyperpigmentation, most often of the face. When occurring in pregnant women, the term "chloasma" is used to describe the hyperpigmented appearance of the face—often referred to as the "mask of pregnancy."

PATHOPHYSIOLOGY

While the disease may appear in any individual, females and those of Asian, Hispanic, and Middle Eastern descent are more commonly affected by melasma than others. The condition is one that typically affects individuals in the second and third decades of life. The hyperpigmentation in melasma is due to the deposition of melanin in the epidermis, dermis, or both. Interestingly, despite the association with several putative etiologic factors that contribute to the development of melasma, the exact pathogenic mechanism remains unknown.

KEY FEATURES

- Melasma is a hormonally related skin hyperpigmentation, most often on the cheeks and upper lip.

- It is often seen during and after pregnancy or with use of oral contraceptives.

- Treatment includes daily sunscreen use and bleaching agents such as hydroquinone.

CLINICAL PRESENTATION

The presence of hyperpigmentation—an increase in pigment deposition resulting in darkening—is most easily apparent against the background of lighter skin tones. However, melasma, a clinical diagnosis based on the presence of acquired hyperpigmentation, may arise in individuals of virtually any baseline skin type. Melasma most commonly is found on sun-exposed areas of skin. There is often a symmetric appearance of the hyperpigmented, which range in color from ashy gray to light- to dark-brown and are nonelevated (Fig. 14-1). The three classic distributions for facial melasma hyperpigmentation are (a) centrofacial, involving the forehead, cheeks, chin and upper lip; (b) malar, involving primarily the cheeks; and (c) mandibular, classically involving the chin and jaw line. Melasma is not limited to the face, and is often seen in the dorsal extremities and sun-exposed areas.

DIAGNOSIS

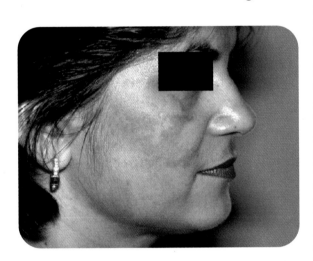

Figure 14-1 Facial melasma. From Goodheart HP. *Goodheart's Photoguide of Common Skin Disorders*, 3rd ed. Philadelphia: Lippincott Williams & Wilkins, 2009.

The diagnosis of melasma is often made clinically based on the physical appearance and patient history. The use of a Wood's lamp (an ultraviolet light source) can aid in determining the level of pigment deposition in melasma. Classically, pigment deposited in the epidermis will result in light brown pigmentation of the affected skin that exhibits enhanced contrast under Wood's lamp examination. Pigment deposition in the dermis often produces ashen or bluish discoloration of the skin that does not change or enhance under Wood's lamp examination. In individuals with pigment deposition in both layers of the skin, the hyperpigmented regions appear an intermediate darker brown in color and will show variable enhancement under Wood's lamp examination. Diagnosis of any of the aforementioned variants may be more complex in individuals with darker background skin complexion. A skin biopsy is not required to make the diagnosis of melasma.

The differential diagnosis for melasma includes other disorders of hyperpigmentation described in this chapter, such as postinflammatory hyperpigmentation, or other inflammatory-based conditions such as contact dermatitis, or drug-related hypersensitivities and photosensitivity. A thorough history is important when melasma is the suspected clinical diagnosis, as several potential underlying causes may be considered (Table 14-1).

TREATMENT

Varying courses of melasma have been reported, from self-resolving episodes to recurrent or chronic hyperpigmentation. Cessation of an obvious external

Table 14-1 Factors Associated with Melasma Development	
Sun exposure	Family history
Pregnancy	Photosensitizing medications
Oral contraceptive/HRT use	Thyroid dysfunction
Cosmetics/topical treatments	Other endocrinologic disorders (e.g., Addison disease)

CHAPTER 14 Pigmentary Disorders

trigger—such as particular contraceptives or topical cosmetics—is indicated when such factors are believed to be part of the causal etiology. Thyroid hormone levels should be checked if there is suspicion of an underlying thyroid disorder, as these states are more common in individuals with melasma. First and foremost, assiduous daily application of a high-number UVA/UVB blocking sunscreen is mandatory if medical therapy or cosmetic procedures are to be undertaken. Months of treatment can be quickly undone by several hours of unprotected sun exposure.

A variety of medical treatments are available to diminish existing hyperpigmentation. Available in 2% or 4% topical cream or topical gel preparation, hydroquinone is the topical medications most commonly prescribed for the treatment of melasma. By inhibiting the action of the enzyme tyrosinase, hydroquinone is effective at blocking a key step in melanin synthesis. For melasma treatment, the 4% hydroquinone is applied twice daily on the affected areas for 2 to 3 months or until results are noted. Preparations of hydroquinone with sunblock are also available by prescription and would be useful for individuals with large sun-exposed areas of hyperpigmentation due to melasma.

Tretinoin 0.05% cream can also be used for the treatment of melasma. Tretinoin acts by increasing the speed of turnover of the stratum corneum (the outermost, keratin-rich layer of the skin) and may be used daily at bedtime for 3 to 6 months for melasma. A more potent preparation of hydroquinone 4%, tretinoin 0.05%, and topical steroid fluocinolone acetonide 0.01% is also available by prescription (Tri-Luma) for the treatment of melasma and can be applied nightly for up to 8 weeks. Another topical hypopigmentation agent that may be used as an alternative to hydroquinone-based preparations is 20% azelaic acid.

Risks of topical hypopigmenting agents include drying of the skin, hypersensitivity reactions, and bleaching of surrounding skin. Hypopigmenting topical agents are relatively contraindicated in the treatment of melasma in pregnant individuals.

Further therapies available for the treatment of refractory melasma include chemical peels. Salicylic acid peels, glycolic acid peels, and trichloroacetic acid peels have been reported to decrease pigmentation in conjunction with the aforementioned depigmenting agents. Other reported modalities include dermabrasion and laser therapy.

"AT A GLANCE" TREATMENT

- All patients with melasma: Daily application of a high SPF sunscreen/block with UVA protection
- Primary medical therapy:
  - Apply 4% hydroquinone BID on the affected areas for 2 to 3 months
  - Tretinoin 0.05% cream QHS for 3 to 6 months
  - A mix of hydroquinone 4%, tretinoin 0.05%, and fluocinolone acetonide 0.01% (Tri-Luma) QHS for up to 8 weeks
- Secondary treatments:
  - Facial chemical peels
  - Dermabrasion
  - Laser therapy

COURSE AND COMPLICATIONS

Melasma is not a life-threatening disease but may cause the sufferer significant concern given its visibility on the face. Despite the incomplete understanding of underlying pathogenesis contributing to melasma, several treatments have evolved to combat the increased pigmentation. Limiting

WHEN TO REFER

- Melasma that is refractory to treatment with topical hypopigmentation agents should be referred to a dermatologist for possible evaluation of alternative treatment modalities.

- Referral to a dermatologist interested in cosmetic procedures is recommended for those desiring chemical peels or laser treatments.

sun exposure and daily use of opaque sunblock regardless of sun exposure should be stressed to the patient to prevent further progression of melasma.

ICD9 Code

709.09   Other dyschromia

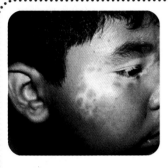

A healthy 28-year-old man presents to your clinic with questions about his skin. Over the past few months he has begun to notice patchy areas of his skin that have become lighter than what he describes as his "normal" skin tone. The areas that he identifies are distributed on his face, trunk, both arms, and fingers (Fig. 14-2). They appear chalk-white in color, and have sharp borders demarcating them from his type IV (olive-brown) colored skin. The patches do not itch and are not painful, but he has become increasingly self-conscious about wearing short sleeves that reveal the discolored patches on his skin. He does note that the light-colored areas appear to be growing in size, and also notes that his sister has some similar patches on her arms as well. He is concerned about the possibility of the patches spreading and affecting his face or other parts of his body. What is his most likely diagnosis? What is the pathologic process at work? What preventative strategies and therapeutic treatments are available for his condition?

Vitiligo

BACKGROUND/EPIDEMIOLOGY

At the opposite end of the spectrum from the hyperpigmented, dark-colored patches of melasma, the tell-tale skin findings in vitiligo are patches of pale skin with a partial or total lack of pigmentation. While not limited to one specific skin type, the lesions of vitiligo are more readily apparent in individuals with darker baseline pigmentation due to the contrast between normal and affected skin. Also known as leukoderma, vitiligo characteristically presents during childhood or early adulthood and may persist throughout an individual's lifetime. The time course for the initial presentation and the chronicity of disease is variable; the depigmentation may be progressive over weeks to months and may continue to expand, remain stable, or even self-resolve in individual cases. Both men and women may be affected by vitiligo, and the disease has been described around the world with a similar prevalence (0.5% to 2.0% of the population). Onset is usually early in life, averaging around age 20 years. Given the easier detection in individuals with darker baseline pigmentation, vitiligo may be more frequently reported—or treatment may be more frequently sought—by individuals with skin of color.

KEY FEATURES

- Vitiligo presents as hypo- or depigmented patches, characteristically symmetric.

- It is caused by death of normal epidermal melanocytes and is associated with thyroid disease and other autoimmune conditions.

- Treatment is often at best partially successful. Topical steroids and tacrolimus may be useful. Narrowband UVB for widespread disease may offer slow improvement.

PATHOPHYSIOLOGY

The underlying etiology of vitiligo is poorly understood. Putative hypotheses have been put forward to explain the pathophysiologic mechanism of the disease, but this remains an area of active research. An understanding of the disease process emerges from the histologic findings seen on microscopic examination of biopsies from vitiligo patches: normal skin but for the total absence of melanocytes.

Prevailing theories about the evolution of vitiligo include a cellular immune-mediated phenomenon (aberrant cytotoxic T-lymphocytes activated against melanocytes), a humoral immune-mediated phenomenon (circulating autoantibodies targeted against melanocytes), a melanin biosynthetic pathway mutation (increased generation of free radicals within melanocytes), as well as combinations of the above postulates. While there is not a direct Mendelian inheritance pattern associated with vitiligo, up to 30% of individuals with the disease will report at first-degree family member with vitiligo as well.

CLINICAL PRESENTATION

An individual with vitiligo often notices the development of focal patches of off-white to chalk-white skin. Often seen in the face (Fig. 14-2), trunk, extensor surfaces, extremities, groin, and axillae, vitiligo is a condition that develops after birth, most commonly presenting in the first three decades of life. The white patches of skin may start as small, millimeter sized areas and expand to involve several square-centimeters of skin. Patients may report a history of trauma, sunburn, or viral illness preceding the onset of depigmentation in vitiligo, though none of these is a necessary prerequisite.

In addition to the dermatologic manifestations of vitiligo, it is important to question about the psychological impact of the disease as well. Vitiligo affects areas of the skin that are easily visible to both the patient and other individuals—such as the face, arms, and hands—the condition may become a source of concern not only for the patient but for those in their immediate surroundings. In addition to the uncertainty of cause underlying the depigmentation that the patient must face, in some cultures there is social stigma to having areas of nonpigmented skin and this generates a psychosocial burden of embarrassment and stress that must also be dealt with.

The physical findings in vitiligo of hypopigmented and depigmented macules may be found distributed throughout the body. The pattern of depigmentation with surrounding hypopigmented patches and normal skin is termed trichrome vitiligo (Fig. 14-3), with a common predilection for the face, trunk, extensor surfaces, extremities, groin, and axillae, as noted above; there is often involvement of peri-orificial tissue such as perioral and perianal regions. The patches of vitiligo retain their normal sensation and do not illicit pain or other discomfort such as itching or burning. Hair growing in the area of depigmentation may turn white (poliosis) due to the loss of melanocytes in these skin appendages as well.

The most common distribution of vitiligo is generalized patches of depigmentation spread throughout the body with relative midline symmetry,

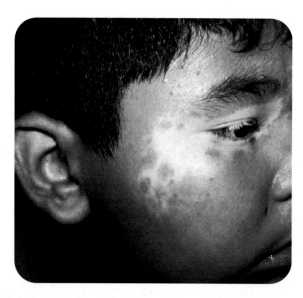

Figure 14-2   Facial vitiligo including pigment loss within the eyelashes. From Goodheart HP. *Goodheart's Photoguide of Common Skin Disorders*, 3rd ed. Philadelphia: Lippincott Williams & Wilkins, 2009.

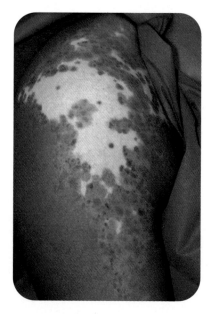

Figure 14-3   Trichrome vitiligo vulgaris.

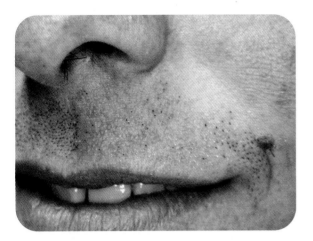

Figure 14-4 Segmental vitiligo.

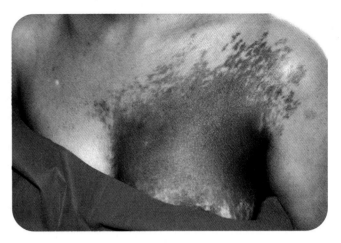

Figure 14-5 Becker's nevus with a small patch of focal vitiligo on the right lateral chest.

termed *vitiligo vulgaris*. Another variant involves primarily the face and distal extremities, so-called *acrofacial vitiligo*. When confined to a single dermatome, the patchy depigmentation is referred to as *segmental vitiligo* (Fig. 14-4), often presenting when the patient is in the first or second decades of life. Finally, an isolated patch of chalk-white depigmentation may be termed *focal vitiligo* (Fig. 14-5). Given the unpredictable nature of the disease, however, it is possible for conversion between distribution subtypes; for example, progression from focal to segmental may occur with time. When the majority of the body surface is involved, the condition is termed *vitiligo universalis*. These categorizations are summarized in Table 14-2.

Additional findings on physical exam that may be present in individuals with vitiligo are related to associated conditions. A significant increase in thyroid abnormalities (both hypothyroidism and hyperthyroidism, with the former being more common) is present in individuals with vitiligo, lending credence to the autoimmune theories of vitiligo etiology. Other autoimmune conditions, such as diabetes mellitus and pernicious anemia, are also found with increased frequency in individuals with vitiligo.

DIAGNOSIS

While the clinical diagnosis of vitiligo is often easily made, the differential diagnosis for vitiligo includes several other depigmenting skin conditions of varying frequency. An important part of the clinical history that distinguishes vitiligo from a genetically inherited, autosomal dominant condition known as piebaldism is the development of depigmented patches after birth. Another important differential diagnosis for vitiligo is chemical-induced depigmentation. A thorough history of exposure to chemicals with depigmenting or

Table 14-2 Classification of Vitiligo Distribution	
Vitiligo vulgaris	Patches throughout body, often symmetric with respect to midline. Most common presentation
Acrofacial vitiligo	Face (often perioral) and distal extremities
Segmental vitiligo	Dermatomal distribution. Often presents at young age
Focal vitiligo	Single patch or area of involvement
Vitiligo universalis	More than half of body surface involved, some patches of normal skin remain

bleaching properties (especially hydroquinones and phenols) is critical for excluding this diagnosis.

Other dermatologic conditions that may present with hypopigmentation include pityriasis alba, morphea, and leprosy. Postinflammatory hypopigmentation can occasionally be so severe that it looks like vitiligo. Pityriasis alba is typically associated with dry, scaly, patches of affected skin followed by hypopigmentation, in contrast to the absence of scale and complete depigmentation seen in vitiligo. Similarly, morphea—hardening of the connective tissue of the skin due to abnormal collagen deposition—may result in patchy hypopigmentation or depigmentation. The involved skin in morphea will be noticeably harder and sclerosed relative to the normal texture of skin seen in vitiligo. Finally, in patients from areas where leprosy is endemic, this disease should be considered in the differential diagnosis. While patches of depigmentation can occur in leprosy as in vitiligo, these patches are characteristically anesthetic—lacking sensation due to neural involvement with the causative mycobacterium.

A diagnosis of vitiligo can often be made with the patient's history and clinical presentation. The use of a Wood's lamp may be helpful to increase the distinction between involved patches and normal skin, particularly in individuals with lighter skin type. If other skin disorders such as morphea or leprosy are in the differential, a skin biopsy may be helpful to rule out these more significant conditions.

In patients diagnosed with vitiligo, screening for associated hyper/hypothyroidism, autoimmune diabetes, and pernicious anemia is warranted given the increased prevalence of these conditions. In the case of vitiligo universalis, the patient should be evaluate for the presence of multiple endocrine neoplasia syndromes, often associated with this severe form of vitiligo.

TREATMENT

Treatment for vitiligo is often determined by the physical and emotional toll on the patient, as well as their willingness to engage in particular therapeutic approaches. For patients with vitiligo in routinely sun-exposed areas, regular sunscreen use over the affected areas must be stressed; the depigmented skin will be at increased risk for sunburn and photodamage relative to the individual's normal skin. Avoidance of sun exposure will also be beneficial to reduce tanning of normal skin, which may increase the contrast with vitiligo patches.

The least-invasive treatment option involves the use of skin tone–matching cosmetics to conceal the involved patches of vitiligo. Over-the-counter cosmetics or self-tanning agents or stains may be used to darken the skin as needed; these will require regular reapplication. It is important that patients recognize these treatments do not affect the actual prognosis of the disease, but offer an easily accessible method for enhanced cosmesis.

Medical therapies for vitiligo are targeted at immune-modulation and anti-inflammatory agents. Corticosteroids are often the first-line treatment of choice in both children and adults with vitiligo. Once-daily application of a medium-potency (adults) or low-potency (children) steroid may be tried for 4 months with intermittent evaluation every 4 to 6 weeks. If there is a repigmentation response, the use of steroids can be continued until the response tapers off or side effects from the corticosteroids limit further usage. Another approach of topical therapy for vitiligo has been the use of immunomodulators such as tacrolimus and pimecrolimus. Tacrolimus 0.1% and pimecrolimus 1% creams, used twice daily over the affected areas, have been shown to result in repigmentation of vitiligo patches in several small clinical trials.

More complex treatment alternatives are available for vitiligo as well. Vitiligo has been successfully treated with the use of ultraviolet light. The most common treatments are with narrow-band UVB (NBUVB). A combination treatment using psoralens, a class of photosensitizing chemical agents, and controlled exposure to UV-A light is known as PUVA. This may also be employed with either topical psoralens applied directly to the involved skin or systemic oral psoralens. Ultraviolet treatment has been demonstrated to be effective but requires patients to undergo treatment sessions multiple times per week, with a minimum of 50 treatments being required. Surgery is also a treatment option, offering the ability to micro-graft normally pigmented tissue into an involved area, leading to a return of pigmentation over time.

For individuals with extensive areas of skin affected by vitiligo, depigmentation of remaining normal skin may be considered as a treatment option after failure of standard therapies. The use of 20% monobenzyl ether of hydroquinone, results in permanent loss of pigmentation. The psychological impact of this treatment must be thoroughly discussed with the patient in advance, as the change in their natural skin tone will be permanent. Such treatment also results in an increased risk of sunburn and photodamage in newly depigmented skin.

"AT A GLANCE" TREATMENT

- Over-the-counter cosmetics or tanning agents
- Topical therapy: corticosteroids or calcineurin inhibitors
  - Moderate potency steroid: triamcinolone 0.1% cream BID × 2 to 3 months
  - Calcineurin inhibitor: pimecrolimus cream or tacrolimus ointment BID × 2 to 3 months
- Narrow-band UVB or Psoralen+UVA offers slow repigmentation for some
- Extensive, recalcitrant vitiligo: 20% monobenzyl ether of hydroquinone, resulting in permanent loss of remaining pigmentation

CLINICAL COURSE

The course of vitiligo is unpredictable. Some patients have rapid and complete response to topical or ultraviolet therapies. Some have slow but incomplete improvement. Others have progressive, treatment-resistant disease.

ICD9 Codes	
709.01	Vitiligo
701.0	Circumscribed scleroderma
030.9	Leprosy, unspecified

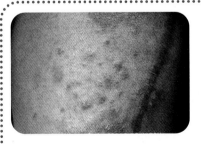

A 52-year-old African American man presents for his annual psoriasis follow-up. He states that he has been in relatively good health over the last year and does not report any major medical illnesses since his last visit. His psoriasis is still active on his outer thighs, but he has noted some improvement (Fig. 14-6). He notes darker skin in the areas in which the psoriasis has cleared and wonders if the pigmentation will ever go away. What is his diagnosis? What treatments are available to help him decrease the prominence of such spots?

Postinflammatory Hyperpigmentation

BACKGROUND/EPIDEMIOLOGY

The activation of the skin's inflammatory response may be initiated by virtually any sort of stress or trauma of either endogenous or exogenous origin. Topical medications, cosmetics, sun exposure, infection, burns, and local or systemic disease can all trigger a discoloration of the skin that fails to self-resolve after the initial healing has taken place or the external stimulus has been removed. When an individual presents with flat area of pigmentation in the distribution of past injury or toxic exposure, the diagnosis of postinflammatory hyperpigmentation (PIH) must be considered.

KEY FEATURES

- Skin darkening following almost any preceding skin inflammation.
- This occurs preferentially in darker skin types, but can occur in any phototype.
- The diagnosis is by clinical history.
- Treatment in all cases is with topical sunscreen use daily. In many cases the pigmentation will fade over time. If topical therapy is desired, hydroquinone 4% may be helpful.

Table 14-3 Common Causes of Postinflammatory Hyperpigmentation

Burns	Photosensitizing medications
Contact allergic reaction	Phototoxic/Phytophototoxic reactions
Cosmetics	Sun exposure
Eczema, lichen planus, psoriasis, or other primary skin eruption	Toxic topical exposure
Inflammatory acne	

PATHOPHYSIOLOGY

As in the case presentation above, stimuli for the development of such hyperpigmented lesions are variable. Table 14-3 lists several common causes of hyperpigmentation that may be considered in an individual presenting for evaluation of persistent pigmented lesions. Given the propensity for various forms of skin cancer to present as pigmented lesions, a thorough history and complete skin examination should always be performed when evaluating hyperpigmentation.

On a cellular level, the darkening seen in postinflammatory hyperpigmentation is attributed to increased melanin production in melanocytes, triggered by a component of the inflammatory response. Possible inducers of upregulated melanin production include various interleukin factors, endocrine mediators, and free-radical ions, such as reactive oxygen species, all of which have been demonstrated to affect melanocyte metabolic activity.

CLINICAL PRESENTATION

While any individual may be affected by postinflammatory hyperpigmentation, the condition affects individuals with darker complexions—skin types IV, V, and VI—more frequently (Figs. 14-6, 14-7). As in the cases of vitiligo and

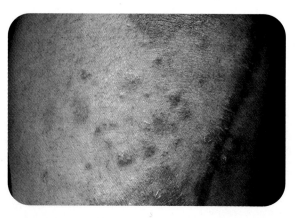

Figure 14-6 Prominent active psoriasis and smaller patches of healed psoriasis with postinflammatory hyperpigmentation.

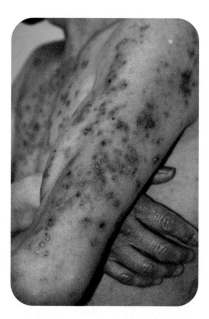

Figure 14-7 Postinflammatory hyperpigmentation and prurigo secondary to allergic contact dermatitis and atopic dermatitis.

melasma, facial involvement is common, particularly in instances of hyperpigmentation secondary to inflammatory acne lesions.

Postinflammatory hyperpigmentation may present in individuals of any age or either gender. The lesions can be persistent, and last up to several years after the resolution of the inciting events. As with other disorders of pigmentation, the psychological and cosmetic impact of the condition is an important consideration when evaluating individuals with postinflammatory hyperpigmentation.

The lesions of postinflammatory hyperpigmentation may be present at any location on the body. Typically, the involved areas are nonelevated patches of skin that are distinctly darker from their surroundings. As in melasma, there may be a range of pigmentary change, from tan to brown to nearly black, as well as grayish- or bluish-tinged coloration pattern.

The regions of hyperpigmentation are within the area of a previous inflammatory response; they may correspond to a geographic distribution such as that of sun exposure or remain more localized to a site of recent injury. The borders of hyperpigmented areas are often described as feathery and poorly demarcated. Additionally, it is important to note that there may be multiple areas of involvement relating to separate prior inflammatory processes that have resulted in similar-appearing hyperpigmented patches.

DIAGNOSIS

A history and physical examination consistent with the findings described above are often enough to make a diagnosis of postinflammatory hyperpigmentation. The use of a Wood's lamp may be employed as in melasma to determine the depth of melanin deposition. Characteristically, dermal melanin will not enhance with Wood's lamp examination while epidermal melanin deposits will become more pronounced.

The clinical history is critical in postinflammatory hyperpigmentation. Because the presence of a pigmented lesion may often raise suspicion of a cutaneous malignant process, a skin biopsy may be helpful in making a specific diagnosis.

TREATMENT

The key concern at the time of presentation is whether the underlying phenomenon responsible for the inflammation has been successfully treated or halted. For endogenous conditions such as psoriasis, eczema, or endocrine disorders that contribute to the causative inflammation, these entities should first be brought under control before the pigmentation itself is addressed. For exogenous factors such as topical medications or cosmetics, the offending agent should be discontinued.

Patients with postinflammatory hyperpigmentation should be counseled about the regular use of sunscreen over affected areas. Sun exposure, with its component UV-radiation, is a well-known hyperpigmenting agent, and can worsen the pigmentation already seen in affected areas. Additionally, patients should be told to avoid physical or chemical trauma to the site by avoiding scratching or rubbing the area and avoiding unnecessary topical chemical applications. For persistent areas of hyperpigmentation that are cosmetically or psychologically displeasing to the patient, various depigmenting agents may be considered as therapies. Hydroquinone, a tyrosinase inhibitor, is available in 2% or 4% topical cream or gel preparation. Use of hydroquinone once or twice daily on the affected areas may to be effective in some patients over a course of 2 to 3 months. Preparations of hydroquinone with sunblock are also

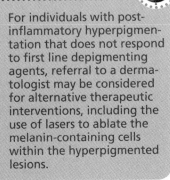

WHEN TO REFER

For individuals with post-inflammatory hyperpigmentation that does not respond to first line depigmenting agents, referral to a dermatologist may be considered for alternative therapeutic interventions, including the use of lasers to ablate the melanin-containing cells within the hyperpigmented lesions.

available by prescription to counter the increased risk of sun-damage associated with depigmentation. Tretinoin 0.05% cream and azelaic acid 20% are other alternative agents causing pigment lightening. Risks of topical hypopigmenting agents include drying of the skin, hypersensitivity reactions, and "bleaching" of surrounding skin.

Another therapeutic option involves the use of mild chemical peels for treating hyperpigmentation. While effective adjuncts, their use may be limited, as they can result in depigmentation of the background skin as well as serve as possible stimuli of an inflammatory reaction.

Finally, the use of cover-up cosmetics may be considered for patients who are able to tolerate the application of these agents, with the understanding that the underlying pigmentation will not be reduced by such approaches but merely camouflaged.

"AT A GLANCE" TREATMENT

- Sunscreen should be used at all times during PIH therapy
- Primary depigmentation: hydroquinone 4% cream QD–BID for 2 to 3 months
- Secondary agents: tretinoin 0.05% cream QHS or azelaic acid 20% gel BID
- Optional use of cover-up cosmetics

COURSE AND COMPLICATIONS

The course of postinflammatory hyperpigmentation is variable from patient to patient. While it is possible for the pigmentation to return to a normal baseline over time, this response cannot be predicted based on a patient's initial presentation.

ICD9 Code

709.00   Dyschromia, unspecified

Other Disorders of Pigmentation

In addition to melasma, vitiligo, and postinflammatory hyperpigmentation, several conditions have been identified that result in either primary or secondary alteration of skin pigmentation. While the topics covered in this chapter are among the most common pigmentary disorders, it is important for the physician to keep in mind a broad range of other possible conditions that may be encountered when examining patients with pigmentary changes.

ALBINISM

Deriving its name from the Latin term for "white," albinism is an inherited disorder of metabolism involving one of several mutations in the synthetic or functional pathway of melanin. The precursor amino acid in the synthesis of melanin is tyrosine, and the gene encoding the tyrosinase enzyme is a common site of mutation in cases of albinism. The inheritance pattern for most forms of albinism is autosomal recessive. Melanin serves as the primary component of pigment in the skin, hair, and irises, and all are typically affected in severe forms of the disease, termed oculocutaneous albinism. The coloration of the skin and hair may vary from completely white to a yellowish tint (Fig. 14-8), depending on the step in the melanin synthesis pathway that is altered in a given variant of the disease; tyrosinase-negative individuals lack any function of this enzyme and have a more complete loss of pigment.

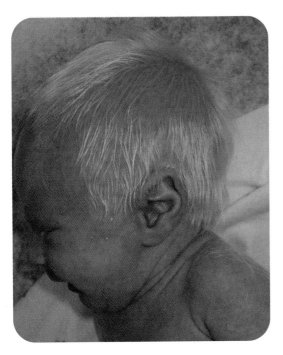

Figure 14-8 Oculocutaneous albinism in an infant. Image provided by Stedman's.

Patients with albinism are at high susceptibility for UV-induced skin damage from solar exposure, and sun protection is a crucial part of preventive health counseling for these individuals. Daily sunscreen use with SPF greater than 40 and minimizing skin exposure to direct daytime sunlight should be stressed. Given the involvement of the skin and the eyes, it is important that individuals with albinism are followed regularly by both a dermatologist and ophthalmologist for monitoring and evaluation as long-term sequelae include increased risks of skin cancers and impaired visual acuity and alignment. Variants of albinism that only affect the eyes are known as ocular albinism and typically have an X-linked pattern of inheritance.

Rarely, albinism may be associated with one of several immune-deficiency disorders. Hermansky-Pudlak syndrome, most prevalent in individuals from Puerto Rico, involves a mutation in subcellular organelle function and manifests as albinism along with increased bleeding times and decreased cell-mediated immunity. Chediak-Higashi syndrome involves a mutation in lysosomal formation and degranulation, resulting in albinism, neutropenia, and increased susceptibility to bacterial infection. Griscelli syndrome is an extremely rare variant of albinism related to microtubule and cytoskeletal transport protein mutations, causing associated secondary neurologic disease and immune deficiency. A summary of various forms of albinism is presented in Table 14-4 (Figs. 14-9 to 14-12).

Table 14-4 Diseases Causing Hypopigmentation

Oculocutaneous albinism (OCA)	
Type 1	Tyrosinase-negative due to mutation in TYR gene; completely white skin and hair, blue-gray irises as adults
Type 2	Most common form; tyrosinase positive; yellowish hair and skin pigmentation
Type 3	Light brownish skin pigment due to abnormal melanin production; common in Africans/African Americans
Type 4	Very rare; seen in East Asian populations. Mutation in protein transport pathway, may improve in early years
Ocular albinism	X-linked recessive inheritance. Only eyes affected
Hermansky-Pudlack	Mutation in subcellular organelle functional activity; common in Puerto Rico; increased bleeding time due to poor platelet function
Chediak-Higashi	Lysosomal transport function impairment; albinism associated with neutropenia and increased susceptibility to bacterial disease. Characteristic silver hair (Fig. 14-9)
Griscelli	Typically presents with silver-colored hair; immune deficiency and neurologic disorder. Due to mutation in microtubule or cytoskeletal transport structure
Tuberous sclerosis	Neurocutaneous disorder, inheritance autosomal dominant (AD). Cutaneous findings: ash-leaf macules (Fig. 14-10); connective tissue nevi; facial angiofibromas (Fig. 14-11); periungual fibromas (Fig. 14-12)
Piebaldism/Waardenburg	AD mutation in the c-kit gene. Multiple subtypes, often presents with white forelock of hair
Phenylketonuria	Deficiency of phenylalanine hydroxylase. Common finding is lighter skin and hair color. May be striking in darker skin phenotypes
Homocystinuria	Autosomal recessive defect in methionine metabolism that is caused by a deficiency in cystathionine synthase. Many systemic findings, cutaneous findings: pale/pink skin
Vitiligo	Discussed above

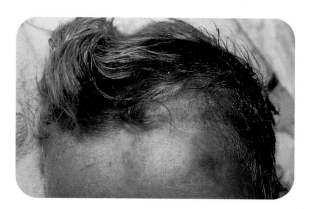

Figure 14-9 Typical silver hair seen in Chediak-Higashi syndrome. From Gold DH, Weingeist TA. *Color Atlas of the Eye in Systemic Disease.* Baltimore: Lippincott Williams & Wilkins, 2001.

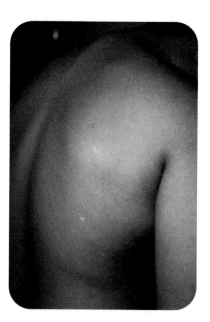

Figure 14-10 Ash-leaf macules of tuberous sclerosis. Courtesy of George A. Datto, III, MD.

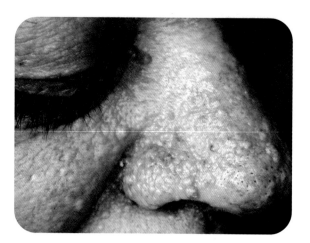

Figure 14-11 Facial angiofibromas of tuberous sclerosis.

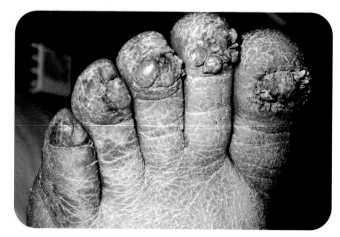

Figure 14-12 Periungual fibromas of tuberous sclerosis.

ACANTHOSIS NIGRICANS

The pigmentation pattern of the skin may at times reflect underlying systemic metabolic processes within the body and aid the observant clinician in the process of a diagnostic evaluation. A common example of this phenomenon is acanthosis nigricans. Acanthosis nigricans is characterized by painless, dense, brown-to-black velvety patches of skin located in the axillae, antecubital fossae, neck, and other flexural surfaces and folds (Fig. 14-13). The skin in these areas is thickened and shows increased markings of the skin lines.

Acanthosis nigricans is a benign skin finding. However, it is often associated with underlying endocrinologic disturbances, most commonly the spectrum of insulin resistance and type 2 diabetes. In addition, the skin changes of acanthosis nigricans may be seen in obese individuals before the development of actual insulin resistance. Rarely, acanthosis nigricans may also be associated with the presence of an internal malignancy; in such cases, the

KEY FEATURES

- Acanthosis nigricans is characterized by painless, dense, brown-to-black velvety patches of skin located in the axillae, antecubital fossae, neck, and other flexural surfaces and folds.
- It is a benign condition that may be associated with insulin resistance, type II diabetes, and rarely internal malignancy.

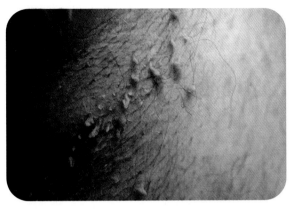

Figure 14-13 Acanthosis nigricans with tags.

malignancy is often found to be of gastrointestinal origin. In an individual who is neither obese nor insulin-resistant, the development of acanthosis nigricans may raise suspicion for an evaluation of occult malignancy risk. In all cases, the disease development process is thought to be mediated through an excess of insulin-like hormonal growth factors. The best treatment for resolution of acanthosis nigricans has been to treat the underling etiologic condition through weight loss or diabetes management in the cases of obesity and insulin resistance, respectively. Other types of endocrinologic disease leading to pigmentary changes are listed in Table 14-5.

METABOLIC DISORDERS AND EXOGENOUS EXPOSURES CAUSING PIGMENTARY DISORDERS

There are a broad spectrum of diseases and exposures, which all have changes in skin pigmentation as one of many manifestations. Systemic conditions lead most commonly to diffuse hyperpigmentation. Other causes of skin darkening are oral medication exposures and nutritional deficiencies. Localized hypopigmentation may be caused by topical exposures. The most frequent causes of chemical leukodermas are products containing hydroquinones, phenols, and sulfhydryl groups. Benzyl alcohol is a preservative added to many topical medicaments and skin products which in rare cases may cause hypopigmentation. Oral medications may also play a role in acquired loss of pigment. Exposures and metabolic causes of pigmentary disorders are summarized in Table 14-5.

Table 14-5 Systemic Causes of Diffuse Hyperpigmentation

SYSTEMIC DISEASE

Wilson disease	Hemochromatosis
Hepatic insufficiency	Hyperthyroid
Biliary cirrhosis	Porphyria cutanea tarda
Rheumatoid arthritis	Scleroderma
Lymphomas	Metastatic melanoma

INGESTIONS

Busulfan	Minocycline
Cyclophosphamide	Clofazimine
5-Fluorouracil	Psoralens
Zidovudine	Hydroxyurea
Methotrexate	Topical nitrogen mustard
Chlorpromazine	Ingested metals: silver (argyria), gold (chrysiasis), bismuth, mercury, inorganic arsenic poisoning
Amiodarone	Antimalarial drugs (i.e., hydroxychloroquine)

NUTRITIONAL

Anorexia nervosa	Bulimia
Folic acid deficiency	Kwashiorkor
Malabsorption syndromes	Marasmus
Pellagra	

Suggested Reading

Cayce KA, McMichael AJ, Feldman SR. Hyperpigmentation: An overview of the common afflictions. *Dermatol Nurs.* 2004;16:401–416.

Epstein JE. Postinflammatory hyperpigmentation. *Clin Dermatol.* 1989;7:55–65.

Grimes PE. Melasma: Etiologic and therapeutic considerations. *Arch Dermatol.* 1995;131:1453–1457.

Grimes PE. New insights and new therapies in vitiligo. *JAMA.* 2005;293:730–735.

Lacz NL, et al. Postinflammatory hyperpigmenation: A common but troubling condition. *Int J Dermatol.* 2004;43:362–365.

Liu JB, et al. Clinical profiles of vitiligo in China: An analysis of 3742 patients. *Clin Exper Dermatol.* 2005;30:327–331.

Ortonne JP, Bissett DL. Latest insights into skin hyperpigmentation. *J Invest Dermatol Symp Proceed.* 2008;13:10–14.

Passeron T, Ortonne JP. Physiopathology and genetics of vitiligo. *J Autoimmun.* 2005;25:63–68.

Rigopoulos D, Gregoriou S, Katsambas A. Hyperpigmentation and melasma. *J Cosmetic Dermatol.* 2007;6:195–202.

Stulberg DL, Clark N, Tovey D. Common hyperpigmentation disorders in adults: Part II. *Am Fam Physician.* 2003;68:1963–1968.

Tunzi M, Gray GR. Common skin conditions during pregnancy. *Am Fam Physician.* 2007;75:211–218.

Victor FC, Gelber J, Rao B. Melasma: A review. *J Cutaneous Med Surg.* 2004;8:97–102.

Wollina, U. The role of topical calcineurin inhibitors for skin diseases other than atopic dermatitis. *Am J Clin Dermatol.* 2007;8:157–173.

CHAPTER 15 Dermatitis

Lilla Landeck and Lynn Baden

Among industrialized countries, *dermatitis* (synonym: eczema) is one of the most frequent dermatologic diagnoses presenting for treatment. By definition, the term dermatitis describes a noncontagious skin disease characterized by inflammation in the epidermis and upper dermis with multiple etiologies. Although the terms dermatitis and eczema are often used interchangeably, "dermatitis" frequently refers to the more acute form of skin inflammation with rapid improvement, while "eczema" tends more to illustrate a chronic relapsing course.

A common term associated with dermatitis is *skin barrier function,* which refers to the damaged skin barrier accompanied by inflammation of the skin and vice versa. The epidermal skin barrier is discussed in detail in Chapter 4. Skin exposure, either to substances that dissolve intercellular lipids (e.g., organic solvents/detergents) or destroy keratinocytes, stresses the skin barrier function. In cases of chronic skin damage, barrier function may be exhausted, resulting in the damage of chronic forms of eczema. Skin inflammation can be classified according to the sequence of inflammation into an acute phase with clinical features such as erythema, edema, exudation, and/or vesiculation and a chronic state that presents clinically with scaling and lichenification. Both can be accompanied by pruritus.

Further attempts to categorize eczema include reference to anatomical localization (e.g., hand, foot, generalized); specific clinical features (nummular, asteatotic); and in some cases, the specific subtype of dermatitis such as shown in Figure 15-1. Because eczema may originate from a mixture of etiological causes with similar morphological/clinical and histopathological appearances, specific differentiation can be difficult. It is possible, especially with hand eczema, for any or all diagnoses to play partial roles in driving the eczema.

Diagnosis of eczema depends on patient's history, clinical distribution, and morphology of skin lesions, and the exclusion of other diagnoses.

Therapy is generally based on three principles: avoidance of possible triggers, restoration of impaired epidermal barrier function with emollients, and treatment with anti-inflammatory therapeutics. The most common first-line anti-inflammatory medications are topical corticosteroids. They are easy to apply and utilized in different potencies and vehicles. Side effects of topical corticosteroids are minimized by appropriate selection and utilization. These will be further discussed in the individual sections below.

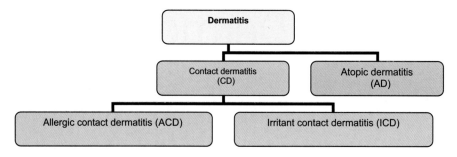

Figure 15-1 Subtypes of dermatitis.

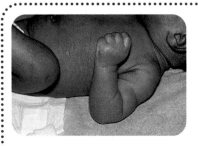

A mother presents with concerns about her 16-month-old son: "Since the beginning of wintertime when we turned on the heat, he scratches himself all night long awaking frequently and crying." Upon examination it is noted that the child is continuously scratching. The skin is erythematous, edematous, and reveals exudative crust and excoriations (Fig. 15-2). The face, the neck, and the flexural areas of the extremities are most prominently affected. Moreover, the mother describes worsening of the skin after giving her son cow's milk or egg-containing foods.

KEY FEATURES

- Atopic dermatitis (AD) is characterized by a pruritic, chronic, relapsing eczema.

- Often, there is a personal and/or family history of atopy and xerosis.

- AD has a genetic basis (filaggrin mutation) with variable expression depending on environmental factors.

- Typically, three stages with different morphologic appearance and anatomic distribution of flares to distinguish them: infantile, childhood, adulthood.

(Continued)

Atopic Dermatitis

BACKGROUND

The word atopy is derived from the Greek word "ατοπία" and depicts a condition "out of place/placelessness," or unusual. From a medical point of view atopy describes a polygenic inherited disposition to develop at least one of the following disorders: atopic dermatitis (AD), allergic rhinitis (AR), or allergic asthma (AA). Atopic disorders (AD, AR, AA) are marked by a manifestation of the interface of the organism to the environment (skin, mucosal skin, lungs) and have in common genetically based increased susceptibility to react to environmental factors. It appears that atopy is more prevalent in highly industrialized societies and higher socioeconomic classes.

AD is characterized by a genetically based hypersensitivity of the skin with predisposition to develop eczema in typical anatomic localizations according to stage. Current estimates show that 15% of schoolchildren and 2% of adults in industrialized countries suffer from AD, with a slight predominance of females. A myriad of possible intrinsic and extrinsic triggers include stress, aeroallergens, microbial products, and/or food allergens. The manifestation of the disease is typically most severe in childhood, with a chronic relapsing course and improvement in most cases occurring during adulthood. Important hallmarks comprise pruritus and xerosis cutis.

PATHOGENESIS

The pathogenesis and etiology of the disease are still not fully understood. Most likely the AD phenotype results from a complex interplay between genetic, immunologic, metabolic, and neuroendocrine alterations and their interaction with the environment.

Genetics

It has long been recognized that inheritance of atopy is on a polygenetic basis with variable expression influenced by environmental factors. Recently, mutations in multiple regions of the filaggrin gene, leading to dysfunction of the filaggrin protein, an essential component in epidermal barrier function, were reported. Not only do filaggrin defects seem to be at least partially responsible

KEY FEATURES (Continued)

- Most often affected individuals are infants and children. Upon reaching puberty, prevalence decreases.

- Mainstays of treatment are the avoidance of triggers, maintenance or restoration of epidermal barrier function with emollients, and topical corticosteroids during flares.

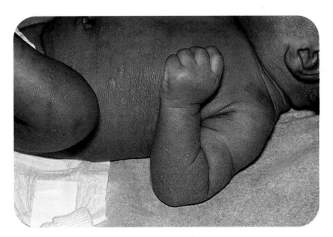

Figure 15-2 Widespread atopic dermatitis on an infant. From Goodheart HP. *Goodheart's Photoguide of Common Skin Disorders*, 3rd ed. Philadelphia: Lippincott Williams & Wilkins, 2009.

for AD, they also play a role in the pathogenesis of ichthyosis vulgaris, a xerotic skin condition seen in conjunction with AD in ~8% of cases.

Barrier-disrupted Skin

AD skin is characterized by severe dryness due to alterations in composition of intercellular lipids and an impaired barrier function of the epidermis, with resulting high transepidermal water loss and lower skin surface hydration levels. A combination of barrier disruption and AD makes the skin highly susceptible to environmental factors such as irritants, allergens, and microbes.

Immunologic Alterations

AD shows a multifaceted immunologic picture with immune deficiency and immune hyperreactivity. Selective immune deficiency is observed by the trend to develop certain skin infections, such as herpes simplex virus. In contrast, approximately 70% of AD patients suffer from increased IgE levels, which were directly correlated to the disease activity. While consensus exists that among atopic individuals there is a heightened tendency to develop IgE-type-I antibodies to environmental factors, some authors have claimed a decreased type-IV cell-mediated immunity, which would lead to the observation of decreased rates of allergic contact dermatitis. However, recent publications showed atopic individuals to be at least as likely to have allergic contact dermatitis as nonatopics, probably because of the increased use of topicals and the eased penetration of allergens due to disrupted skin barrier.

CLINICAL PRESENTATION

The majority of patients are infants and children. Up to 90% of cases arise before the age of 5 years. At each stage AD may show acute, subacute, or chronic skin changes. However, certain presentations are more common in specific stages. AD of infants and children is predominately an acute, exudative inflammation, with secondary excoriations. In adulthood, chronic inflammation with hyperkeratotic skin-thickening, lichenification (accentuated skin markings), and scaling are more prominent. Postinflammatory pigment changes, either hyper- or hypopigmentation, can be observed. Pruritus is almost always present. The typical anatomic distribution of AD varies by stages, changing over lifetime. AD lesions of infants are predominantly located on the face and the extensor surface of the extremities, while the childhood pattern is typified by flexural

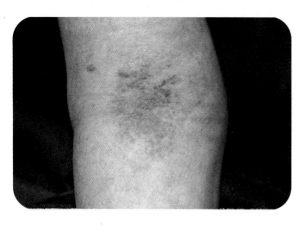

Figure 15-3 Atopic dermatitis in the popliteal fossa of an elderly woman.

involvement. For the adult with atopic dermatitis, the earlier classic locations are often involved, such as flexural areas (Fig. 15-3). There also is more frequent facial (especially eyelid) and hand/foot eczema.

DIAGNOSIS

Diagnostic criteria for AD are based primarily on clinical presentation, patients/family history, and the exclusion of other disease entities. Hanifin and Rajka compiled, in the early 1980s, important diagnostic features, which attained international recognition. Since that time, the criteria have evolved into the current schema. A consensus conference, convened by the American Academy of Dermatology (AAD) suggested the clinical criteria for the diagnosis of AD given in Table 15-1.

Diagnosis is made using the above-mentioned criteria. In questionable cases, a supportive biopsy with histopathologic interpretation may help, especially when other differential diagnoses, such as cutaneous T-cell lymphoma must be excluded. Biopsy is not appropriate to classify the eczema according to a specific etiology because of many histologic similarities between eczema types. Analytical measurement of total IgE is used to distinguish between intrinsic and extrinsic forms of AD. Extrinsic AD, with elevated serum IgE, is characterized by a personal or family history of respiratory allergy and can be found in 70% of AD individuals. Patients without IgE reactivity or obvious allergic respiratory conditions have intrinsic AD.

Differential Diagnoses

In children: seborrheic dermatitis, contact dermatitis (allergic or irritant), psoriasis, scabies, familial keratosis pilaris, Langerhans cell histocytosis, congenital ichthyosis

In adults: seborrheic dermatitis, contact dermatitis (allergic or irritant), psoriasis, scabies, familial keratosis pilaris, tinea manuum, asteatotic eczema, cutaneous T-cell lymphoma, secondary syphilis

THERAPY

The inherited hypersensitivity and the disposition of the skin to develop eczema is a lifelong condition. Thus, whether disease is active or not, avoidance of potential triggers and maintenance of physiologic skin barrier function with hydration (e.g., with urea 3% to 5% as an ingredient) and thick

Table 15-1	Diagnostic Features of Atopic Dermatitis as Suggested by the AAD Consensus Conference
Essential (must be present)	Pruritus, eczematous changes, chronic or relapsing course
Important (for support of diagnosis)	Early age of onset, atopy (IgE reactivity, personal and/or family history), xerosis
Associated (indicative)	Atypical vascular responses, keratosis pilaris/hyperlinear palms/ichthyosis vulgaris, ocular/periorbital changes, other regional findings (perioral/periauricular changes), perifollicular accentuation/lichenification/prurigo

emollients is essential. Generally, patients with AD should limit potentially skin-irritating activities such as wet work and contact to chemicals/detergents. Moreover the use of mild, perfume-free, nonalkali soaps is recommended. Although bathing dries the skin, patients often sense a general relief and reduction of pruritus while immersed. Hence recommendation for bathing patients includes the immediate reapplication of moisture. Use of a cream containing ceramides (either prescription or over-the-counter) is helpful for many patients.

Reduction of house dust mites with vacuum cleaning, removal of carpets and curtains, and the use of special bed covers seems to improve the skin condition as well. Cotton clothing is preferred to wool and synthetics. Avoidance of specific food products such as eggs, milk, or nuts in those patients who experience a flare when eating them can be helpful too.

In case of active flares, intensity and distribution of skin lesions, as well as specific symptoms, determine the therapeutic choices. The mainstay of treatment for pruritus is antihistamines whereas corticosteroids are used to gain control of skin inflammation. Advantages of topical corticosteroids include ease of application, possibility of combination with other therapies (e.g., phototherapy), and the opportunity of choices with regard to ingredient potency. Rapid flares are best treated with 5 days of a medium- to high-potency topical corticosteroid ointment. Application should be once to twice a day. Once disease control is achieved, the topical corticosteroid can be tapered to a less-potent class and eventually withdrawn. Adjustment of steroid class when used in the groin area and the face should be considered, as these areas are more vulnerable for cutaneous atrophy. Alternating therapy with topical immunomodulators (calcineurin inhibitors tacrolimus and pimecrolimus, FDA approved for patients > 2 years) or days of therapeutic pause decrease the risk of cutaneous atrophy. Especially for moderate to severe AD, phototherapy in combination with topical therapy can improve AD. Appropriate regimens comprise narrow-band UVB and PUVA (Psoralen + UVA). Disadvantages of phototherapy are the inconvenience of traveling to clinic for tri- or bi-weekly treatments, as well as the risk of photoaging and/or induction of cutaneous malignancies and sunburns.

If a patient is not already applying topical corticosteroid twice daily to all affected areas, a regimen of triamcinolone 0.1% cream dispensed in a 454-g jar often is helpful. This allows aggressive application topically as in many cases patients do not have enough to adequately treat affected areas (see Chapter 2). Using triamcinolone 0.1% in conjunction with open wet dressings (Table 15-2) is very helpful for patients able to apply them once or twice daily.

For severe, unresponsive AD, systemic use of corticosteroids may be employed judiciously. Chronic utilization of oral corticosteroids should be avoided because of possible systemic complications. Tapering should be done carefully, because abrupt cessation of therapy may be associated with a rebound flaring.

Another helpful systemic medication in severe AD is systemic cyclosporine in daily dosage of 2 to 5 mg/kg. It can improve the condition quickly, but its usefulness may be limited by side effects. Less often used systemic treatments include methotrexate and azathioprine.

Systemic antistaphylococcal therapy is helpful for all stages of infected AD. Antibiotics of choice are oral cephalosporin and dicloxacillin in doses of 250 mg four times daily for adults, or 125 mg twice a day (25 to 50 mg/kg/day divided into two doses) for young children. Future treatments may include the use of IgE-binding biologics for a subgroup of patients. A simple method to reduce bacterial colonization is bleach baths. These are simple and cost effective. In a standard 40-gallon bathtub, fill with comfortable temperature (not hot) water. Add ½ cup bleach (such as Clorox). Soak for ~10 minutes. Gently

Table 15-2 Open Wet Dressings

These dressings are useful for any body surface area other than the face or scalp. Necessary items include thin cotton cloth material such as a flat sheet or t-shirt material in a size large enough to wrap around the affected area, warm to hot water, and a topical steroid cream. The choice of steroid depends on the severity of the dermatitis. For acute moderate to severe dermatitis, a moderate potency steroid such as triamcinolone 0.1% cream is adequate. For more chronic, severe, lichenified dermatitis a super-potent steroid such as clobetasol propionate 0.05% cream may be a more helpful choice.

Application:

1. Soak the cloth in hot water
2. While the cloth is soaking, apply a thick layer of the corticosteroid cream on the affected area(s)
3. Remove the cloth from the water, wring out excess water leaving the cloth wet but not dripping
4. Wrap the affected area(s) with the cloth or multiple pieces if necessary for several body sites
5. Leave the cloth on until it is too cold for comfort, usually 30–60 minutes, then remove the cloth
6. Pat the treated area dry
7. Reapply another layer of the steroid cream
8. Repeat the process above 2–3 times daily as necessary

rinse the face with a washcloth, keeping eyes closed. Repeat this as maintenance 2 to 3 times weekly.

"AT A GLANCE" TREATMENT

- Maintenance therapy:
  - Patients with AD should limit potentially skin-irritating activities such as wet work and contact to chemicals/detergents.
  - Use mild, perfume free, nonalkali soaps.
  - Bleach baths 2 to 3 times weekly.
  - Following bathing, patients must moisturize immediately.
  - Apply cream containing ceramides (either prescription [Atopiclair/Mimyx] or over-the-counter [Cerave]).
  - Topical mild or moderate potency corticosteroid application immediately with dermatitis flare, after resolution return to moisturizing regimen as above.
  - Alternate maintenance: topical tacrolimus (Protopic) to AA BID × 1 to 6 weeks until dermatitis clear, then apply as maintenance to prior AA twice weekly.
- Mild or moderate active flares:
  - The mainstay of treatment for pruritus is antihistamines whereas corticosteroids are used to gain control of skin inflammation.
  - Rapid flares are best treated with 5 days of a medium-to high-potency topical corticosteroid ointment. Application should be once to twice a day. Once disease control is achieved, the topical corticosteroid can be tapered to a less potent class and eventually withdrawn.
  - Adjustment of steroid class when used in the groin area and the face should be considered, as these areas are more vulnerable for cutaneous atrophy.
  - Alternating therapy with topical immunomodulators (calcineurin inhibitors tacrolimus and pimecrolimus, FDA approved for patients >2 years) may be helpful.
  - Moderate to severe AD: consider combination topical and ultraviolet therapy.
    - Narrow-band UVB and PUVA (Psoralen + UVA).

- Severe, unresponsive AD:
  - Topical triamcinolone cream: dispense 454-g jar. Advise open wet dressings to affected areas as described.
  - Systemic use of corticosteroids may be employed judiciously. Chronic utilization of oral corticosteroids should be avoided. Taper carefully.
  - Systemic cyclosporine in daily dosage of 2 to 5 mg/kg.
  - Less often used systemic treatments include methotrexate and azathioprine.
- Systemic antistaphylococcal therapy is helpful for all stages of infected AD:
  - Antibiotics of choice are oral cephalosporin and dicloxacillin in doses of 250 mg four times daily for adults, or 125 mg twice a day (25 to 50 mg/kg/day divided into two doses) for young children.
  - Bleach baths 2 to 3 times weekly: put ¼ to ½ cup bleach in a standard bathtub. Soak for at least 10 minutes.

COURSE AND COMPLICATIONS

In most affected infants and children, the frequency of active inflammatory flares decreases with age until the teens. Around two thirds of childhood AD cases clear in early adolescence or become symptom free. Of note, patients with childhood AD are at risk for the later development of hand eczema, allergic rhinitis, and/or asthma. A minority of patients show a chronic relapsing course beyond puberty. Frequently these patients develop a moderate-severe AD accompanied by other atopic features such as allergic rhinitis and/or allergic asthma.

Even with diminution of active AD skin lesions, the inherited hypersensitivity and the disposition of the skin to develop eczema is a lifelong condition. This can be important when choosing a profession. Avoidance of potential triggers such as frequent contact to water, detergents, and chemicals is a lifelong necessity.

Infections

Patients with AD are prone to develop skin infections. One specific feature of AD is dense colonization with *Staphylococcus aureus*. In addition to bacterial infections, patients with AD show an increased prevalence of viral infections from herpes-, pox-, and papillomavirus groups. Typical viral infections include eczema herpeticum, molluscum contagiosum, and flat warts. There is also an increased susceptibility to superficial fungal infections, especially *Trichophyton rubrum* and *Pityrosporum ovale*.

Erythroderma

In severe cases of AD, a significant exacerbation may lead to an erythrodermic skin condition possibly complicated by cardiac and renal compromise.

Neuropsychiatric Changes

The intractable course of AD may result in a diminished sense of personal well-being and self-esteem, leading to depressive mood and withdrawal from social interaction.

Complication of Treatments

The use of topical immunosuppressive therapy can worsen skin infections. Moreover the chronic use of topical corticosteroids leads to poor wound healing, skin atrophy, and telangiectasias. Regular application of corticosteroids to the face can cause rosacea, acneiform skin eruptions, and hypertrichosis.

WHEN TO REFER

- Dermatologic referral becomes useful when skin lesions do not resolve or when they exacerbate with common treatment options.
- In cases of severe infections, (e.g., zoster ophthalmicus); systemic involvement (e.g., erythroderma); neuropsychiatric impairment (e.g., depression); or when side effects of pharmacotherapy are unacceptable, consultation with the appropriate specialist is essential.

CHAPTER 15 Dermatitis

NOT TO BE MISSED

- Staphylococcal colonization and infection can drive chronic AD. Be sure to assess and treat skin infection.

- For spreading, painful dermatitis consider eczema herpeticum.

- Open wet dressings are exceedingly helpful for acute, severe dermatitis.

Allergic reactions to vehicles in products, such as wool alcohols or preservatives, are also possible. Oral immunosuppressive steroid therapy may lead to osteoporosis, Cushing syndrome, and hip necrosis, and the use of cyclosporine can lead to hypertension and renal failure.

ICD9 Codes

706.8	Other specified diseases of sebaceous glands
372.53	Conjunctival xerosis
691.8	Other atopic dermatitis and related conditions
692.0	Contact dermatitis and other eczema due to detergents
692.1	Contact dermatitis and other eczema due to oils and greases
692.2	Contact dermatitis and other eczema due to solvents
692.3	Contact dermatitis and other eczema due to drugs and medicines in contact with skin
692.4	Contact dermatitis and other eczema due to other chemical products
692.5	Contact dermatitis and other eczema due to food in contact with skin
692.6	Contact dermatitis and other eczema due to plants (except food)
692.70	Unspecified dermatitis due to sun
692.71	Sunburn
692.72	Acute dermatitis due to solar radiation
692.73	Actinic reticuloid and actinic granuloma
692.74	Other chronic dermatitis due to solar radiation
692.75	Disseminated superficial actinic porokeratosis (dsap)
692.76	Sunburn of second degree
692.77	Sunburn of third degree
692.79	Other dermatitis due to solar radiation
692.81	Dermatitis due to cosmetics
692.82	Dermatitis due to other radiation
692.83	Dermatitis due to metals
692.84	Contact dermatitis and other eczema due to animal (cat) (dog) dander
692.89	Contact dermatitis and other eczema due to other specified agents
698.9	Unspecified pruritic disorder

CONTACT DERMATITIS

Dermatitis resulting from skin contact to exogenous substances is termed contact dermatitis (CD). There are two major forms of CD each with a different etiology: irritant contact dermatitis (ICD) and allergic contact dermatitis (ACD). ICD is more frequent than ACD (ratio 4:1) and results from a localized toxic effect following contact with irritants such as acids, alkalis, and soaps (Fig. 15-4). In contrast, ACD is a delayed allergen-specific type IV-hypersensitivity reaction elicited upon reapplication of a chemical to the skin after previous immunologic sensitization (Fig. 15-5).

Clinical and histological cutaneous responses of both forms of CD, particularly in the chronic stage, are similar. While the acute phase is predominated by erythema, edema, and vesiculation, characteristic clinical features of the chronic phase are scaling and lichenification. Localization of lesions generally corresponds specifically to the site of contact, with well-defined margins. In ACD the skin involvement may extend beyond the margins of the contact. Clinical features are described in Table 15-3.

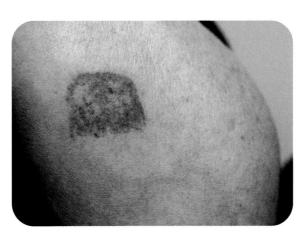

Figure 15-4 Acute irritant contact dermatitis following exposure to a strong acid.

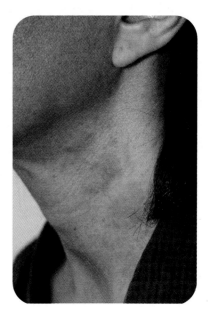

Figure 15-5 Acute allergic contact dermatitis from poison ivy exposure. The patient's dog rubbed her neck and face.

Table 15-3 Comparison of Important Features of ACD and ICD

CONTACT DERMATITIS

	Allergic contact dermatitis (ACD)	Irritant contact dermatitis (ICD)
Ratio of contact dermatitis	20%	80%
Course	Acute, (subacute) chronic	Acute, (subacute) chronic
Culprits	Allergens, e.g., metals, preservatives, fragrances	Water, acids, alkalis, soaps, solvents
Onset	48–96 hours in clinically sensitized	Strongly depending on irritants potency, ranging from rapid to late (weeks/months)
Course of healing	*Transient increase* in the reaction after removal of offending agent before healing occurs (crescendo phenomenon)	Healing starts *immediately* after removal of offending agent (decrescendo phenomenon)
Affected individuals	Only sensitized	Everyone who is exposed to the noxa, if duration and concentration is sufficient
Number of necessary contacts to develop dermatitis	Delayed reaction, only when re-exposition to a sensitized (2nd time of exposition)	Dermatitis can occur at the 1st time of exposition, previous contact is not necessary
Distribution	Localized with possible spreading	Localized
Diagnosis	Patient's history patch test	Exclusion of other entities, no specific diagnostic test
Differential diagnoses	AD, ICD, tinea	AD, ACD, tinea
Therapy	Avoidance of *allergens* anti-inflammatory therapy, restoration of diminished skin barrier function, e.g., moisturizers, ointments	Avoidance of *triggers* anti-inflammatory therapy, restoration of diminished skin barrier function, e.g., moisturizers, ointments

As there is no single diagnostic feature, diagnosis of CD is based on the detailed exploration of patients' history, evaluation of morphology, and distribution of skin lesions in addition to the exclusion of other dermatologic entities. Patch testing allows the identification of causative allergens, which helps differentiate ACD from ICD. It is common for eczema to arise from a combination of factors (e.g., ICD with a decreased skin barrier function is frequently affected by secondary ACD due to facilitated absorption of allergens).

Mainstays of treatment are primarily the avoidance of the eliciting allergen/irritant, temporary anti-inflammatory treatment, and restoration of physiologic skin barrier function with appropriate skin care. When using topical therapy, a decision regarding the appropriate active ingredient, as well as the vehicle, must be considered. Selection of the vehicle is based on the type of skin inflammation. Exudative skin lesions respond best to less occlusive vehicles, such as solutions or gels, while chronic, dry skin does will with occlusive ointments, such as petrolatum. Furthermore, patients have to be enlightened that significant improvement may take several weeks to months, and patients should be counseled that they must be patient and adhere to the chosen regimen.

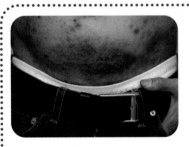

A 53-year-old man presents with sharply demarcated, pruritic erythematous scaling plaques on his abdomen near the umbilicus and a generalized dermatitis. Further examination reveals similar skin lesions on his arms, legs, and back. He described flaring of his dermatitis after starting to take a chromium dietary supplement. His lower abdomen has had dermatitis for several years as shown in Figure 15-6. He has always worn a belt similar to the one shown. Patch testing reveals 2+ reactions to potassium dichromate and nickel sulfate.

Allergic Contact Dermatitis (ACD)

BACKGROUND

ACD is a frequently observed skin condition caused by a delayed allergen-specific type IV hypersensitivity reaction to low-molecular-weight haptens that is elicited when a chemical is reapplied to the skin after previous exposure and immunological sensitization. Risk factors include the inherent sensitization potential of an allergen, allergen concentration, frequency and time of exposure, occlusion, the presence of penetration enhancing factors, and an altered skin barrier function.

Data from the 2006 National Ambulatory Medical Care Survey revealed an estimated 9.5 million outpatient visits yearly to U.S. physicians for "contact dermatitis and other eczema," of which 20% are likely allergic in nature with the remaining classified as irritant related. This suggests that ~2 million visits per year are allergic in origin.

PATHOGENESIS

ACD is a type IV, delayed, allergen-specific hypersensitivity response of an individual to a chemical. The pathogenesis involves an initial sensitization when the patient first comes in contact with the chemical, which penetrates the stratum corneum of the skin and is processed by Langerhans cells in the epidermis. Antigen-coupled Langerhans cells then leave the epidermis and migrate to the regional lymph nodes via the afferent lymphatics, where they present the antigens to naive CD4+ positive cells. The responding T cells are stimulated via a complex immunologic process to proliferate into memory and affector T cells. The subsequent re-exposure of the skin leads to the presentation of the responsible allergen to an already primed T-cell milieu, ending in the release of numerous cytokines and chemotactic factors that result in the clinical picture.

KEY FEATURES

- Allergic contact dermatitis (ACD) is an eczematous skin reaction resulting from an immunologic reaction following re-exposure to allergens.

- ACD represents the immunological model for delayed type IV hypersensitivity reactions.

- Clinically, ACD presents with demarcated plaques according to the site of contact, but may show some spreading reaction as well.

(Continued)

KEY FEATURES (Continued)

- The gold standard of diagnosis is patch testing.

- The most important sensitizers include metals (nickel, cobalt); fragrances (fragrance, balsam of Peru); preservatives (formaldehyde, quaternium-15, diazolidinyl urea, DMDM hydantoin and imidazolidinyl urea); and topical antibiotics (neomycin, bacitracin).

- Mainstays of therapy are avoidance of allergens and restoration of physiologic skin barrier function in times of acute inflammation.

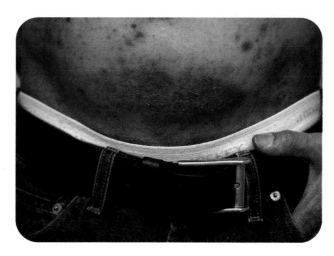

Figure 15-6 Nickel allergic contact dermatitis from the patient's metal belt buckle.

Once sensitized, only a low amount of causative chemical is necessary to elicit the reaction that typically occurs within 48 to 96 hours after re-exposure.

CLINICAL PRESENTATION

Clinically, ACD presents as a well-demarcated, pruritic eczematous eruption, typically localized to the area of contact. Spreading of the eruption slightly beyond the borders of the area of contact may be seen. Three clinical stages can be observed: acute, subacute, and chronic ACD.

Acute ACD is dominated by erythema, edema, possible vesiculation, and significant pruritus. In case of ongoing exposure to the allergen, skin changes consistent with chronic disease can be seen. This transitional stage is called subacute ACD and presents with erythema, crusts, and hyperkeratosis. With progression of inflammation acute exudative inflammation decreases while epidermal disorganized thickened skin, fissures, and lichenification appear, marking chronic dermatitis.

DIAGNOSIS

Careful evaluation of patient's history with special regard to the working and hobby environment is necessary and appropriate. Enquire about frequent exposure to products from everyday life, such as cosmetics, metals, topical medication, earlier treatments, and the course of skin inflammation when avoiding ACD-suspicious allergens. Localization of skin lesions according to anatomical body sites may also be helpful to find causing allergens, as certain body sites are differently exposed to certain chemicals.

Patch Testing

Patch testing is the gold standard for the diagnosis of ACD (Fig. 15-7). Most common allergens that react at rates of > 0.5% to 1.0% in routine testing of patients with suspected contact dermatitis are summarized in a "standard" or baseline series. Numbers and allergens that are included in this tray may vary according to regulations of local patch test societies, which are based on the occurrence of potential allergens from regional habits and governmental regulations. Beside the standard tray, there are various other test trays (e.g., cosmetics/preservative, metals, textile dyes, dental material) for specific occupations or exposures.

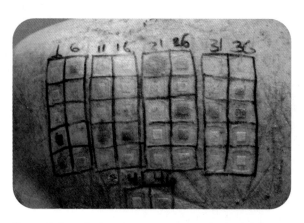

Figure 15-7 Multiple positive reactions on the back following patch testing.

Testing can be conducted with commercially available preimpregnated tests (TRUE Test) or with tests that are prepared at the physicians' office. The most common test site is the upper back (Fig. 15-7). Test sites have to be free of inflammation for most accurate reading. Systemic and/or local anti-inflammatory treatments that may decrease the immunologic reaction should be stopped prior patch testing, for example, a 1-week pause for local corticosteroids, phototherapy, or after sunburns. One to 2 weeks off of systemic corticosteroids should be observed.

Differential Diagnosis

The differential diagnosis of ACD includes other forms of dermatitis such as irritant contact dermatitis (discomfort rather than pruritus dominates), atopic dermatitis (other associated atopic features, distribution of skin lesions), and seborrheic dermatitis (located in areas of sebaceous glands). Hand-and-foot dermatitis needs to be distinguished from psoriasis and fungal infections. In case of widespread ACD, consider a medication-induced dermatitis or additional causes of erythroderma.

THERAPY

The most important therapeutic intervention is the identification of causative allergens, and subsequent education of the patient as to which substances to avoid. Clinical interventions depend on stage of inflammation and morphologic at presentation.

Acute ACD and AD respond to cool, wet compresses, and the use of local corticosteroids for rapid diminution of inflammation. A very helpful method for doing wet dressings is presented in Table 15-2 in the atopic dermatitis section.

In contrast, preferred treatment of subacute/chronic stages with symptoms of dry hyperkeratosis include the application of occlusive ointments and creams. Anti-inflammatory treatment with corticosteroids (local and/or systemic) helps to limit inflammation. In some cases of flared atopic dermatitis, open wet dressings are also helpful to calm the flare without using an oral corticosteroid. In severe cases of ACD in areas where a strong corticosteroid would not be desired, such as the anogenital skin or facial skin, consider prescribing pimecrolimus cream or tacrolimus ointment.

"AT A GLANCE" TREATMENT

- Acute ACD will resolve in 1 to 3 weeks in absence of continued allergen exposure without therapy.
- Identify causative allergens through avoidance and challenge or through patch testing.
- Acute ACD and AD responds to cool, wet compresses and the use of local corticosteroids for rapid diminution of inflammation.
- For eyelid or anogenital dermatitis, consider usage of tacrolimus ointment or pimecrolimus cream to avoid topical steroid side effects.

COURSE AND COMPLICATIONS

Clearing of acute skin lesion might take up to several weeks and requires patience and adherence to treatment plans. In case of ubiquitously occurring contact allergens and severe allergy the difficulty in avoiding causative allergens completely may lead to chronic disease.

WHEN TO REFER

When skin lesions do not improve, despite avoidance of allergens and/or appropriate anti-inflammatory treatment, patients should be introduced to a specialist. Also if identification of rare allergens not included in commercially available trays may be suspected, particularly those chemicals that need to be produced/diluted, patients should be referred.

NOT TO BE MISSED

- Have a high index of suspicion for allergy with recurrent dermatitis in areas that topical products are applied.
- Consider irritant dermatitis for palmar dermatitis in addition to ACD.

ICD9 Codes

692.0	Contact dermatitis and other eczema due to detergents
692.1	Contact dermatitis and other eczema due to oils and greases
692.2	Contact dermatitis and other eczema due to solvents
692.3	Contact dermatitis and other eczema due to drugs and medicines in contact with skin
692.4	Contact dermatitis and other eczema due to other chemical products
692.5	Contact dermatitis and other eczema due to food in contact with skin
692.6	Contact dermatitis and other eczema due to plants (except food)
692.70	Unspecified dermatitis due to sun
692.71	Sunburn
692.72	Acute dermatitis due to solar radiation
692.73	Actinic reticuloid and actinic granuloma
692.74	Other chronic dermatitis due to solar radiation
692.75	Disseminated superficial actinic porokeratosis (dsap)
692.76	Sunburn of second degree
692.77	Sunburn of third degree
692.79	Other dermatitis due to solar radiation
692.81	Dermatitis due to cosmetics
692.82	Dermatitis due to other radiation
692.83	Dermatitis due to metals
692.84	Contact dermatitis and other eczema due to animal (cat) (dog) dander
692.89	Contact dermatitis and other eczema due to other specified agents
691.8	Other atopic dermatitis and related conditions
692.9	Contact dermatitis and other eczema, unspecified cause

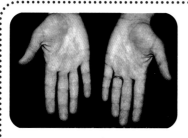

A 28-year-old mother presents for treatment of severe hand eczema characterized by fissures and skin thickening (Fig. 15-8). Seven months before, she had delivered twins, subsequently washing, changing diapers, preparing food, and other housework. She reports having sensitive skin in the past, but never had such severe eczema before. She is otherwise healthy. Patient's history and further dermatologic exam was unremarkable. Now she is seeking treatment as her hands are getting more and more painful and she is becoming less able to do her regular tasks.

Irritant Contact Dermatitis (ICD)

BACKGROUND

Irritant contact dermatitis is the most common form of contact dermatitis, including a number of subtypes that contribute to different clinical presentations. Irritants cause cell damage in different ways. In the acute forms of ICD, exposure to strong irritants (e.g., acids, alkalis) damage keratinocytes with direct cytotoxic effects. As strong irritants are usually recognized as such, protection is generally used and acute ICD occurs accidentally. In contrast, repeated, long-term exposure to weak irritants (e.g., wet work) in chronic ICD removes surface lipids and water-retaining substances, followed by impaired cell membrane function. When the cumulative exposure to irritants exceeds a threshold unique for each individual, overwhelming the repair capacity of the skin, ICD manifests. Elicitation threshold often decreases with progression of disease. Because of frequent exposure for chronic ICD

KEY FEATURES

- ICD is a circumscribed inflammatory reaction resulting from a single or repeated application of a chemical substance to the skin.

- Anyone exposed may be affected if duration/concentration of the irritant is sufficient.

- The most commonly affected anatomical site is the hands.

- In acute ICD *strong* irritants (e.g., alkalis, acids) predominate, while chronic ICD results from repeated exposure to *low-grade* irritants (e.g., water, soap).

- The most common irritant is wet work; it is often seen in the occupational setting.

- Severity is determined by the irritating substance, host/environmental factors, and exposure parameters such as concentration, pH, temperature, occlusion, and duration of contact.

- The diagnosis of ICD is often the diagnosis of exclusion in the case of suspected ACD with negative patch testing; there is no readily available diagnostic test.

- Therapy includes the avoidance of triggering irritants, anti-inflammatory therapy, and restoration of diminished skin barrier function with moisturizers.

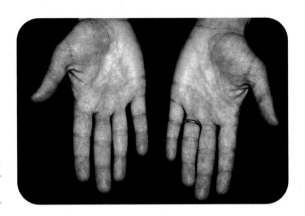

Figure 15-8 Irritant hand eczema.

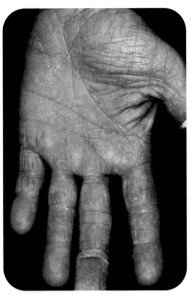

Figure 15-9 Irritant hand eczema.

hands are the most affected anatomic site (Fig. 15-9). A summary of common irritants is presented in Table 15-4.

Forms of ICD are determined by the characteristics of the irritating substance, host features, such as individual's age (susceptibility to irritants is inversely proportional to age); race; sex (increased risk for women); pre-existing

Table 15-4 Overview of Important Irritants

IRRITANT	MECHANISM OF TOXICITY	
Acids e.g., sulfuric, nitric, hydrochloric, chromic	Protein denaturation, cytotoxicity coagulation of skin proteins impedes further penetration	<u>Stron</u>g irritant, important role in *acute* ICD
Alkalis or bases e.g., sodium, calcium, potassium hydroxides, wet concrete	Protein denaturation and lipid degradation with saponification of the resulting fatty acids form soaps which aid penetration of alkalis deeper into the deeper skin	<u>Stron</u>g irritant, important role in *acute* ICD, clinical reaction is more painful and severe in damage than most acids, no vesicles, but rather necrotic skin
Organic solvents	Solubilization of membrane lipids, membrane toxicity, dissolvation of the intercellular lipid barrier	Irritating capability is attributed mainly to their lipophilicity: aromatic > aliphatic > chlorinated > turpentine > alcohols > esters > ketones
Detergents and cleansers	Solubilization and/or disruption of barrier lipids and natural moisturizing factors in the stratum corneum, protein denaturation membrane toxicity	Often causes *chronic* forms of ICD
Water	Universal solvent, ubiquitous skin irritant, irritancy of water is exacerbated by occlusion	<u>Weak</u> irritant, in *chronic* forms of ICD

skin disease; and anatomic region exposed. Moreover environmental factors such as the concentration, molecular size, ionization state and fat solubility of the irritant, mechanical pressure, temperature, humidity, pH, and duration of contact play an important role.

PATHOGENESIS

Currently, numerous pathogenic mechanisms are linked to ICD and include the denaturation of epidermal keratins, disruption of the permeability barrier, damage to cell membranes, and direct cytotoxic effects. The general mechanisms eliciting acute or chronic ICD are different. Acute ICD involves direct cytotoxic damage to keratinocytes with a following release of mediators of inflammation with resultant T-cell activation. In contrast, in chronic ICD, repeated irritant-exposures cause slow damage to the stratum corneum lipids. Lipids play a major role in the maintenance of skin barrier function and displacement of those is associated with a loss of corneocyte cohesion, desquamation, and increase in transepidermal water loss. Finally the stratum corneum as a barrier is disrupted.

CLINICAL PRESENTATION

ICD can be divided into acute, subacute, and chronic forms. Beyond those, because of lacking standard classification, some authors prefer to differentiate further clinical types.

Acute (toxic) ICD is observed when skin comes into contact with a strong irritant (e.g., acids, alkalis). The skin is damaged within a short period of time. When the exposure is stopped, an immediate healing begins. This is called the decrescendo phenomenon and can be a helpful sign to differentiate it from ACD, where a transient increase in the reaction before healing occurs (crescendo phenomenon). Clinical symptoms include burning, stinging, soreness. Signs of ICD are bright erythema, edema, bullae, and possible necrosis of the skin. Lesions are restricted to the area of exposure delineated by sharply demarcated borders.

Subacute ICD generally occurs in individuals exposed to wet chemical environments. Morphologically it is a transitional stage between acute and chronic phases, with clinical signs of both, such as darker erythema, edema, vesicles, crusts, and scaling.

Chronic (cumulative) ICD results from chronic, repeated subthreshold skin insults. This is the most prevalent form encountered in clinical practice, especially in the realm of occupational ICD. Between the exposures, there is not enough time for a complete restoration of skin barrier function. Chronic lesions of ICD present with less sharply demarcated and more indistinct borders. Predominant signs are lichenification and hyperkeratosis, xerosis, erythema, and vesiculation. Itching and pain due to fissures are further symptoms.

Special Variants of ICD

Asteatotic eczema is mainly seen during the winter months in elderly individuals who frequently bathe without restoring skin moisture. Intensive pruritus is common as well as dry skin with ichthyosiform scaling. It often presents with nummular (coin-shaped) scaling plaques on the legs and trunk.

Airborne ICD develops in sensitive skin of the face, neck, and periorbital regions exposed to irritants.

DIAGNOSIS

Patient's history, particularly to habits in working and hobby environments, is key to the appropriate diagnosis. History should include occupation, course of inflammation (recovery in leisure/weekends/vacation suggests an occupational background), commonly used chemicals, detergents, soaps, cosmetics, special hobbies, and previous treatments and their efficacy.

Diagnostic Methods

Diagnosis of ICD is based on patient's history, clinical appearance, and on the exclusion of other dermatologic entities. There is no specific diagnostic test.

Differential Diagnoses

Most common differential diagnoses include allergic contact dermatitis (ACD). Differentiation can be done by patch testing and on clinical features. In comparison to ACD, ICD is more frequently accompanied by pain than pruritus. Also in ICD, the decrescendo phenomenon (immediate healing when irritant exposure is stopped) in the course of healing may help to differentiate from ACD, where typically a crescendo phenomenon with transient increase in reaction before healing occurs. Further common differential diagnoses are atopic dermatitis, seborrheic dermatitis, psoriasis, and tinea.

THERAPY

Primary treatment of all ICD stages is the avoidance of causative irritants. Additional therapeutic interventions are based on stage and morphologic characteristics at presentation. In the acute stage, thorough removal of the irritant is essential. Exudative acute forms are treated with thinner creams, if necessary with an anti-inflammatory ingredient, while the occlusion effect of thick ointments is avoided. For chronic stages, when severe dryness, scaling, and hyperkeratosis predominate, nonallergic fatty substances (e.g., petrolatum) restores barrier function the best.

Photochemotherapy (PUVA) may be considered for chronic dermatitis. Hyperkeratotic palmoplantar dermatitis from chronic ICD may benefit from the adjunctive use of systemic retinoids such as acitretin. Once the skin lesions are cleared further strategies focus on the prevention of ICD, such as reduction of exposure to identified irritants, educational programs in the utilization of personal protective equipment (e.g., gloves, special clothing), and the application of ointments/creams for restoration/maintenance of the skin barrier function.

"AT A GLANCE" TREATMENT

- Primary treatment is avoidance of irritants.
- Exudative acute ICD: treat with thinner creams, if necessary with a corticosteroid, while the occlusion effect of thick ointments is avoided.
- Chronic ICD with severe xerosis, scaling and hyperkeratosis: petrolatum repairs barrier function best.
- Consider PUVA for chronic recalcitrant ICD.
- Systemic retinoids (acitretin) may be helpful in severe cases.

COURSE AND COMPLICATIONS

Course and possible complications of ICD are determined by a myriad of factors. In acute ICD caused by strong irritants, characteristics of irritants as well as host and environmental factors influence the degree of damage. According to the intensity of reaction, possible complications are erythema, erosions, necrosis, superinfections, postinflammatory hypo-/hyperpigmentation, scarring, and keloid formation. When repeatedly exposed to weak irritants, skin

WHEN TO REFER

When skin inflammation, despite avoidance of irritants and/or appropriate anti-inflammatory treatment does not improve, patients should consult a specialist for treatment and for exclusion of other entities.

CHAPTER 15 Dermatitis

NOT TO BE MISSED

- Always consider allergic contact dermatitis as a primary or secondary diagnosis in cases suspected of ICD.

- Consider addition of ultraviolet light or systemic retinoids in recalcitrant cases.

lesions can become chronic. With progress of ICD, barrier function may be exhausted completely. As a result, patients are unable to perform their occupation. Occupational disability due to ICD is common in health care employees, hairdressers, caterers, and housekeepers/cleaning lines of work.

ICD9 Codes

692.9	Contact dermatitis and other eczema, unspecified cause
706.8	Other specified diseases of sebaceous glands
372.53	Conjunctival xerosis

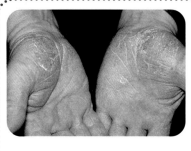

A 47-year-old woman presents with hand issues. On exam, she shows you initially hyperkeratotic scaling plaques on her palms (Fig. 15-10), fingers, and on some knuckles bilaterally. There are no nail changes, no muscle weakness, and no eyelid dermatitis. Her feet are clear. She has a history of atopic dermatitis and asthma. She relates chronic pain and itch from this. She has treated her hands with a variety of topical steroids without success. Her labs are unremarkable including CBCl, complete metabolic panell, ANAl, double stranded DNAl, anti-Jo1 and Mi2 antibodies. Patch testing is negative. You perform a complete skin exam and find subtle hyperkeratotic plaques on her elbows and gluteal pinking, as well as a 3-cm hyperkeratotic plaque with micaceous scale in the upper gluteal cleft. What is her diagnosis? How would you treat her?

Figure 15-10 Psoriatic hand eczema. From Goodheart HP. *Goodheart's Photoguide of Common Skin Disorders,* 3rd ed. Philadelphia: Lippincott Williams & Wilkins, 2009.

Hand and Foot Dermatitis

BACKGROUND

The ubiquitous use of one's hands as essential "tools in everyday life" and their role in sensation, communication, and aesthetics attests to the significance of hand dermatitis. Besides the difficulty of performing job and household responsibilities, hand eczema may lead to a diminution of the sense of well-being and self-esteem. Thus, hand eczema is an important and frequently occurring disease, particularly in the realm of occupational dermatology.

Because of similar anatomic skin structures of the palms and soles, hand and foot dermatitis has similar etiologic causes. Also, these particular anatomic features impact the etiology and treatment of palmoplantar dermatitis. First, the thicker epidermis presents an increased physical barrier (several millimeters versus 50 μm). Moreover, the palmoplantar skin has the highest concentration of eccrine sweat glands ($400/cm^2$ vs. $80/cm^2$ at the legs). Because the effect of sweat on chemicals is the release of ions, an increased risk of penetration of these and subsequent irritants or allergic reaction is seen.

Palmoplantar eczema results from three major etiologies including exogenous and endogenous exposures and infection or a combination of these factors.

CLINICAL PRESENTATION

An overview of the various types/causes of hand-and-foot dermatitis is presented in Fig. 15-11.

Exogenous-Contact Dermatitis

Clinical appearance relates to stage of disease. In the acute phase, erythema, induration, edema, and vesiculation are prominent features. In contrast, chronic stages present

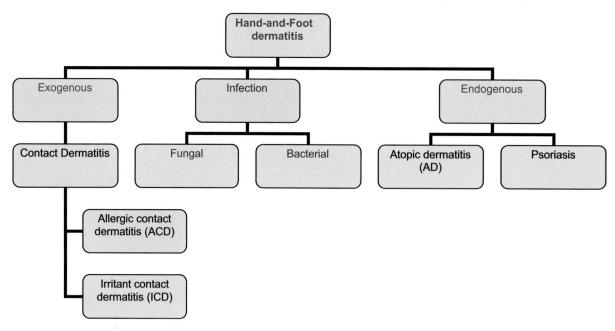

Figure 15-11 Hand and foot dermatitis.

with hyperkeratosis, scaling, and lichenification. Skin lesions are sharply limited to the site of contact. The most common external cause of hand eczema is contact with irritants, while allergic contact dermatitis of the hands is much less frequent. Allergic contact dermatitis of the hands is most commonly due to fragrances, preservatives, metals, acrylates, rubber accelerators, and topical antibiotics. In contrast, frequent allergens in ACD of the feet are dichromates, rubber accelerators, colophony, formaldehyde, or dyes.

Endogenous

Atopic dermatitis frequently affects the hands, particularly the distal fingers and fingertips. Hyperlinearity of the palms is a common feature. Clinical symptoms are scaling, dryness, fissures, and erythema. Hyperkeratosis is observed in severe and chronic stages. Psoriasis presents in the palmoplantar area with thick, dry adherent scales and hyperkeratoses on an erythematous basis. Fissures may be present. Frequently nails are affected, resulting in nail pitting, discoloration, dystrophy, and onycholysis.

Infection

Palmoplantar dermatophyte infection may involve only one hand and both feet. In some cases an "id" reaction occurs and the hands are hyperkeratotic, without dermatophyte reaction. Occasionally, a focal or generalized dermatitis may accompany this reaction. Tinea of the hands may be either intertriginous or palmar. Plantar tinea extends up the lateral aspects of the feet. Erythematous skin lesions are often well demarcated with circinate scaling borders. Nails may also be affected. Bacterial infection presents with pustules or crusts on an erythematous base.

DIAGNOSIS

Correct diagnosis for hand and/or feet eczema includes the identification of the causing agent and/or exclusion of other causes. The following algorithm may simplify the way to final diagnosis (Table 15-5).

Table 15-5 Algorithm for Diagnosis of Hand and/or Feet Dermatitis

TO DO	GOAL
1. Ascertainment of **detailed patient and family history**	Supports endogenous cause or contact dermatitis
2. Careful **investigation of further skin:** → Looking for psoriatic plaques elsewhere, check common places: belly button, rima ani, upper gluteal cleft and extensor sites of extremities, nails, joint involvement	Exclude psoriasis
→ Looking for eczematous lesion in the flexor sites of extremities	Exclude atopic dermatitis
3. **KOH, fungal culture**	Exclude tinea
4. **Gram stain, culture**	Exclude bacterial infection Patients with atopic dermatitis have an increased colonization with *S. aureus*.
5. **Patch test**	Identification of relevant allergens confirm allergic contact dermatitis
6. Everything above: negative	Consider irritant contact dermatitis
7. None of the diagnoses above seems to be reasonable: **biopsy**	Exclude other syndromes that include involvement of hands and refer to specialist

Differential Diagnoses

The following diseases and syndromes affect the hands or the feet and may mimic a palmoplantar dermatitis:

- **Inherited entities:** ichthyosis, palmoplantar keratodermas (PPK), Darier disease, epidermolysis bullosa, pityriasis rubra pilaris
- **Acquired entities:** hypothyroidism, lichen planus
- **Infections:** scabies, secondary syphilis, warts
- **Malignancies:** sézary syndrome

WHEN TO REFER

- Patients should be referred in cases where the diagnosis is unclear, when therapeutic options fail, or the dermatitis progresses.
- If ultraviolet light therapy is necessary, refer to dermatology.

THERAPY

Refer to the treatment section appropriate for the diagnosis.

COURSE AND COMPLICATIONS

Hand eczema/dermatoses are often particularly challenging to cure. Marked improvement often is achieved with appropriate therapy, but the patient often will have flares/recurrence of almost every diagnosis considered above. Chronic management/therapy is necessary for most.

NOT TO BE MISSED

- Always consider psoriasis and atopic dermatitis in addition to an exogenous infection or contact dermatitis; more than one cause of hand/foot dermatitis may be present.

ICD9 Codes

692.0	Contact dermatitis and other eczema due to detergents
692.1	Contact dermatitis and other eczema due to oils and greases
692.2	Contact dermatitis and other eczema due to solvents
692.3	Contact dermatitis and other eczema due to drugs and medicines in contact with skin
692.4	Contact dermatitis and other eczema due to other chemical products

692.5	Contact dermatitis and other eczema due to food in contact with skin
692.6	Contact dermatitis and other eczema due to plants (except food)
692.70	Unspecified dermatitis due to sun
692.71	Sunburn
692.72	Acute dermatitis due to solar radiation
692.73	Actinic reticuloid and actinic granuloma
692.74	Other chronic dermatitis due to solar radiation
692.75	Disseminated superficial actinic porokeratosis (DSAP)
692.76	Sunburn of second degree
692.77	Sunburn of third degree
692.79	Other dermatitis due to solar radiation
692.81	Dermatitis due to cosmetics
692.82	Dermatitis due to other radiation
692.83	Dermatitis due to metals
692.84	Contact dermatitis and other eczema due to animal (cat) (dog) dander
692.89	Contact dermatitis and other eczema due to other specified agents
692.9	Contact dermatitis and other eczema, unspecified cause
696.1	Other psoriasis and similar disorders
691.8	Other atopic dermatitis and related conditions
684	Impetigo
110.2	Dermatophytosis of hand
110.4	Dermatophytosis of foot

Suggested Reading

Belsito DV. Occupational contact dermatitis: etiology, prevalence, and resultant impairment/disability. *J Am Acad Dermatol.* 2005;53(2):303–313.

Brown SJ, Irvine AD. Atopic eczema and the filaggrin story. *Semin Cutan Med Surg.* 2008;27(2):128–137.

Bruze M, Conde-Salazar L, Goossens A, et al. Thoughts on sensitizers in a standard patch test series. *Contact Dermatitis.* 1999;41:241–250.

Burt CW, McCaig LF, Rechtsteiner EA. Ambulatory medical care utilization estimates for 2005. *Adv Data.* 2007;388:1–15.

Coenraads PJ. Hand eczema is common and multifactorial. *J Invest Dermatol.* 2007;127:1568–1570.

Eichenfield LF, Hanifin JM, Luger TA, et al. Consensus conference on pediatric atopic dermatitis. *J Am Acad Dermatol.* 2003;49:1088–1095. Review.

Ellis C, Luger T, Abeck D, et al. ICCAD II Faculty. International Consensus Conference on Atopic Dermatitis II (ICCAD II): Clinical update and current treatment strategies. *Br J Dermatol.* 2003;148(Suppl 63):3–10.

ESSCA Writing Group. The European Surveillance System of Contact Allergies (ESSCA): results of patch testing the standard series, 2004. *J Eur Acad Dermatol Venereol.* 2008;22:174–181.

Hanifin J, Rajka G. Diagnostic features of atopic dermatitis. *Acta Derm Venereol.* 1980;92;44–47.

Hanifin JM, Cooper KD, Ho VC, et al. Guidelines of care for atopic dermatitis, developed in accordance with the American Academy of Dermatology (AAD)/American Academy of Dermatology Association "Administrative Regulations for Evidence-Based Clinical Practice Guidelines." *J Am Acad Dermatol.* 2004;50:391–404.

Hanifin JM. Epidemiology of atopic dermatitis. *Immunol Allergy Clin North Am.* 2002;22:1–24.

Kedrowski DA, Warshaw EM. Hand dermatitis: a review of clinical features, diagnosis, and management. *Dermatol Nurs.* 2008;20:17–25.

Mortz CG, Andersen KE. New aspects in allergic contact dermatitis. *Curr Opin Allergy Clin Immunol.* 2008;8:428–432. Review.

Mowad CM, Marks Jr JG. Allergic Contact Dermatitis. In: Bolognia JL, Jorizzo JL, Rapini RP, editors: *Dermatology Vol I*, 1st ed: Mosby Philadelphia; 2003:227–240.

Robinson MK, Gerberick GF, Ryan CA, et al. The importance of exposure estimation in the assessment of skin sensitization risk. *Contact Dermatitis.* 2000;42:251–259.

Sidbury R, Hanifin JM. Systemic therapy of atopic dermatitis. *Clin Exp Dermatol.* 2000;25:559–566.

Simpson EL, Hanifin JM. Atopic dermatitis. *J Am Acad Dermatol.* 2005;53:115–128.

Slodownik D, Lee A, Nixon R. Irritant contact dermatitis: A review. *Australas J Dermatol.* 2008;49:1–9.

Smith HR, Basketter DA, McFadden JP. Irritant dermatitis, irritancy and its role in allergic contact dermatitis. *Clin Exp Dermatol.* 2002;27:138–146.

Williams HC. Epidemiology of atopic dermatitis. *Clin Exp Dermatol.* 2000;25:522–529.

Zug KA, Kornik R, Belsito DV, et al. North American Contact Dermatitis Group. Patch-testing North American lip dermatitis patients: Data from the North American Contact Dermatitis Group, 2001 to 2004. *Dermatitis.* 2008;19:202–208.

CHAPTER 16 Skin of Color

Evelyn Lilly and Ellen K. Roh

"Ethnic skin" is generally defined as nonwhite darker skin types that fall into Fitzpatrick skin types IV, V, and VI. Patients from many racial groups may have "ethnic skin," including blacks, Asians, and Hispanics. In 2000, the U.S. Census Bureau found that nonwhites accounted for 25% of the U.S. population. In addition, it predicted that by 2050, nonwhites would no longer constitute the minority and will comprise 54% of the population. These changing demographics highlight the growing importance of familiarity with skin problems that are more prominent in ethnic patients. The following disorders are found predominantly in patients with ethnic skin and thus will become more prominent with the changing demographics.

Until recently, there were few studies on people with skin of color. What has been found is that there are some differences in the structure and function of ethnic skin that contribute to its unique features. These differences are found in the production and distribution of melanin, distribution of dermal collagen, number and size of fibroblasts, and structure of hair. Though light and dark skins have the same number of melanocytes, darker skin has larger melanosomes that are distributed throughout the entire epidermis, unlike in lighter skin, where the melanosomes are concentrated at the basal layer. These larger melanosomes are thought to be more photoprotective, which may explain why darker-skinned patients have less actinic damage than their lighter-skinned counterparts. Analyses of the dermis of people of African descent has revealed more closely packed collagen bundles and collagen fragments, as well as increased numbers of larger fibroblasts, possibly accounting for the increased incidence of keloid formation seen in black individuals. Finally, ethnic patients, especially those of African descent, often have helical or spiral curls as a result of curved terminal hair follicles, which are more likely to repenetrate the skin, causing an inflammatory response.

Normal Changes in Pigmentation of Ethnic Skin

FUTCHER OR VOIGT LINES (FIG. 16-1)

- Vertical pigmentary demarcation line between darker skin laterally and lighter skin anteromedially
- Well-defined hypopigmented patches on the lower leg, arm, or sternum that may extend laterally and inferiorly onto the abdomen
- Found most commonly in blacks, but can also affect Asians and darker-skinned whites
- Often evident at birth, tends to darken with time

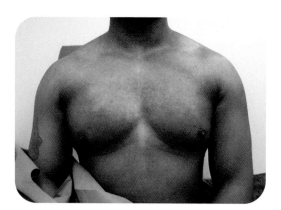

Figure 16-1 Voigt line on the central chest.

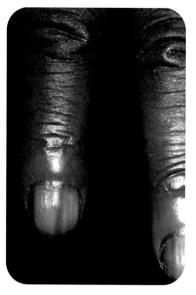

Figure 16-2 Longitudinal melanonychia.

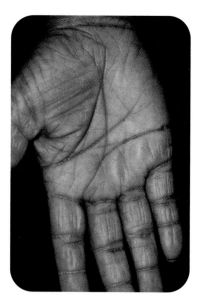

Figure 16-3 Palmar crease hyperpig-mentation.

ORAL HYPERPIGMENTATION

- Pigmented areas range in color from brown to bluish black
- Develops in childhood
- Affects gingivae, but may include tongue and rest of oral mucosa as well

NAIL PIGMENTATION (MELANONYCHIA) (FIG. 16-2)

- May be either diffuse or a longitudinal band, often bilateral
- Affects at least 50% of African Americans, increases with age
- Due to increased melanin deposition in the nail plate
- Must be differentiated from a subungual melanoma (solitary lesion, occurs at a young age, very dark or varied in color, spills over the nail)

PALMAR HYPERPIGMENTATION (FIG. 16-3)

- Creases in the palms are darker than the skin on the remainder of the palms

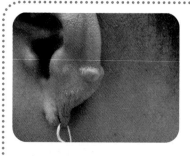

A 25-year-old Dominican female student presents to the office with large, well-defined, tuberous lesions on both of her ear lobes (Fig. 16-4). The lesions are 1 centimeter in diameter, firm, and smooth. The last time she was home, the areas on both ears were excised, but the large scars regrew. According to the patient, the lesions seem to have gotten bigger since she first noticed them. She reports no previous history of these lesions and no other medical problems.

DERMATOSES THAT OCCUR MORE FREQUENTLY IN ETHNIC SKIN

Keloids

BACKGROUND

Keloids are more common among darker-skinned patients such as African Americans, Asian Americans, and Latin Americans, who have more pigmented skin. Up to 15% of the population is at risk, although there appears to be genetic loci linked to increased susceptibility to keloid formation. Keloids occur most often in the second and third decade of life. Men and women are equally affected but women have a higher reported incidence.

KEY FEATURES

- A keloid is excessive scar growth at areas of self-inflicted or surgical trauma.

- The scar enlarges beyond the original border of injury compared to a hypertrophic scar, which does not.

- Keloids occur more frequently in places with increased tension, such as the sternum, shoulder, earlobe, and cheek.

- Patients may present with lesions that also cause pain, burning, itching, and restriction of movement.

- Treatment is most effective with intralesional triamcinolone.

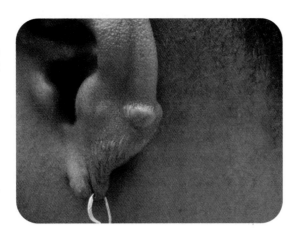

Figure 16-4 Keloid on the helix.

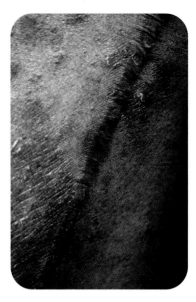

Figure 16-5 Old hypertrophic surgical scar with active psoriasis surrounding.

PATHOGENESIS

Keloids result from pathologic wound healing after injury to the skin. They may occur after local skin trauma such as ear piercing, surgery, injection, burn, or cut, or after local inflammatory skin problems, such as acne, bites, or infectious abscesses. Keloids occur more frequently in places with increased tension, such as the sternum, shoulder, earlobe, and cheek. Patients may present with lesions that also cause pain, burning, itching, and restriction of movement. It is unknown why certain individuals develop keloids. Current theories include intrinsically abnormal fibroblasts and increased growth factor receptors.

CLINICAL PRESENTATION

Keloids are generally firm nodules, with a smooth but irregular border (Fig. 16-4). Initially, they may appear erythematous, but can become paler or red-brown with time. Alibert coined the term "cheloid" in 1806 from the Greek word for "crab's claw" because the lesions push beyond the borders of the original wound. Keloids also do not regress, and usually recur after excision. In contrast, hypertrophic scars (Fig. 16-5) do not extend beyond the borders of the original wound, retain their shape over time, and can occasionally partially regress.

DIAGNOSIS

The diagnosis is generally a clinical one; however, a skin biopsy may be helpful for confirming the diagnosis. Most often, the differential diagnosis is a hypertrophic scar. Keloids and hypertrophic scars are distinct entities. Clinically, hypertrophic scars grow intensely and then regress, whereas keloids may grow indefinitely. Histologically, collagen fibers in keloids are larger, thicker, and have a wavy random pattern, whereas collagen fibers in hypertrophic scars lie parallel to the epidermis. Biopsy is not recommended, as the procedure can worsen the keloid.

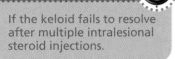

WHEN TO REFER

If the keloid fails to resolve after multiple intralesional steroid injections.

TREATMENT

Unfortunately, no single effective therapeutic exists for keloids. Thus, prevention is all-important, as patients with one keloid are predisposed to other keloids with future skin injury. These patients should be encouraged to minimize elective skin injury, such as ear piercings, tattoos, and elective mole

NOT TO BE MISSED

- Differentiate between keloids and hypertrophic scars; the latter will involute on its own, while keloids may benefit from therapy.
- Avoid further skin trauma/surgery/biopsy if possible in keloid patients as they likely will again form keloids.

removals. Additionally, causes of inflammation, such as acne and infections, should be treated quickly and aggressively to minimize scarring.

Intralesional steroid injections are the mainstay of treatment. Triamcinolone acetonide (10 mg per linear centimeter of keloid) is injected every 2 to 6 weeks until the keloid involutes. Steroids inhibit the proliferation of fibroblasts and collagen synthesis, increase collagenase production, and reduce levels of collagenase inhibitors. Surgery can be attempted, but patients must be closely followed to prevent recurrence. Radiation therapy can reduce keloid recurrence, but the risk of inducing malignancy has dampened its use. Silicone gel sheeting can be used alone or as an adjuvant therapy, but requires patient compliance, as the sheets must be worn 12 to 24 hours/day for at least 2 to 3 months. Pressure therapy has been found to be effective for earlobe keloids. Patients can be instructed to wear compression earrings after keloid excision. Cryosurgery, interferon therapy, intralesional bleomycin or 5-FU, imiquimod, and laser therapy are helpful, at times using more than one treatment modality concurrently.

"AT A GLANCE" TREATMENT

- No clearly effective single therapy which is uniformly beneficial
- The most effective treatment is intralesional triamcinolone acetonide (10 mg per linear centimeter of keloid) injected every 2 to 6 weeks until the keloid involutes
- Other second-line treatments: silicone gel sheeting, excision, cryosurgery, interferon therapy, intralesional bleomycin or 5-FU, imiquimod, and laser therapy

CLINICAL COURSE AND COMPLICATIONS

Keloids can have a variable clinical course. Most will continue to grow for weeks to months, though some may grow for years. Growth tends to be slow, and once stopped, keloids remain stable. At this stage, they usually do not cause symptoms. Intralesional steroid injections may be started as soon as possible after keloid formation, which can lead to symptomatic relief in 72% of patients and complete flattening in 64% of lesions.

ICD9 Code	
701.4	Keloid scar

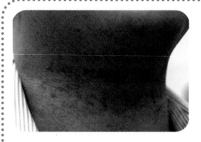

A 30-year-old black man presents to the office with painful red bumps on his lower face and neck (Fig. 16-6). When you examine him, you find nodular scars mixed in with the inflammatory pustules.

He has always shaved regularly, but these "razor bumps" have gotten worse lately. Upon questioning, he recalls that he has recently switched to a "nicer, four blade" razor. He does not feel comfortable having a beard at his work place, and would like to know what alternative treatments are available.

Pseudofolliculitis Barbae
BACKGROUND

Pseudofolliculitis barbae (PFB), also known as barber's itch or razor bumps, is a chronic inflammation of shaved skin. PFB is the most common dermatologic complaint of African American males. The U.S. Army, which requires clean shaven faces, found that 83% of their black recruits had PFB. Occasionally, white men and hirsute black women can also be affected.

PATHOGENESIS

PFB is mostly seen in people with tightly curled hair and occurs when the newly

KEY FEATURES

- Pseudofolliculitis barbae (PFB) presents as inflammatory papules and pustules limited to the beard area.

- PFB is the most common dermatologic complaint of African American males.

- Caused by curled, newly shaved hair coiling upon itself and penetrating the skin.

- PFB is best treated by prevention: not shaving and allowing hair growth. Beards can be neatly maintained with clippers.

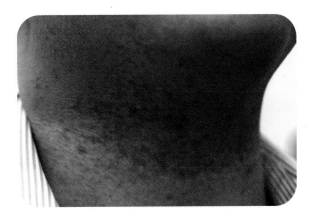

Figure 16-6 Pseudofolliculitis barbae papules on the neck.

cut, sharp tip of hair coils upon itself and penetrates the skin. Patients present with painful papules and pustules in the beard and neck area. Two alternatives for PFB caused by curving shaved hairs are presented in Figure 16-7.

CLINICAL PRESENTATION

Follicular-based papules and pustules are found in the beard area (Fig. 16-6). They may be pruritic, erythematous, and hyperpigmented. Generally, one finds more papules than pustules in PFB. However, intraepidermal micro-abscesses may form, accompanied by foreign-body giant cell immune reaction. Long term, these inflammatory sites may scar, forming small hard bumps all over the affected area.

DIAGNOSIS

The diagnosis is generally clinical. If performed, biopsies will show inflammation and abscess formation. Cultures are usually sterile or have only normal skin flora. Unlike true folliculitis, a pathogenic microorganism is not involved in PFB unless secondary infections have occurred.

TREATMENT

PFB is best treated by prevention: not shaving and allowing hair growth. Beards can be neatly maintained with clippers. Hair-releasing techniques, such as washing the affected area with warm water and soap in a circular manner, may speed recovery.

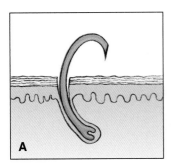
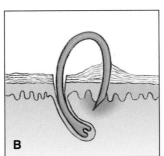
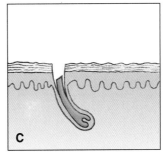
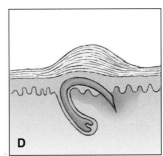

Figure 16-7 Pseudofolliculitis barbae: extrafollicular penetration. **(A)** A curly hair grows from a sharply curved follicle. When shaved, the hair is left with a sharp point. **(B)** As this hair grows, the sharp tip curves back and pierces the skin. Right: Transfollicular penetration. **(C)** Alternatively, when hairs are cut too closely, the hairs penetrate the side of the follicle. **(D)** Both types of follicular reentry cause a foreign body-like reaction (papule). Modified from Crutchfield CE 3rd. The causes and treatment of pseudofolliculitis barbae. *Cutis* 1998;61:351–356, with permission.

WHEN TO REFER

If the patient chooses more invasive treatment techniques such as laser hair removal, referral to a dermatologist expert in laser surgery is indicated.

If hair or beard growth is not possible, other removal options are available. Chemical depilatories remove hair without leaving sharp ends, and may prevent PFB. However, depilatories cause irritation if used too frequently or left on the skin for too long. A hair removal product, eflornithine hydrochloride cream 13.9%, inhibits an enzyme required for hair growth. It needs to be applied twice a day and washed off 4 hours after application. Like depilatories, a side effect of this cream is local irritation. Electrolysis has been shown to be ineffective and may even cause hyperpigmentation. Laser hair removal is the definitive treatment, and its use in the treatment of PFB is increasing. Patients need to know that laser hair removal requires multiple visits, and is the only treatment that results in long-term diminution of hair growth. It is essential that long-wavelength lasers, such as the Nd:YAG or diode, be used for this therapy.

If none of these options is possible, the patient needs to be counseled on shaving techniques. Razors with a foil guard, such as the Bump Fighter Razor™ and a single blade prevent close shaves that exacerbate PFB. Topical regimens, such as steroid application in the morning and retinoid application at night, may help. Finally, topical antibiotics can treat ongoing inflammatory pustules.

"AT A GLANCE" TREATMENT

- PFB is best treated by prevention: not shaving and allowing hair growth.
- Eflornithine hydrochloride cream 13.9% BID, inhibits an enzyme required for hair growth.
- Laser hair removal is effective for most PFB patients.
- Use a single blade razor and avoid close shaving of the beard area.

CLINICAL COURSE AND COMPLICATIONS

PFB is a chronic disorder that is challenging to cure. With treatment, inflammatory pustules and papules may resolve in a few weeks, but the underlying predisposition remains.

ICD9 Codes	
704.8	Other specified diseases of hair and hair follicles
704.8	Other specified diseases of hair and hair follicles

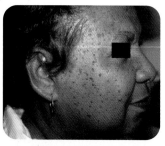

A 65-year-old African American woman has had small raised black bumps on her cheeks and forehead for years (Fig. 16-8). She remembers that her late mother may have had similar lesions. She is bothered by these spots, wants to know if they might be cancerous, and how she can get rid of them.

Dermatosis Papulosa Nigra

BACKGROUND

Dermatosis papulosa nigra (DPN) is commonly found on the cheeks, forehead, and sometimes neck, chest, and upper back of people with Fitzpatrick skin type IV or greater. It occurs in up to 35% of African Americans, and can also be seen in Asian Americans. Women are more frequently affected than men.

PATHOGENESIS

The cause is unknown, but there is a strong genetic influence. Up to 50% of people with dermatosis papulosa nigra have a family history of this disorder.

KEY FEATURES

- Dermatosis papulosa nigra are multiple small dark papules most commonly on the face.

- The lesions occur most often in individuals of African descent.

- No treatment is necessary unless cosmetic removal is desired.

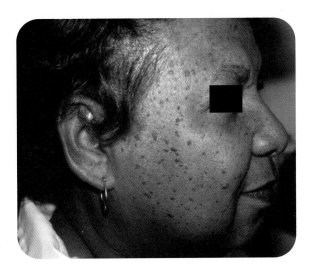

Figure 16-8 Dermatosis papulosa nigra. From Goodheart HP. *Goodheart's Photoguide to Common Skin Disorders*, 3rd ed. Philadelphia: Lippincott Williams & Wilkins, 2009.

Some hypothesize it to be a nevoid developmental defect of the pilosebaceous follicle.

CLINICAL PRESENTATION

Dermatosis papulosa nigra is characterized by multiple, small (usually 1 to 2 mm), firm, smooth, brown to black papules (Fig. 16-8). Lesions appear most often on the central face but also occur on the rest of the face, neck, and upper chest.

DIAGNOSIS

Diagnosis is by clinical exam. There is no need for a skin biopsy unless a lesion is rapidly changing or behaving in an otherwise clinically alarming manner. Histopathology of DPN lesions resembles seborrheic keratosis.

TREATMENT

Treatment is not necessary because the lesions are benign. If patients request cosmetic removal, options include gentle use of cryosurgery, curettage, and electrocautery, taking care to minimize scarring or pigment changes. 532 nm and 1,064 nm lasers can be used and give good cosmetic results.

"AT A GLANCE" TREATMENT

- Treatment is necessary only for cosmetic reasons.
- Cosmetic removal options include cryosurgery, curettage, and electrocautery.
- All options for removal have risks of pigmentary change and scarring of the treated area.

CLINICAL COURSE AND COMPLICATIONS

Lesions often begin during puberty, increasing in size and number as the patient ages.

WHEN TO REFER

Refer to a dermatologist if the patient wants to remove lesions for cosmetic purposes and they respond to skin injuries with hypertrophic scars, keloids, or pigmentation changes.

NOT TO BE MISSED

- DPN lesions are stable in size and color unless newly appeared; consider a melanocytic premalignancy or malignancy for changing lesions.

ICD9 Code	
709.8	*Other specified disorders of skin*

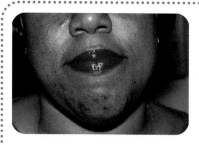

A 28-year-old African American woman comes to your office with acne that has not improved with the many over-the-counter remedies that she has tried. She reports that her blemishes heal with "dark spots" and scarring (Fig. 16-9). She seeks treatment for both the acne and pigmentation.

Acne

BACKGROUND/EPIDEMIOLOGY

Acne vulgaris is one of the most common skin conditions in all ethnic and racial groups. For a detailed discussion of acne, see Chapter 6.

PATHOGENESIS

The pathogenesis of acne is a multifactorial one with four key events: (a) excessive sebum production; (b) abnormal follicular keratinization and plugging; (c) growth of *Propionibacterium acnes*; and (d) inflammation. Androgen hormones are considered to be the initial trigger of the disease process, as they stimulate sebaceous gland size and sebum production. Genetics also plays a large role, as family history is associated with an increased risk of developing acne.

CLINICAL PRESENTATION

Acne vulgaris most commonly involves the face, and to a lesser degree the chest, back, and shoulders. There are multiple lesion types, and it is not uncommon for several types to co-exist. Acne can be comedonal (open/"blackhead" or closed/"whitehead"), papular, pustular, and nodular. It has been shown that acne lesions in darker skin show significant inflammation histologically even in lesions that do not clinically appear erythematous. This may help explain the high prevalence of postinflammatory hyperpigmentation (Fig. 16-9) found in darker-skinned patients. In a study of ethnic skin, at least one-third of acne patients had resulting hyperpigmentation, which lasted 4 months or more.

DIAGNOSIS

The diagnosis of acne vulgaris is a clinical one that is usually made from seeing the different types of acne lesions on the face, back, and/or chest. The patient should also be assessed for any scarring and hyperpigmentation. Lab work is not necessary, except when hyperandrogenism/virilization is suspected.

KEY FEATURES

- Acne occurs in all racial and ethnic groups.

- The characteristic lesions are papules, pustules, and open comedones.

- Acne can heal with hyperpigmentation and scarring in darker-skinned patients.

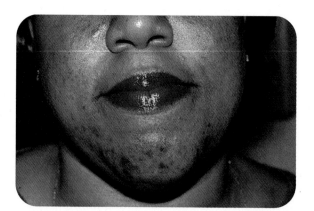

Figure 16-9 Postinflammatory hyperpigmentation in an acne patient. From Goodheart HP. *Goodheart's Photoguide to Common Skin Disorders*, 3rd ed. Philadelphia: Lippincott Williams & Wilkins, 2009.

TREATMENT

Treatment planning is central for acne in darker skin tones, and the goals should include the prevention of hyperpigmentation and scarring. One needs to first elucidate the history of past and current acne treatments as well as all skin and hair-care products to ensure that they are oil-free/noncomedogenic. Half of patients with skin of color report hair oil or pomade use, which is strongly associated with forehead acne. These patients should be counseled to stop using these products or to use them sparingly on the distal ends of the hair away from the scalp. Furthermore, one should also place the patient in a skin type category—dry/sensitive, normal, or oily—to determine topical agents and formulation of choice to minimize irritant contact dermatitis. Cream or lotion formulations of less concentrated agents are a better choice for sensitive dry skin, especially in winter months. The concentration of the agent can then be increased until both acne and irritant contact dermatitis are minimized.

Topical therapies often include retinoids and antimicrobials. Retinoids decrease hyperkeratinization, comedogenesis, inflammation, and fibroblast formation. Formulation, concentration, and frequency of retinoid use can slowly be increased to minimize irritation. Additionally, patient education on correct retinoid use is important. Rather than thinking that more is better, the patient ought to use a pea-sized amount evenly. Antimicrobial agents, such as clindamycin, are also anti-inflammatory and shown to be effective in treating acne. Combination with benzoyl peroxide is recommended to minimize potential antibiotic resistance. Azelaic acid is another therapeutic option. It is generally nonirritating, and has keratolytic, antimicrobial, and anti-inflammatory properties. Additionally, it is effective in treating postinflammatory hyperpigmentation. Hydroquinone 4% and topical retinoids are also effective in treating postinflammatory hyperpigmentation. Patients should be counseled on sunscreen use, as UV rays are thought to exacerbate hyperpigmentation.

For severe acne, systemic therapies should be considered. Oral antibiotics are the first-line systemic option. The tetracyclines (tetracycline, doxycycline, and minocycline) are most commonly used, though trimethoprim-sulfamethoxazole and azithromycin can be alternatives. Hormonal therapy can also be effective in females with acne that worsens with menses. Pharmacologic agents include oral contraceptives and spironolactone. Isotretinoin is a highly effective oral retinoid that is considered by many medical professionals to be the "gold standard" of acne therapy, as it can produce a long-lasting remission in the great majority of patients. It is reserved for severe recalcitrant acne because of a significant side effect profile, most notably that it is teratogenic.

Some alternative therapies may also help. Manual comedone extraction can be performed by dermatologists for retinoid-resistant acne. Chemical peels are common, but darker-skinned patients should be warned to start with low concentrations and frequencies to minimize contact irritation and postinflammatory hyperpigmentation. Microdermabrasion and laser therapies are often used to treat past deep acne scars and to resurface the skin. Again, darker-skinned patients are at increased risk with these procedures for postinflammatory hyperpigmentation.

"AT A GLANCE" TREATMENT

- First-line topical for all patients (other than pregnant women): use topical retinoids such as tretinoin 0.05% cream QHS.
- First-line oral therapy: antibiotics such as minocycline or doxycycline 100 mg PO BID for at least 2 months, then consider tapering doses. Low-dose (40 mg doxycycline) therapy may also be considered.
- Treat hyperpigmentation with hydroquinone 4% for up to 2 to 3 months.

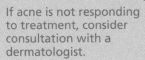

WHEN TO REFER

If acne is not responding to treatment, consider consultation with a dermatologist.

NOT TO BE MISSED

- Distinguish between acne vulgaris and rosacea based on the presence or absence of comedones (acne has them).
- In patients with signs of virilization, consider evaluation for polycystic ovarian syndrome.

CHAPTER 16 Skin of Color

CLINICAL COURSE AND COMPLICATIONS

Acne vulgaris follows a similar clinical course regardless of skin type. Because the after-effects of acne in ethnic skin can be long lasting, treatment should begin quickly and effective therapy should be achieved.

ICD9 Codes	
706.1	Other acne
709.00	Dyschromia, unspecified

Alopecia

Alopecia, both scarring and nonscarring, is discussed in detail in Chapter 24 as well as in respective sections throughout the book. In this section, aspects of hair loss relevant to skin types IV to VI are briefly discussed.

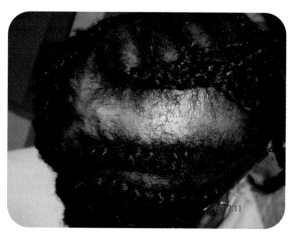

Figure 16-10 Traction alopecia. Courtesy of Carrie Ann Cusack, MD.

TRACTION ALOPECIA

Some cultural practices may contribute to alopecia. Traction alopecia occurs after prolonged tension on the hair, and is most often seen in patients who braid their hair tightly or wear ponytails (Fig. 16-10). It can also be seen with hair extension or hair roller use. Possible sequelae include inflammation, pustules, and even permanent hair loss. Follicular degeneration syndrome (also known as central centrifugal cicatricial alopecia) is characterized by decreased numbers of hair follicles due to scarring. The vertex scalp is involved, with slow outward progression. Historically, this syndrome was thought to occur because of the use of hot combs, though this has been disputed. It is currently thought to be a result of chronic chemical and/or physical trauma.

DISSECTING CELLULITIS (SEE CHAPTER 6)

Dissection cellulitis is a chronic disorder of the scalp which begins with pustules most commonly on the vertex and occiput that progress to abscess and sinus tract formation. It is most prevalent in young adult black men, and is associated with acne conglobata, hidradenitis suppurativa, and pilonidal cysts. Treatment is challenging, and options include oral antibiotics, isotretinoin, CO_2 laser ablation, intralesional steroids, and surgical excision.

TINEA CAPITIS (SEE CHAPTER 9)

As the name suggests, tinea capitis is a fungal infection of the scalp that primarily affects children, especially black and Hispanic children in urban areas. In the United States, *Trichophyton tonsurans* is the predominant causative organism. It begins as erythematous follicular papules, which become scaly, ring-like areas of alopecia, as the fungal infection causes the hair to fracture. Often, these residual hair stubs result in "black dot" alopecia. Other subtypes include noninflammatory seborrheic dermatitis-like infection, kerion, and favus. Noninflammatory tinea capitis is characterized by perifollicular scaling often accompanied by broken gray hairs in the affected areas. The kerion subtype is more serious, presenting with follicular pustules, edema, abscesses, and plaques. Patients may feel pain in the affected areas, and report systemic inflammatory symptoms such as fever and lymphadenopathy. Favus is an uncommon presentation with adherent yellow crusting that has a distinctive "mousy" odor.

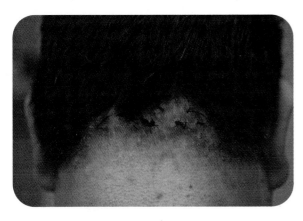

Figure 16-11 Acne keloidalis in a Hispanic man. Note inflammatory, scarred papules on lateral borders.

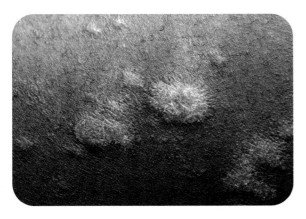

Figure 16-12 Hypertrophic lichen planus: deep purple lesions with surrounding hyperpigmentation on the shins.

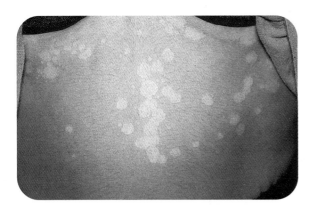

Figure 16-13 Tinea versicolor. Hypo- or hyperpigmented patches instead of the tan patches seen on lighter skin. From Goodheart HP. *Goodheart's Photoguide to Common Skin Disorders*, 3rd ed. Philadelphia: Lippincott Williams & Wilkins, 2009.

Tinea capitis can be diagnosed by microscopy with KOH-prepared slides or fungal culture. Wood's lamps, which can fluoresce certain fungal organisms, are unfortunately often not useful, as *T. tonsurans* does not fluoresce. Griseofulvin for 6 to 8 weeks is the most common therapy used in children with tinea capitis. Other treatment options include terbinafine, itraconazole, and fluconazole. Selenium sulfide shampoo can be used as an adjunctive treatment.

ACNE KELOIDALIS NUCHAE (SEE CHAPTER 6)

Acne keloidalis nuchae (AKN) is a form of chronic folliculitis that results in scarring on the occipital scalp and posterior neck. It is most commonly seen in young adult black men, though it is also seen in Hispanic and Asian men (Fig. 16-11). Despite its name, it is not a result of acne vulgaris, and is thought to be a result of follicular occlusion. Patients present first with a group of firm papules on the neck. These lesions may develop into larger inflamed pustules that cause scarring and alopecia. As short hair cuts and close shaving can aggravate the condition, it is important to educate patients. Mild cases can be treated with topical steroids and retinoids. Topical and systemic antibiotics should be prescribed for inflammatory disease. Intralesional steroids, cryosurgery, laser ablation, and radiation therapy may be used with some success.

Hidradenitis Suppurativa

Hidradenitis suppurativa is a chronic inflammatory disorder of the apocrine sweat glands occuring more frequently in African Americans. It is characterized by chronic follicular occlusive disease of the intertriginous skin of axillary, groin, perianal, perineal, and inframammary regions followed by inflammation, secondary adnexal involvement, fibrosis, and scarring. It is discussed in depth in Chapter 6.

Differential Presentation and Effects of Common Dermatoses in Ethnic Skin

Because of the increased melanin in darker skin, some skin lesions may appear different on patients with ethnic skin. Inflammatory conditions such as lichen planus (Fig. 16-12), tinea versicolor (Fig. 16-13), and pityriasis rosea (Fig. 16-14), or acne rosacea may appear different when compared to lighter skin types due to the lack of "characteristic" erythema.

LICHEN PLANUS (FIG. 16-12)

Deep purple lesions with surrounding hyperpigmentation are seen on the shins.

TINEA VERSICOLOR (FIG. 16-13)

Hypo- or hyperpigmented patches instead of the tan patches seen on lighter skin are seen.

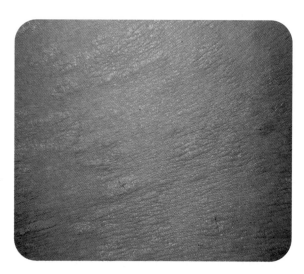

Figure 16-14 Pityriasis rosea. A range of brown to black, more papular lesions with white scales without necessarily seeing the characteristic pink erythema. From Fleisher GR, Ludwig S, Baskin MN. *Atlas of Pediatric Emergency Medicine.* Philadelphia: Lippincott Williams & Wilkins, 2004.

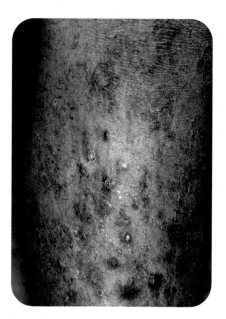

Figure 16-15 Postinflammatory hyperpigmentation secondary bed bug bites. Note prominent lichenification from excoriation.

PITYRIASIS ROSEA (FIG. 16-14)

A range of brown to black, more papular lesions are present, with white scales without necessarily seeing the characteristic pink erythema.

Pigmentary Disorders

Pigmentary disorders are discussed in detail in Chapter 14. A brief summary of relevant conditions and features relating to ethnic skin is presented here.

POST-INFLAMMATORY HYPERPIGMENTATION

Post-inflammatory hyperpigmentation (PIH) is more pronounced and enduring in patients with darker skin, and can be a more distressing problem than the initial skin disorder. It may be caused by eczema, contact dermatitis, acne, or any inflammatory dermatosis (Fig. 16-15). Thus, treatment for any inflammatory dermatosis in patients prone to PIH should be prompt and aggressive. Any existing PIH may be treated with hydroquinone, which reduces melanin production and degrades melanosomes. Sun exposure exacerbates hyperpigmentation, so sunblock must be used during treatment.

MELASMA

Melasma is characterized by well-demarcated hyperpigmented patches that can occur in a centrofacial, malar, or mandibular pattern. It is more apparent and frequent in individuals with darker skin (Fig. 16-16). It can be precipitated by oral contraceptive use, hormone therapy, and pregnancy. Hydroquinone is the mainstay of therapy (either alone or in combination with tretinoin and steroid). Other options include tretinoin, chemical peels, azelaic acid, and

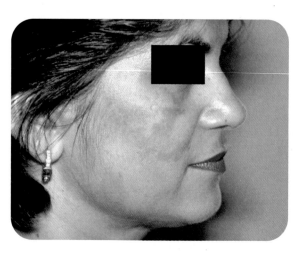

Figure 16-16 Melasma. From Goodheart HP. *Goodheart's Photoguide to Common Skin Disorders,* 3rd ed. Philadelphia: Lippincott Williams & Wilkins, 2009.

laser therapy. Patients must also be counseled on concurrent broad-spectrum sun protection, even for darker-skinned individuals who normally would not consider using a sunscreen.

POST-INFLAMMATORY HYPOPIGMENTATION

Post-inflammatory hypopigmentation is often secondary to dermatoses such as tinea versicolor, pityriasis alba, and seborrheic dermatitis, and can be very prominent and troubling to patients with darker skin. Post-inflammatory hypopigmentation (Fig. 16-17) generally improves over time in most skin types, but may be more enduring in darker skin types. Corticosteroids, tars, and laser therapy may help stimulate melanogenesis.

VITILIGO

Although vitiligo occurs in all racial groups equally, it is significantly more noticeable and psychologically devastating in individuals with darker skin. Furthermore, cultural stigma such as associations with leprosy in India should be taken into account for some ethnic patients. Individuals with vitiligo, especially those who formerly depended on their skin's melanin protection, should be counseled to increase sun protection in the depigmented areas. Vitiligo is discussed in more detail in Chapter 14.

CONFLUENT AND RETICULATED PAPILLOMATOSIS (CRP)

CRP is a papulosquamous disorder seen in individuals of African descent. It presents as asymptomatic confluent scaling plaques, most often on the neck, trunk, and extremities (Fig. 16-18). The cause of this condition is unknown. Diagnosis is generally clinical, but skin biopsy may be helpful in unclear cases. Treatment is often successful with minocycline 100 mg PO BID for 2 to 3 months. Other options include topical retinoids such as Tazarotene 0.1% gel QD to affected areas. The course is generally self-limited.

CHAPTER 16 Skin of Color

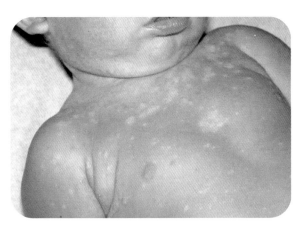

Figure 16-17 Postinflammatory hypopigmentation in an infant with atopic dermatitis. From Goodheart HP. *Goodheart's Photoguide to Common Skin Disorders,* 3rd ed. Philadelphia: Lippincott Williams & Wilkins, 2009.

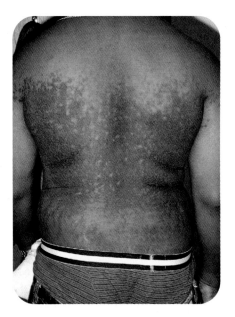

Figure 16-18 Confluent and reticulated papillomatosis.

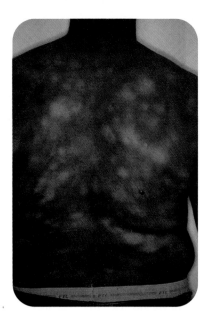

Figure 16-19 Hypopigmented mycosis fungoides.

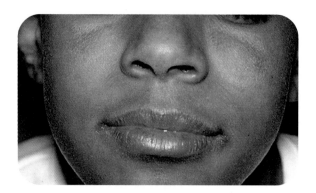

Figure 16-20 Pityriasis alba. From Goodheart HP. *Goodheart's Photoguide to Common Skin Disorders,* 3rd ed. Philadelphia: Lippincott Williams & Wilkins, 2009.

HYPOPIGMENTED MYCOSIS FUNGOIDES

Hypopigmented mycosis fungoides (MF) is a subtype of cutaneous T-cell lymphoma (CTCL) most commonly seen in darker-skinned individuals. Presentation is with hypopigmented discreet and confluent patches (Fig. 16-19), which may or may not coincide with typical MF lesions. Diagnosis is challenging and should be considered when considering vitiligo or pityriasis alba (Fig. 16-20) and any other diffuse hypopigmented dermatosis. Biopsy is essential for confirming diagnosis. Treatment is based on the extent of the lymphoma and ranges from topical corticosteroids such as clobetasol propionate to phototherapy to systemic chemotherapy. This condition should be managed by a hematologist/oncologist or dermatologist with a special interest in CTCL.

Suggested Reading

Al-Attar A, Mess S, Thomassen JM, et al. Keloid pathogenesis and treatment. *Plastic Reconstr Surg.* 2006;117: 286–300.

Alibert JLM. Description des maladies de la peau observees a l'hopital Saint-Louis et exposition des meilleures methods suives pour leur traitment. *Barrois l'aine et fils.* 1806;113.

Arndt, KA (ed). *Scar Revision.* Philadelphia: Elsevier Saunders; 2006:138.

Bigby ME, David AK, Brown AE. Recognition and management of skin diseases in people of color. Boston: Harvard School of Public Health. 1994.

Bridgeman-Shah S. The medical and surgical therapy of pseudofolliculitis barbae. *Dermatol Ther.* 2004:17: 158–163.

Butler P, Longaker M, Yang G. Current progress in keloid research and treatment. *J Am Coll Surg.* 2008;206:731–741.

Callender VD. Acne in ethnic skin: special considerations for therapy. *Dermatol Ther.* 2004;17:184–195.

Hairston MA Jr, Reed RJ, Derbes VJ. Dermatosis papulosa nigra. *Arch Dermatol.* 1964;89:655–658.

Halder, Nootheti PK. Ethnic skin disorders overview. *J Am Acad Dermatol.* 2003;48:S143–148.

Halder RM, Holmes YC, Bridgeman-Shah S, et al. A clinical pathological study of acne vulgaris in black females. *J Invest Dermatol.* 1996;106:888.

Halder RM, Richards GM. Therapeutic approaches for pseudofolliculitis barbae. *Cosmetic Dermatol.* 2003: 15:42–45.

Leyden JJ. New understandings of the pathogenesis of acne. *J Am Acad Dermatol.* 1995;32:S15–25.

Louw L. The keloid phenomenon: Progress toward a solution. *Clinical Anatomy.* 2007;20:3–14.

Perry PK, Cook-Bolden FE, Rahman Z, et al. Defining pseudofolliculitis barbae in 2001: A review of the literature and current trends. *JAAD.* 2002;46:s113–119.

Schweiger ES, Kwasniak L, Aires DJ. Treatment of dermatosis papulosa nigra with a 1064 nm Nd:YAG laser. *J Cosmet Laser Ther.* 2008;10(2):120–122.

Taylor SC, et al. Acne vulgaris in skin of color. *J Am Acad Dermatol.* 2002;46(2 Suppl Understanding):S98–106.

Taylor SC. Skin of color: Biology, structure, function, and implications for dermatologic disease. *J Am Acad Dermatol.* 2002;46:S41–62.

CHAPTER

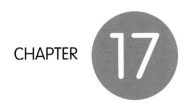

17 Geriatric Dermatology

Gregory L. Wells and Peter C. Schalock

With advances in medicine and nutrition, the aging population continues to grow. Common causes of geriatric dermatologic visits include a multitude of dermatoses that are related to the aging of the skin and human body. Some common causes of geriatric skin problems are benign keratoses such as seborrheic keratoses and cherry angiomas, as well as neoplastic problems such as basal cell/squamous cell carcinomas and melanomas. These are reviewed in their respective chapters. Other conditions that are seen more commonly in the older individual will be reviewed here and include angular cheilitis, generalized pruritus, Grover disease, xerosis, and neoplasm-related dermatoses. Stasis dermatitis and skin ulcerations are also frequently encountered in older individuals. These topics are covered in Chapter 20.

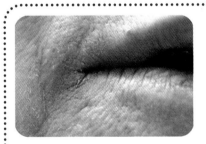

A 72-year-old man describes a painful rash at the corners of the mouth (Fig. 17-1). During examination, it is noted that he has fissured pink patches affecting the bilateral angles of the mouth. He describes poor-fitting dentures. What is the most likely diagnosis?

Angular Cheilitis

BACKGROUND

Angular cheilitis (AC) is a common dermatosis affecting the corners of the lips and adjacent skin. The causes of this condition are multifactorial. AC is most commonly seen in older individuals, though any age may be affected. The risk of developing AC is three times higher for those wearing dentures, and it is estimated that 30% to 50% of those with upper and lower dentures will develop AC. Another group at higher risk for developing AC is acquired immunodeficiency syndrome (AIDS) patients with lower CD4+ counts, thus allowing more frequent candidal infections. Patients with anemia, malignancy, or diabetes mellitus are also at higher risk for developing this condition.

KEY FEATURES

- Angular cheilitis (AC) is a reaction due to excessive wetness or dryness.
- Presentation is with fissured pink-red to gray-white papules and plaques at the angles of the mouth.

(Continued)

PATHOGENESIS

Angular cheilitis results from chronic inflammation most often caused by saliva contacting the angles of the mouth (maceration/irritant dermatitis also known as perlèche). In elderly patients, ill-fitting dentures or resorption and atrophy of the alveolar bone may lead to poor occlusion of the lips, allowing chronic saliva leakage. In many, a fine crease at the corners of the mouth allows saliva to move out of the mouth by capillary action, thus creating a moist

KEY FEATURES (Continued)

- Perform a potassium hydroxide (KOH) exam to rule out *Candida* or culture to rule out *Staphylococcus aureus* infection.

- Treat with antifungals or antibacterials and consider low- to mid-potency topical steroids or emollients if necessary.

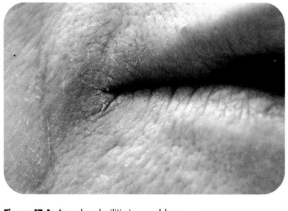

Figure 17-1 Angular cheilitis in an older man.

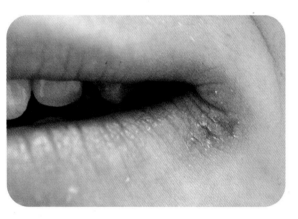

Figure 17-2 Angular cheilitis secondary to allergic contact dermatitis to applied neomycin.

environment that is conducive for fungal or bacterial growth. The most commonly encountered organisms in AC are *S. aureus* and *Candida albicans*.

Another consideration is allergic contact dermatitis, often secondary to products being used to treat the primary AC. An example would be the patient who uses a neomycin and bacitracin-containing ointment to treat her AC, and who then develops pruritic dermatitis in addition to the primary AC (Fig. 17-2). Causes of AC are summarized in Table 17-1.

CLINICAL PRESENTATION

Angular cheilitis initially presents as bilateral fissuring, erythematous plaques, and scaling at the corners of the mouth (Figs. 17-1, 17-2). These changes sometimes extend laterally and inferiorly. In many cases, the cutaneous lip and cheek skin are fissured. Depending on the process causing this condition, there are often other findings. Honeycomb crusting would suggest bacterial impetigo, while satellite pustules and a deep red appearance and fine scale suggest a fungal infection. Symptoms include pain, pruritus, or burning.

Table 17-1 Causes of Angular Cheilitis
Allergic contact dermatitis
Atopic dermatitis
C. albicans infection
Iron deficiency
Irritant contact dermatitis
Mechanical trauma (lip licking/frequent flossing)
Plummer-Vinson syndrome (upper esophageal web, iron deficiency anemia, glossitis, cheilitis)
Poorly fitting dentures
Retinoid therapy (isotretinoin/acitretin, etc.)
S. aureus infection
Vitamin deficiency (folate, B12, riboflavin)

DIAGNOSIS

Angular cheilitis is a clinical diagnosis. To evaluate for fungal infection, one should consider a KOH preparation or send a culture for fungus/yeast. Bacterial infection is appropriately evaluated by taking a swab for culture. In general, a skin biopsy or further invasive testing is not indicated.

In patients in whom an underlying systemic cause is suspected, appropriate further workup is recommended. Consider checking a complete blood count, blood glucose, vitamin levels, and in patients with risk factors, a human immunodeficiency virus (HIV) test. Nutritional status should be evaluated. If allergic contact dermatitis is suspected, simply discontinuing all topical medications other than white petrolatum for at least 3 weeks should show considerable improvement. If definite identification of an allergen is necessary, the patient should be referred to a dermatologist for patch testing.

THERAPY

Therapy is based on the underlying cause of AC. In the patient with dentures, refitting problematic/ill-fitting prostheses should be helpful. Treat infections appropriately with agents such as topical antifungals (i.e., ketoconazole, clotrimazole, miconazole); topical antibiotics (i.e., mupirocin); or topical anti-inflammatory agents such as calcineurin inhibitors (i.e., tacrolimus and pimecrolimus). If there is a component of atopic or allergic dermatitis, the mainstay of therapy is low- to mid-potency topical steroids (i.e., desonide or triamcinolone acetonide). In cases of recalcitrant yeast infection, consider oral fluconazole therapy.

Once the acute dermatitis is controlled, one may consider zinc oxide or white petrolatum as a barrier for maintenance. In difficult cases, one may consider treating with injectable intradermal fillers such as hyaluronic acid to reshape the oral commissures.

"AT A GLANCE" TREATMENT

- Refit ill-fitting dentures.
- Treat based on etiology of infection or irritation:
  - Bacterial infection: mupirocin ointment BID × 1 to 2 weeks then PRN
  - Atopic or allergic dermatitis: desonide 0.05% cream BID for up to 3 weeks
  - Fungal: ketoconazole 2% cream BID × 1 to 2 weeks then PRN
  - Recalcitrant yeast: fluconazole PO

COURSE AND COMPLICATIONS

Angular cheilitis generally follows a benign course without significant complication. Identification of the underlying cause of AC is essential to prevent acute cases from becoming chronic and also treating/curing chronic cases of AC.

ICD9 Codes	
528.5	*Diseases of lips*
692.0	*Contact dermatitis and other eczema due to detergents*
692.1	*Contact dermatitis and other eczema due to oils and greases*
692.2	*Contact dermatitis and other eczema due to solvents*
692.3	*Contact dermatitis and other eczema due to drugs and medicines in contact with skin*
692.4	*Contact dermatitis and other eczema due to other chemical products*
692.5	*Contact dermatitis and other eczema due to food in contact with skin*

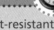

WHEN TO REFER

- Refer treatment-resistant AC.
- Cases where ACD is suspected should be referred to dermatology if the allergen cannot be identified by avoidance regimens.
- Ill-fitting dentures should be refit by the prosthodontist.

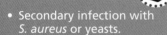

NOT TO BE MISSED

- Secondary infection with *S. aureus* or yeasts.
- Poor fitting dentures need to be refit.
- Consider secondary allergic contact dermatitis to topical medicaments.

CHAPTER 17 Geriatric Dermatology

692.6	Contact dermatitis and other eczema due to plants (except food)
692.70	Unspecified dermatitis due to sun
692.71	Sunburn
692.72	Acute dermatitis due to solar radiation
692.73	Actinic reticuloid and actinic granuloma
692.74	Other chronic dermatitis due to solar radiation
692.75	Disseminated superficial actinic porokeratosis (dsap)
692.76	Sunburn of second degree
692.77	Sunburn of third degree
692.79	Other dermatitis due to solar radiation
692.81	Dermatitis due to cosmetics
692.82	Dermatitis due to other radiation
692.83	Dermatitis due to metals
692.84	Contact dermatitis and other eczema due to animal (cat) (dog) dander
692.89	Contact dermatitis and other eczema due to other specified agents

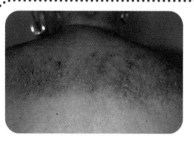

A 52-year-old woman with chronic kidney disease secondary to diabetic nephropathy presents with a several-month history of diffuse pruritus. She has been on hemodialysis for the last 5 years. She denies any rash but has been scratching her skin uncontrollably (Fig. 17-3). What is the most likely diagnosis? What tests can support the diagnosis?

KEY FEATURES

- Pruritus is the most common skin symptom.
- It can be caused by cutaneous and systemic disease or xerosis.
- Generalized pruritus without primary skin lesion merits laboratory investigation.
- Treatment includes topical and systemic antipruritics.

Generalized Pruritus

BACKGROUND

Pruritus or *itch* is the most common symptom of the skin. It can be caused by both cutaneous and systemic disorders. Systemic generalized pruritus is defined by the underlying disease that causes the symptom of cutaneous itch. Fifty percent of dialysis patients report cutaneous pruritus, as do 25% of those with jaundice. A thorough workup of primary pruritus patients is essential, considering an underlying systemic illness is found in 10% to 50% of primary pruritus patients. General categories of systemic pruritus include renal pruritus, cholestatic pruritus, hematologic pruritus, endocrine pruritus, pruritus related to malignancy, and idiopathic generalized pruritus.

PATHOGENESIS

Unmyelinated C and A-delta neurons in the epidermis respond to pruritogenic and thermal stimuli. These neurons synapse with central neurons in the dorsal ganglia and travel through the spinothalamic tracts to the thalamus and cerebral cortex. These signals are processed in various areas of the brain. Multiple mediators of pruritus are responsible for the cutaneous sensation of itch. These mediators include histamine, tryptase, prostaglandin E, substance P, opioid peptides, nerve growth factor, and interleukin-2. The pathogenesis of systemic pruritus is related to the underlying cause (Table 17-2).

CLINICAL PRESENTATION

Patients with pruritus may have a primary dermatologic disease or a systemic disease leading to itch. In patients with generalized pruritus, or pruritus affecting the entire body, the practitioner must rule out a systemic source

Table 17-2 Pathogenesis of Systemic Pruritus

SYSTEM	POTENTIAL PATHOGENESIS
Renal	Possibly due to increased blood histamine levels, increased levels of calcium/magnesium, increased parathyroid hormone levels
Cholestatic	Unknown. Possibly due to elevated systemic levels of bile salts, histamine, and opioid levels
Hematologic	**Iron deficiency** may contribute to pruritus. **Polycythemia vera** patients have increased mast cells and basophils. Degranulation causes increased levels of serotonin (an itch mediator in the skin).
Endocrine	**Hyperthyroid** and **hypothyroid** states both are more susceptible to pruritus due to activated kinins and increased xerosis respectively. **Diabetes mellitus** increase pruritus but the mechanism is not known.
Malignancy-related	**Hodgkin disease:** increased leukopeptidase and bradykinin **Carcinoid syndrome:** increased serum serotonin levels Almost any other malignancy can cause generalized pruritus through unclear mechanisms.
Idiopathic generalized	Idiopathic

for the sensation. Clinical findings may include skin without a primary lesion, or may demonstrate cutaneous changes due to scratching or rubbing, as shown in Figure 17-3, or prurigo nodularis/lichen simplex chronicus, as shown in Figure 17-4. These skin findings may include multiple crusted papules, plaques, and ulcers with surrounding or overlying erosions and excoriations. Affected areas may include the arms, legs, abdomen, chest, and buttocks with sparing of the back or other unreachable body sites.

DIAGNOSIS

The differential diagnosis of generalized pruritus is large and covers a wide range of systemic illness (Table 17-3).

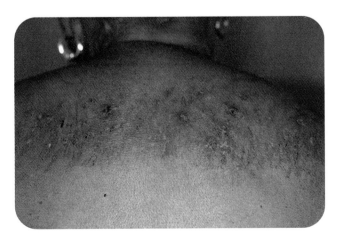

Figure 17-3 Excoriations and postinflammatory hyperpigmentation on the upper back of an elderly woman.

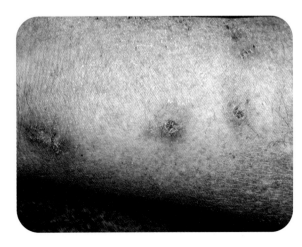

Figure 17-4 Prurigo nodularis.

Table 17-3 Differential Diagnosis of Generalized Pruritus

- Uremia
- Cholestasis
- Primary biliary cirrhosis
- Viral hepatitis
- Hodgkin disease
- Non-Hodgkin lymphoma
- Hyperthyroidism
- Hypothyroidism
- Iron deficiency anemia
- Systemic carcinoma
- Diabetes mellitus
- Leukemia
- Polycythemia vera

- HIV
- Brain abscess
- Multiple sclerosis
- Drug hypersensitivity reactions
- Psychogenic pruritus
- Pregnancy
- Xerosis
- Carcinoid syndrome
- Multiple myeloma
- Sjögren syndrome
- Gastrointestinal parasite infection

In a patient where all cutaneous sources of pruritus have been eliminated, one must consider a systemic etiology. Guided by the history and physical exam, one should consider the following laboratories and studies to assist in diagnosis (Table 17-4).

Table 17-4 Possible Laboratory and Studies in the Diagnostic Evaluation of Generalized Pruritus

INITIAL STUDIES

- Complete blood cell count with differential (CBC with differential)
- Renal function tests (electrolytes, BUN/Cr)
- Liver function tests
- Thyroid and parathyroid function tests (TSH, T3/T4, calcium, phosphate)

- Fasting glucose
- Iron studies (iron, TIBC, ferritin)
- Antinuclear antibody (ANA)
- Serum IgE

ADDITIONAL STUDIES IF NECESSARY

- Stool for ova and parasites
- Stool guaiac
- Urinalysis
- Erythrocyte sedimentation rate
- Viral hepatitis screen
- HIV
- Chest x-ray or other imaging studies
- Antimitochondrial and antismooth muscle antibodies
- Prick testing

- Patch testing for allergic contact dermatitis
- Serum tryptase
- Serum histamine
- Serum chromogranin-A
- 24-hour urine for 5-HIAA or MIAA
- Serum protein electrophoresis
- Urine protein electrophoresis
- Tissue transglutaminase antibody

CHAPTER 17 Geriatric Dermatology

Table 17-5 Treatment of Generalized Pruritus

TOPICAL THERAPY

Emollients	Ointments may worsen pruritus, but are excellent for xerosis. Consider thicker cream such as Cerave or Elta crème.
Menthol/camphor- or pramoxine-containing lotions	Over-the-counter (OTC) Sarna lotion or other pramoxine-containing anti-itch products
Topical corticosteroids	Triamcinolone 0.1% cream BID to affected areas as necessary. Comes in 454-g jar for larger areas
Topical tar derivatives	LCD 10%
Topical anesthetics	Lidocaine cream or gel by RX or benzocaine OTC
Colloidal oatmeal bath	OTC colloidal oatmeal in a cool bath; follow with application of topical emollient

SYSTEMIC THERAPIES

Nonsedating antihistamines	OTC loratadine or cetirizine
Sedating antihistamines	Diphenhydramine, hydroxyzine
Tricyclic antidepressants	Doxepin is a potent antihistamine. Start at 10 PO qhs, taper up slowly for maximum dose of 50 qhs.
Ultraviolet light therapy	Narrowband UVB is extremely helpful beginning at three times weekly.
Opioid antagonists	Naltrexone 50 mg PO QD may be helpful, especially for cholestatic pruritus.

WHEN TO REFER

- When unable to determine the etiology of generalized pruritus, consider referral to a dermatologist.
- Phototherapy is desired for symptom relief. In most cases, these units are available in medical dermatology practices.
- Refer patients for age-or symptom-appropriate malignancy screening (i.e., colonoscopy).

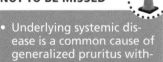

NOT TO BE MISSED

- Underlying systemic disease is a common cause of generalized pruritus without rash.
- In the elderly, xerosis causes low-grade pruritus, especially in winter.
- Supplement iron-deficient patients.

THERAPY

Treatment of generalized pruritus includes both topical and systemic therapies. These are summarized in Table 17-5. If a systemic cause of pruritus is identified, therapy should be tailored to treat the underlying etiology. In most cases, therapy of the underlying cause will lead to remission of pruritus.

"AT A GLANCE" TREATMENT

- First-line: start with a topical emollients and a menthol/camphor containing topical PRN as well as a nonsedating antihistamine for daytime and a sedating antihistamine for nighttime.
- Assess potential systemic causes of itch.
- Alternate therapies: consider referral for ultraviolet (UV) light therapy in recalcitrant cases.

COURSE AND COMPLICATIONS

Patients generally follow a chronic relapsing course with pruritus controlled by the topical and/or systemic treatments. Treatment of underlying disease often will bring remission. Some patients with severe unremitting pruritus may benefit from psychiatric care to help control depression.

ICD9 Code

698.9   *Unspecified pruritic disorder*

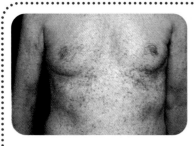

A 69-year-old man presented with a pruritic rash affecting his upper chest and back (Fig. 17-5). The rash began 3 months ago and has been unresponsive to over-the-counter hydrocortisone cream. On examination, he has multiple crusted red and flesh-colored papules on the upper torso with many erosions. What is the most likely diagnosis? What test is required to confirm the diagnosis?

KEY FEATURES

- Grover disease is common in white men over the age of 40.

- Presentation is with pruritic red and flesh-colored crusted papules on the mid- and upper torso.

- For definitive diagnosis, a skin biopsy is necessary.

- Treatment is with topical or oral corticosteroids, ultraviolet therapy, or systemic retinoids; often these are not completely successful.

Grover Disease (Transient Acantholytic Dermatosis)

BACKGROUND

Grover disease was originally described in 1970 by Ralph Wier Grover, MD. He published a cases series of six patients and named the condition transient acantholytic dermatosis, but since that time the condition is more commonly referred to as Grover disease. The frequency of disease is not known, but it is considered a relatively common finding on exam in the older male white population. Despite being named a "transient dermatosis," this condition tends to be chronic in nature and recalcitrant to therapy.

PATHOGENESIS

The etiology of Grover disease is unknown, but exacerbating factors include occlusion, sweating, ultraviolet (UV) light exposure, and friction. Patients tend to have a history of atopic or asteatotic eczema. Linkages to bacterial and viral infections have been postulated but no evidence has yet supported this. Often, patients will report sunlight exposure and sweating before the onset of disease. Despite this linkage to sunlight exposure, artificial UV sources are often used as a successful therapy.

CLINICAL PRESENTATION

Grover disease most commonly affects white men over the age of 40. It is characterized by flesh-colored to red papules on the anterior mid- to upper chest and back (Fig. 17-5). The lower trunk and extremities are less commonly affected. Often, the first signs of this condition are pruritus, which is followed by development of crusted, pruritic papules. Other less typical morphologies include acneiform, vesicular, pustular, or bullous lesions. The typical distribution is

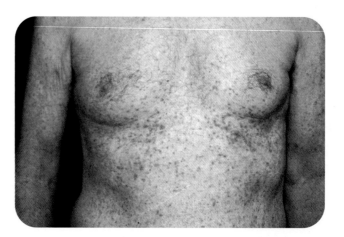

Figure 17-5 Grover disease on the trunk of an elderly man.

that of discrete to coalescing papules, though a zosteriform or unilateral distribution is infrequently seen.

DIAGNOSIS

The differential diagnosis of Grover disease includes: miliaria rubra, folliculitis, arthropod bite reactions, drug eruption, scabies, papular pityriasis rosea, and other rare blistering disorders such as pemphigus foliaceus or dermatitis herpetiformis. Secondary syphilis and disseminated herpes simplex/zoster should be clinically distinct but in mild forms may be considered on the differential. Definitive diagnosis requires skin biopsy.

THERAPY

Grover disease in many cases does not require therapy and when resolution is desired, it can be difficult to treat. Asymptomatic disease in patients who do not desire therapy can simply be followed.

Most patients respond to moderate-potency topical corticosteroids such as fluocinonide 0.05% cream applied twice daily as necessary. Symptomatic relief for pruritus in many cases may be achieved with camphor/menthol containing lotions such as Sarna or anti-itch creams containing pramoxine. Emollients may be a useful adjunctive topical therapy. For persistent cases, consider UV therapy (narrow-band UVB) or systemic retinoids such as isotretinoin or vitamin A. Other treatment options include Psoralen+UVA.

"AT A GLANCE" TREATMENT

- Mild disease or first-line therapy (Step 1):
  - Topical emollients
  - Menthol/camphor-containing lotions
  - Pramoxine-containing lotions

- Moderate disease or second-line therapy (Step 2):
  - Mild topical therapies as above
  - Potent topical corticosteroids: fluocinonide 0.05% cream BID or clobetasol 0.05% lotion (for hair-bearing areas)

- Recalcitrant disease:
  - Systemic corticosteroids (prednisone taper over 2 to 3 weeks, 60-40-20-10 mg each morning, each step for 4 to 5 days)
  - Phototherapy: narrow-band UVB primary or Psoralen+UVA secondary
  - Systemic retinoids (vitamin A 50,000 units 3 times a day for 2 weeks then daily for up to 12 weeks or isotretinoin 40 mg/d for 2 to 12 weeks)

COURSE AND COMPLICATIONS

Despite the name, transient acantholytic dermatosis, the majority of patients with Grover disease suffer a prolonged or persistent course that may relapse, requiring chronic therapy. While the chronic pruritus may decrease quality of life, this condition is essentially benign.

WHEN TO REFER

Refer if skin lesions do not resolve with topical corticosteroids.

NOT TO BE MISSED

- Secondary syphilis.
- Disseminated herpes simplex or zoster.
- Dermatitis herpetiformis or pemphigus foliaceus.

ICD9 Code	
694.8	*Other specified bullous dermatoses*

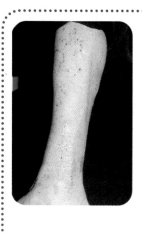

An 87-year-old woman presents with diffuse generalized pruritus. She bathes daily with a bar soap and hot water. She relates that the hot showers help relieve the itch temporarily. She complains of very dry skin. On clinical exam she has diffuse xerosis of the trunk, extremities, face, and scalp with white scale (Fig. 17-6A). What is the diagnosis? What will improve the patient's condition?

Xerosis

BACKGROUND

Xerosis or dry skin is the most common cause of generalized pruritus in geriatric population. It is commonly seen on the lower legs of the elderly but in more severe cases, it may be generalized. Causation is multifactorial, including decreased sebaceous and eccrine gland activity with aging. Symptoms tend to worsen as ambient humidity decreases and living spaces are heated (winter).

PATHOGENESIS

Cutaneous atrophy secondary to age with changes in lipid composition and moisture retention of the skin may lead to scaling and xerosis in elderly patients. Xerosis in other age groups may be due to lipid depletion, genetic predisposition, and lack of moisture retention due to frequent bathing and/or lack of moisturization. Some forms of xerosis are genodermatosis and generally fall within the family of ichthyosis (Table 17-6). The most common ichthyosis is ichthyosis vulgaris, which is often associated with atopic dermatitis.

CLINICAL PRESENTATION

On clinical exam, patients demonstrate diffuse xerosis or dry skin with fine white scale on the trunk, face, and extremities (Figs. 17-6A, B). The intertriginous areas are generally spared. An inflammatory variant of xerosis is erythema craquelé. In this condition, the skin is cracked in appearance, similar to dried mud in a creek-bed with considerable erythema and often surrounding excoriation (Fig. 17-7). This is most commonly seen on the lower legs/shins.

The family of genodermatoses with increased scaling, often with plate-like characteristics similar to fish scales is called *ichthyoses*. The most commonly

KEY FEATURES

- Xerosis is the most common cause of pruritus in elderly.
- Clinical exam reveals xerosis with fine white scale.
- Topical emollients are the mainstay of therapy.

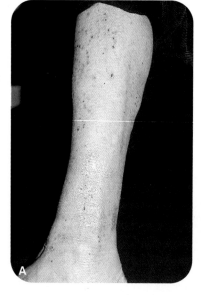

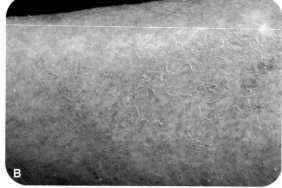

Figure 17-6 (A) Xerosis on the lower legs of an older woman. From Goodheart HP. *Goodheart's Photoguide of Common Skin Disorders*, 3rd ed. Philadelphia: Lippincott Williams & Wilkins, 2009. **(B)** Clinical presentation of xerosis on the leg of an elderly man.

Table 17-6	Causes of Xerosis

Aging/decreased sebaceous and eccrine gland function

Medications (especially oral retinoids)

Vitamin deficiency (A/C/zinc/essential fatty acids)

Genodermatoses (ichthyosis vulgaris, etc.)

Atopy (h/o asthma, seasonal allergies, eczema)

Sjögren syndrome

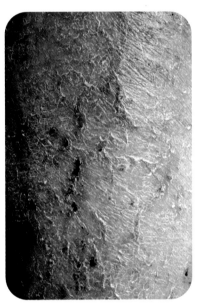

Figure 17-7 Erythema craquelé.

seen is ichthyosis vulgaris. Compared to acquired xerosis, it is a usually more defined/apparent fine white scale with characteristic sparing of the popliteal fossae (Fig. 17-8). Another occasionally seen ichthyosis is X-linked ichthyosis (steroid sulfatase deficiency ichthyosis)(Fig. 17-9). This condition presents with generalized platelike scales with characteristic sparing of the antecubital fossae (Fig. 17-9). Other less commonly seen ichthyoses include lamellar ichthyosis, epidermolytic hyperkeratosis, Harlequin fetus, as well as many others.

DIAGNOSIS

Xerosis is a clinical diagnosis. The differential diagnosis of xerosis includes generalized pruritus and xerotic eczema. Rarely is a biopsy indicated. Patients with recalcitrant lower extremity xerosis may have ichthyosis vulgaris.

THERAPY

Topical emollients are the mainstay of therapy for xerosis. The various forms of ointments, creams, and lotions are discussed in detail in Chapter 2. Creams or ointments should be applied daily, especially after bathing and

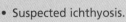

WHEN TO REFER

- Xerosis unresponsive to conservative therapy.
- Suspected genodermatosis or Sjögren disease.
- Suspected ichthyosis.

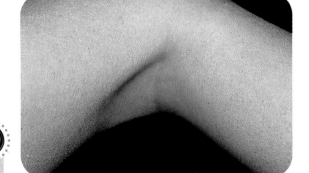

Figure 17-8 Ichthyosis vulgaris. This patient has atopic dermatitis and ichthyosis vulgaris. There is characteristic sparing of the popliteal fossa. From Goodheart HP. *Goodheart's Photoguide of Common Skin Disorders*, 3rd ed. Philadelphia: Lippincott Williams & Wilkins, 2009.

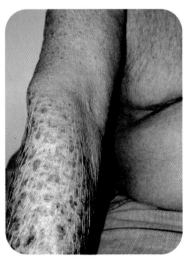

Figure 17-9 X-linked ichthyosis in a man in his 60s. This was an incidental finding on this man's exam.

CHAPTER 17 Geriatric Dermatology

NOT TO BE MISSED

- Ichthyosis vulgaris or X-linked ichthyosis.
- Nutritional deficiency (vitamin A/C/zinc/essential fatty acids).
- Sjögren disease.

more frequently if necessary. Ceramide-containing creams are helpful for repairing the damaged skin barriers by providing the necessary fats for barrier repair. There are several prescription creams and one over-the-counter cream now available if this is desired. In recalcitrant cases, patients should be advised to bathe only once or twice a week in lukewarm water using a synthetic detergent with a moisturizer. Patients should not routinely scrub their skin while bathing.

"AT A GLANCE" TREATMENT

- Apply topical emollients such as white petrolatum or a ceramide-containing cream (i.e., Cerave brand cream) applied at least once daily after bathing.
- Decrease frequency of bathing; recommend using lukewarm water only.
- Avoid harsh soaps/cleansers; instead recommend a synthetic detergent with an added moisturizer (i.e., Dove bar soap).
- Do not scrub skin while bathing.

COURSE AND COMPLICATIONS

Xerosis is characterized by a chronic course for the majority of patients. When severe, it may result in xerotic eczema/erythema craquelé requiring topical corticosteroids to treat the inflammation. Ichthyoses are chronic and respond at best partially to topical therapy.

ICD9 Codes

706.8	Xerosis cutis
757.1	Ichthyosis congenita

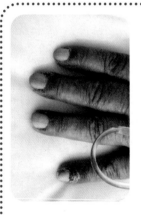

An 83-year-old man with a several-year history of alcohol and tobacco abuse presented with a 4-month history of hyperkeratotic and psoriasiform papules and plaques on the ears, nose, and multiple paronychia on the fingers (Fig. 17-10). A skin biopsy was nonspecific and topical steroids were initiated. At a 2-month follow-up visit, the patient had worsening of his rash despite treatment and now complained of dysphagia. What is the diagnosis? What is the typical location of the malignancy associated with this dermatosis?

Acrokeratosis Paraneoplastica and Other Paraneoplastic Syndromes

BACKGROUND

In 1965, André Bazex, MD and others described acrokeratosis paraneoplastica or Bazex syndrome. Since his original description, over 140 cases of Bazex syndrome have been published in the literature. The stereotypical patients are older men, with an average age of presentation being 61 years.

PATHOGENESIS

The etiology of acrokeratosis paraneoplastica is unknown, however it has been hypothesized that it may be related to underlying cytokines, growth factors, or hormones associated with the primary tumor. Some suggest AN results from an immune reaction in which tumor antigens share similar structure to an unknown cutaneous antigen. The most common associated neoplasm is squamous cell carcinoma of the aerodigestive tract, although other cancers can cause this skin reaction.

KEY FEATURES

- Acrokeratosis paraneoplastica (AN) is usually associated with cancers of the upper aerodigestive tract.

- Clinically, AN demonstrates hyperkeratotic plaques on acral sites (ears, nose, fingers, and toes).

- There are many different rare paraneoplastic dermatoses that mostly affect the geriatric population.

- Successful therapy requires treatment of the underlying malignancy.

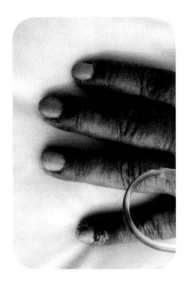

Figure 17-10 Multiple paronychias associated with acrokeratosis neoplastica.

CLINICAL PRESENTATION

Acrokeratosis paraneoplastica is characterized by pink/red scaly papules and plaques that affect acral surfaces. The most common sites of involvement include the ears, nose, fingers, toes, hands, and feet. It commonly begins distally and progresses proximally with time. Multiple acute paronychias may be seen with AN (Fig. 17-10). It is often recalcitrant to topical therapy and can be mistaken for other common skin dermatoses. Consider papulosquamous conditions such as psoriasis, lichen planus, discoid lupus erythematosus, or eczematous conditions such as allergic contact dermatitis on the differential.

DIAGNOSIS

The diagnosis of acrokeratosis paraneoplastica requires a clinical picture consistent with a coexisting malignancy. Table 17-7 shows diagnostic labs and studies, which can be helpful in finding the most common types of malignancy associated with acrokeratosis paraneoplastica.

Other Paraneoplastic Dermatoses

In addition to acrokeratosis paraneoplastica, there are many other paraneoplastic dermatoses that can affect the geriatric population. These are summarized in Table 17-8 (Figs. 17-11 to 17-14).

Table 17-7 Diagnosis of Malignancy Associated with Acrokeratosis Paraneoplastica

- Detailed history and physical including cervical lymph nodes
- Basic labs (CBC, BMP, ESR, stool guaiac)
- Chest x-ray
- Referral to otolaryngologist for examination
- Endoscopy and/or colonoscopy
- Computed tomography of the chest, abdomen, pelvis
- Repeat exam every 3 months while clinical suspicion present

Table 17-8 Paraneoplastic Dermatoses

DISORDER	CLINICAL FINDINGS	ASSOCIATED MALIGNANCY
Strong association with malignancy		
Acrokeratosis paraneoplastica	Psoriaform scaling of acral surfaces, ears, nose, keratoderma	Upper aerodigestive tract cancers
Carcinoid syndrome	Episodic flushing	Carcinoid tumor
Erythema gyratum repens	Migrating bands of wood-grain-like erythema	Lung, esophageal, and breast carcinoma
Hypertrichosis lanuginosa acquisita	Fine, downy hair on the face	Colorectal, lung, and breast carcinoma
Hypertrophic osteoarthropathy	Clubbing, periosteal bone formation	Lung cancer
Necrobiotic xanthogranuloma	Yellowish plaques and nodules	Plasma cell dyscrasia, multiple myeloma
Necrolytic migratory erythema	Superficial erosions, vesicles, and bullae	Glucagonoma
Paraneoplastic pemphigus	Stomatitis and other mucosal erosions with flaccid bullae	Non-Hodgkin lymphoma, chronic lymphocytic leukemia, Castleman disease
Primary amyloidosis	Purpura, waxy papules, and macroglossia	Plasma cell dyscrasia, multiple myeloma
Scleromyxedema	Symmetric waxy papules that may progress to leonine facies	Plasma cell dyscrasia
Moderate association with malignancy		
Dermatomyositis	Proximal muscle weakness, heliotrope rash (Fig. 17-11), Gottron papules (Fig. 17-12), shawl sign, mechanic's hands	Ovarian, lung, gastrointestinal carcinomas
Multicentric reticulohistio-cytosis	Papules on hands, arthritis	No predominant cancer type
Pityriasis rotunda	Scaling patches on the trunk	Hepatocellular carcinoma
Sweet syndrome	Edematous mammillate plaques often on the head and neck (Fig. 17-13)	Acute myelogenous leukemia, other hematologic and solid organ tumors
Less likely to be associated with malignancy		
Acanthosis nigricans	Velvety or verrucous hyperpigmentation in interginous areas (Fig. 17-14). Acanthosis nigricans on the palms is most suggestive of malignancy.	Gastric adenocarcinoma
Acquired ichthyosis	Fine scaling of arms and legs	Hodgkin disease
Cushing syndrome	Hyperpigmentation, edema, proximal muscle weakness	Oat cell carcinoma of the lung
Erythroderma	Generalized erythema with desquamation	Cutaneous T-cell lymphoma
Pruritus	No abnormality	Hodgkin disease
Scleredema	Nonpitting edema around neck and upper back	Lymphomas and multiple myeloma
Sign of Leser-Trélat	Diffuse abrupt onset of multiple inflamed seborrheic keratoses	Adenocarcinoma of stomach, colon, and breast
Vasculitis	Palpable purpura	Hematologic malignancies

*Modified from Pikin CA, Lio PA. Cutaneous manifestations of internal malignancies: An overview. Dermatol Clin. 2008;26:1–15.

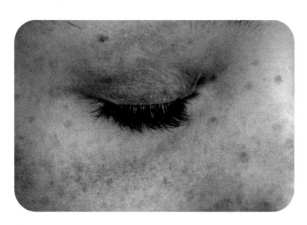

Figure 17-11 Heliotrope rash on the upper eyelid of a woman with dermatomyositis, also note the similar dermatitis on her cheek.

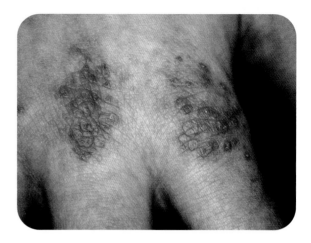

Figure 17-12 Gottron papules on the knuckles, a typical presentation of dermatomyositis.

WHEN TO REFER

- Most cases of acrokeratosis paraneoplastica are difficult to diagnose. If concerned that a patient may have the condition refer to a dermatologist for confirmation of the cutaneous findings.
- Once a malignancy is identified, referral to the appropriate oncology team is necessary.

NOT TO BE MISSED

- Nonneoplastic–related dermatoses such as psoriasis or tinea.

THERAPY

The dermatologic manifestations of acrokeratosis paraneoplastic do not usually respond to any topical or systemic therapy. The cutaneous manifestations resolve on treatment of the underlying malignancy by surgery, chemotherapy, or radiation therapy.

"AT A GLANCE" TREATMENT

- Acrokeratosis paraneoplastica and other malignancy-related dermatoses respond to treatment of the underlying malignancy.
- Rarely is topical or systemic therapy successful.

COURSE AND COMPLICATIONS

The skin disease of acrokeratosis paraneoplastica continues to advance, with skin involvement progressing from acral sites proximally until the malignancy is treated. Successful treatment and potential cure depends on the specific type of underlying malignancy.

ICD9 Code	
701.1	Keratoderma, acquired

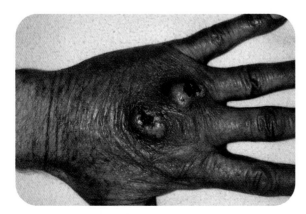

Figure 17-13 Sweet syndrome on the hand. This man had a new onset of myelodysplastic syndrome.

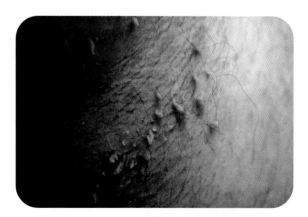

Figure 17-14 Acanthosis nigricans in the axilla. In this case, it was associated with insulin resistance and not a neoplasm.

Suggested Reading

Bolognia JL, Brewer YP, Cooper DL. Bazex syndrome (acrokeratosis paraneoplastica). An analytic review. *Medicine (Baltimore)*. 1991;70:269–280.

Butler DF, Lund JJ. Pruritus and systemic disease. Available at: http://emedicine.medscape.com/article/1098029-overview. Accessed December 11, 2009.

Gonsalves WC, Wrightson AS, Henry RG. Common oral conditions in older persons. *Am Fam Physician*. 2008;78:845–852.

Jainkittivong A, Aneksuk V, Langlais RP. Oral mucosal conditions in elderly dental patients. *Oral Dis*. 2002;8:218–223.

Pipkin CA, Lio PA. Cutaneous manifestations of internal malignancies: An overview. *Dermatol Clin*. 2008;26:1–15, vii.

Simion FA, Abrutyn ES , Draelos ZD. Ability of moisturizers to reduce dry skin and irritation and to prevent their return. *J Cosmet Sci*. 2005;56:427–444.

Sommer F, Hensen P, Bockenholt B, et al. Underlying diseases and co-factors in patients with severe chronic pruritus: A 3-year retrospective study. *Acta Derm Venereol*. 2007;87:510–516.

Stander S, Weisshaar E, Mettang T, et al. Clinical classification of itch: A position paper of the International Forum for the Study of Itch. *Acta Derm Venereol*. 2007;87:291–294.

Villalon G, Martin JM, Monteagudo C, et al. Clinicopathological spectrum of chemotherapy induced Grover's disease. *J Eur Acad Dermatol Venereol*. 2007;21:1145–1147.

Zirwas MJ, Seraly MP. Pruritus of unknown origin: A retrospective study. *J Am Acad Dermatol*. 2001; 45:892–896.

CHAPTER 18 Dermatoses of Pregnancy

Katrina Abuabara and Ellen K. Roh

Skin changes during pregnancy are common and range from physiologic changes to specific dermatoses of pregnancy. Some are well-defined conditions, such as pemphigoid gestationis, that can be diagnosed via direct immunofluorescence staining, while the etiology of many others remains poorly understood. There is a great deal of overlap in the terminology and diagnostic criteria for the dermatoses of pregnancy and even experienced dermatologists may have difficulty differentiating among some of the pruritic conditions. The information in this chapter is grouped into four categories: intrahepatic cholestasis of pregnancy, pemphigoid gestationis, polymorphic eruption of pregnancy (also commonly known as pruritic urticarial papules and plaques of pregnancy), and atopic eruptions of pregnancy, which includes eczema, prurigo of pregnancy, and pruritic folliculitis. Table 18-1 lists these categories with synonymous terms and associated conditions. Table 18-2 summarizes the three main conditions seen during pregnancy.

When evaluating a pregnant patient with a dermatologic complaint, physicians should inquire about gestational age, possibility of a twin pregnancy, parity, dermatologic changes in previous pregnancies, and a family history of pregnancy dermatoses. In addition to differentiating among dermatoses of pregnancy, the physician must rule out other common causes of cutaneous eruptions, such as allergic contact dermatitis, drug reactions, and insect bites. The physician should also be prepared to counsel the patient regarding potential effects to the fetus, cosmetic appearance, expected timing of resolution, and reoccurrence in subsequent pregnancies.

PHYSIOLOGIC SKIN CHANGES DURING PREGNANCY

Hormonal and endocrine factors trigger a number of physiologic skin (Table 18-3), hair, connective tissue, and vascular changes during pregnancy. Hyperpigmentation affects up to 90% of pregnant women and includes darkening of the areolae, nipples, genital skin, axillae, and face (otherwise known as melasma or the "mask of pregnancy"). Melasma may also occur among women on oral contraceptives and can be exacerbated by sunlight. Patients should be advised to use sunscreen and to avoid excessive sun exposure. The linea alba becomes the linea nigra (Fig. 18-1) in the second trimester. Historically, it was assumed that darkening moles were also a physiologic, common change; however, it has recently been found that melanocytic nevi do not typically change during pregnancy. Therefore, any changing nevus in a pregnant patient should be closely observed and possibly biopsied.

Table 18-1 Dermatoses of Pregnancy and Common Synonyms

Intrahepatic cholestasis of pregnancy (ICP)
- Cholestasis of pregnancy/obstetric cholestasis
- Pruritus/prurigo gravidum
- Jaundice of pregnancy

Pemphigoid gestationis (PG)
- Herpes gestationis (HG)

Polymorphic eruption of pregnancy (PEP)
- Pruritic urticarial papules and plaques of pregnancy (PUPPP)
- Toxic erythema of pregnancy
- Bourne's toxemic rash of pregnancy
- Linear IgM dermatosis of pregnancy
- Nurse's late-onset prurigo

Atopic eruption of pregnancy
- Prurigo of pregnancy (prurigo gestationis of Besnier)
- Early-onset prurigo of pregnancy
- Popular dermatitis of pregnancy
- Pruritic folliculitis
- Eczema of pregnancy

Adapted from Ambros-Rudolph CM, Mullegger RR, Vaughn-Jones SA, et al. The specific dermatoses of pregnancy revisited and reclassified: Results of a retrospective two-center study on 505 pregnant patients. *J Am Acad Dermatol.* 2006;54:395–404.

Table 18-2 Differentiating the Dermatoses of Pregnancy

	ONSET (MEAN)	DESCRIPTION	DIAGNOSTIC STUDIES	RECURS IN SUBSEQUENT PREGNANCIES	FETAL EFFECTS	ASSOCIATED CONDITIONS
ICP	3rd tri (31 wks)	Generalized pruritis, no primary lesions	Serum bile acid levels	Occasionally	Placental anoxia, fetal distress	Cholesterol gallstones
PG	2nd tri (21 wks)	Polymorphic: urticarial papules and plaques that may progress into vesicles and tense bullae, beginning around the umbilicus and spreading to the trunk and extremities	DIF	Common	Risk of preterm delivery and slow intrauterine growth	Autoimmune disease involving HLA D3 and D4
PEP	3rd tri (34 wks)	Polymorphic: pruritic urticarial papules and plaques beginning in the abdominal striae	Diagnosis of exclusion	Rare	None	Primiparous women and multiple gestation births

Table 18-3 Common Skin Changes in Pregnancy

- Skin hyperpigmentation: especially areolae, nipples, genital skin, axillae, and face
- Linea nigra: linear hyperpigmentation along the center of the abdomen
- Hirsutism
- Diffuse alopecia/telogen effluvium
- Striae distensae
- Spider telangiectasias
- Palmar erythema
- Nonpitting edema
- Hyperemia of gingival mucosa

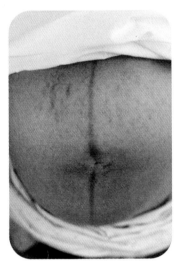

Figure 18-1 Linea nigra.

Hirsutism, which is common on the face and occasionally on the extremities and back, affects many women during pregnancy. It typically resolves by the third trimester or in the postpartum period. Diffuse alopecia, or telogen effluvium, may begin a month or two postpartum and persist for up to a year. Striae distensae, "stretch marks," appear as purple atrophic bands most commonly on the abdomen in the majority of women. Vascular changes such as spider telangiectasias; palmar erythema; nonpitting edema of the face, eyelids, and extremities; and hyperemia of the gums may also occur.

A 25-year-old G1P1 white woman presents at 34 weeks of pregnancy with severe pruritus, especially of her hands and feet. She reports that she feels "exhausted," though she thinks that it is because she has been unable to sleep the past few nights. She has also noticed that her urine is darker than usual. Her past medical history is notable for hepatitis C, treated with interferon. Physical examination reveals no primary lesions, only multiple excoriations.

Intrahepatic Cholestasis of Pregnancy (ICP)

BACKGROUND/EPIDEMIOLOGY

Intrahepatic cholestasis of pregnancy (ICP) is characterized by a generalized pruritus and elevated bile acid levels consistent with cholestasis. It is unique in that there are no primary skin lesions associated with the condition, however, women may present with excoriations from scratching due to the intense pruritus. It is a rare condition; prevalence estimates range from 1 in 1,000 to 1 in 10,000 pregnancies, though rates are much higher in some geographic areas including Sweden and Chile.

PATHOGENESIS

The etiology is heterogenous and thought to be caused by a combination of genetic, hormonal, and environmental factors. Multiple pregnancies and a history of liver damage are also thought to be risk factors.

CLINICAL PRESENTATION

ICP typically presents during the third trimester of pregnancy as a generalized pruritus that may begin in the palms and soles and is usually more

KEY FEATURES

- ICP presents as severe pruritus, particularly on hands and feet.
- There are no primary skin lesions, only secondary change such as excoriations/crusts.

(Continued)

KEY FEATURES (Continued)

- Other common features of presentation include dark urine color and light-colored feces.

- Presents most commonly in the third trimester of pregnancy.

- Treatment is with topical antipruritics for mild cases. Moderate or severe cases often improve with ursodeoxycholic acid therapy.

severe at night. Patients can also have dark-colored urine, light-colored stool, and symptoms of fatigue, loss of appetite, and depression. Jaundice is present in about 20% of cases, and is associated with the development of cholesterol gallstones. In rare cases, ICP can cause steatorrhea, leading to decreased absorption of fat-soluble vitamins, vitamin K deficiency, and subsequent hemorrhage.

ICP can be very uncomfortable because of severe pruritus, but poses few risks to the mother except in rare cases of steatorrhea and postpartum hemorrhage. It has been shown, however, to cause placental anoxia leading to fetal distress, meconium staining, preterm delivery, and even intrauterine fetal death.

DIAGNOSIS

Liver function tests should be ordered for all pregnant women who experience pruritus. A rise in serum bile acid levels is the most sensitive indicator of ICP, and mild increases in alkaline phosphatase and transaminase levels occur in up to 60% of patients. ICP is a diagnosis of exclusion, therefore hepatitis panels should be sent to rule out a viral cause of liver disease. An abdominal ultrasound should be considered in patients with right upper quadrant symptoms to rule out cholelithiasis. Histopathology from skin biopsies are nonspecific and liver biopsy reveals nondiagnostic cholestatic changes.

THERAPY

Given the hypoxic risks to the fetus, women should undergo early intrauterine fetal monitoring. Labor induction is recommended in weeks 36 to 38 of pregnancy depending on the severity of the case.

Symptomatic treatment for the mother includes emollients and topical antipruritics. Antihistamines have not been found to be effective aside from their sedative properties that may help women with severe nighttime pruritus to sleep. Ursodeoxycholic acid should be considered a first-line treatment for moderate-severe cases. Although not yet approved by the FDA for treatment of ICP, it has been shown to improve the biochemical abnormalities associated with ICP and may reduce fetal mortality. The bile resin cholestyramine has been used to treat ICP in the past, but it is less effective than ursodeoxycholic acid and may precipitate vitamin K, thereby elevating the risk for bleeding.

"AT A GLANCE" TREATMENT

- Early intrauterine fetal monitoring is recommended. Labor induction is recommended in weeks 36 to 38 of pregnancy.
- Initiate symptomatic treatment including topical antipruritics.
- Oral antihistamines are not effective.
- Ursodeoxycholic acid should be first-line therapy for moderate to severe cases.

COURSE AND COMPLICATIONS

ICP typically presents during the third trimester of pregnancy (mean 31 weeks). It resolves during the first month postpartum, often within 1 to 2 days after delivery. It recurs in 60% to 70% of pregnancies. Given the hypoxic risks to the fetus, women should undergo early intrauterine fetal monitoring. Labor induction is recommended in weeks 36 to 38 of pregnancy depending on the severity of the case.

WHEN TO REFER ❓

All women diagnosed with ICP should be referred to an obstetrician or maternal and fetal care specialist for fetal monitoring.

NOT TO BE MISSED 🚧

- Signs of placental anoxia or fetal distress.

ICD9 Codes	
698.9	*Unspecified pruritic disorder*
V22.0	*Supervision of normal first pregnancy*
V22.1	*Supervision of other normal pregnancy*
576.8	*Other specified disorders of biliary tract*

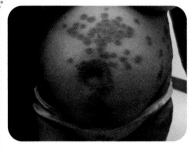

A 33-year-old G2P1 Asian woman presents at 21 weeks of pregnancy to the emergency room with a severely pruritic rash on her abdomen (Fig. 18-2). She has also noticed several blisters in her umbilicus. This is her second pregnancy, and she reports having no complications with her first. On physical exam, there are confluent erythematous urticarial papules and plaques primarily on her abdomen, but also slightly involving her back and upper legs. There are tense bullae in the periumbilical area.

Pemphigoid Gestationis (PG)

BACKGROUND/EPIDEMIOLOGY

Pemphigoid gestationis (PG) is a rare bullous disease estimated to occur in approximately 1 in 50,000 pregnancies. It typically presents in the second or third trimester, though there have been rare reports of occurrences in the first trimester. Complications can include possible autoimmune disease in the mother and blistering lesions in the neonate, however, fortunately, there is no increase in fetal or maternal mortality.

CHAPTER 18 Dermatoses of Pregnancy

KEY FEATURES

- PG presents during the second or third trimester.
- Blisters are caused by the same autoantibody pathogenic in bullous pemphigoid—BPAG2.
- Presentation is with pruritic urticarial papules and plaques beginning on abdomen, often with periumbilical bullae.
- Treatment during pregnancy is with topical and/or oral corticosteroids; following delivery, the condition resolves.

PATHOGENESIS

Pemphigoid gestationis is an autoimmune disease. Patients develop antibodies to a hemidesmosomal protein, the 180-kd protein bullous pemphigoid antigen 2 (BPAG2). The binding of this antibody to the skin's basement membrane triggers an inflammatory response, resulting in the disease's cutaneous features. These antibodies are capable of crossing the placenta. Hence, the infant may occasionally also have transient lesions that dissipate as the mother's antibodies are catabolized.

There is a genetic disposition toward the development of PG; 60% to 80% of patients have the HLA-DR3 MHC class II molecule and 50% are HLA-DR4 carriers. Women with PG are more likely to develop other autoimmune conditions associated with HLA-DR3 and 4, including Graves disease and pernicious anemia.

CLINICAL PRESENTATION

PG is often polymorphic in presentation. The lesions may begin as urticarial papules and plaques and progress into vesicles and tense bullae (Fig. 18-2). They usually appear first around the umbilicus, and then spread peripherally to the rest of the abdomen and thighs. The palms, soles, back, chest, and extremities can be affected but mucosal and facial involvement is rare. Of note, the outbreak of cutaneous symptoms may be preceded by days to weeks of pruritus.

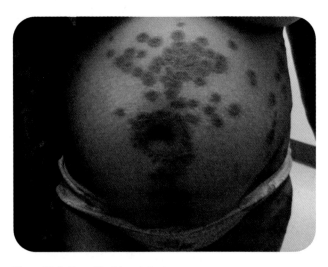

Figure 18-2 Pemphigoid gestationis.

Although an early study suggested an increase in fetal mortality rates, most experts agree there is only a greater risk of preterm delivery and small for gestational age births. A bullous eruption occurs in 5% to 10% of newborns and resolves spontaneously within a few weeks after birth as the mother's antibodies disappear from the fetal circulation.

DIAGNOSIS

Direct immunofluorescence is essential for the diagnosis of PG. It will show complement deposition along basement membrane in samples of perilesional skin (specifically, C3). Histology will show a characteristic but nonspecific pattern: subepidermal separation and vesicle formation with a perivascular infiltrate composed predominantly of eosinophils.

THERAPY

Left untreated, pemphigoid gestationis will spontaneously resolve weeks to months postpartum. The goals of treatment are to relieve pruritus and avoid new blister formation. Mild cases of PG can be treated with topical corticosteroids and antihistamines. Most cases will require oral corticosteroids, which can be tapered over the course of the pregnancy as clinically tolerated. Recommended dosing for prednisone is 20 to 60 mg PO QD. If there is no improvement with 4 to 7 days of therapy, consider a 50% increase in dose every 3 to 5 days until improvement. The use of corticosteroids has not been shown to affect fetal outcomes. Rare bullous eruptions in infants are self-limiting and do not require treatment.

"AT A GLANCE" TREATMENT

- Untreated PG will spontaneously resolve weeks to months postpartum.
- Mild cases: topical corticosteroids and antihistamines
- Moderate to severe cases: oral corticosteroids in addition to topical therapy

COURSE AND COMPLICATIONS

Most cases present during the second trimester (mean 21 weeks), though onset can vary and may not occur until immediately after delivery in 20% of cases. A flare in symptoms at the time of delivery occurs in 75% of patients. Most lesions spontaneously heal without scarring within 3 months after delivery, and the duration of symptoms may be shorter among women who breastfeed. PG may recur with menses, oral contraceptive use, or in subsequent pregnancies, though recurrence is very common but not uniform with every subsequent pregnancy.

WHEN TO REFER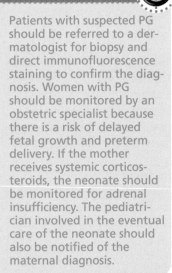

Patients with suspected PG should be referred to a dermatologist for biopsy and direct immunofluorescence staining to confirm the diagnosis. Women with PG should be monitored by an obstetric specialist because there is a risk of delayed fetal growth and preterm delivery. If the mother receives systemic corticosteroids, the neonate should be monitored for adrenal insufficiency. The pediatrician involved in the eventual care of the neonate should also be notified of the maternal diagnosis.

NOT TO BE MISSED

- Diagnosis must be made on the basis of immunofluorescence studies as described above.

ICD9 Codes	
698.9	Unspecified pruritic disorder
694.5	Pemphigoid

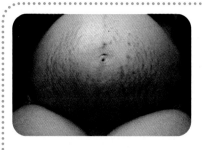

A 28-year-old G1P0 woman presents at 39 weeks of pregnancy to your office with an extremely pruritic rash of several weeks' dura-tion. Her pregnancy has been complicated by gesta-tional diabetes and a 55-pound maternal weight gain. She is visibly scratching her abdomen as she speaks with you, and on examination, there are multiple erythematous papules and plaques on her abdomen, legs, and arms. The lesions are predominantly located within striae (Fig. 18-3).

Polymorphic Eruption of Pregnancy (PEP)

BACKGROUND/EPIDEMIOLOGY

Polymorphic eruption of pregnancy (PEP) is the most common dermatitis of preg-nancy, estimated to affect approximately 1 in 160 deliveries. It usually presents late in the third trimester, most often affecting primigravidas. This condition is also commonly known as pruritic and urticarial papules and plaques of preg-nancy (PUPPP).

PATHOGENESIS

The etiology remains poorly understood; it has been hypothesized that connec-tive tissue damage secondary to abdominal distension, high progesterone lev-els, or the migration of fetal cells to the skin during the third trimester could trigger a localized inflammatory reaction. Risk factors are thought to include multiple gestation pregnancies, male gender of the fetus, and excessive mater-nal and fetal weight gain, though this has been debated.

CLINICAL PRESENTATION

The hallmark of PEP is the development of urticarial papules and plaques along abdominal striae during late pregnancy (Fig. 18-3), though it may begin in the immediate postpartum period. The eruption may spread to the thighs and extremities, but typically spares the umbilicus, palms, soles, and face. It is poly-morphic in presentation, especially later in its course, and may include ery-thema, wheals, vesicles, and targetoid lesions (Aronson). Resolving lesions may appear eczematous with scaling and crusting.

DIAGNOSIS

PEP is primarily a clinical diagnosis of exclusion. Other potential causes for the eruption should be considered including drug-induced reactions, contact or atopic dermatitis, infection, or other dermatoses of pregnancy. A direct immuno-fluorescence study should be performed if there is any question of pemphigoid

KEY FEATURES

- PEP presents late in preg-nancy, during the mid- to late-third trimester.

- It most often affects primi-gravid women.

- Skin lesions are erythema-tous urticarial papules and plaques within striae on the abdomen with charac-teristic sparing of the area surrounding the umbilicus.

- PEP is self-limited and poses no long-term compli-cations or potential harm to the fetus.

- Treatment is with topical emollients, corticosteroids, or small doses of oral anti-histamines.

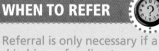 **WHEN TO REFER**

Referral is only necessary if a skin biopsy for direct immunofluorescence is nec-essary to rule out pem-phigoid gestationis.

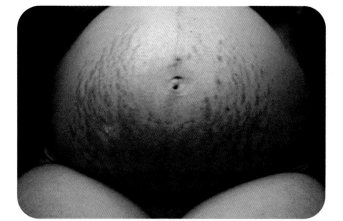

Figure 18-3 Polymorphic eruption of pregnancy.

NOT TO BE MISSED

- Due to its polymorphic appearance, PEP may be mistaken for pemphigoid gestationis; it is important to differentiate PEP from pemphigoid gestationis.

gestationis. No linear deposits of complement should be found in the basement membrane zone in PEP. Skin biopsy is likely to be nonspecific showing upper dermal edema and perivascular infiltrate with varying numbers of eosinophils.

THERAPY

Women should be reassured that PEP is a relatively common and well-defined dermatitis of pregnancy that is self-limited and poses no long-term complications or potential harm to the fetus. Symptomatic treatment may include emollients, topical corticosteroids, or small doses of antihistamines. Severe cases with intractable pruritus can be managed with a short course of oral corticosteroids.

"AT A GLANCE" TREATMENT

- No treatment is required, though symptomatic treatment of pruritus is often desired
- Symptomatic treatments: emollients, topical corticosteroids such as triamcinolone 0.1% cream BID, or small doses of oral antihistamines such as diphenhydramine
- Severe cases with intractable pruritus can be managed with a short tapering course of oral prednisone.

COURSE AND COMPLICATIONS

Most cases present in the third trimester (mean 34 weeks), and resolve a few days after delivery. PEP is unlikely to occur in subsequent pregnancies.

ICD9 Code

692.72   Acute dermatitis due to solar radiation

Atopic Eruption of Pregnancy

Atopic eruption of pregnancy is a new category that was suggested when the results of a large retrospective trial showed that two classically described dermatoses of pregnancy, prurigo of pregnancy and pruritic folliculitis of pregnancy, showed considerable clinical overlap with eczema in pregnancy. Atopic eruptions of pregnancy are all characterized by relatively early onset (before the third trimester of pregnancy) with both truncal and limb involvement. They resolve spontaneously after delivery and present no serious risk to the mother or fetus. They can be treated symptomatically with topical emollients such as Cerave cream or corticosteroids such as triamcinolone 0.1% cream bid PRN.

PRURIGO OF PREGNANCY

Prurigo of pregnancy is relatively common, occurring in up to 1 in 300 pregnancies. It has been reported in all trimesters, and is characterized by discrete erythematous papules and nodules on the extensor surfaces. It is not unusual for most lesions to be excoriated at presentation. An association with intrahepatic cholestasis of pregnancy has been reported, and some experts believe that the two disorders may be related.

PRURITIC FOLLICULITIS OF PREGNANCY

Pruritic folliculitis of pregnancy typically presents between the fourth and ninth months of pregnancy with small erythematous follicular-based papules or sterile pustules. It typically begins on the upper trunk, and spreads peripherally to include the extremities. The etiology is unknown but some authors have postulated that it may be a type of hormonally induced acne.

ECZEMA IN PREGNANCY

Eczema in pregnancy is characterized as a pruritic skin eruption occurring primarily on the flexors. Patient often have a personal or family history of atopy. Most women present with a new lesion; only a minority of women with eczema during pregnancy experience an exacerbation of a pre-existing atopic dermatitis.

Suggested Reading

Ahmadi S, Powell FC. Pruritic urticarial papules and plaques of pregnancy: Current status. *Aus J Derm.* 2005;46:53–60.

Ambros-Rudolph CM, Mullegger RR, Vaughn-Jones SA, et al. The specific dermatoses of pregnancy revisited and reclassified: Results of a retrospective two-center study on 505 pregnant patients. *J Am Acad Dermatol.* 2006;54:395–404.

Aronson IK, Bond S, Fiedler VC, et al. Pruritic urticarial papules and plaques of pregnancy: Clinical and immunopathologic observations in 57 patients. *J Am Acad Dermatol.* 1998;39:933–939.

Driscoll MS, Grant-Kels JM. Hormones, nevi and melanoma: An approach to the patient. *J Am Acad Dermatol.* 2007;57:919–931.

Engineer L, Bhol K, Ahmed AR. Pemphigoid gestationis: A review. *Am J Obstet Gynecol.* 2000;183:483–491.

Kroumpouzos G, Cohen LM. Dermatoses of pregnancy. *J Am Acad Dermatol.;*2001;45:1–19.

Kroumpouzos G, Cohen LM. Pruritic folliculitis of pregnancy. *J Am Acad Dermatol.* 2000;43(1 Pt 1):132–134.

Kroumpouzos G. Intrahepatic cholestasis of pregnancy: What's new. *Eur Acad Dermatol Venerol.* 2002; 16:316–318.

Lammert F, Marschall H-U, Glantz A, et al. Intrahepatic cholestasis of pregnancy: Molecular pathogenesis, diagnosis and management. *J Hepatol.* 2000;33:1012–1021.

Petropoulou H, Georgala S, Katsambas AD. Polymorphic eruption of pregnancy. *Int J Dermatol.* 2006; 45(6):642–648.

Regnier S, Fermand V, Levy P, et al. A case-control study of polymorphic eruption of pregnancy. *J Am Acad Dermatol.* 2008;58(1):63–67. Epub September 19, 2007.

Reyes H. Intrahepatic cholestasis: A puzzling disorder of pregnancy. *J Gastroenterol Hepatol.* 1997;12:211.

Rudolph CM, Al-Fares S, Vaughan-Jones SA, et al. Polymorphic eruption of pregnancy: Clinicopathology and potential trigger factors in 181 patients. *Br J Dermatol.* 2006;154:54–60.

Saleh MM, Abdo KR. Intrahepatic cholestasis of pregnancy: Review of the literature and evaluation of current evidence. *J Womens Health.* 2007;16:833–841.

Shimanovich I, Broker EB, Zillikens D. Pemphigoid gestationis: New insights into the pathogenesis lead to novel diagnostic tools. *BJOG.* 2002:109:970–976.

Weatherhead S, Robson SC, Reynolds NJ. Eczema in pregnancy. *BMJ.* 2007;335(7611):152–154.

CHAPTER 19 Newborn Skin Conditions

Khanh P. Thieu

The newborn skin is target to a host of cutaneous conditions that, thankfully, are often benign and self-limiting. However, common neonatal skin conditions can be a source of significant consternation for first-time families due to lack of recognition and awareness. Understanding the clinical presentation and course of common skin diseases will help clinicians reassure parents, institute appropriate therapy as needed, and avoid unwarranted workup and treatment of presumed serious diseases. This chapter is designed to provide a succinct discussion of the most common skin conditions affecting neonates. While the conditions discussed below are generally benign and usually merit only nominal interventions, clinicians should maintain a low threshold for referrals when the diagnosis is uncertain or when lesions do not resolve as expected with appropriate therapy. A summary of these conditions is presented in Table 19-1.

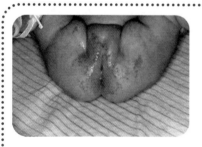

A 10-month-old female infant presents to the pediatric clinic for evaluation of a rash in her inguinal region. Her mother relates that she recently hired a new nanny and feels that the baby's diaper has not been changed as regularly as before. On physical exam, erythematous, confluent areas of shiny erythema over labia majora and buttocks is noted (Fig. 19-1). The inguinal folds are relatively spared. The mother is concerned that this may represent a fungal infection.

Diaper Dermatitis

BACKGROUND

Diaper dermatitis entails all cutaneous eruptions in areas covered by the diaper. Prototypically, diaper dermatitis refers to conditions that are caused or exacerbated by the wearing of diapers, but it can also include skin diseases that have a predilection for the diaper area whether or not diapers are worn. The term will be used in this chapter to refer to the two most commonly encountered form of diaper dermatitis: irritant diaper dermatitis and candidiasis.

Diaper dermatitis is seen commonly in infants, with peak incidence occurring between 6 and 12 months. Boys and girls are affected equally. The condition is prevalent and can be seen in up to 50% of infants in mild forms. Diaper dermatitis is not limited to infants and can affect anyone who wears a diaper, especially elderly patients.

PATHOGENESIS

The etiology of diaper dermatitis is multifactorial. Wetness from urine and occlusion with diapers causes the skin to be overhydrated, making it more susceptible to friction and maceration. Prolonged contact with urine and feces

KEY FEATURES

- Diaper dermatitis is a cutaneous eruption in the diaper area arising usually in setting of prolonged contact with urine and feces ± *Candida albicans* infection.

(Continued)

Table 19-1 Summary of Common Newborn Skin Conditions

CONDITION	FREQUENCY	TYPICAL AGE OF ONSET	DURATION	MORPHOLOGY	AREAS COMMONLY AFFECTED	THERAPY
Irritant diaper dermatitis	Up to 30%–50% of infants	3–18 mo	<1 wk (if treated)	Erythematous, scaly plaque	Convex surfaces of diaper area; inguinal and gluteal creases are spared	Frequent diaper change, emollients, zinc oxide, topical steroids
Candidal diaper dermatitis	~3% of infants	2–6 mo	1–2 wk (if treated)	Erythematous patch with peripheral scale, or tiny pink papules topped with scale	Inguinal and gluteal creases, genitalia, perineal area	In addition to above: topical antifungals (e.g., nystatin, ketoconazole)
Erythema toxicum neonatorum	30%–70% of full-term newborns; 5% of premature newborns	48–72 hr (up to 2 wk of life)	<1 wk	Discrete papules, vesicles, or pustules surrounded by erythematous wheals	Face, trunk, proximal extremities	Reassurance
Transient neonatal pustular melanosis	4%–5% of black newborns; 0.6% of white newborns	Present at birth	<48 hr for initial lesions; up to several months for resolution of macular pigmentation	1. Superficial pustules or vesicles 2. Ruptured pustules with collarette of scale 3. Hyperpigmented macules without scale	Forehead, chin, retroauricular area, neck, chest, and back	Reassurance
Milia	40%–50% of infants	Birth–48 hrs (but can occur at any time in infancy)	<3–4 wk	Discrete, smooth, pearly-white papules	Face: nose, periocular area, cheeks, forehead	Reassurance; incision and expression if needed
Infantile seborrheic dermatitis	Very common (exact incidence unknown)	4–6 wk (up to 1 yr of age)	2–3 wk (if treated); several months if untreated	Yellow, greasy scales on erythematous background	Scalp, glabella, eyebrows, nasolabial folds, ears, skin folds	Keratolytics (tar shampoo, oatmeal baths, mineral oil), mild topical steroid
Infantile hemangioma (superficial type)	Up to 10%–13% of full-term infants	2 wk–1 yr of age	~2–10 yr (depending on rate of involution)	Well-circumscribed, bright red, lobulated plaques	Scalp, face, neck	Reassurance; corticosteroids, interferon α, pulsed-dye laser, surgical excision

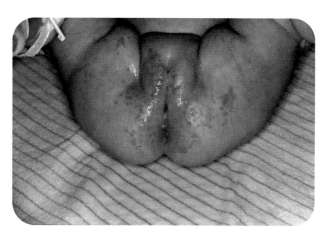

Figure 19-1 Primary irritant diaper dermatitis. Confluent areas of shiny erythema over labia majora and buttocks (Courtesy of Jan E. Drutz, MD).

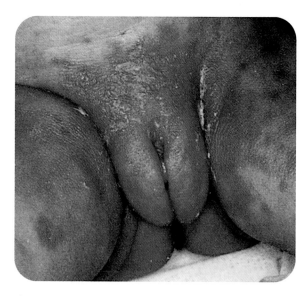

Figure 19-2 Candidal diaper dermatitis. This bright red rash involves the intertriginous folds, with small "satellite lesions" along the edges. From Fletcher M. *Physical Diagnosis in Neonatology.* Philadelphia: Lippincott-Raven Publishers, 1998.

further damages the epidermis due to activity of fecal proteases and lipases and contamination from bacteria. Frequent diarrhea and antibiotic use have been shown to be independent risk factors. Last, *Candida albicans* is believed to play a major role in diaper dermatitis and has been isolated from the perineum in up to 90% of children with diaper dermatitis. The warmth and moistness provided by diapers make the perineum particularly hospitable for *Candida*, and some infants lack the developed immune systems needed to ward off candidal infections. About 3% of infants develop candidiasis in the diaper area from the 2nd to 4th month of life.

CLINICAL PRESENTATION

Irritant Diaper Dermatitis

The initial eruption consists of erythema and scaling on the convex surface of the lower abdomen, inner thigh, and buttock area (Fig. 19-1). The genitocrural creases are typically spared. Fissures, erosions, bullae, and vesicles can sometimes be seen in the involved areas. Symptoms can range from relatively asymptomatic presentation to striking discomfort from soreness and inflammation, especially following bowel movements or urination.

Candida Diaper Dermatitis

Candidiasis in the diaper area can present with either diffuse erythema in the perineal area (including creases) with peripheral scaling and satellite pustules, or coalescing small pink papules, topped with scales, in the perineal area (Fig. 19-2). Unlike in irritant diaper dermatitis, the inguinal folds are usually involved.

DIAGNOSIS

The diagnosis is made clinically based on history, appearance, and location. Candidal diaper dermatitis can be confirmed with a potassium hydroxide (KOH) preparation, although this is usually not necessary. An algorithm for diagnosis of diaper area dermatitis is presented in Figure 19-3.

KEY FEATURES (*Continued*)

- Skin findings.
  - Irritant diaper dermatitis: erythema and scaling on the convex surfaces of diaper area with sparing of inguinal folds.
  - Candidal diaper dermatitis: diffuse erythema in the perineal area, or coalescing small pink papules topped with scale.
- Treatment: frequent diaper change, bland emollients, topical steroids (irritant diaper dermatitis), topical antifungals (candidal diaper dermatitis).
- Clinical course: most cases generally resolve within 1 to 2 weeks.

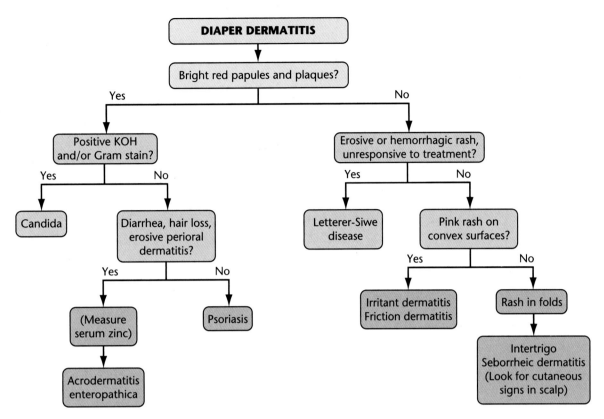

Figure 19-3 An algorithm for diagnosis of diaper area dermatitis.

Differential Diagnosis

Diaper dermatitis can be confused with atopic dermatitis, acrodermatitis enteropathica, and psoriasis. Atopic dermatitis tends to be pruritic and is associated with other rashes in the typical atopic distribution: face and extensor limb surfaces. Acrodermatitis enteropathica is a rare, autosomal recessive disorder characterized by marked perioral dermatitis, diarrhea, hair loss, and failure to thrive, in addition to the diaper-area rash. Psoriasis typically also demonstrates involvement outside of the diaper area, including scalp and nails.

TREATMENT

Irritant Diaper Dermatitis

Prevention of exacerbating factors is the key to successful treatment. The goal is to restore the skin's barrier function and keep the area dry. Key factors are outlined below:

- Diaper change: Frequent diaper changes and gentle cleansing of the diaper area with each change will minimize the skin's contact with feces and urine. Cleaning is best achieved with lukewarm water, followed by a gentle but complete drying of the area. Harsh brushing should be avoided.
- Emollients: Bland emollients are the first-line topical therapy. Topical zinc oxide or petrolatum helps provide a barrier against urine and feces. Apply emollients frequently and especially after bathing.
- Corticosteroids: Moderate or severe cases may benefit from a low-potency topical steroid (e.g., hydrocortisone 1%). The steroid may be applied three times a day, covered by emollients to improve absorption. Strong corticosteroids or extended duration of steroid use beyond several days should be avoided to prevent skin atrophy and striae.

WHEN TO REFER

- Rash does not improve with above treatment.
- If the patient has history of rashes outside the diaper area, which may indicate an alternative diagnosis.

CHAPTER 19 Newborn Skin Conditions

NOT TO BE MISSED

- For dermatitis lasting more than a week, consider candidal infection.
- While unlikely other than in cases of abuse, secondary infection such as herpes simplex virus (HSV) should be considered with appropriate morphology.
- If there is diarrhea, hair loss, and periorificial dermatitis, consider checking a zinc level to rule out acrodermatitis enteropathica.

Candidal Diaper Dermatitis

Treatment consists of minimizing moisture to the diaper area by frequent diaper changes and use of emollients as outlined above. In addition, topical antifungal agents such as nystatin or ketoconazole two to three times daily are effective and typically lead to resolution by 2 weeks. If inflammation is significant, consider adding a short course of topical hydrocortisone 1% to reduce skin inflammation.

"AT A GLANCE" TREATMENT

- Irritant diaper dermatitis:
  - Frequent diaper changes and gentle cleansing
  - Bland emollients are the first-line topical therapy. Topical zinc oxide or petrolatum helps provide a barrier against urine and feces. Apply emollients frequently and especially after bathing.
  - Moderate or severe cases may benefit from a low-potency topical steroid (e.g., hydrocortisone 1% TID PRN). Strong corticosteroids or extended duration of steroid use beyond several days should be avoided to prevent skin atrophy and striae.
- Candidal diaper dermatitis:
  - Minimize moisture by frequent diaper changes.
  - Emollients
  - Nystatin cream or ketoconazole cream BID–TID for 2 weeks
  - If inflammation is significant, consider adding a short course of topical hydrocortisone 1% to reduce skin inflammation.

CLINICAL COURSE AND COMPLICATIONS

Irritant diaper dermatitis generally resolves within several days after initiating treatment. Candidal diaper dermatitis follows a more protracted course but usually resolves within 1 to 2 weeks. Complications most frequently arise from secondary bacterial superinfections, in which case an appropriate topical antibiotic may be added to the skin care regimen.

ICD9 Codes

692.9	Contact dermatitis and other eczema, unspecified cause
112.3	Candidiasis of skin and nails

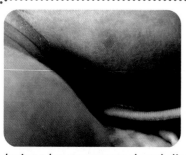

A first-time mother brings in her 10-day old baby boy to the pediatric clinic for evaluation of a rash on the baby's back. The rash started on the back 6 days after the baby was born, and crops of lesions have appeared and disappeared over the past several days. On physical examination, scattered discrete pustules and papules, with surrounding erythema are seen on the baby's back (Fig. 19-4). The mother is concerned that this may represent some kind of infection, although her baby has not exhibited any concerning symptoms.

Erythema Toxicum Neonatorum (ETN)

BACKGROUND

Erythema toxicum neonatorum (ETN) is a common, benign, self-limited cutaneous eruption affecting healthy newborns. The condition's prevalence is positively correlated with birth weight and gestational age, and thus, is rarely seen in significantly premature infants. ETN is present in approximately 30% to 70% of full-term newborns and affects different sexes and races equally.

PATHOGENESIS

The underlying pathogenesis of ETN remains unknown. Although the lesions characteristically contain an eosinophilic infiltrate, an allergic or hypersensitivity-related etiology has not been confirmed.

CLINICAL PRESENTATION

Classically, the eruption consists of scattered, small, discrete papules and pustules surrounded by irregular erythematous macules or erythematous wheals measuring 1 to 3 cm in diameter (Figs. 19-4 and 19-5). The individual papules and pustules are discrete, although the background areas of erythema may become confluent. The lesions are asymptomatic and can be found anywhere but have a predilection for the face, trunk, and proximal extremities.

DIAGNOSIS

Diagnosis is usually based on clinical appearance. Microscopic examination of the pustular contents can provide diagnostic confirmation. A Gram stain or Wright stain of the contents will show a predominance of eosinophils. Peripheral eosinophilia is observed in approximately 15% of newborns with ETN.

Differential Diagnosis

Erythema toxicum can be confused with herpes simplex infection, impetigo, or miliaria rubra (heat rash). Herpes simplex lesions tend to have a more vesicular appearance rather than pustular and require a history of herpes from the mother. Impetigo usually has more developed pustular lesions and can be differentiated based on Gram stain of intralesional contents. Presence of neutrophils on Wright stain or presence of organisms on Gram stain is suggestive of bacterial impetigo. Diagnosis of miliaria rubra typically follows from a history of excessive warming, either from occlusive clothing or from an incubator. Lesions are usually more confluent than those seen in ETN and demonstrate a lymphocytic infiltrate on Wright stain.

CHAPTER 19 Newborn Skin Conditions

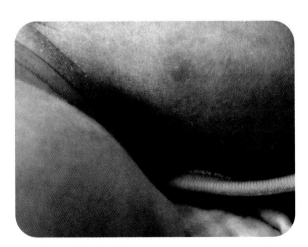

Figure 19-4 Erythema toxicum neonatorum on the shoulder of a 10-day-old infant.

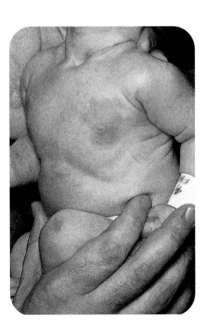

Figure 19-5 Erythema toxicum on the trunk of a neonate. From O'Doherty N. *Atlas of the Newborn.* Philadelphia: JB Lippincott, 1979.

WHEN TO REFER

Refer to a specialist if the rash is associated with any systemic symptoms or does not resolve as expected after several weeks.

NOT TO BE MISSED

- Disseminated HSV or bacterial infection.

KEY FEATURES

- Pathology: benign, self-limiting inflammatory skin condition commonly seen in infants of African heritage.

- Skin findings: 3 stages of lesions: (a) pustules without underlying erythema; (b) ruptured pustules with collarette of scale; (c) residual hyperpigmented macules with no scale.

- Treatment: reassurance.

(Continued)

TREATMENT

Provide reassurance to the family regarding the benign nature and self-limiting course of the eruption.

"AT A GLANCE" TREATMENT

- Reassurance. ETN is a self-limited, benign condition.

CLINICAL COURSE AND COMPLICATIONS

Crops of lesions wax and wane before disappearing after several days, although they can rarely persist for up to a few weeks. The lesions resolve without any residual sequelae.

ICD9 Codes	
778.8	*Other specified conditions involving the integument of fetus and newborn*
705.1	*Miliaria rubra (aka prickly heat)*
684	*Impetigo*

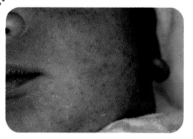

A 2-week-old African-American baby girl presents to the clinic with her father for evaluation of "brown spots" on her forehead and neck. The father reports that the baby's mother remembered seeing "white pimples" on the baby's forehead and neck at birth that changed to "dark spots" after a few days. On physical examination, clusters of several 2 to 3 mm hyperpigmented macules are observed on the infant's forehead and on the neck under the chin (Fig. 19-6). The infant's father wants to know if the brown spots will be permanent.

Transient Neonatal Pustular Melanosis

BACKGROUND AND PATHOGENESIS

Transient neonatal pustular melanosis (TNPM) is a benign, self-limiting skin condition characterized by superficial vesicopustules and pigmented macules. Lesions are always present at birth. TNPM affects approximately 0.2% to 4% of all term newborns but is seen most commonly in African American infants. One report suggests a prevalence of 4.4% of black newborns compared to 0.6% of white infants. The cause of TNPM is not known.

CLINICAL PRESENTATION

TNPM is characterized by three stages: initial inflammatory pustules, rupture of pustular lesions, and finally, postinflammatory hyperpigmentation (Fig. 19-6).

The initial lesions are superficial pustules or vesicles with little or no surrounding erythema. These lesions may be clustered or solitary, typically measure around 2 to 10 mm, and are always present at birth. Because of their superficial nature, the initial lesions are very fragile and often are destroyed at birth during the cleaning of the infant. The second stage of lesions exists as ruptured pustules, appearing as hyperpigmented macules with surrounding fine collarettes of scale. The last stage consists of resolving hyperpigmented macules without scale. Infants may have lesions from different stages at a given point in time. TNPM commonly appears on the forehead, chin, retroauricular area, neck, chest, and back, although any part of the body can be affected, including palms and soles.

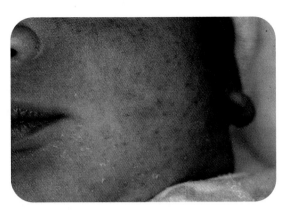

Figure 19-6 *Transient neonatal pustular melanosis. Courtesy of Paul S. Matz, MD.*

DIAGNOSIS

Diagnosis is made on clinical grounds. A Wright stain of pustular contents reveals a predominance of neutrophils with occasional eosinophils. Gram stain is negative for bacteria; Tzanck smear lacks evidence of viropathic changes; and KOH prep fails to reveal hyphae or spores. Tissue biopsy is not needed for diagnosis, but if performed, will demonstrate subcorneal pustules comprised of neutrophils and fibrin.

Differential Diagnosis

TNPM can be confused with erythema toxicum neonatorum (ETN), miliaria, staphylococcal infection, neonatal candidiasis, and viral infections. Cutaneous infections of bacterial, viral, or fungal etiologies can often cause pustules similar to TNPM. Smear preparations of pustular contents with Wright stain, Gram stain, Tzanck smear, or KOH preparation should be performed to rule out suspicion for infection. Miliaria has a later onset, is associated with heat and sweating, and typically would not leave postinflammatory hyperpigmentation. ETN usually appears a few days after birth and demonstrates eosinophil-predominant pustular contents, whereas TNPM is always present at birth and has pustules containing predominantly neutrophils.

KEY FEATURES *(Continued)*

- Clinical course: spontaneous resolution of initial pustules within 48 hours. Residual hyperpigmentation may take months to fade away.

WHEN TO REFER ?

Refer to a specialist if lesions do not follow the expected course or if clinical suspicion for another diagnosis is high.

NOT TO BE MISSED

- Disseminated herpes simplex infection.
- Miliaria rubra.
- Impetigo/bacterial folliculitis.

TREATMENT

No therapy is necessary because the condition is benign and transient. Families should be reassured that the postinflammatory hyperpigmentation may take weeks to months to resolve.

"AT A GLANCE" TREATMENT

- No therapy is necessary because the condition is benign and transient.

CLINICAL COURSE AND COMPLICATIONS

The initial superficial vesicles and pustules of TNPM usually resolve within 48 hours. However, the residual hyperpigmentation may take up to several months to fade away.

ICD9 Code

709.09   *Other dyschromia*

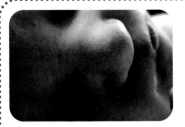

A 2-week-old baby boy comes with his mother to the pediatric clinic for a regular check-up. The baby's mother expresses concern regarding several white spots on the baby's face (Fig. 19-7). She would like to know if the spots can be treated or removed. On physical examination, clusters of tiny 1 to 2 mm smooth, white papules are observed on the central forehead and nose.

Milia

BACKGROUND AND PATHOGENESIS

Milia are common, benign inclusion cysts filled with keratin. Primary milia arise from the pilosebaceous apparatus of vellus hair. Primary milia can occur in all ages, but is typically found in infants, where approximately one-half of term newborns are affected.

More rarely, secondary milia can appear after blistering or trauma to the

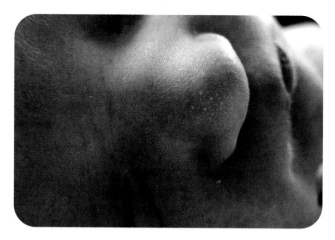

Figure 19-7 Milia on the nose of a 2-week-old neonate.

skin. These lesions originate from the damaged sweat ducts or sebaceous ducts induced by the trauma.

CLINICAL PRESENTATION

Milia can be present at birth or manifest later in the neonatal period. Lesions appear as discrete small (1 to 2 mm), smooth, pearly-white, dome-shaped papules occurring typically on the face of newborns (Fig. 19-7). The lesions are asymptomatic and can number from a few to several hundred. Milia is most prominently featured on the nose of infants, but also have predilection for the cheeks, chin, and forehead. In children and adults, the lesions are most commonly seen around the eyes.

DIAGNOSIS

Diagnosis is based on clinical appearance. For confirmation, a #11 blade or a small-gauge needle can be used to create a small incision in the lesion, releasing the smooth keratinous contents inside.

Differential Diagnosis

Milia are most commonly confused with sebaceous hyperplasia. Sebaceous hyperplasia also occurs commonly on the nose of term newborns and typically spontaneously resolves within the first few weeks of life. These lesions usually manifest as a cluster of multiple tiny, yellow, follicular papules. They are typically smaller, more yellow, and clustered in distribution compared to milia.

TREATMENT

There are no effective topical or systemic medications for milia. If removal is desired, then lesions can be incised with a needle to allow contents inside to be manually expressed.

"AT A GLANCE" TREATMENT

- No treatment is required, but the lesions can be incised with a needle to allow contents inside to be manually expressed.

CLINICAL COURSE AND COMPLICATIONS

Milia in infants typically resolve spontaneously within the first several weeks of life, whereas milia in older children and adults tend to persist. There are no complications associated with persistent lesions. Treatment with incision and expression of intralesional contents is offered to adults who desire cosmesis.

ICD9 Code	
706.2	Milia

KEY FEATURES

- Pathology shows inclusion cysts filled with keratin.
- Skin findings: discrete, smooth, pearly-white papules occurring on the face of newborns.
- Treatment: conservative management or removal with incision and manual expression if cosmesis is desired.
- Clinical course: spontaneous resolution within the first several weeks of life.

WHEN TO REFER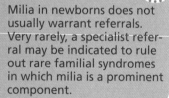

Milia in newborns does not usually warrant referrals. Very rarely, a specialist referral may be indicated to rule out rare familial syndromes in which milia is a prominent component.

NOT TO BE MISSED

- In general, this is a benign, self-limited condition needing no specific treatment other than reassurance of concerned parents.

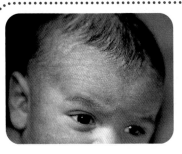

A 1-month-old baby boy presents to the pediatric clinic with his mother for a regular check-up. In the course of the check-up, the mother expresses concern regarding a scaly rash on the baby's scalp (Fig. 19-8). The rash appeared gradually 2 weeks ago and has persisted despite meticulous application of moisturizing lotion to the area. On physical examination, an erythematous rash with yellow, greasy scale is noted covering the infant's vertex. There is some fine scaling on the infant's eyebrows and behind the ears. The mother is concerned that the rash may lead to hair loss on the scalp.

Infantile Seborrheic Dermatitis

BACKGROUND AND PATHOGENESIS

Infantile seborrheic dermatitis (SD) is characterized by an erythematous, scaly, greasy eruption occurring on sebum-rich areas of the scalp, face, and skin folds. It most commonly occurs during an infant's first 6 weeks of life and typically not any later than after 1 year of age. Because the condition is common and usually mild, an exact frequency of infantile seborrheic dermatitis is not known. Although seborrheic dermatitis also occurs in adults—where its mild form is commonly known as "dandruff"—there is no evidence to suggest that having infantile seborrheic dermatitis predicts development of the same condition as an adult.

The pathogenesis of infantile seborrheic dermatitis is unclear. Several lines of evidence suggest a role for the fungus *Malassezia furfur* in the development infantile seborrheic dermatitis.

CLINICAL FEATURES

Infantile SD classically manifests first on the scalp, appearing as yellow, greasy scales on a background of erythema (Fig. 19-8]). This common presentation has coined the term "cradle-cap." The degree of scaling on the scalp can vary from fine scales to plates of thick crust-like scale. Other common areas of involvement include the face (particularly forehead, eyebrows, retroauricular areas, and nasolabial folds); diaper area; and skin folds (neck, axillae, cubital fossa, popliteal fossa). Scaling on the face tends to be less thick compared to the scalp. Due to maceration of skin, SD in the skin creases is often more erythematous with less scaling compared to its counterpart on the face and scalp.

KEY FEATURES

- Pathology: common, benign eruption seen in infants' first year of life thought to be due to the fungus *Malassezia furfur*. Also appears in adults, where it is commonly known as "dandruff".

- Skin findings: erythematous plaque with yellow, greasy scale occurring most commonly on the scalp, face, and skin folds.

- Treatment: mild tar shampoo, mineral oil for scalp, oatmeal baths for body, mild topical corticosteroids, or conservative management.

- Clinical course: often resolves spontaneously by 6 to 12 months of age; responds well to topical treatment.

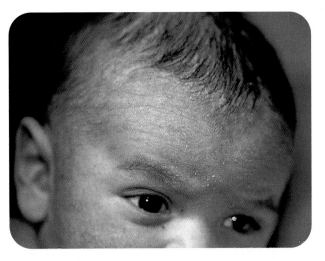

Figure 19-8 Seborrheic dermatitis (cradle cap) on the scalp and face. From Fleisher GR, Ludwig S, Baskin MN. *Atlas of Pediatric Emergency Medicine*. Philadelphia: Lippincott Williams & Wilkins, 2004.

Secondary bacterial infection may occur and will be evidenced by presence of pustules or honey-colored crusts over involved areas.

DIAGNOSIS

A diagnosis of seborrheic dermatitis is usually made on clinical grounds. Histopathologic findings of seborrheic dermatitis are nonspecific, thus making tissue biopsies unhelpful except in cases where the intent is to exclude psoriasis. There are no laboratory markers to support this diagnosis.

Differential Diagnosis

Seborrheic dermatitis is most often confused with psoriasis and atopic dermatitis. In infants, both psoriasis and AD are characterized by scaly, erythematous plaques and can occur in areas overlapping those affected by seborrheic dermatitis. Psoriasis typically does not have prominent greasy scale and tends to preferentially target diaper areas whereas SD most often affects the scalp and face. Unlike SD, atopic dermatitis generally is associated with pruritus and xerosis and tends to also involve extensor surfaces on arms and legs.

TREATMENT

Topical therapy is sufficient for most cases of infantile seborrheic dermatitis. Treatment consists of bathing with a mild agent such as mild tar shampoo, mineral oil, or oatmeal baths, to remove the scales followed by application of a topical corticosteroid to affected areas. A weak steroid cream, such as hydrocortisone 1%, can be applied to affected areas three times a day. Stronger topical steroids should be avoided unless the lesions have been unresponsive to hydrocortisone and are located on the trunk and limbs. Combination therapy with an antifungal therapy is also effective although usually not necessary for resolution. Full recovery usually occurs in a few weeks.

"AT A GLANCE" TREATMENT

- Topical therapy:
  - Bathing with a mild agents such as mild tar shampoo, mineral oil, or oatmeal baths to remove the scales
  - Follow bathing with application of a topical hydrocortisone 1% applied to affected areas three times a day.
  - An antifungal cream (i.e., ketoconazole 2% cream) is not required, but may be added if desired.

WHEN TO REFER

Referral is indicated if lesions do not resolve after several weeks of topical therapy or if involvement is widespread.

NOT TO BE MISSED

- Tinea capitis.
- Psoriasis.
- Eczema/Atopic dermatitis.

CLINICAL COURSE AND COMPLICATIONS

Infantile seborrheic dermatitis often resolves spontaneously by 6 to 12 months of age. The vast majority of infantile SD responds well to topical therapy. There are no long-term sequelae of the condition. Scalp involvement in infants does not adversely affect hair growth. There is no evidence currently to suggest a link between infantile SD and later development of atopic dermatitis or psoriasis.

ICD9 Code	
690.10	Seborrheic dermatitis, unspecified
690.11	Seborrhea capitis
690.12	Seborrheic infantile dermatitis
690.18	Other seborrheic dermatitis

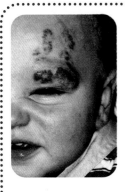

A concerned mother presents to the pediatric clinic with her 6-month-old baby boy for evaluation of a "red area" on her baby's forehead. The lesion appeared about 2 months ago and has since grown rapidly and become more "fleshy." Her relatives and friends have started to question her about it, and she is now concerned that the lesion may represent a serious congenital defect. On physical examination, the infant is a well-appearing white baby. A single 5-cm, well-demarcated cherry red plaque is noted on the infant's left lower forehead (Fig. 19-9). There are no other lesions noted on the skin or mucous membranes. Abdominal exam was negative for organomegaly. The mother is concerned that the lesion will eventually start bleeding and wants to know about treatments to stop its expansion. The lesion is partially blocking vision from mass effect.

Infantile Hemangioma

BACKGROUND

Infantile hemangiomas are benign tumors, comprised of proliferating endothelial cells, which are commonly observed in neonates. These vascular neoplasm are characterized by a rapid growth phase after birth followed by spontaneous regression or involution. In contrast, other vascular malformations (e.g., port-wine stains, stork bites, etc.) are generally already present at birth and usually grow in proportion to the infant rather than regress.

Infantile hemangiomas are among the most common tumors of the neonatal period, occurring in up to 10% of infants. Certain risk factors have been observed to increase the incidence of infantile hemangiomas:

- White, non-Hispanic ethnicity
- Female gender (2 to 5 times more common in female versus male infants)
- Prematurity, especially if birth weight <1,500 g

CHAPTER 19 Newborn Skin Conditions

KEY FEATURES

- Pathology: hemangiomas are benign tumors arising from proliferation of endothelial cells.

- Skin findings: usually well-circumscribed, bright red, plaques with lobulated surface texture.

- Treatment: conservative management is preferred in most cases. Other options include corticosteroids, interferon alpha (if steroid-refractory), pulsed-dye laser, propranolol, and surgical excision.

- Clinical course: rapid growth in first 6 months of life, followed by gradual involution over a variable number of years after 1 year of age.

- Multiple gestations
- Advanced maternal age
- Pre-eclampsia
- Placenta previa

PATHOGENESIS

The exact mechanism of hemangioma formation is not known. Various cellular markers of angiogenesis, such as basic fibroblast growth factor (BFGF), vascular endothelial growth factor (VEGF), and type IV collagenase have been demonstrated to be increased within proliferating hemangiomas. Programmed cell death (i.e., apoptosis) is theorized to be responsible for the involution of hemangiomas.

CLINICAL PRESENTATION

Common Hemangiomas

Classically, hemangiomas are absent at birth and later become apparent within the few weeks of life, corresponding temporally with its rapid growth phase during this period. Lesions are localized and solitary in four out of five cases. Infantile hemangiomas preferentially target the head and neck region in 60% of the cases, although they can occur anywhere on the body and can affect mucous membranes and visceral organs. Size of lesions can vary widely, although the typical maximum diameter ranges from 0.5 to 5 cm. The color of lesions depends on the depth of involvement. Based on their clinical morphology, hemangiomas are classified into superficial, deep, or combined (i.e., mixed) subtypes.

- Superficial hemangiomas are most common and are characterized by well-circumscribed, bright red, lobulated plaques. The lobulated texture of these lesions has led to the informal use of term "strawberry hemangioma" to describe superficial hemangiomas (Fig. 19-9).
- Deep hemangiomas generally appear as swelling of the skin or subcutaneous masses. The raised skin is often normal or may exhibit subtle changes, such

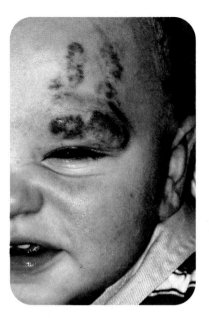

Figure 19-9 Superficial hemangioma on the forehead of a young boy. Note the ptosis with impaired vision of the left eye.

as a bluish hue or central telangiectasias, due to the vascular proliferation underneath. Deep lesions typically have a firm, rubbery consistency and are nontender to palpation.
- Combined hemangiomas exhibit characteristics of both superficial and deep subtypes. Combined lesions are the second most common, behind superficial hemangiomas.

Segmental Hemangiomas

Segmental hemangiomas are large, plaque-like lesions that cover a broader geographic area of skin. The territory does not necessarily follow known dermatomal patterns. Large segmental hemangiomas usually lead to more complications than their localized counterparts, due to their faster growth rate and wider area of involvement. Facial segmental hemangiomas have been associated with congenital anomalies, especially PHACE syndrome (Posterior fossa abnormalities, Hemangiomas, Arterial abnormalities, Cardiac abnormalities, and Eye abnormalities). Female infants have a higher risk of developing segmental hemangiomas.

Multiple Hemangiomas

Multiple hemangiomas are defined as more than five small lesions occurring in a localized distribution, rather than the linear or geographic area seen in segmental lesions. Rarely, infants with multiple hemangiomas also have visceral involvement. Hepatic hemangiomas are the most common form of visceral hemangiomas and are usually asymptomatic. Gastrointestinal (GI) or central nervous system (CNS) involvement are much less frequent but can lead to more potential complications, including GI bleeding and CNS mass effect, respectively. Very rarely, diffuse hemangiomas can result in high-output congestive heart failure due to massive shunting of blood across the vascular tumors.

Hemangioma Precursors

Approximately one-third to one-half of hemangiomas are preceded by a precursor lesion. The herald lesions can have varied appearances: telangiectasias on large area of pallor, a slightly erythematous patch, or an ecchymosis-like patch. Most of these precursor lesions develop into full hemangiomas.

DIAGNOSIS

Diagnosis is typically made on the basis of history and clinical appearance. Careful inspection of the mucous membranes as well as palpation of the liver for hepatomegaly should be included as part of the physical exam. Tissue biopsy may be necessary to differentiate deep hemangiomas from other mesenchymal tumors. Histologic examination generally reveals aggregates of endothelial cells with varying density, depending on whether the lesion is growing or involuting.

Imaging studies such as ultrasound, computed tomography (CT), or magnetic resonance imaging (MRI) may help delineate the location and extent of complicated or visceral hemangiomas. They can also help differentiate infantile hemangiomas from other vascular anomalies, although tissue biopsy is the preferred diagnostic test if readily attainable.

Differential Diagnosis

Superficial infantile hemangiomas are most frequently confused with capillary vascular malformations (e.g., port-wine stains, nevus flammeus) or pyogenic granulomas. Vascular malformations such as port-wine stains are congenital and fully developed at birth, as opposed to hemangiomas, which typically become conspicuous only after a period of rapid growth in the first few weeks of life. Additionally, vascular malformations expand only in proportion to the growth of the infant's body, in contrast to the brisk expansion seen in hemangiomas. Pyogenic granulomas are generally small subcentimeter lesions that develop later in life, typically after preschool years. The lesions are friable and may bleed periodically, which is generally not seen in uncomplicated superficial hemangiomas.

Deep hemangiomas are often harder to recognize, especially when overlying skin changes are absent. The differential includes soft-tissue tumors (e.g., fibrosarcomas, rhabdomyosarcoma, etc.), and a tissue biopsy may be necessary to exclude these malignancies.

TREATMENT

Typically, infantile hemangiomas resolve spontaneously and do not require intervention. For uncomplicated hemangiomas, the cosmetic results of spontaneous involution are typically superior to those produced by excisional surgery or laser therapy. Thus, reassurance and observation are preferred means of management for the vast majority of hemangiomas. If ulcerations occur, they should be treated promptly with occlusive dressings and topical antibiotics to prevent infections.

In the event treatment is pursued, therapeutic options include corticosteroids, pulsed dye laser, recombinant interferon alpha, and surgical excision (Table 19-2).

Table 19-2 Therapeutic Options for Infantile Hemangiomas

THERAPEUTIC MODALITY	ADVANTAGES/INDICATIONS	ADVERSE EFFECTS
Systemic steroids	Highest response rates among all modalities of steroid treatment; may induce early regression, effective for multiple lesions; most effective during proliferative stage	Cushingoid facies, delayed skeletal growth, GI upset, adrenal suppression
Intralesional steroids	Effective for small lesions that are actively growing	Skin atrophy, skin necrosis, bleeding, infection, adrenal suppression. Extra caution is needed for periocular lesions due to rare risk of eyelid necrosis and central retinal artery occlusion.
Topical steroids	May be useful for very early, superficial hemangiomas; only anecdotal evidence for efficacy	Skin atrophy, adrenal suppression from systemic absorption
Interferon alpha	Second-line agent for treatment of complicated hemangiomas refractory to corticosteroids; usually reserved for vision-threatening periorbital lesions	Transient fever, irritability, neutropenia, severe neurotoxicity (permanent spastic diplegia)
Surgery	Well-demarcated, pedunculated hemangiomas; small, localized lesions refractory to nonsurgical treatments; slowly involuting hemangiomas in cosmetically unacceptable locations	Surgical scarring
Pulsed-dye laser	Superficial hemangiomas with ulceration; residual erythema or telangiectasias after involution	Hypopigmentation, surface textural changes

"AT A GLANCE" TREATMENT

- Treatment options are summarized in Table 19-2.

CLINICAL COURSE AND COMPLICATIONS

The natural history of hemangiomas involves a brief phase of rapid growth followed by a phase of gradual involution. Classically, hemangiomas exhibit their most rapid growth in the first 6 months of life. The rate of growth then slows down, and lesions typically reach maximal size between 9 and 12 months of age. Many lesions, unfortunately, do not conform to this time frame. Moreover, the morphology of hemangiomas may affect the growth rate; in general, segmental and deep hemangiomas may proliferate for longer periods of time.

Involution of hemangiomas typically starts at around 1 year of age. The involution is often signaled by a color change from bright red to dull purple, beginning centrally in the tumor. The lesion also flattens, softens, and becomes less warm as involution progresses. The duration of involution depends on the size of the tumor and also varies with each patient. Approximately 50% of hemangiomas have completely involuted by 5 years of age, and 90% have finished involuting by 9 years of age. Unfortunately, involution does not necessarily always give rise to normal skin. Residual skin changes, such as scarring, atrophic wrinkling, residual telangiectasia, and pigmentary changes, affect around 20% to 50% of children.

The vast majority of infantile hemangiomas are uncomplicated. The most common complications include ulceration, bleeding, scarring, and infection. Ulceration is the most common complication and can cause pain, infection, and scarring. Meticulous wound care and analgesia are the mainstays of therapy. Bleeding is a common concern among parents, but fortunately, occurs infrequently and is rarely profuse. Parents should be reassured that bleeding can usually be stopped with application of pressure. The most severe complications, such as vision impairment, airway obstruction, or visceral involvement are seen in hemangiomas with specific morphology or anatomic locations (Table 19-3).

WHEN TO REFER

- Refer to a specialist when hemangiomas have a high risk for severe complications.
- If the parents wish to discuss therapeutic modalities other than watchful waiting.
- Morphology and anatomic location of hemangiomas are the most important factors in predicting risk for complications (Table 19-3). Refer lesions with potential for causing long-term damage/disfigurement.

Table 19-3	Concerning Locations for Presentation of Hemangiomas
ANATOMIC LOCATION	**ASSOCIATED COMPLICATIONS**
Periorbital	Amblyopia, astigmatism, tear-duct occlusion, exophthalmos
Trigeminal V3 distribution ("beard area")	Upper airway involvement and occlusion (stridor, hoarseness, etc.)
Periauricular	Impingement of auditory canal, involvement of parotid gland
Perioral, lips, nasal tip	Permanent scarring and disfigurement
Lumbosacral back	Occult spinal dysraphism (e.g., tethered cord syndrome), genitourinary anomalies
Perianal, axilla, trauma-prone regions	Ulceration
Multiple hemangiomas (≥5 small, localized lesions)	Visceral organ involvement (e.g., liver, gastrointestinal, brain)
Segmental facial	PHACE syndrome

NOT TO BE MISSED

- Rapidly growing lesions on areas with potential for causing long-term damage/disfigurement.

- Beard-area hemangiomas should be evaluated for potential airway involvement.

- Multiple hemangiomas in a neonate may have risk for high-output heart failure; these infants should be evaluated by cardiology.

- Lumbar lesions should be evaluated for occult spinal dysraphism.

ICD9 Codes

| 228.01 | *Hemangioma of skin and subcutaneous tissue* |
| 228.01 | *Hemangioma of skin and subcutaneous tissue* |

Suggested Reading

Bound JP. Thrush napkin rashes. *Br Med J.* 1956;1:782.

Broberg A, Faergemann J. Infantile seborrheic dermatitis and Pityrosporum ovale. *Br J Dermatol.* 1989;120:359–362.

Campbell RL, Bartlett AV, Sarbaugh FC, et al. Effects of diaper types on diaper dermatitis associated with diarrhea and antibiotic use in children in day-care centers. *Pediatr Dermatol.* 1988;5:83–87.

Haggstrom AN, Drolet BA, Baselga E, et al. Prospective study of infantile hemangiomas: Demographic, prenatal, and perinatal characteristics. *J Pediatr.* 2007;150(3):291–294.

Liu C, Feng J, Qu R. Epidemiologic study of the predisposing factors in erythema toxicum neonatorum. *Dermatology.* 2005;210(4):269–272.

Rammurthy RS, Reveri M, Esterly NB, et al. Transient neonatal pustular melanosis. *J Pediatr.* 1976;88:831–835.

Ruiz-Maldonado R, Lopez-Matinez R, Chavarria P, et al. Pityrosporum ovale in infantile seborrheic dermatitis. *Pediatr Dermatol.* 1989;6:16–20.

CHAPTER 19 Newborn Skin Conditions

Leg Ulcers and Decubitus Ulcers

Gregory L. Wells and Jane Barry

An ulcer is defined as a wound with full epidermal involvement and some level of dermal loss. Partial-thickness wounds involve the epidermis and part of the dermis while full-thickness wounds extend through the dermis and may expose muscle, tendon, or bone. Chronic wounds are defined as those of over 6 weeks' duration.

In the United States, it is estimated that 2.5 million people have leg ulcers with venous ulceration accounting for around 70% to 80%. Although venous disease, arterial disease, and neuropathy account for the majority of leg ulcers, there is a long list of possible diagnoses that should be considered including infection, neoplasia, medication, pyoderma gangrenosum, necrobiosis lipoidica, vasculitis, calciphylaxis, panniculitis, hypercoagulable states, and hematologic disorders. Other factors that should be taken into account for chronic ulcers are those that affect wound healing. These include age, nutritional status, continued pressure, shear and frictional forces, chronic illness, inflammatory or autoimmune conditions, immunosuppression, reduced oxygenation of tissues, bacterial load, stress, contact dermatitis, and noncompliance with treatment.

A detailed history and physical exam are essential to aid diagnosis of the etiology of the ulcer, to assess factors that affect healing and to form a comprehensive management plan for each patient (Table 20-1) (Appendix A). Furthermore, there should be regular assessments to monitor healing progress. Body drawings, wound tracings, and photography aid both assessment and documentation.

Approach to the Patient with an Ulcer

MEASURING THE WOUND

For length, the longest distance is measured top to bottom regardless of orientation. Width is the longest distance side to side perpendicular to the length. To measure depth, a cotton-tipped swab is inserted into the deepest portion of the wound. The swab is grasped by its handle flush with the wound margins and is removed. The distance between the tip of the swab and the fingers is then measured. This technique may also be used to measure tunneling and undermining.

DESCRIBING THE WOUND

- The percentages of red healthy granulation tissue, yellow fibrinous slough, and black necrotic tissue should be documented. Dead tissue serves as a medium for microorganism proliferation and may slow healing.

Table 20-1 Key Points in the Assessment of Leg Ulcers

HISTORY	PHYSICAL EXAM
Duration, onset, precipitating factors, and clinical course	Anatomic location
Associated symptoms: ulcer, neuropathy, vascular insufficiency	Size: length, width, depth, shape
Alleviating and exacerbating factors	Edge: punched out, sloping, indurated, presence of new epithelial tissue
Previous treatments and effects	Undermining/tunneling: depth and location
Pain assessment Assessment of nutrition	Wound bed: granulation tissue, fibrin slough, necrotic tissue, black eschar (percentage involvement of each)
Previous treatments and effect	Exudate: amount and type, odor
Full past medical history: diabetes, atherosclerotic disease, lower limb surgery, trauma or radiation, previous ulceration (also see above)	Partial thickness (to dermis) versus full thickness. Presence of exposed tendon, ligament, muscle, or bone
Medications, including anti-inflammatory and immuno-suppressant, hydroxyurea, illegal drug use, all topical treatments	Surrounding skin: erythema, callosity, maceration, scarring, dermatitis, lower limb edema, signs of venous hypertension or arterial insufficiency
Family history of chronic wounds	Peripheral pulses, capillary refill time
Social history (e.g., occupation, smoking, alcohol use, impact on quality of life, home environment, travel history)	Neurologic exam Cardiovascular exam Abdominal exam

CHAPTER 20 Leg Ulcers & Decubitus Ulcers

- Drainage can be serous, serosanguineous, sanguineous, or purulent:
  - Is the dressing saturated or dry?
  - Is the wound oozing over the ulcer edge?

INVESTIGATION

The etiology of the ulcer can often be determined by clinical assessment alone. Additional tests, such as ultrasound, arterial and venous duplex, and ankle-brachial indices (ABI) are useful in selected cases. ABI is calculated by dividing the ankle systolic pressure by the higher of the two systolic pressures obtained from the brachial arteries in both arms. Normally the ankle pressure should be equal to the arm pressure. ABIs in diabetics or in those with calcified vessels can be falsely elevated. Laboratory investigations may also be indicated by assessment and include: complete blood count and differential, fasting glucose and lipids, serum albumin, ferritin and zinc, inflammatory markers, hypercoagulability screen, rheumatoid factor, cryoglobulins, and hepatitis screen. Specimens for cultures should be obtained by biopsy or following wound debridement to aid differentiation between colonization and infection. When the diagnosis is still unclear or the ulcer is unresponsive to therapy, a biopsy and fungal and mycobacterial cultures should be considered to rule out other causes of chronic leg ulcers. Either multiple sampling biopsies or preferably a deep-wedge biopsy including the ulcer bed and edge are required for histopathology. Patch testing may be considered if a contact allergic component is suspected and plain film, blood cultures +/− more specific investigations if an underlying osteomyelitis is suspected.

TREATMENT

Treatment of leg ulcers is dependent on identifying and treating the cause and exacerbating factors and meticulous wound care (Appendix B). Management of leg ulcers can be difficult and requires significant dedication from the patient and the provider. Healing is evidenced by a decrease in ulcer dimensions, an increase in granulation tissue, and re-epithelialization. An approach to a chronic wound or skin ulceration is presented in Figure 20-1. Specific dressing types and examples are mentioned in Figure 20-1 as well as in more detail in Table 20-2.

For most wounds, an occlusive dressing will maintain adequate moisture and may permit a patient to have a dressing on for more than 24 hours. The interval in dressing changes depends on the type and quality of the wound. There are five main types of dressing available (Table 20-2) (Figs. 20-2 to 20-6).

Good Wound Care

The basic principles of wound care include keeping the wound clean, keeping the wound moist, and keeping the tissue well nourished.

CLEAN WOUND

Maintaining a clean wound is essential for the healing process. Depending on the wound, this can be accomplished by mild soap and water or with saline.

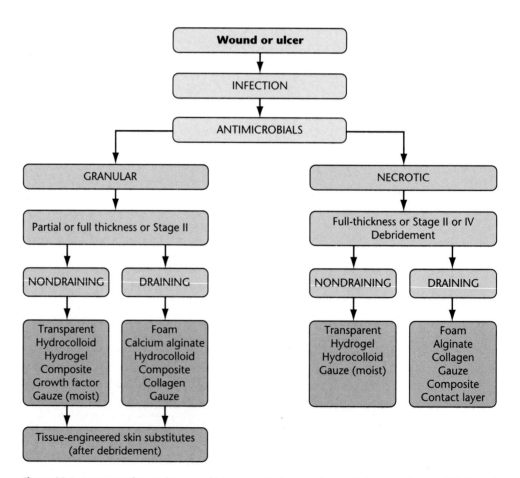

Figure 20-1 An approach to a skin wound/ulceration. Redrawn with permission from Baranoski S. Wound and skin care: Choosing a wound dressing, part 1. *Nursing* 2008;38(1):60–61.

Table 20-2 Dressing Types

Type	FILMS	HYDROCOLLOIDS	FOAMS	HYDROGELS	ALGINATES	COMPOSITES
Image	Fig. 20-2	Fig. 20-3	Fig. 20-4	Fig. 20-5	Fig. 20-6	
Characteristics	Thin, transparent, semipermeable, nonabsorbent	Adherent, opaque, gas impermeable, absorbent. Ability to conform to different body areas. Available as a paste or granules for deeper wounds. Can be left in place for several days. May accumulate a yellow gel material that smells.	Moist environment, absorbent, nonadherent. Require a secondary dressing to be held in place.	Semitransparent, absorbent, nonadherent. Feel cool. Desiccate easily. Avoid in extremely exudative wounds.	Biodegradable dressings made from seaweed. High absorption capacity.	A single dressing which combines two or more of the other dressing materials
Use for these wound types	Superficial wounds with minimal drainage: Decubitus ulcers (I & II), thin burns, skin graft donor sites	Ulcers with low to moderate drainage: Decubitus ulcers (I–IV), any thickness wound, dermal ulcers, necrotic wounds. May also be placed under wraps to help prevent ulceration.	Ulcers with drainage: Decubitus ulcers (III&IV), partial to full thickness ulcers with draining (light or heavy). Useful under compression wraps.	Useful to rehydrate wound base. Absorptive. Useful in: Decubitus ulcers (II–IV); any thickness wound, following dermabrasion, radiation burns or necrotic wounds. OK to use on infected ulcers in most cases.	Cavities, sinuses, undermining stage IV ulcers. Ideal for heavy draining wounds. Require a secondary dressing to keep in place.	Depending on composition
Examples	Tegaderm	Tegasorb hydrocolloid, Comfeel, Replicare hydrocolloid	Allevyn polyurethane, Copa foam	Vigilon, Hollister Restore	Algosteril, Comfeel Alginate, Kaltostat and Sorbsan	Coversite Plus, Allevyn composite

Modified from Baranoski S. Wound and skin care: Choosing a wound dressing, part 1. *Nursing.* 2008:38(1):60–61 and Baranoski S. Wound and skin care: Choosing a wound dressing, part 2. *Nursing.* 2008:38(2):14–15.

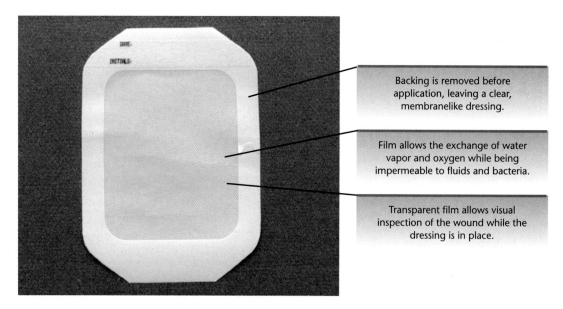

Backing is removed before application, leaving a clear, membranelike dressing.

Film allows the exchange of water vapor and oxygen while being impermeable to fluids and bacteria.

Transparent film allows visual inspection of the wound while the dressing is in place.

Figure 20-2 Transparent film dressings. Springhouse. *Lippincott's Visual Encyclopedia of Clinical Skills.* Philadelphia: Wolters Kluwer Health, 2009.

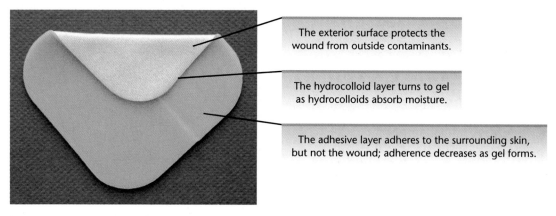

The exterior surface protects the wound from outside contaminants.

The hydrocolloid layer turns to gel as hydrocolloids absorb moisture.

The adhesive layer adheres to the surrounding skin, but not the wound; adherence decreases as gel forms.

Figure 20-3 Hydrocolloid dressings. Springhouse. *Lippincott's Visual Encyclopedia of Clinical Skills.* Philadelphia: Wolters Kluwer Health, 2009.

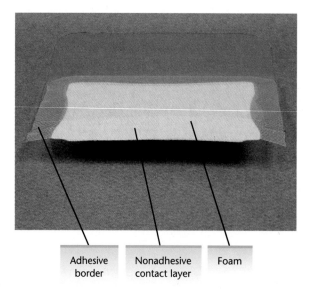

Adhesive border   Nonadhesive contact layer   Foam

Figure 20-4 Foam dressings. Springhouse. *Lippincott's Visual Encyclopedia of Clinical Skills.* Philadelphia: Wolters Kluwer Health, 2009.

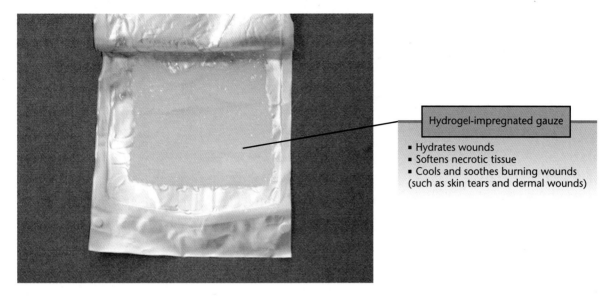

Hydrogel-impregnated gauze

- Hydrates wounds
- Softens necrotic tissue
- Cools and soothes burning wounds
  (such as skin tears and dermal wounds)

Figure 20-5 Hydrogel dressings. Springhouse. *Lippincott's Visual Encyclopedia of Clinical Skills*. Philadelphia: Wolters Kluwer Health, 2009.

This should be performed on a regular basis to ensure that the wound continues to be clean. Depending on the patient and the location of the wound, patients may need assistance with this. If patients develop an infection, this will increase healing time for the wound and may lead to cellulitis, sepsis, osteomyelitis, or other complications. Usage of hydrogen peroxide solution, povidone iodine, or acetic acid solutions is contraindicated, as they are cytotoxic to migrating/dividing keratinocytes in the wound base.

MOIST WOUND

Wounds re-epithelialize more rapidly when the wound bed is kept moist (not wet) due to enhanced keratinocyte migration. Moist wounds can be maintained with topical ointments such as white petrolatum. Many patients will heal only

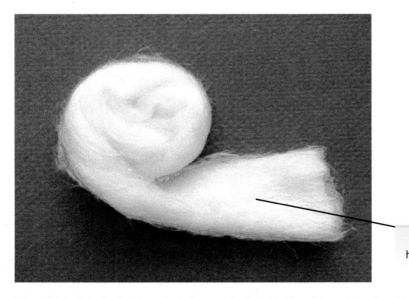

Fibers encourage
hemostasis in minimally
bleeding wounds.

Figure 20-6 Alginate dressings. Springhouse. *Lippincott's Visual Encyclopedia of Clinical Skills*. Philadelphia: Wolters Kluwer Health, 2009.

using white petrolatum. An antibacterial ointment is not necessary in most cases. Some patients may need topical antibiotics due to infection; however a few may become sensitized to these products or other preservatives in topical medicaments. This leads to an allergic contact dermatitis and complicates the healing process. Also, allergy to topical antibiotics such as neomycin or bacitracin may develop in chronic ulcer patients. In addition to topical ointments, dressings are essential to maintaining a moist wound.

TISSUE NOURISHMENT

The first consideration in healing an ulcer is to assess the nutritional status of the patient. A malnourished and/or vitamin-deficient patient will heal more slowly. Assessing levels of vitamin A, C, E, and zinc as well as a prealbumin level are helpful. Keeping the tissue nourished is challenging for many ulcer patients. Essentially, this means increasing the oxygen available to the wound base through improved blood flow or by adding pressure on the leg to decrease edema and improve venous flow. For arterial ulcers, vascular bypass may be necessary to heal recalcitrant ulcerations.

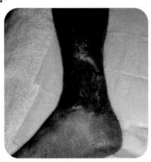

An 71-year-old man presents with a 3-year history of a nonhealing ulcer located over the medial malleolus on his right ankle (Fig. 20-7). He gives a history of a right deep venous thrombosis 5 years previously. His right leg is edematous and the ulcer is large and irregularly shaped, measuring 4 cm × 6.5 cm. The wound bed is covered with fibrous slough and the surrounding skin is macerated. Granulation tissue is seen in 10% of the wound bed. Exudation is moderate in amount and serous. Hemosiderin deposition, atrophie blanche, and a venous flare are seen in the surrounding skin. The ankle brachial index is 0.9. What is the diagnosis? What treatment will be most beneficial to this patient?

Venous Leg Ulceration
BACKGROUND/EPIDEMIOLOGY

Skin ulcerations caused by venous insufficiency are common in the general population and are the most commonly encountered leg ulceration. The overall prevalence of vascular ulcers is not known, but it is estimated at ~1% of the population. Eighty percent of these ulcers are thought to be venous ulcers with the remaining 20% being arterial or mixed venous and arterial in nature.

Venous ulcers are associated with chronic venous insufficiency. Normally during exercise, leg muscle contraction increases venous return and decreases venous pressure in the legs. In patients with incompetent venous valves, venous pressure remains high despite exercise and muscle contraction. Though the pathophysiology of venous ulceration is not fully elucidated, it is known to be related to multiple predisposing factors, presented in Table 20-3. These elements may contribute to incompetence of the perforating and deep vein valves or calf muscle pump dysfunction. Venous hypertension results in inflammation leading to capillary damage, capillary leakage, and edema.

KEY FEATURES

- Venous ulceration is often large, irregular in shape, and often located over the medial malleolus.

- Signs of venous hypertension (edema/stasis dermatitis/varicosities) are common.

- Compression of the lower leg and good wound care form the cornerstone of treatment.

PATHOGENESIS

With chronic venous hypertension, multiple cytokines and fibrinogen are released leading to more inflammation. In time, remodeling leads to capillary proliferation and a fibrous fibrinogen cuff in the vessel, impeding oxygen delivery. Alternately, some believe that ulcerations are caused by pressure-related vessel damage, leading to leaking of proteolytic enzymes and free radicals into the dermis. These processes lead to chronic inflammation resulting in stasis

Table 20-3 **Risk Factors for Venous Ulceration**	
Obesity	History of deep venous thrombosis
Traumatic leg injury	Factor V Leiden mutation
Absent valves (inherited defect)	Neuromuscular disease
Disuse/atrophy of the calf muscles	

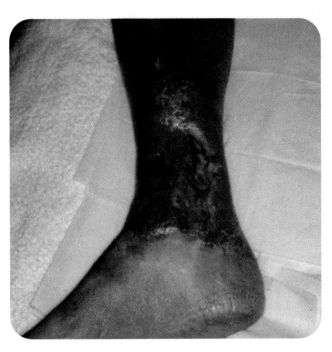

Figure 20-7 Venous ulceration on the medial malleolus. From Nettina SM. *The Lippincott Manual of Nursing Practice,* 7th ed. Philadelphia: Lippincott Williams & Wilkins, 2001.

dermatitis, lipodermatosclerosis, and eventually venous ulceration.

CLINICAL PRESENTATION

Venous ulcers are located most commonly around the medial malleolus (the gaiter area) and vary considerably in size and shape (Fig. 20-7). They are often large and shallow. They may be single or multiple. The ulcer margin is well defined but not raised or undermined. The ulcer base may show yellow and doughy or healthy red hemorrhagic granulation tissue.

Other features to look out for in the surrounding skin:

- Stasis dermatitis is common and presents with scale, erythema, and itch
- Signs of venous hypertension:
  - Pitting edema
  - Varicosities, which are tortuous, dilated veins. They may cause discomfort on prolonged standing and during pregnancy
  - Venous flares: dilated veins around the ankles
- Extravasation of red blood cells leading to hemosiderin deposition and melanin deposition following inflammation lead to petechiae and brownish pigmentation of coalescing macules.
- Atrophie blanche: a term describing ivory-white atrophic sclerotic plaques with a red stippling at the periphery. These are also found in certain hypercoagulable states.
- Lipodermatosclerosis describes the condition when the subcutaneous tissue of the lower extremity becomes woody, indurated, sclerodermatous, and fibrotic. Early on it may be mistaken for cellulitis, later on it results in the appearance of an inverted champagne bottle with tapering distally at the ankle and proximal swelling.
- If dermatitis is well demarcated or does not respond to traditional treatment a contact dermatitis may be present. This can be caused by components of topically applied medications (antibiotics, preservatives, anesthetics), dressings, or rubber in elastic stockings.
- Pseudo-Kaposi's sarcoma: an exaggerated stasis dermatitis presenting as purple well-defined plaques
- Look for signs of co-existing arterial disease (see next section).

SYMPTOMS

Venous ulcers are often painless. There may be a sensation of heaviness or aching or swelling of the lower leg particularly after prolonged standing. A history of preceding minor injury or infection may be elucidated.

CHAPTER 20 Leg Ulcers & Decubitus Ulcers

DIAGNOSIS

Ankle brachial indices should be measured before compression therapy to assess for arterial disease. It should be noted that values are not reliable in diabetics. Compression is contraindicated if the value is less than 0.5 and a value less than 0.8 indicates arterial disease and caution should be used. A vascular surgery opinion should be sought in cases with decreased values. Venous duplex ultrasound allows visualization of the veins and flow through the valves. Patch tests should be performed if a component of contact dermatitis is suspected. The ulcer should be measured carefully (length, width, and depth). Consider photographing the ulceration at each visit to aid assessment of progress.

TREATMENT

- The patient should be counseled regarding duration of treatment. Fifty percent heal in 6 months and most are healed at 1 year
- General advice:
  - Rest is an important part of the treatment regimen. Antigravity measures include limiting prolonged standing. When seated, the feet should be raised above the level of the heart and the end of the bed may also be raised in the absence of breathing difficulties/orthopnea.
  - Exercise should be encouraged to maintain the calf muscle pump.
  - Weight reduction advice may be appropriate.
- Compression therapy is the mainstay of treatment. Graduated sustained compression decreases pressure in the superficial venous system. The optimal pressure is 35 to 40 mm Hg at the ankle. This improves edema and the effect of the muscle pump. Non-elastic or elastic systems may be used. Non-elastic bandages require muscle activity in order to work and are thus not recommended in immobile patients. Options for compression include Unna boots (moist zinc impregnated nonelastic bandages); multilayer elastic bandaging (which maintain a constant pressure for 7 days); orthotic devices; and compression pumps.
- Patients should wear compression stockings for the rest of their lives. These are put on before rising from bed in the morning and kept on until bedtime.
  - There are four classes of stocking depending on the pressure at the ankle:
    - 20 to 30 mm Hg for aching and mild edema
    - 30 to 40 mm Hg for moderate edema and venous hypertension/severe varicosities
    - 40 to 50 mm Hg for severe edema and venous hypertension
    - 50 to 60 mm Hg for elephantiasis
  - The stockings should be replaced every 6 months.
- Dermatitis affecting surrounding skin should be treated with topical corticosteroids such as triamcinolone 0.1% cream twice daily as necessary, taking care to avoid the ulcer base and edge.
- Wound dressings as appropriate to the patient's ulcer

"AT A GLANCE" TREATMENT

- Fifty percent heal in 6 months and most are healed at 1 year
- Lifestyle modification:
  - Rest and antigravity measures include limiting prolonged standing.
  - Exercise should be encouraged to maintain the calf muscle pump.
  - Weight reduction advice as appropriate
- Compression therapy: patients should wear compression stockings for the rest of their lives.
- Wound dressings

WHEN TO REFER

- Patients with ABI values less than 0.8 should be evaluated by vascular surgery.
- For chronic/recalcitrant ulcers, consider referral to a wound specialist or dermatologist for consideration of Unna boot application.

NOT TO BE MISSED

- For recalcitrant lesions, evaluation for a secondary complicating diagnosis should be undertaken, especially evaluation of infection with bacteria, fungi, or mycobacteria.
- Skin cancers may present as chronic ulcerations, both melanoma and non-melanoma types.
- Consider allergic contact dermatitis to topically applied medicaments or the dressings themselves, especially in cases with acute dermatitis and/or pruritus.

- Dermatitis affecting surrounding skin should be treated with topical corticosteroids such as triamcinolone 0.1% cream twice daily as necessary, taking care to avoid the ulcer base and edge.

COURSE AND COMPLICATIONS

The recurrence rate is high: 70% in ulcers that have been present for over 1 year. Poor prognostic factors include wound chronicity, large surface area, history of venous ligation, fibrin slough affecting over half of the wound area, and a compromised arterial supply.

ICD9 Codes

459.81	Venous (peripheral) insufficiency, unspecified
707.00	Pressure ulcer, unspecified site
707.01	Pressure ulcer, elbow
707.02	Pressure ulcer, upper back
707.03	Pressure ulcer, lower back
707.04	Pressure ulcer, hip
707.05	Pressure ulcer, buttock
707.06	Pressure ulcer, ankle
707.07	Pressure ulcer, heel
707.09	Pressure ulcer, other site
707.10	Unspecified ulcer of lower limb
707.11	Ulcer of thigh
707.12	Ulcer of calf
707.13	Ulcer of ankle
707.14	Ulcer of heel and midfoot
707.15	Ulcer of other part of foot
707.19	Ulcer of other part of lower limb
707.20	Pressure ulcer, unspecified stage
707.21	Pressure ulcer stage I
707.22	Pressure ulcer stage II
707.23	Pressure ulcer stage III
707.24	Pressure ulcer stage IV
707.25	Pressure ulcer, unstageable
707.8	Chronic ulcer of other specified sites
707.9	Chronic ulcer of unspecified site
701.3	Striae atrophicae
681.00	Unspecified cellulitis and abscess of finger
681.01	Felon
681.02	Onychia and paronychia of finger
681.10	Unspecified cellulitis and abscess of toe
681.11	Onychia and paronychia of toe
681.9	Cellulitis and abscess of unspecified digit
682.0	Cellulitis and abscess of face
682.1	Cellulitis and abscess of neck
682.2	Cellulitis and abscess of trunk
682.3	Cellulitis and abscess of upper arm and forearm
682.4	Cellulitis and abscess of hand, except fingers and thumb
682.5	Cellulitis and abscess of buttock
682.6	Cellulitis and abscess of leg, except foot
682.7	Cellulitis and abscess of foot, except toes
682.8	Cellulitis and abscess of other specified sites
682.9	Cellulitis and abscess of unspecified sites

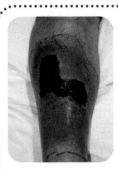

A 66-year-old smoker presents with a recent history of a large painful ulcer on the central shin (Fig. 20-8). His medical history is notable for hypertension and angina pectoris, which are controlled on medication. He describes a cramping pain in his left calf on walking and more recently pain in the dorsum of his foot at night. His lower leg is cold, dusky red, and the skin on his left calf is smooth and hairless. The ulcer is ~5 cm × 7 cm and punched out, with surrounding erythema. There is no exudate and the base is pale with no necrosis or granulation tissue. What is your approach to management?

Arterial Leg Ulcerations

BACKGROUND/EPIDEMIOLOGY

Arterial ulcers are most often caused by atherosclerotic plaques, which result in progressive narrowing of the lumen and a reduction of oxygenated arterial blood flow to the tissues. Distal tissue ischemia, necrosis, and ulceration result. Minor trauma (frequently related to footwear) may precipitate ulceration due to increasing oxygen demands. As noted previously, vascular ulcerations are estimated to be present in about 1% of the general population, of which 20% are likely arterial ulcerations. Risk factors for developing arterial ulcerations are summarized in Table 20-4.

PATHOGENESIS

Arterial ulcerations are simply caused by tissue hypoxia and death due to an inadequate blood supply. Interruption in supply may cause these ulcers. Causes of a reduced arterial supply are summarized in Table 20-5.

CLINICAL PRESENTATION

Symptoms

- Arterial ulcers are frequently painful, especially when the limb is elevated. The pain can be severe and persistent.
- Other symptoms of ischemia include a sensation of coldness, numbness, burning, or paresthesia.
- There is often a history of preceding minor trauma.
- Intermittent claudication is a symptom of arterial insufficiency. It manifests as pain, burning, cramping, or weariness in the calf, thigh, buttock, or foot on walking (increased oxygen demand) which is relieved by less than 5 minutes rest. The pain occurs distal to the site of arterial narrowing.
- Rest pain is associated with more severe critical obstruction and occurs at night in the feet when the legs are elevated. The pain may be relieved by placing the legs in a more dependent position.
- Pain may not be a feature in patients with diabetes due to peripheral neuropathy.

Ulcer Morphology

Arterial ulcers are located at pressure sites, usually below the malleoli, particularly over bony prominences such as on the toes, ankles, shins (Fig. 20-8)

KEY FEATURES

- Painful punched-out ulcers on pressure points.
- Atherosclerosis or arterial embolism are common causes.
- Revascularization is cornerstone of treatment.

Table 20-4 Risk Factors for Atherosclerotic Arterial Ulceration	
Age >40	Family history of cardiovascular disease
Cigarette smoking	Hypertension
Diabetes mellitus	Male gender
Hyperlipidemia	Sedentary lifestyle
Ischemic heart disease, cerebrovascular disease, peripheral vascular disease	Homocysteinemia

Table 20-5 Causes of Reduced Arterial Blood Supply

- Atherosclerosis +/− thrombosis
- Trauma (open or closed)
- Vasospasm
- Cholesterol emboli
- Arteriovenous malformations
- Hypothermia

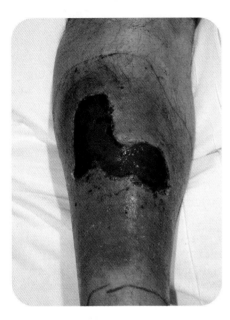

Figure 20-8 Arterial insufficiency ulceration on the shin of a 66-year-old man with secondary cellulitis.

or the lateral aspect of the foot. They are typically small in size and deep. They are commonly rounded or may reflect the shape of a traumatic injury. The borders are sharply demarcated giving the ulcer a punched-out appearance. The ulcer base is dry with minimal drainage or exudate and may be necrotic. The wound bed is pale gray or yellow. There is little or no granulation tissue. Tendons and deeper tissue may be exposed. If the wound is debrided, the base is usually does not bleed.

Other characteristic features:

- Normal, cool, dry, shiny, thin, atrophic, hairless skin affecting the surrounding skin or the distal lower limb
- Pale, cyanosed, or blotchy erythematous skin on the lower leg
- Weak or absent peripheral pulses; pulse examination in diabetics is less reliable due to calcification of the arteries.
- Prolonged capillary refill time, more than 3 to 4 seconds (the tip of the big toe is compressed until it blanches and the time taken for it to refill is measured)
- Pallor on limb elevation to 45 degrees for 1 minute and rubor starting distally following a delay of 10 to 15 seconds when leg is replaced in a dependent position)
- Thickened distorted nail plates
- Bruits over the femoral arteries
- Signs of infection including erythema, edema, increased temperature, pain, and/or discharge

INVESTIGATION

- Full physical examination including cardiovascular, abdominal, and examination of the fundi should be performed to look for evidence of cardiovascular disease.
- A noninvasive Doppler device is used to measure the ABI (ankle-brachial index).
- Doppler segmental studies compare systolic pressures at various locations along the limb and can identify the location of arterial disease.
- Transcutaneous oxygen measurements assess the degree of microvascular perfusion in the absence of infection. A reading of less than 20 mm Hg indicates marked ischemia and decreased propensity for healing.
- Conventional contrast angiography or magnetic resonance angiography may be performed in patients who will undergo revascularization procedures.
- A complete cardiovascular examination, full blood count, renal profile, fasting glucose and cholesterol, and an electrocardiogram are recommended.

PATIENT ASSESSMENT

- The importance of risk factor modification such as quitting smoking and controlling cholesterol levels.
- Light exercise helps build a good collateral supply.
- Support stockings and compression are contraindicated.
- Avoid constrictive clothing.
- Signs and symptoms of infection, gangrene, and progressive arterial insufficiency should be discussed.

ABI	SYMPTOMS	ARTERIAL COMPROMISE
1 or slightly >1	None	None
0.5–0.8	Claudication	Narrowing of lumen with arterial insufficiency
<0.5	Pain at rest, tissue loss	Severe occlusive disease

THERAPY

The primary therapeutic aim is to achieve revascularization and to restore arterial oxygen supply. This can be achieved either by angioplasty or bypass surgery. General measures include pain control and elevation of the head of the bed to improve arterial flow, adequate nutrition to promote healing, and a supervised exercise regimen to improve collateral circulation.

Risk factors for atherosclerotic disease should be addressed including smoking cessation, weight loss, and good control of hypertension, hyperlipidemia, and diabetes.

The wound should be cleaned with normal saline and an appropriate occlusive dressing such as hydrogel should be applied. Dressings protect the ulcer from trauma and infection, reduce pain, debride, and maintain a moist wound environment. Necrotic tissue may be carefully debrided taking care not to disturb the already compromised arterial supply. Removing eschar from heels and toes in the absence of infection should be avoided. Hyperbaric oxygen therapy can be used to improve tissue perfusion if the ulcer is slow to heal or the patient is not suitable for revascularization.

"AT A GLANCE" TREATMENT

- The most effective therapy is to achieve revascularization and restore arterial oxygen supply. This can be achieved either by angioplasty or bypass surgery.
- Good wound care is essential, as with all ulcerations.
- Hyperbaric oxygen therapy may be beneficial for those not suitable for revascularization surgery.

COURSE AND COMPLICATIONS

Arterial ulcerations tend to be chronic, recalcitrant, and/or recurrent without treatment of the underlying vascular insufficiency.

ICD9 Codes	
707.10	Unspecified ulcer of lower limb
443.9	Peripheral vascular disease, unspecified

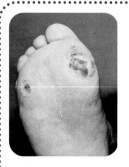

A 63-year-old man with a 25-year history of insulin-dependent diabetes comes into your clinic with asymptomatic ulcerations on the ball of his foot (Fig. 20-9). These ulcerations have been present for about 6 months. He first noticed the ulcers after finding a stone in his shoe. He has tried to treat them himself but they have not improved. How would you proceed with assessment and management in this case?

Neuropathic Ulcerations

ETIOLOGY/PATHOGENESIS

Neuropathy can result in sensory loss, motor dysfunction, and autonomic dysfunction. Loss of protective pain sensation results in an under-appreciation of repetitive trauma, pressure, frictional, and shearing forces. Motor neuropathy preferentially affects the small intrinsic muscles of the foot. Extrinsic muscles overpower the atrophied intrinsic muscles leading to foot deformity including cocked-up claw toes and prominent metatarsal heads. The newly uneven pressure distribution throughout the forefoot coupled with the thinning and displacement of the protective fat pads leaves the skin overlying bony prominences more susceptible to tissue damage. Autonomic dysfunction leads to hypohidrosis and dry, brittle skin

KEY FEATURES

- The most common cause of neuropathic foot ulcers in the United States is diabetes mellitus.

- The ulcer has a punched-out appearance surrounded by a rim of callus and occurs over pressure points.

- Management involves offloading of pressure, good wound care, good foot care, and treatment of associated atherosclerotic disease if present.

Table 20-6 Causes of Neuropathic Foot Ulcers	
• Diabetes mellitus	• Syringomyelia
• Spinal cord lesions	• Alcohol abuse
• Tabes dorsalis	• Medications
• Spina bifida	• Leprosy

prone to fissures and callus formation. Callosities can be responsible for a 30% increase in local pressure. Causes of neuropathic foot ulcerations are discussed in Table 20-6.

The most common cause of neuropathic foot ulcers in the United States is diabetes mellitus. One in 20 diabetics in the United States will develop a foot ulcer and one in 100 will require amputation annually (http://www.emedicine.medscape.com/article/460282-followup). Neuropathy, peripheral arterial disease, and impaired wound healing, as well as increased susceptibility to infection, are important factors in the development and management of diabetic ulcers. Risks include male sex, diabetes for more than 10 years, poor glucose control, associated cardiovascular, retinal, or renal complications. In addition, arterial ulcers occur more frequently and at an earlier age in diabetics than in the general population.

CLINICAL PRESENTATION

Neuropathic ulcers are usually asymptomatic. There are often features of peripheral neuropathy and/or peripheral vascular disease.

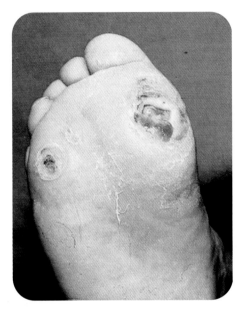

Figure 20-9 Neuropathic ulceration on the ball of the foot in a patient with peripheral neuropathy. From Bates BB. *A Guide to Physical Examination and History Taking,* 6th ed. Philadelphia: JB Lippincott, 1995.

Ulcer Location and Morphology

Ulcers occur at sites of pressure such as the plantar surfaces overlying the metatarsal heads, the toes and the heels, and over altered areas of increased pressure due to structural deformity. The edge often has a punched-out appearance. A thick rim of callus may be seen surrounding the ulcer (Fig. 20-9).

Other Characteristic Features

- Dryness/fissuring of surrounding skin
- Hypo- or anhidrosis
- Callosities occurring on other areas of pressure
- Peripheral neuropathy with loss of protective sensation. The Semmes-Weinstein monofilament can be used to test cutaneous perception.
- Foot deformity with cocked-up claw toes and prominent metatarsal heads
- Previous amputation alters the pressure distribution and may predispose to ulceration.
- While peripheral vascular disease is an important etiologic factor in the diabetic foot, pulse examination is less reliable due to calcification of the arteries. It is important to look for other symptoms and signs of poor perfusion as discussed previously. Occlusion of the tibial and peroneal arteries is common resulting in an ischemic foot in the presence of a strong popliteal pulse. The dorsalis pedis is typically spared.
- Increased drainage, erythema, pain, temperature, foul odor, and lymphangitis suggest infection, which should be recognized early to prevent progression to gangrene.

- It is important to take note of the condition of the nails, and to assess mobility and the condition and type of footwear.

TREATMENT

Management includes:

- Offloading of pressure and reducing trauma and friction at the site of the wound is critical. This may involve a strict non–weight-bearing regimen, orthotic devices, cushioning inserts, total contact casting, or special therapeutic footwear. In addition, calluses should be removed regularly.
- Clinical, +/− microbacterial, +/− radiological assessment for infection with empiric antibiotic therapy if indicated. If severe or there is bone, joint, or systemic involvement the patient should be admitted to the hospital.
- Meticulous wound care is critical. The wound is cleaned with normal saline. Devitalized, infected, and necrotic tissue and callus should be removed by mechanical debridement or enzymatic debriding agents and should be performed until good granulation tissue is seen. The appropriate sterile dressing should then be applied. Hydrocolloid dressings and hydrogels maintain a moist environment and provide some autolytic debridement for dry necrotic ulcers. Alginates and absorptive dressings are useful for moist granulating ulcers.
- Treatment of arterial disease and risk factors, if present, as appropriate.
- Good foot care should be a lifelong commitment and should include daily washing, drying, moisturizing, and self-examination. Walking barefoot should be avoided, shoes should be checked carefully for foreign objects, and water temperature should be tested before bathing. It may be prudent for a podiatrist to be responsible for nail and callus care. The nail should be cut straight across and should be smooth without sharp edges. Shoes and orthotics should fit correctly and offer support and protection from trauma and friction.
- Adequate nutrition is essential to promote wound healing.
- Wound dressings as appropriate to the patient's ulcer

Consider hospital admission for patients with acute infections or infected gangrene and those with penetration of infection into the deeper foot, including involvement of the plantar fascia.

"AT A GLANCE" TREATMENT

- Offloading of pressure and reducing trauma and friction at the site of the wound is critical
- Clinical, +/− microbacterial, +/− radiological assessment for infection with empiric antibiotic therapy if indicated
- Meticulous wound care and debridement
- Appropriate sterile dressings:
  - Dry ulcerations: hydrocolloid or hydrogel dressings
  - Moist/granulating ulcerations: alginates and absorptive dressings
- Treatment of arterial disease and risk factors, if present, as appropriate
- Good foot care
- Adequate nutrition to promote wound healing

COURSE AND COMPLICATIONS

Management of these patients requires long-term attention. Acutely, appropriate ulcer care and treatment is essential. In the long term, addressing the underlying cause, such as diabetes, is essential. Everyone with decreased sensation should perform good foot care as outlined above.

WHEN TO REFER

- Managing those with decreased foot sensation in conjunction with a podiatrist is often helpful.
- Consult a dermatologist or a wound care specialist for recalcitrant/nonhealing ulcerations.
- Consider endocrinology consultation for those patients with hard-to-control diabetes.

Complications include progression of ulceration to involve deeper structures and further compromise of function. Progressive infections can lead to gangrene and the necessity for amputation. Systemic sepsis may also occur.

ICD9 Codes

356.9	*Unspecified idiopathic peripheral neuropathy*
707.10	*Unspecified ulcer of lower limb*
250.00	*Diabetes mellitus without mention of complication, type II or unspecified type, not stated as uncontrolled*
250.01	*Diabetes mellitus without mention of complication, type I (juvenile type), not stated as uncontrolled*
250.02	*Diabetes mellitus without mention of complication, type II or unspecified type, uncontrolled*
250.03	*Diabetes mellitus without mention of complication, type I (juvenile type), uncontrolled*

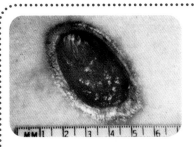

An 82-year-old man was recently hospitalized for community-acquired pneumonia. His hospitalization was complicated by respiratory failure requiring intubation. During the second week of his stay he developed an ulcerated area on his sacrum (Fig. 20-10). Subcutaneous fat was visible in the ulcer base but no muscle, tendon, or bone. What is the most likely diagnosis? What grade of ulcer does he have? How could it have been prevented?

Pressure/Decubitus Ulcerations

BACKGROUND

Pressure ulcers are also known as bedsores or decubitus ulcers. They affect 3% to 14% of acutely hospitalized patients and 15% to 25% of long-term patients. Patients are usually elderly and immobilized (bed bound or chair bound). Other risk factors include limited mobility, altered sensory perception, poor nutritional status, incontinence, compromised circulatory status, inadequate nursing or home care.

PATHOGENESIS

Pressure ulcers are caused by compression of the soft tissues between bony prominences and external surfaces for prolonged periods. Pressure occludes blood vessels resulting in tissue anoxia with subsequent necrosis and tissue loss. The tissue damage is proportional to the extent and duration of pressure. Other contributory factors include shearing forces, friction, moisture, and heat.

CLINICAL PRESENTATION

Symptoms

These ulcerations are painful unless the patient is sensation impaired. They usually occur over bony prominences including the sacral and coccygeal areas (Fig. 20-10), ischial tuberosities, greater trochanters, heels, lateral malleoli, elbows, and occiput (Fig. 20-11). Sixty-five percent of pressure ulcers occur in the sacral/pelvic area and 30% in the lower extremities.

Ulcer Staging

Wounds are classified according to the depth of tissue damage that is visible (Table 20-7) (Figs. 20-12 to 20-15). Necrotic tissue must be removed before

KEY FEATURES

- Areas of soft-tissue destruction caused by pressure.
- Risk factors include prolonged immobility, sensory deficits, circulatory deficits, and poor nutrition.
- Most commonly located on the sacral area and lower extremities over bony prominences.
- There can be extensive necrosis underlying a small skin defect.
- Treatment involves a multidisciplinary team, and goals include pressure reduction, adequate nutrition, and good wound care.

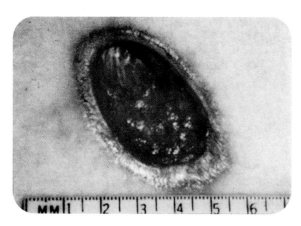

Figure 20-10 Stage III pressure ulceration. Source of photo: National Pressure Ulcer Advisory Panel. Reston, VA.

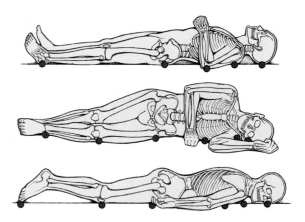

Figure 20-11 Most common decubitus ulcer sites due to proximity of bone to skin. Courtesy of Neil O. Hardy, Westport, CT.

Stage I

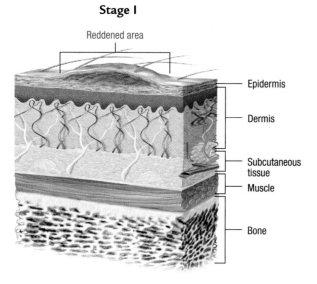

Figure 20-12 Staging pressure ulcers. Stage I. Asset provided by Anatomical Chart Co.

Stage II

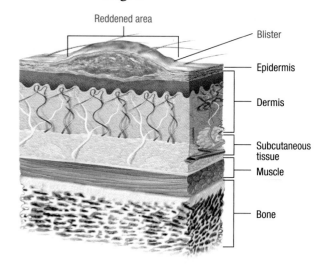

Figure 20-13 Staging pressure ulcers. Stage II. Asset provided by Anatomical Chart Co.

Stage III

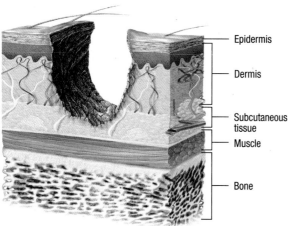

Figure 20-14 Staging's pressure ulcers. Stage III. Asset provided by Anatomical Chart Co.

Stage IV

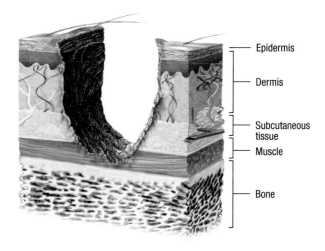

Figure 20-15 Staging pressure ulcers. Stage IV. Asset provided by Anatomical Chart Co.

Table 20-7 Decubitus Ulcer Staging

STAGE	IMAGE	MORPHOLOGY
Suspected deep-tissue injury		• Purple or maroon localized patch with intact skin • Blood-filled blister
Stage I	Fig. 20-12	• Intact skin • Nonblanchable localized erythema • +/− pain, induration, temperature change
Stage II	Fig. 20-13	• Partial thickness loss of dermis presenting as a shallow open ulcer with a red or pink wound bed without slough • Intact or ruptured serum filled bulla
Stage III	Fig. 20-14	• Full-thickness tissue loss. Subcutaneous fat may be visible but muscle, tendon, and bone are not visible. There may be undermining and tunneling.
Stage IV	Fig. 20-15	• Full-thickness tissue loss with exposed bone, tendon, or muscle. Slough or eschar may be present on wound bed and there is often undermining and tunneling.

staging is attempted. The stage of an ulcer does not change as healing occurs. What is seen at the level of the skin is often the tip of the iceberg. Well-established ulcers are widest at the base and there can be extensive necrosis underlying a small skin defect. The diagnosis is usually made clinically. Other causes other than pressure include infections, malignant ulcers, fistulae, and pyoderma gangrenosum.

TREATMENT

Management and prevention involves a multidisciplinary team, as well as input from the patient and caregivers. The team may include physician, nurse, physical therapist, occupational therapist, dietitian, social services, and pharmacist. All patients should have a risk assessment performed upon entry to an institution or hospital and again periodically throughout their stay. At-risk patients may be identified by assessing sensory perception, exposure of the skin to moisture, degree of physical activity, mobility, nutrition, friction, and shear. Prevention should focus on pressure reduction, nutritional assessment, good skin care, and education of both the patient and caregiver. Techniques necessary for preventing pressure ulcerations are summarized in Table 20-8. Treatment of these ulcerations include good prevention techniques, wound dressing and debridement, and potentially surgical full-thickness skin grafting. It is important to remember that healed decubitus ulcers remain significantly more fragile than the surrounding "normal" skin.

"AT A GLANCE" TREATMENT

- Pressure, friction, shearing, and moisture reduction methods, nutrition, and general skin care are managed as above
- Wound care:
  - Analgesia may be taken 30 to 60 minutes before dressing changes if required

Table 20-8 Techniques to Prevent Pressure Ulcerations

PRESSURE REDUCTION

- Patient repositioning should occur at regular intervals both when lying down (2 hourly) and sitting (at least hourly). A 30-degree side-lying position should be used in bed. Sitting should be limited to a 2-hour period.
- Special support surfaces (mattresses, overlays, and cushions)
- Pillows should be placed under the calves (not under the knees) to protect the heels when lying on his/her back and between the bony prominences of the heels and knees. Doughnut pillows may reduce blood flow to the tissues.
- Patients should be encouraged to mobilize and perform daily exercise

Decrease frictional and shearing forces by the use of proper repositioning and transfer techniques. The head of the bed should be raised no more than 30 degrees to reduce shearing forces on the coccyx and sacrum.

Nutritional status may be monitored with serial weights, an intake diary +/− albumin levels. Consider nutritional, vitamin and mineral supplementation as needed. A dietician should be consulted as required.

Good skin care involves the use of mild cleansing agents, bland emollients, and protection of the skin from moisture (incontinence, sweat, and wound drainage). The use of diapers should be limited.

Education should include both written and verbal instructions.

- The pressure sore should be cleaned at each dressing change. Irrigation with normal saline and gentle wiping away of debris with gauze.
- Debridement removes dead tissue and debris that can lead to infection and delay wound healing. This can be achieved by mechanical or surgical debridement, rinsing of the wound, enzyme medications, or specialized dressings.
- Dressings should provide a moist environment.
- Stage IV ulcers may require surgical intervention.
- Once healed, it must be remembered that an old pressure ulcer remains fragile.

WHEN TO REFER

A multidisciplinary team, as well as input from the patient and caregivers, is required. The team may include physician, nurse, physical therapist, occupational therapist, dietitian, social services, pharmacist.

COURSE AND COMPLICATIONS

Decubitus ulcerations are challenging to heal once established. The best treatment is initial prevention through the techniques described above. In the early stages, simple therapy usually will reverse the course of the ulceration. For deeper, longstanding ulcerations, some form of surgical therapy is often necessary, ranging from a simple debridement to skin grafting. Complications include infections, and ulceration/involvement of deeper structures such as blood vessels, muscles, and tendons.

NOT TO BE MISSED

- Secondary wound infections (gram-positive bacteria) or viral infections (HSV).
- Prevention by assiduous pressure off-loading of pressure bearing areas is essential and should never be missed for immobile patients.

ICD9 Codes	
707.00	Pressure ulcer, unspecified site
707.01	Pressure ulcer, elbow
707.02	Pressure ulcer, upper back
707.03	Pressure ulcer, lower back
707.04	Pressure ulcer, hip
707.05	Pressure ulcer, buttock
707.06	Pressure ulcer, ankle
707.07	Pressure ulcer, heel
707.09	Pressure ulcer, other site

Other Causes of Lower Limb Ulceration

- Connective tissue disease/vasculitis:
  - Lupus erythematosus, scleroderma, Raynaud disease, rheumatoid arthritis, small vessel vasculitis, livedoid vasculopathy, polyarteritis nodosa, Wegener granulomatosis
- Inflammatory disease:
  - Pyoderma gangrenosum, necrobiosis lipoidica, panniculitis
- Hematologic disease:
  - Sickle cell disease, thalassemia, lymphoproliferative and myeloproliferative disorders, hypercoagulable disorders
- Infection:
  - Bacterial, deep fungal, Buruli ulcer, *Mycobacteria*, leishmaniasis, syphilis
- Drugs/treatment:
  - Hydroxyurea, radiation therapy, intravenous drug abuse
- Neoplasia:
  - Basal cell carcinoma, squamous cell carcinoma, melanoma, lymphoma, Kaposi sarcoma
- Trauma:
  - Including dermatitis artefacta
- Other:
  - Lymphedema, insect bites, calciphylaxis, perniosis, Klinefelter syndrome, prolidase deficiency

Appendix A Clinical Comparison of Common Leg Ulcers

Types	VENOUS	ARTERIAL	NEUROPATHIC
Associated symptoms	Aching and swelling legs (improved with elevation)	Painful ulcer (worse when elevated), claudication, rest pain	Lower extremity pain, paresthesia, or anesthesia; burning sensation at ulcer
Significant history	Obesity, previous leg injury, history of deep vein thrombosis or phlebitis	Peripheral vascular disease, hyperlipidemia, atherosclerosis, smoking, diabetes mellitus	Peripheral neuropathy, diabetes mellitus, poor glucose control, complications of diabetes, alcohol abuse, spinal cord lesions, other causes of neuropathy
Location	Medial malleoli	Pressure points, areas of trauma, and distal sites (e.g., toes)	Heel, plantar metatarsal area, great toe
Appearance	Irregular, ragged border	"punched out" with sharply demarcated border, dry appearing with gray or black base, possibly covered in necrotic debris	Deep ulcer surrounded by thick callus
Adjacent skin	Brown to brown-red pigmentation and purpura, eczematous changes (stasis dermatitis), induration and fibrosis (lipodermatosclerosis), white scar tissue (atrophie blanche)	Hair loss, atrophic shiny skin, dystrophic nails	Anesthetic skin
Associated findings on exam	Lower extremity edema, varicosities	Diminished to absent peripheral pulses, bruits in femoral arteries, prolonged capillary refill	Sensation loss (light touch, vibration, proprioception), impaired reflexes

Appendix B Treatment of Leg Ulcers

VENOUS	ARTERIAL	NEUROPATHIC
Compression*	Revascularization	Proper foot wear
Wound care	Wound care	Non-weight bearing
Antibiotics	Lipid-lowering agents	Wound care
Topical corticosteroids	Antiplatelet agents	Antibiotics
Venous surgery		Improved control of diabetes

*Avoid if there is co-existing arterial insufficiency

Suggested Reading

Baranoski S. Wound and skin care: Choosing a wound dressing, part 1. *Nursing* 2008:38(1):60–61.

Baranoski S. Wound and skin care: Choosing a wound dressing, part 2. *Nursing* 2008:38(2);14–15.

Bergan JJ, Schmid-Schonbein GW, Smith PDC, et al. Chronic venous disease. *N Engl J Med.* 2006;355(5): 488–498.

Bergstrom N, Allman RM, Alvarez OM, et al. Treatment of pressure ulcers. *Clinical Practice Guideline*, no 15. publication No. 95-0652, Dec 1994. Rockville, MD: US Department of Health and Human Services.

Boulton AJM, Kirsner RS, Vileikyte L. Neuropathic diabetic foot ulcers. *N Engl J Med.* 2004;351(1):48–55.

Brown P. *Quick Reference to Wound Care.* 2009. Canada: Jones and Bartlettt Publishers.

Fonder MA, Lazarus GS, Cowan DA, et al. Treating the chronic wound: A practical approach to the care of nonhealing wounds and wound care dressings. *J Am Acad Dermatol.* 2008;58(2):185–206.

Grey JE, Harding KG, Enoch S. ABC of wound healing. Venous and arterial leg ulcers. *BMJ.* 2006;332(7537): 347–350.

Hiatt WR. Medical treatment of peripheral arterial disease and claudication. *N Engl J Med.* 2001;344(21):1608–1621.

Kanj LF, Wilking SVB, Phillips TJ. Pressure ulcers. *J Am Acad Dermatol.* 1998;38(4):517–536.

Naik J, Bello AM, Scriven JM, et al. Lower limb unceration: A detailed study of aetiology in 555 patients. *Br J Surg.* 2000;87(4);502.

O'Meara S, Cullum NA, Nelson EA. Compression for venous leg ulcers. *Cochrane Database of Systematic Reviews.* 2009, Issue 1. Art. No.: CD000265.

Pham HT, Rich J, Veves A. Wound healing in diabetic foot ulceration: a review and commentary. *Wounds.* 2000;12:79–81.

Philips T, Staunton B, Provan A, et al. A study of the impact of leg ulcers on quality of life: Financial, social and psychologic implications. *J Am Acad Dermatol.* 1994;31(1):49–53.

Phillips TJ, Machado F, Trout R, et al. The Venous Ulcer study Group. Prognostic indicators in venous ulcers. *J Am Acad Dermatol.* 2000; 43(4):627–630.

Sarkar PK, Ballantyne S. Management of leg ulcers. *Postgrad Med J.* 2000;76:674–682.

Simon DA, Dix FP, McCollum CN. Management of venous leg ulcers. *BMJ.* 2004;328(7452):1358–1362.

Sumpio BE. Foot ulcers. *N Engl J Med.* 2000;43(11):787–793.

Valencia IC, Falabella A, Kirsner RS, et al. Chronic venous insufficiency and venous leg ulceration. *J Am Acad Dermatol.* 2001;44(3):401–421.

CHAPTER 21 Urticaria

Susan J. Huang and Arturo Saavedra-Lauzon

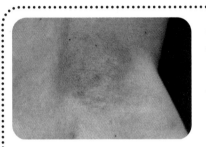

Mary is a 21-year-old student who presents to the university health services. She complains that she developed numerous itchy hives all over her body a half hour ago after a clambake.

She reports a history of hives after eating shellfish. On examination, there are multiple well-circumscribed pink plaques over the arms, trunk, and legs (Fig. 21-1). She has no involvement of the lips or around the eyes. Her vital signs are stable and she has no other findings. You recommend avoidance of shellfish to prevent future episodes and prescribe fexofenadine for daytime use and, as necessary, diphenhydramine at bedtime. You instruct her to return to the clinic if her symptoms progress or last for more than 24 hours.

Acute and Chronic Urticaria

BACKGROUND/EPIDEMIOLOGY

Urticaria is more commonly referred to as hives or wheals. It is a fairly common condition, affecting up to 20% of the general population at some time in their lifetime. There is no predominant gender for acute urticaria, but more females have the chronic form of urticaria. Its distribution is worldwide.

PATHOGENESIS

Urticaria is frequently caused by allergic triggers, which lead to mast cell degranulation of histamines, cytokines, and other vasoactive substances. While angioedema and anaphylaxis are separate entities, all three conditions reflect edema caused from leaky endothelium of differing depth and with differing distribution of involvement. Urticaria involves edema of the epidermis and dermis and affects the skin only. Individual lesions are usually pruritic, marked by rapid onset and resolve in less than 24 hours. Systemic symptoms including fatigue, sweats, chills, and joint pain may accompany severe attacks of urticaria.

Angioedema involves edema of the dermis, subcutaneous tissues, and/or submucosal tissues. Unlike urticaria, lesions usually are not pruritic, but rather, are painful. Lesions favor the eyelids, lips, genitalia, palms, and soles; commonly last between 24 and 48 hours.

Causes of angioedema include food exposures, or medications including nonsteroidal anti-inflammatory drugs (NSAIDs), sulfa medications, penicillins, or anticholinesterase (ACE) inhibitors. Angioedema is frequently accompanied by urticaria. Angioedema without urticaria should increase suspicion of C1 esterase inhibitor deficiency. Anaphylaxis involves edema of the skin and mucosa and involves multiple organ systems. It may lead to cardiovascular and respiratory decompensation. It is caused by a systemic allergic reaction, most commonly to a food, medication, insect bite, or other exposure. Primary evaluation of the patient's vital signs is essential.

KEY FEATURES

- "Hives" are common, affecting up to 20% of the population during a lifetime.

- Most episodes resolve within 6 weeks (acute urticaria). Continued episodes beyond 6 weeks are defined as chronic urticaria.

- Cause of urticaria is identified in acute urticaria (40%–60%) more commonly than in chronic urticaria (10%–20%).

(Continued)

327

KEY FEATURES (*Continued*)

- Therapy is with oral antihistamines, topical antipruritics, and oral immunosuppressive medications. Ideally, the cause is identified and the etiology appropriately treated or exposure eliminated.

- For patients with anaphylaxis, consider prescribing an EpiPen (epinephrine autoinjector).

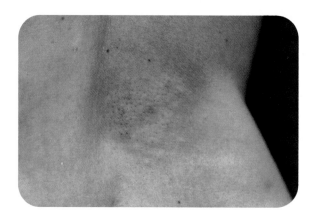

Figure 21-1 Urticarial wheal on the lower back

CLINICAL PRESENTATION

In this section, we will discuss two patterns of urticaria: acute and chronic (Table 21-1) (Figs. 21-2 to 21-6). We will discuss physical urticaria in the next section. Acute urticaria lasts for under 6 weeks, whereas chronic urticaria is marked by onset of lesions for more than two times per week for 6 or more weeks without treatment. The most common known causes of acute urticaria and chronic urticaria are presented in Table 21-2 (Figs. 21-7 to 21-9). Some important causes are upper respiratory tract infections medications (Table 21-3), and foods. However, many cases are idiopathic or autoimmune. Chronic urticaria can have a profound negative affect on a patient's quality of life. The cause of urticaria is identified in acute urticaria (40%–60%) more commonly than in chronic urticaria (10%–20%).

Given the prevalence of idiopathic cases, this condition is often difficult to treat. Conditions associated with chronic urticaria include autoimmune

Table 21-1 Classification of Urticaria*

TYPE	TRIGGERS
Spontaneous urticaria:	
Acute	Idiopathic, viral infections, foods, medications
Chronic	Idiopathic, autoimmune, infections
Physical urticaria:	
Cholinergic urticaria (Fig. 21-3)	Increased core body temperature
Heat urticaria	Contact with heat
Exercise-induced urticaria or anaphylaxis	Physical exercise
Cold urticaria (Fig. 21-6)	Cold temperature
Aquagenic urticaria	Water contact
Dermographic urticaria (Figs. 21-2, 21-4)	Mechanical shearing forces
Delayed pressure urticaria	Pressure
Solar urticaria (Fig. 21-5)	UV or light exposure
Contact urticaria	Contact with allergens
Vibratory urticaria	Vibration

*Adapted from Zuberbier T, Maurer M. Urticaria: Current opinions about etiology, diagnosis and therapy. *Acta Derm Venereol.* 2007;87:196–205.

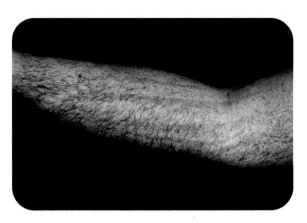

Figure 21-2 Dermographism following excoriation

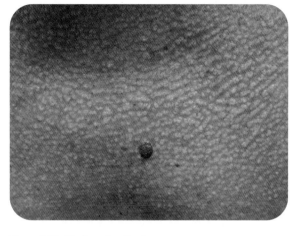

Figure 21-3 Cholinergic urticaria

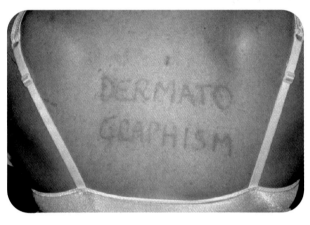

Figure 21-4 Dermatographism from stroking the skin with a cotton applicator. From Goodheart HP. *Goodheart's Photoguide to Common Skin Disorders.* 3rd ed. Philadelphia: Lippincott Williams & Wilkins, 2009.

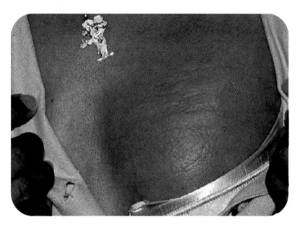

Figure 21-5 Solar urticaria following exposure to 15 minutes of sunlight through a glass window. From Goodheart HP. *Goodheart's Photoguide to Common Skin Disorders.* 3rd ed. Philadelphia: Lippincott Williams & Wilkins, 2009.

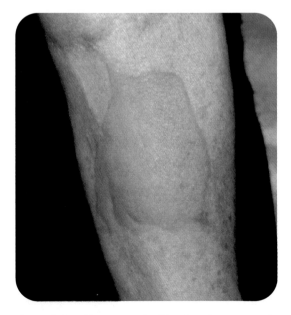

Figure 21-6 Cold urticaria–wheal forming after exposure to an ice cube. From Goodheart HP. *Goodheart's Photoguide to Common Skin Disorders.*3rd ed. Philadelphia: Lippincott Williams & Wilkins, 2009.

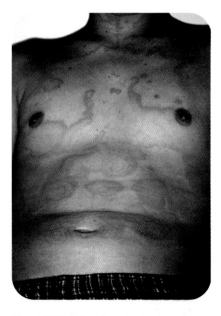

Figure 21-7 Polycyclic urticaria secondary to *M. pneumoniae* pneumonia.

Table 21-2 Precipitants of Acute and Chronic Urticaria (Adapted from Linscott, 2009)

ACUTE

Viral infections	Upper/lower respiratory, human immunodeficiency virus
Bacterial infections	Dental abscesses, *Mycoplasma pneumonia* (Fig. 21-7), other bacterial infections
Parasitic infections	Amebiasis, ascariasis, strongyloidiasis, trichinosis, malaria
Latex exposure	Consider both natural rubber latex exposure and foods (below)
Foods	Shellfish, fish, eggs, cheese, chocolate, nuts, berries, tomatoes For latex-allergic individuals: avocado, banana, chestnut, kiwi, potato

CHRONIC

Autoimmune disorders • Systemic lupus erythematosus (Fig. 21-8), rheumatoid arthritis, polymyositis, thyroid autoimmunity, and other connective tissue diseases	Around 50% of chronic urticaria is autoimmune
Cholinergic urticaria	Induced by emotional stress, heat, or exercise
Chronic medical illness	Hyperthyroidism, amyloidosis, polycythemia vera, malignant neoplasms, and lymphoma
Cryoglobulinemia/cryofibrinogenemia	
Mastocytosis	
Muckle-Wells syndrome	
Familial cold autoinflammatory syndrome	
Syphilis	
Urticaria pigmentosa	Purple macules, single or multiple (Fig. 21-9) that urticate with stroking (the Darier sign)

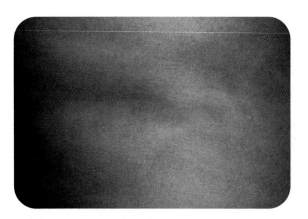

Figure 21-8 Wheal on the back of a woman with active systemic lupus erythematosus.

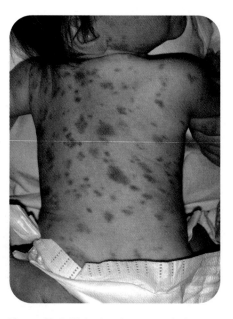

Figure 21-9 Urticaria pigmentosa lesions on the back of an infant (Photo Credit: James GH Dinulos, MD).

Table 21-3 Some Medications Causing Urticaria (Linscott, 2009)

Antiepileptic agents	Isoniazid
Aspirin	Morphine/codeine derivatives
Bromides	Nonsteroidal anti-inflammatory drugs (NSAIDs)
Cephalosporins	Penicillins
Chloroquine	Quinidine
Diuretics	Sulfas
Intravenous radiocontrast media	Vancomycin
Iodides	

hypothyroidism, parasitic and *Helicobacter pylori* infections, systemic lupus erythematosus, and hematologic malignancies. It is estimated that approximately 50% of chronic urticaria is autoimmune related.

Differential diagnoses of ordinary urticaria include urticarial vasculitis, C1 esterase deficiency, insect bites, Sweet syndrome, and contact dermatitis. Individual lesion should not last for more than 24 hours; although new hives may continue to occur and crops in various stages of evolution may be present. Lesions most commonly occur on the face and extremities, although they may occur anywhere on the body. Individual wheals lasting more than 24 hours and associated with high fevers, arthralgias, ecchymoses, and pigmentary changes should increase suspicion of urticarial vasculitis.

PHYSICAL FINDINGS

Individual wheals develop rapidly and present as pruritic, well-circumscribed edematous, blanching pink plaques of variable size (Figs. 21-1, 21-8). Individual lesions may coalesce with other lesions, forming polycyclic urticarial plaques (Fig. 21-7).

Anaphylaxis is frequently accompanied by cutaneous findings. Cutaneous reactions include erythema, urticaria, pruritus, and angioedema. These may be accompanied by upper and lower respiratory symptoms. Nasal congestion, sneezing, and coryza are early symptoms. Cough, hoarseness, and a sensation of a "tight throat" often precedes partial airway obstruction and true dyspnea. Lower respiratory symptoms may include chest pain, either due to bronchospasm or actual myocardial ischemia. In some cases, crampy abdominal pain, nausea, vomiting, or diarrhea may accompany these symptoms.

DIAGNOSIS

The diagnosis of urticaria is clinical. In straightforward cases that respond to treatment, no further workup is necessary. In chronic cases and in nonresponders, an individualized workup may include complete blood cell count with differential; stool ova and parasite exam to evaluate for parasitic infections; erythrocyte sedimentation rate (ESR) and C-reactive protein (CRP) to evaluate for urticarial vasculitis; thyroid-stimulating hormone (TSH) to evaluate for associated thyroid disease; physical or dietary challenges or changes; food diary; skin prick testing; patch testing; radioallergosorbent test (RAST) testing; biopsy to evaluate for urticarial vasculitis; and C4 levels in cases of angioedema without wheals and suspected C1 esterase inhibitor deficiency.

One consideration for diagnosis of chronic urticaria is patch testing. In general, patch testing is used to diagnose delayed type hypersensitivity, not immediate type IIgE-mediated reactions. However, in a single study, patients with chronic urticaria were patch tested and those who were allergic avoided all of their allergens, both topically and through ingestion. These individuals had 100% clearance of their urticaria, with recurrence on oral challenge. The majority

WHEN TO REFER

- Patients who do not respond to conventional therapy and/or need phototherapy may be referred to a dermatologist or allergist.
- If patch testing is desired, referral to a patch-testing expert is helpful (see http://www.contactderm.org). Patients with anaphylaxis should receive emergent care.

of these patients had nickel allergies. While patch testing is certainly not recommended for all chronic urticaria patients, for those with chronic, recalcitrant, longstanding hives it may be a useful addition to the diagnostic workup.

TREATMENT

If the agent inciting urticaria can be identified, it should be avoided to prevent further episodes. Following development of lesions, antihistamines and H2 blockers may be used as first-line agents. Newer H1-specific antihistamines may be preferred due to less sedation. However, older antihistamines are more effective (i.e., diphenhydramine, hydroxyzine). H2 blockers may be taken in conjunction with antihistamines. Second-line agents include doxepin, prednisone, epinephrine, nifedipine, leukotriene receptor antagonists, colchicine, sulfa drugs, and NSAIDs. Psoralen + ultraviolet A (PUVA), induction of tolerance through repeated challenges in cases of known offenders, methotrexate, and cyclosporine may be used in patients refractory to the above treatments. Topical therapy includes emollients, topical antipruritics such as menthol/camphor, or pramoxine-containing lotions.

Treatment of angioedema can be managed similarly. However, hereditary angioedema does not respond to the above treatments and should be acutely treated with intravenous fresh frozen plasma or C1 inhibitor concentrate. In cases of anaphylaxis, the patient should be advised to seek emergency treatment. Patients may autoinject epinephrine if they have an autoinjector available (e.g., EpiPen for adults or EpiPen Jr for children). Antihistamines should also be administered. Corticosteroids and H2 blockers may have an additional beneficial effect.

"AT A GLANCE" TREATMENT

Urticaria

- First-line therapy: antihistamines and H2 blockers
  - Nonsedating antihistamines (cetirizine, fexofenadine, loratadine)
  - Sedating antihistamines (diphenhydramine, hydroxyzine, doxepin)
  - H2 blockers (cimetidine, famotidine)
- Second-line agents:
  - Doxepin, prednisone, epinephrine, nifedipine, leukotriene receptor antagonists, colchicine
  - Psoralen + UVA
  - Methotrexate and cyclosporine for those refractory to the above treatments

Angioedema

- Treat with same agents as urticaria.
- Hereditary angioedema does not respond to the above treatments and should be acutely treated with intravenous fresh frozen plasma or C1 inhibitor concentrate.

Anaphylaxis

- **Seek emergency care immediately.**
- Patients may autoinject epinephrine if they have an autoinjector available (e.g., EpiPen for adults or EpiPen Jr for children).
- Antihistamines (diphenhydramine or hydroxyzine)
- Corticosteroids and H2 blockers may have an additional beneficial effect

NOT TO BE MISSED

- Anaphylaxis, including exercise-induced anaphylaxis.
- C1 esterase inhibitor deficiency (hereditary angioedema).
- Urticarial vasculitis/urticarial syndrome.
- Associated syndromes such as autoimmune hypothyroidism.

COURSE AND COMPLICATIONS

Individual lesions resolve within 24 hours without residual hyperpigmentation or ecchymoses. In chronic urticaria, half of the cases resolve spontaneously within 6 months but 20% will continue to be symptomatic 20 years later. Chronic urticaria may follow a waxing and waning course.

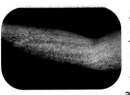

Sam is a 24-year-old man who comes to your office for an annual checkup. He feels well except that he complains of swelling and irregular itchy red wheals on his skin after scratching (Fig. 21-2) or toweling after a shower. He first noticed these episodes a few months ago. You suspect dermographism, the most common form of physical urticaria, and proceed to test this hypothesis in the clinic. You pre-scribe nonsedating antihistamines and ask him to follow-up with you in a few weeks.

Physical Urticaria
BACKGROUND/EPIDEMIOLOGY

Physical urticarias are those provoked by physical stimuli. These include hot and cold temperatures, increased body temperature, contact with water or light, physical pressure, vibration, and exercise. Most episodes tend to be brief and usually last less than an hour. Physical urticarias without an identified source likely account for a proportion of chronic urticaria.

KEY FEATURES

- Physical urticarias are those provoked by physical stim-uli. These include hot and cold temperatures, increased body tempera-ture, contact with water or light, physical pressure, vibration, and exercise.

- Reactions are brief, often lasting around 60 minutes.

- The exact mechanism is unknown.

- Therapy is similar to urticaria, with antihista-mines; often hydroxyzine orally is very helpful.

PATHOGENESIS

The exact mechanism of these various types of urticaria is unclear. It is believed that both mast cell activation and histamine release play a role, but why the physical contacts cause a reaction in some individuals is unknown.

CLINICAL PRESENTATION

Physical urticarias are summarized in Table 21-4. **Dermographism** is the most common physical urticaria. It presents as wheals that arise after mechanical shearing on the skin after activities such as scratching, stroking, or toweling. Pruritic wheals occur at sites of trauma (Fig. 21-2). The most common form of dermographism is symptomatic dermographism, which occurs within minutes after skin trauma. Wheals can last for a few hours. Delayed dermographism is rare, and presents as burning and deep swelling occurring 30 minutes to hours after skin trauma. Lesions do not last for more than 2 days.

Cholinergic urticaria is a fairly frequently occurring urticaria, which appears with a rise in core body temperature brought about by bathing, sweating, alcohol consumption, eating spicy foods, having intense emotions, or exercising. In min-utes, small papular wheals arise in a symmetric distribution (Fig. 21-3). Lesions often last for about 30 minutes and may be accompanied by angioedema, syncope, headaches, nausea, and abdominal pain.

Heat urticaria differs from cholinergic urticaria in that it develops after expo-sure to a localized source of heat. Another important differential diagnosis is exer-cise-induced urticaria or anaphylaxis. Here, the urticaria is due to physical exer-cise itself and not the rise in core temperature. Pruritic wheals arise during or after exercise and can last for hours. In cases of anaphylaxis, the individual may expe-rience compromised cardiorespiratory function, necessitating prompt evaluation.

Acquired **cold urticaria** arises from contact with a cold object or cold air. Localized pruritic wheals present within minutes of exposure. Rewarming may lead to pruritus and burning wheals. Headache, flushing, syncope, and abdom-inal pain may accompany the wheals.

Aquagenic urticaria arises after exposure to water. Onset is on the order of minutes, and lesions may develop up to 30 minutes after exposure. Papular pruritic wheals resembling those in cholinergic urticaria favor the upper body. Lesions disappear without further contact with water. It is important for patients with this condition to not swim alone. In rare cases, anaphylaxis has occurred while swimming.

CHAPTER 21 Urticaria

Table 21-4 Physical Urticarias

Type	TRIGGER	SKIN FINDINGS	CHALLENGE TESTING
Cholinergic urticaria	Increased core body temperature, e.g., bathing, exercising, emotions, spicy foods	Monomorphic papular pruritic wheals	Exercise, bathing
Heat urticaria	Contact with hot object	Pruritic wheals	Hot compress
Exercise-induced urticaria or anaphylaxis	Physical exercise	Pruritic wheals	Exercise testing, patients may experience cardiorespiratory compromise with anaphylaxis
Acquired cold urticaria	Contact with cold object or air	Pruritic wheals	Cold water, cold beaker, cold air
Aquagenic urticaria	Water contact	Monomorphic papular pruritic wheals	Water
Dermographic urticaria	Mechanical shearing forces, e.g., stroking, scratching	Pruritic wheals in areas of trauma	Stroking
Delayed pressure urticaria	Pressure	Localized edema and erythema	Weights
Solar urticaria	UV or visible light exposure	Pruritic wheals	Light
Contact urticaria	Direct contact with allergens, e.g., chemicals, foods, plants, medications, cosmetics	Pruritic wheals	Specific allergen
Vibratory urticaria	Vibration	Angioedema	Vibration source

Delayed **pressure urticaria** presents as diffuse edema and erythema at points of pressure such as the buttocks and thighs after sitting, the feet after walking, the hands after carrying groceries, and under seat belts, waistbands, and bras. Symptoms can arise hours after the pressure occurs. Edema can last from 8 hours to 2 days. Sixty percent of cases are associated with chronic idiopathic urticaria. Individuals with delayed pressure urticaria are more likely to have delayed dermographism.

Solar urticaria arises after exposure to either ultraviolet radiation or visible light. Pruritic wheals arise within minutes of exposure and can last from minutes to several hours.

DIAGNOSIS

The classic wheals of urticaria are pruritic, well-circumscribed edematous, blanching pink plaques of variable size. Such pruritic wheals may be seen in cold, heat, exercise-induced, and solar urticaria. Cholinergic and aquagenic urticaria tend to present with pruritic monomorphic papular wheals (Fig. 21-3). Wheals of immediate dermographism follow the pattern of skin trauma. Pressure urticaria presents with diffuse tender edema and erythema in areas exposed to pressure.

Diagnostic Methods

In cases without clear identifiable triggers, additional tests may be helpful. To evaluate for cholinergic urticaria, the patient can be challenged with methacholine chloride injection, exercise, or a bath in hot water. To evaluate for heat urticaria, exposure to a warm compress can be used. For cold urticaria, exposure to cold water, a cold beaker, or cold air can tested. To evaluate for exercise-induced urticaria or anaphylaxis, exercise testing can be performed in a controlled environment. In anaphylaxis, the patient may present with cardiorespiratory compromise marked by wheezing and hypotension. To elicit dermographism, the skin can be scratched and then observed. Weights can be used to elicit pressure urticaria. Exposure to light can be used to evaluate for solar urticaria.

TREATMENT

If a trigger is identified, it should be avoided to prevent future episodes. After symptoms develop, antipruritic topical medications may be helpful.

Oral antihistamines and H2 blockers may be used (as discussed in the acute and chronic urticaria section). Often, the sedating H2 blocker hydroxyzine is quite helpful for both symptomatic relief as well as preventing further outbreaks. The nonsedating variant of hydroxyzine is cetirizine, which is often appropriate for daytime use. A regimen that is often helpful is to take cetirizine 10 mg every morning and hydroxyzine 25 mg at bedtime. An alternate to hydroxyzine is doxepin. In addition to its norepinephrine and serotonin reuptake inhibition, it has significant H2 blocking activity at very low doses. A common dose for pruritus and urticaria would be 10 mg at bedtime.

For heat and cold contact urticaria, desensitization can be attempted. In aquagenic urticaria, individuals can apply an oil barrier before exposure to water. In pressure urticaria, antihistamines are not helpful, but steroids may be helpful if avoidance of the trigger is not possible.

"AT A GLANCE" TREATMENT

- Identify and avoid triggers of the specific physical urticaria.
- Topical antipruritics (i.e., menthol/camphor-containing lotions [Sarna OTC], benzocaine or lidocaine creams, pramoxine)
- Oral antihistamines: first-line—cetirizine 10 mg every morning and hydroxyzine 25 mg at bedtime
- Heat and cold contact urticaria—desensitization can be attempted.
- Aquagenic urticaria—apply an oil barrier (i.e., white petrolatum) before exposure to water.
- Pressure urticaria:
  - Antihistamines are not helpful
  - Oral steroids may be helpful if avoidance of the trigger is not possible.

COURSE AND COMPLICATIONS

The clinical course of individual lesions varies depending on the specific trigger. Avoidance of the trigger is crucial in preventing further episodes.

ICD9 Codes	
708.9	Unspecified urticaria
287.0	Allergic purpura

WHEN TO REFER

Patients who need desensitization or are unresponsive to treatment may be referred to a dermatologist or allergist.

NOT TO BE MISSED

- Anaphylaxis, including exercise-induced anaphylaxis.
- C1 esterase inhibitor deficiency.
- Urticarial vasculitis/urticarial syndrome.

Suggested Reading

Greaves M. Chronic urticaria. *J Allergy Clin Immunol.* 2000;85:521–544.

Guerra L, Rogkakou A, Massacane P, et al. Role of contact sensitization in chronic urticaria. *J Am Acad Dermatol.* 2007;56(1):88–90.

Guldbakke KK, Khachemoune A. Etiology, classification, and treatment of urticaria. *Cutis.* 2007;79:41–49.

LaShell MS, Tankersley MS, Kobayashi M. Cold urticaria: A case report and review of the literature. *Cutis.* 2005;76:257–260.

Linscott, MS. Urticaria. Available at: http://emedicine.medscape.com/article/762917-overview. Accessed May 12, 2009.

Negro-Alvarez JM, Miralles-Lopez JC. Chronic idiopathic urticaria treatment. *Allergol Immunopathol (Madr).* 2001;29:129–132.

Varadarajulu S. Urticaria and angioedema: Controlling acute episodes, coping with chronic cases. *Postgraduate Medicine.* 2005;117:25–31.

Zuberbier T, Maurer M. Urticaria: Current opinions about etiology, diagnosis and therapy. *Acta Derm Venereol.* 2007;87:196–205.

CHAPTER 22 Ultraviolet Light Reactions

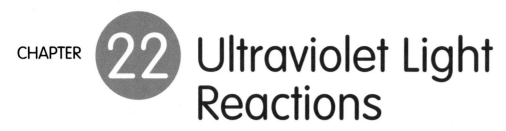

My-Linh T. Nguyen

Sunburn is acute inflammation of the skin in response to ultraviolet (UV) damage. Its characteristic erythema and pain are well known to many patients. Sunburns present a problem not only because of their immediate symptomatology, but also because they are a marker of excessive sun exposure and thus cancer risk. Patients with a history of sunburn carry a twofold relative risk of developing melanoma versus patients with no sunburn history. Treatment for sunburns involves symptomatic relief, fluid replacement, prophylaxis for possible infection, and preventative counseling.

There are many other reactions to the sun that may mimic sunburn or have more of an eczematous nature. Commonly encountered conditions would include polymorphous light reaction, photoallergic contact dermatitis, and phytophotodermatitis. These will be discussed in further detail.

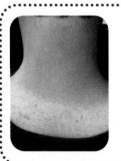

A 23-year-old white man presents with sharply demarcated, uniform erythema with pain on his neck (Fig. 22-1). History reveals that he had been skiing earlier in the day. What is the most likely diagnosis? How should he be treated? What counseling should he be given?

KEY FEATURES

- Sunburn is caused by excessive UV radiation causing delayed, sharply demarcated, uniform edema in exposed skin with possible pain, pruritus, edema, and vesicles/bullae.

- Predisposing factors include: light skin, light hair, and photosensitizing medications.

(Continued)

Sunburn

BACKGROUND/EPIDEMIOLOGY

For lighter-skinned individuals, most have experienced sunburn as a result of prolonged sunlight exposure. In the United States, 30% to 40% of adults and 83% of children report at least one sunburn in the preceding year. Individuals with darker skin types are less likely to burn, but occasionally may experience sunburn while on a photosensitizing medication or in some cases as a result of a systemic illness that includes photosensitivity. In general, sunburns are classified as a superficial or first-degree burn. Sunburns are more common in men and, in general, children are burned more frequently than adults.

PATHOGENESIS

The exact mechanisms leading to the sunburn reaction are not fully known. Current evidence suggests that UV irradiation leads to cutaneous vasodilation, causing erythema, edema, and neutrophilic infiltration. UVB radiation causes apoptosis through a variety of pathways, including DNA mutagenesis, direct activation of membrane-bound death receptors, and generation of intracellular reactive oxygen species.

KEY FEATURES (Continued)

- Treatment:
  - Symptomatic therapy (cold compress, moisturizing lotion, nonsteroidal anti-inflammatory drugs [NSAIDs], corticosteroids).
  - Fluid replacement.
  - Infection prophylaxis (topical antibiotic if vesicles/bullae present).
  - Sun avoidance during healing.
  - Preventative counseling.

Table 22-1 Fitzpatrick's Skin Phototypes

SKIN TYPE	BASELINE COLOR BEFORE SUN EXPOSURE	RESPONSE TO SUN EXPOSURE AS ESTIMATED BY PATIENT
I	Pale white	Does not tan; burns easily
II	White	Tans with difficulty; burns easily
III	White to olive	Tans gradually; burns minimally
IV	Light brown	Tans easily; burns minimally
V	Brown	Tans easily; rarely burns
VI	Black	Becomes darker; never burns

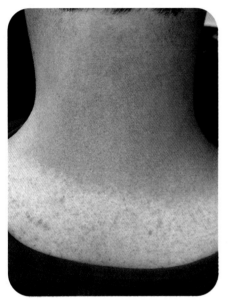

Figure 22-1 Acute sunburn on the neck. Note the sharp cutoff where the shirt protected the skin.

CLINICAL PRESENTATION

Manifestation

The presentation of sunburn can range from mild (sharply demarcated, uniform erythema on sun-exposed areas with sparing of covered skin [Fig. 22-1]) to severe (erythema accompanied by edema, vesicles, bullae, pain, and/or pruritus). Erythema typically arises 6 hours after sun exposure, peaks at 12 to 24 hours, and resolves after 72 hours. In severe cases, fever, fatigue, headache, and tachycardia may be present.

History and Risk Factors

- UV exposure: the amount of UV exposure correlates with severity of sunburn. Low latitude, high altitude, and midday exposure (11 AM to 4 PM) represent the greatest risk for skin damage. Sunburns can occur on cloudy days, as UV radiation penetrates cloud cover, and in the shade, because UV can reflect off of snow, water, and concrete to reach skin.
- Skin type: the Fitzpatrick skin phototypes scale (Table 22-1) classifies skin based on its baseline color and reaction to sun exposure. Skin types I and II are at greatest risk for sunburns.
- Hair color: lighter hair such as blonde, red, or light brown is associated with increased risk of sunburns.
- Photosensitizing medications: summarized in Table 22-2.

Table 22-2 Medications Associated With Photosensitivity

Amiodarone	Psoralens
Antifungals (itraconazole, voriconazole)	Quinolones
Diltiazem	Retinoids (isotretinoin, acitretin)
Furosemide	Sulfonylureas (glipizide, glyburide)
NSAIDs (ibuprofen, diclofenac, piroxicam, naproxen)	Tetracyclines (tetracycline/doxycycline)
Phenothiazines	Thiazides

Table 22-3 Differential Diagnosis of Sunburn Reactions

CONDITION	NOTES
Systemic lupus erythematosus	Obtain antinuclear antibody (ANA) level if suspected. Often presents as malar ("butterfly") rash.
Drug-induced photosensitivity	Reaction may be more severe with limited sun exposure. History reveals exposure to photosensitizing drugs or other chemicals. See Table 22-2 for a summary of important causes of photosensitivity. Systemic photosensitizing drugs cause an exaggerated sunburn reaction in all areas of sun-exposed skin, whereas topical drugs cause the reaction in areas where the drug was applied.
Photoallergic contact dermatitis	Occurs due to reaction between a topically applied products (such as sunscreen) which is modified by UV exposure, subsequently causing a delayed type hypersensitivity
Phototoxic reaction	Most commonly caused by plant exposures, as discussed in the following section.
Polymorphous light eruption	Presents as rash rather than uniform erythema.
Solar urticaria	Wheals/erythema after minutes of sun exposure
Xeroderma pigmentosum	Presents in early childhood after minimal sun exposure.
Erythropoietic protoporphyria	Rare autosomal dominant disease that presents in early childhood after minimal sun exposure.

DIAGNOSIS

Diagnosis is relatively straightforward given a history of recent sun exposure and physical exam showing characteristic skin reaction in sun-exposed areas.

- History: UV exposure 3 to 6 hours before onset of erythema
- Physical exam:
  - Skin: uniform erythema in sun-exposed areas with sharp demarcation versus nonexposed areas. In severe sunburn, erythema may be accompanied by edema, vesicles, and bullae.
  - General: in severe cases, fever, malaise, and rapid pulse may be present.
  - Mucous membranes: rarely, tongue may be sunburned if mouth is open during physical activity

The differential diagnosis of sunburn reactions is broad. Causes range simply from prolonged UV exposure to systemic illnesses, which cause increased sensitivity to the sun. This differential is summarized in Table 22-3.

TREATMENT

Sunburn is managed through symptomatic treatment, fluid replacement, prophylaxis for infection if needed, and avoidance of sun exposure during recovery. Currently, there are no recommended therapies that significantly shorten recovery time or reduce epithelial injury.

For hyperpigmentation following phytophotodermatitis, hydroquinone 4% cream may be useful in lightening the dark pigment.

Symptomatic Treatment

- The patient may find moisturizing lotion, aloe vera gel, cool water soaks, and/or cold compresses helpful in relieving discomfort.
- Topical or oral NSAIDs decrease erythema if used before or immediately after UV exposure, but their benefits drop off 24 hours after UV exposure. One exception is topical diclofenac 0.1% gel (5 mg/cm^2), which, when applied 6 and 10 hours after UV exposure, can relieve pain and erythema for up to 48 hours.

- Topical corticosteroids may boost the benefits of NSAIDs if applied shortly after UV exposure. They do not provide clinically significant benefit after 30 hours post-UV exposure or when used without NSAIDs.
- Antihistamines are *not* recommended, as they have not been shown to produce clinically significant benefits.
- Although there is little published evidence documenting the efficacy of topical anesthetics in sunburn, some patients may find relief with agents such as benzocaine. Benzocaine may cause allergic contact dermatitis.

Fluid replacement: oral rehydration is recommended to compensate for increased fluid loss through the injured skin.

Infection prophylaxis: if vesicles/bullae are present, a topical antibiotic such as silver sulfadiazine or bacitracin may be used to decrease the risk of infection.

Sun avoidance during healing: further sun exposure should be avoided for 1 to 2 weeks, as the injured skin is more susceptible to sunburns during this time. See "Prevention" below.

"AT A GLANCE" THERAPY

Symptomatic Treatment

- Moisturizing lotion, aloe vera gel, cool water soaks, and/or cold compresses
- Topical (diclofenac 0.1% gel applied 6 and 10 hours after UV exposure) or oral NSAIDs
- Topical corticosteroids should be used in conjunction with topical NSAIDs
- Antihistamines produce clinically significant benefits.
- Although there is little published evidence documenting the efficacy of topical anesthetics in sunburn, some patients may find relief with agents such as benzocaine. Benzocaine use may cause allergic contact dermatitis.

Prevention

To avoid further sunburns as well as to reduce chronic sun damage and cancer risk, UV exposure should be limited using the following techniques:

- Avoid sun exposure between 10 AM to 4 PM, and especially between 11 AM to 2 PM. This should be done even on cloudy days, as UV radiation penetrates cloud cover.
- Wear sunglasses, a wide-brimmed hat, and dark, loose-fitting clothing.
- Wear sunscreen with at least an SPF (sun protection factor) of 30. SPF is the factor by which a substance prolongs the minimal duration of UV exposure required to produce erythema. If a patient normally develops erythema after 10 minutes of exposure, for instance, then with SPF-15 sunscreen, he/she would theoretically develop erythema after 150 minutes of UV exposure. However, this is an overestimate, as most people significantly under-apply sunscreen (recommended application is 2 mg/cm^2 or 30 to 35 mL/body application) and realistically achieve only 20% to 50% of the expected SPF. Sunscreen should be applied 15 to 30 minutes before sun exposure and re-applied every 2 to 3 hours.
- Oral and topical antioxidants such as vitamins A, C, and E help protect against sunburns. However, antioxidants should be used in conjunction with sunscreen, not as a replacement.
- Although tanning through gradual sun exposure or tanning beds can decrease the risk of sunburn, it is *not* recommended as a preventative technique, because tanning may not prevent chronic sun damage and skin cancer and may carry its own negative risks. Artificial "sunless" tanning uses dyes to give the appearance of tanned skin and does not confer sunburn protection.

COURSE AND COMPLICATIONS

- Rupturing of vesicles and bullae can lead to infection.
- Severe sunburns can damage melanocytes, leading to mottled depigmentation, or induce melanocyte proliferation, causing solar lentigines.
- Sunburns are a marker of excessive UV exposure and indicate increased risk of dermatoheliosis, actinic keratoses, and skin cancer. A history of sunburn confers a 2.0 relative risk of developing melanoma versus no sunburn history.

ICD9 Codes	
692.71	Sunburn
692.72	Acute dermatitis due to solar radiation
692.72	Acute dermatitis due to solar radiation

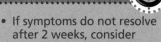

WHEN TO REFER

- If symptoms do not resolve after 2 weeks, consider consulting a dermatologist.
- When the eyes are affected, consider ophthalmology consultation.

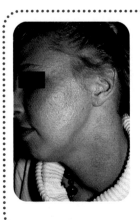

A 44-year-old woman complains of a rash following a trip to the beach. She is taking piroxicam for knee pain. Her forehead, cheeks, and neck are erythematous and edematous (Fig. 22-2). She is surprised that the moderate amount of sun she received yesterday could have caused such a severe reaction. She has a long history of hypertension, and was started on furosemide a few weeks ago.

KEY FEATURES

- *Phototoxic and photoallergic* reactions to UV radiation, which occur in the presence of an exogenous agent. The agent absorbs UV radiation to cause the skin reaction. Phototoxic lesions represent tissue injury *directly inflicted* by the agent, whereas photoallergic lesions are *immune reactions* against the agent.

- *Presentation:*

  - *Phototoxicity:* patient is exposed to a phototoxin and then exposed to the sun. Minutes to hours later, *painful, sunburn-like* lesions arise in photodistributed areas.

(Continued)

Phototoxic and Photoallergic Dermatitis

BACKGROUND/EPIDEMIOLOGY

Exogenous agents can cause UV skin reactions through either the phototoxic or photoallergic pathway. Almost 400 different drugs can act as phototoxins, photoallergens, or both. Of the many known agents, only a few are frequently found to cause UV skin reactions (Tables 22-4, 22-5). The actual incidence of phototoxicity and photoallergy in the general population is not known, but phototoxicity is, in general, more common than photoallergy. While both conditions can result from systemic or topical agents, phototoxicity is more often caused by systemic agents (usually oral medications), while photoallergy is more often caused by topical agents (sunscreens, fragrances, topical NSAIDs). There is no association with gender or age. Unsurprisingly, lighter skin types are more susceptible to developing phototoxic dermatitis, as they are to developing ordinary sunburns.

PATHOGENESIS

In phototoxic dermatitis, the phototoxin, upon reaction with UV radiation, acquires the ability to inflict cell damage through mechanisms such as generating reactive oxygen species, cross-linking DNA, or activating complement. Ultimately, these injuries lead to cell death. Because the phototoxin itself injures the skin, phototoxic reactions are dose dependent, and a significant amount of toxin is required to produce a clinically evident lesion.

In photoallergic dermatitis, absorption of UV radiation by the photoallergen (a hapten) allows it to conjugate with a carrier protein, producing a complete, T-cell recognizable antigen. The antigen is taken up by Langerhans cells and brought to regional lymph nodes. Should the patient possess T-cells that specifically recognize this antigen, an immune reaction is launched. Initial exposure to an allergen may yield a weak, clinically imperceptible reaction. However, clonal expansion and memory cell production allow subsequent exposures to induce stronger type-IV hypersensitivity responses, yielding

KEY FEATURES (Continued)

- *Photoallergy*: a patient is exposed to a photoallergen and then to the sun. One to two days later, a *pruritic, eczematous rash* arises in areas exposed to both the allergen and the sun.

- Phototoxicity is more common than photoallergy, as it can occur in anyone given a sufficient dose of phototoxin and UV radiation.

- Photoallergy is idiosyncratic, only occurring in individuals who possess immune recognition for a photoallergen and who are subsequently sensitized to it by repeat exposure.

- *Diagnosis*: by history and exam. Additionally, phototesting and photopatch testing can help identify the causative agent, distinguish phototoxicity from ordinary sunburn, or distinguish photoallergy from contact dermatitis.

- *Treatment*: identify and discontinue the offending drug/agent. UV protection. Treat symptoms if necessary.

Table 22-4 Common Phototoxic Agents

TOPICAL AGENTS	Rose bengal	Eye drops used in ophthalmologic exams
	Tar	Roofing and roadwork materials
	Plants containing furocoumarins ("phytophoto-dermatitis")	• Limes, lemons • Celery • Carrots • Parsley • Parsnips • Figs • Burning bush (red berries appear only in the fall) • Pomelo (large citrus fruit native to Asia)
SYSTEMIC AGENTS	Antimicrobial drugs	• Antifungal: griseofulvin • Antibacterial: quinolones, sulfonamides, tetracyclines • Antimalarial: chloroquine, quinine
	Cardiac drugs	Amiodarone, quinidine
	Chemotherapeutic drugs	Dacarbazine, fluorouracil, methotrexate, vinblastine
	Dermatologic drugs	Isoretinoin, psoralens
	Diuretics	Furosemide, thiazides
	NSAIDs	Diclofenac, piroxicam, naproxen, nabumetone (Relafen, often used in rheumatoid arthritis)
	Psychiatric drugs	• Anxiolytics: alprazolam, chlorpromazine • Tricyclic antidepressants: amitriptyline, desipramine, imipramine • Antipsychotics: chlorpromazine, prochlorperazine
	Plants	• St. John's wort (hypericin) • Excessive ingestion of any of the plants listed under topical agents above

cutaneous lesions within 24 to 48 hours. Thus, in sensitized patients, even a tiny amount of photoallergen can cause a clinically significant lesion. In both phototoxic and photoallergic dermatitis, the action spectrum (type of UV radiation responsible for producing symptoms) is mostly UVA (wavelength 315 to 400 nm).

Table 22-5 Common Photoallergic Agents

TOPICAL AGENTS	Sunscreens	Those containing benzophenones, PABA, or cinnamates
	Fragrances	Those containing musk ambrette, sandalwood oil, or 6-methylcoumarin
	NSAIDs	Ketoprofen, diclofenac
SYSTEMIC AGENTS	Antimicrobial drugs	• Antifungal: griseofulvin • Antibacterial: quinolones, sulfonamides • Antimalarial: quinine
	Cardiac drugs	Quinidine
	NSAIDs	Ketoprofen, piroxicam
	Vitamins	B6

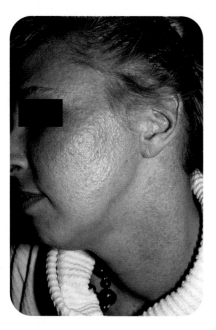

Figure 22-2 Photoallergic dermatitis on the face of a woman taking piroxicam following a trip to the beach. From Goodheart HP. *Goodheart's Photoguide to Common Skin Disorders*, 3rd ed. Philadelphia: Lippincott Williams & Wilkins, 2009.

CLINICAL PRESENTATION

History

Exposure history: history may reveal exposure to an agent from Tables 22-4 or 22-5. Inquire about oral and topical medications, skin products (sunscreen, perfumed products), eye drops or recent eye exams, contact with or ingestion of fruits or other plants, and occupational exposure to tar. Phototoxic reactions are dependent on toxin dose, while photoallergic reactions can arise from even minimal allergen exposure.

When did the skin lesions occur? Phototoxic lesions arise minutes to hours after sun exposure. Photoallergic lesions are caused by delayed-type hypersensitivity reactions and thus arise 1 to 2 days after sun exposure.

Are the lesions pruritic or painful? Phototoxic lesions burn or sting. Photoallergic lesions itch.

Exam

Distribution: lesions should be confined to photoexposed skin, sparing shaded regions such as the nasolabial folds or the submental area. Widespread lesions across photoexposed areas suggest a systemic phototoxin or photoallergen, while bizarrely shaped distributions suggest a topical agent.

Appearance: phototoxicity usually yields sunburn-like lesions (affected skin is erythematous and edematous, and may form vesicles/bullae in severe reactions). More rarely, phototoxicity can simply yield a blue-gray coloring to photodistributed areas; this is called "slate gray pigmentation," and can be caused by the phototoxins amiodarone, chlorpromazine, or diltiazem. Additionally, phototoxicity can mimic the lesions of the metabolic disease porphyria cutanea tarda. This presentation is called "pseudoporphyria" and can be caused by phototoxins such as furosemide or NSAIDs. Here, bullae develop on affected skin, often on the dorsal surface of hands. When the bullae rupture, erosions are left behind that scar with healing. Affected skin is quite fragile, and can become denuded with minor trauma. Milia (tiny white papules) can also develop following bulla/erosion healing. Photoallergic lesions resemble eczema (erythematous, scaly, sometimes crusty plaques/papules).

DIAGNOSIS

Diagnosis is usually clinical, by history and full skin exam as above. The differential diagnosis is summarized in Table 22-6.

Phototesting can help identify systemic phototoxins and photoallergens. Measuring the MED (minimal erythema dose, the lowest dose of UV radiation that yields erythema at the irradiated skin site 24 hours later) while the patient is on the culprit drug/agent yields a low value. If UVA and UVB radiation are tested separately, the MED is decreased for UVA but may be normal for UVB. Repeat testing once the drug is excreted yields a higher MED.

Photopatch testing can help identify topical photoallergens. In this test, topical agents are applied in identical configurations to two sites on the body. One site is irradiated with UVA. Reaction at the irradiated site but not the other site confirms photoallergy. Reaction at both sites suggests allergic contact dermatitis not requiring sun exposure.

Skin biopsy may be helpful. Phototoxic lesions show apoptotic or necrotic keratinocytes (similar to ordinary sunburn). Photoallergic lesions show spongiosis (intercellular edema between keratinocytes) and a prominent lymphocytic infiltrate; these features are also seen in allergic contact dermatitis.

Table 22-6 Differential Diagnosis of Phototoxic and Photoallergic Dermatitis

CONDITION	RESEMBLES	CHARACTERISTICS
Sunburn	Phototoxicity	Requires larger dose of UV radiation to develop, as there is no phototoxin to act as a photosensitizer. MED often normal.
Porphyria cutanea tarda	Phototoxicity (pseudoporphyria)	Elevated plasma porphyrin level
Toxic/irritant contact dermatitis	Phototoxicity from topical agent	Affects sun-protected skin as well
Allergic contact dermatitis	Photoallergy from topical agent	Affects sun-protected skin as well
Airborne allergic contact dermatitis	Photoallergy from systemic agent	Can affect exposed but sun-protected areas such as nasolabial folds or submental area. Normal MED
Chronic actinic dermatitis	Photoallergy	Lichenified plaques induced by UVA, UVB, and even visible light. No exogenous agent necessary. Lesions may be chronic. May have long history of recurrent phototoxic or photoallergic dermatitis, but skin lesions now arise in absence of inducing agent. More common in elderly men.
Polymorphic light eruption	Both	No exogenous-inducing agent
Solar urticaria	Both	Develops within minutes of sun exposure and rapidly disappears with termination of exposure.

TREATMENT

- Identify and discontinue exposure to the inducing agent. Phototesting can help identify systemic agents, while photopatch testing can help identify topical photoallergens.
- UV protection. Counsel patients to use sunscreens that have an SPF of at least 30, broad-spectrum UVA and UVB coverage, and ingredients such as ecamsule or avobenzone that further enhance UVA protection. Additionally, wearing a wide-brimmed hat and dark, loose clothing while outdoors and keeping a distance from windows while indoors can help (UVA penetrates window glass).
- Symptomatic therapy. Cold compresses and topical steroids may help alleviate symptoms. Oral corticosteroids should only be used in severe cases.

COURSE AND COMPLICATIONS

- Most acute eruptions will resolve after discontinuing the inducing agent.
- Phototoxic lesions may desquamate as they resolve, and may leave behind hyperpigmentation that lasts months to years. The special presentations of phototoxicity (slate-gray pigmentation, pseudoporphyria) may resolve more slowly over months. Repeated phototoxic injury can predispose to premature photoaging and skin cancer.
- A small number of patients (5% to 10%) may develop an exquisite sensitivity to light that persists even after cessation of the inducing agent. This is called chronic actinic dermatitis, persistent light reaction, actinic reticuloid, or photosensitive eczema. It is more commonly seen in elderly men following a history of recurrent phototoxic, photoallergic, contact, or atopic dermatitis. In this condition, minimal exposure to UVA, UVB, and even visible light can induce pruritic, erythematous, lichenified plaques.

WHEN TO REFER

- The eruption does not improve 2 weeks after discontinuing the inducing agent.
- The identity of the inducing agent is unclear.
- The patient experiences severe or recurrent eruptions.
- New "moles" develop on affected skin.

ICD9 Codes

692.72	Acute dermatitis due to solar radiation
693.0	Dermatitis due to drugs and medicines taken internally
692.71	Sunburn
708.9	Urticaria, unspecified

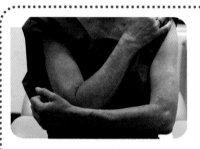

A 20-year-old woman presents with small, erythematous papules on the extensor surface of both upper arms in early spring (Fig. 22-3). There is associated pruritus. She is wearing a t-shirt and comments that she has been enjoying the newly warm weather. She had a similar rash last year that disappeared on its own.

Polymorphous Light Eruption

BACKGROUND/EPIDEMIOLOGY

Sometimes called "sun poisoning," polymorphous light eruption (PMLE) affects 10% of North Americans. Possibly due to the phenomenon of "hardening," the prevalence of PMLE increases with distance from the equator, ranging from an estimated less than 1% in Singapore to 21% in Sweden. Eruptions are more common in the spring or early summer. PMLE preferentially affects young patients younger than 30 years of age and females two to three times more often than males. While more common among fair-skinned patients, it can affect all skin types. A positive family history is found in approximately 15% of cases, but no associated single gene locus has yet been identified.

PATHOGENESIS

While the pathogenesis of PMLE is still incompletely understood, evidence suggests that it may result from a delayed-type hypersensitivity reaction to UV-modified auto-antigens. Histologic examination of affected skin lesions demonstrates an inflammatory infiltrate dominated by T cells, primarily CD4+ cells within hours after UV exposure and CD8+ cells within days of exposure. Both UVA (wavelength 315 to 400 nm) and UVB (280 to 315 nm) radiation can cause the symptoms of PMLE, but UVA seems to be more effective. Because UV radiation is known to have immunosuppressive effects, periods of frequent UV exposure may eventually reduce inflammation, possibly explaining the "hardening" phenomenon observed in PMLE.

KEY FEATURES

- Polymorphous light eruption (PMLE) is a cutaneous rash in response to UV radiation, possibly autoimmune in nature.

- Presents with pruritic, erythematous rash (papular, papulovesicular, or plaques) on photoexposed areas starting hours after sun exposure and lasting 7 to 10 days.

- Rash often occurs in spring or early summer of each year, triggered by patient's first significant episode of sun exposure after a prolonged period of low exposure.

(Continued)

CLINICAL PRESENTATION

History

Symptoms typically occur in the setting of intense UV exposure after a prolonged period of low exposure (i.e., during spring or early summer, while vacationing in a sunny locale, after tanning bed use). Risk factors include age less than 30, female sex, light skin, family history, and primary residency at a northern latitude. Patients may have history of similar rashes. Recurrent eruptions of PMLE tend to have the same appearance and general distribution as prior eruptions. Rarely, systemic symptoms may occur including malaise, fever/chills, headache, and nausea.

Dermatitis develops within 30 minutes to days after sun exposure. Associated pruritus may be present. Rash can affect any sun-exposed area, but sometimes prefers areas that were previously covered (i.e., trunk, arms, legs) while sparing areas that receive more constant sun exposure (face or neck). In

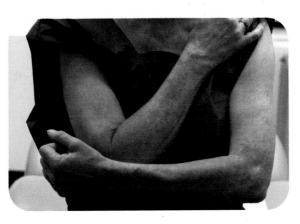

Figure 22-3 Polymorphous light eruption. Note the sharp cutoff on the upper arms.

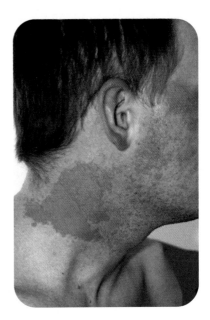

Figure 22-4 Papulovesicular polymorphous light eruption.

KEY FEATURES (*Continued*)

- Risk factors:
  - Northern latitude (long "winter" periods of low sun exposure).
  - Young, age <30.
  - Female.
  - Light skin.
  - Positive family history.
  - Exclude SLE, erythropoietic protoporphyria, and solar urticaria.

a subtype of PMLE termed "juvenile spring eruption," the rash affects helices of the ears in young children, usually boys. With avoidance of UV radiation, the rash resolves without scarring in 7 to 10 days.

"Hardening" may be observed, whereby continuous UV exposure gradually reduces the frequency/severity of eruptions, such that lesions may disappear by late summer (however, with interruption of UV exposure during the winter months, symptoms often recur the following spring).

Exam

Photodistributed, symmetric dermatitis is the most common appearance (Fig. 22-3). The skin lesions are erythematous and take on one of many possible appearances (hence the name "polymorphous"). The three most common forms are papular, papulovesicular (Fig. 22-4), and plaques. More rarely, rashes can be vesiculobullous or resemble insect bites or erythema multiforme. The rashes of an individual patient will usually take on one consistent form rather than be a combination of multiple forms. There is no known difference in prognosis between the various rash morphologies.

DIAGNOSIS

- Diagnosis is usually clinical, by history and examination as above.
- Differential diagnosis: see Table 22-7. Importantly, SLE, erythropoietic protoporphyria, and solar urticaria should be excluded.
- Skin biopsy is helpful but not diagnostic. Negative direct immunofluorescence (staining for presence of immunoreactants such as IgG or IgM deposited in skin) helps exclude SLE.
- Standard phototesting is not particularly useful, and may reveal a normal or decreased MED (minimal erythema dose, the lowest dose of UV radiation that will cause erythema at the irradiated skin site 24 hours postexposure).
- Provocative phototesting can help confirm the diagnosis of PMLE. Normal-appearing skin sites are irradiated daily for 7 to 10 days with increasing doses of UV radiation. The diagnosis is confirmed when irradiation produces lesions similar to those of the patient's original rash. However, note that sensitivity is poor, and testing will be positive in only about 50% of PMLE cases.

Table 22-7 Differential Diagnosis of Polymorphous Light Eruption

CONDITION	NOTES
Systemic lupus erythematosus	Cutaneous lesions can mimic PMLE (subacute cutaneous lupus can yield erythematous papules/plaques like those of PMLE; malar rash can resemble PMLE facial rash). If suspicion exists, obtain ANA, SSA, and SSB titers.
Erythropoietic protoporphyria	Rare autosomal dominant disease that typically presents in early childhood. In contrast to PMLE, skin lesions are painful, and scar with healing. If suspicion exists, obtain erythrocyte protoporphyrin levels.
Solar urticaria	Wheals/erythema appear within minutes of sun exposure and rapidly disappear with termination of exposure.
Phototoxic dermatitis	History reveals exposure to drug/chemical or plants listed in Table 22-4. Lesions are painful rather than pruritic.
Photoallergic dermatitis	History reveals exposure to drug/chemical listed in Table 22-5. Photo-patch testing can help elucidate diagnosis.
Xeroderma pigmentosum	Recessive trait; cellular DNA repair defect. Presents in early childhood after minimal sun exposure with multiple skin cancers, lentigines, photosensitivity, and early skin aging.

TREATMENT

Therapy is indicated when the patient desires treatment. Aside from cosmetic concerns, symptoms such as intense pruritus may be especially bothersome. Treatment may be offered in the following suggested order:

1. Decreased UV exposure. Patient should be counseled to avoid sun exposure and to wear a wide-brimmed hat and dark, loose-fitting clothing. A sunscreen should be used that fulfills three criteria. First, it should have an SPF of at least 30. Second, it should have broad-spectrum UVA and UVB coverage. Third, it should contain either ecamsule (trade name Mexoryl SX) or avobenzone, ingredients that specifically enhance UVA protection.

2. Basic symptom management. Patients may find symptomatic relief with over-the-counter NSAIDs, hydrocortisone lotion, or cold compresses.

3. Topical corticosteroids. For treatment of mild PMLE eruptions. Class VI to VII steroids (desonide 0.05% cream BID) should be used for facial lesions, while more potent class II–IV (triamcinolone 0.1% or mometasone 0.1% cream BID) steroids may be used elsewhere. These topicals can be combined with phototherapy.

4. Systemic corticosteroids. Appropriate for treatment or prophylaxis of acute, *infrequent* PMLE eruptions such as those that arise during vacation travel. Prednisolone 20 to 30 mg PO daily for 4 to 5 days at first onset of symptoms (for prophylaxis, give 2 days before starting sun exposure followed by another 2 days) can decrease the duration of pruritus and rash. Given side effects of systemic steroid use, treatment course should not be repeated more often that every few months.

5. Phototherapy. Appropriate for prophylaxis in patients who experience frequent eruptions each spring/summer despite adequate sun protection. Phototherapy is given early each spring, with the goal of inducing "hardening" before the symptomatic season begins. Treatments are typically three times a week for 5 to 6 weeks with either PUVA (UVA irradiation combined with psoralens, an oral UV-sensitizing agent) or narrow-band UVB irradiation (311 nm). Both have similar efficacy, but given lower cost and better safety profile of narrow-band UVB, it is emerging as the preferred option.

6. Drugs with low or uncertain efficacy. These drugs have demonstrated only mild benefit or have shown benefit in only small or uncontrolled trials.

• Consider consulting a dermatologist:
  • If the dermatitis does not resolve after 2 weeks of sun avoidance.
  • Treatment with first-line therapy (UV avoidance, topical corticosteroids) fails to improve symptoms.
  • Skin lesions involve significant blistering with or without mucous membrane involvement.

a. Nicotinamide. 2 to 3 g taken daily before sun exposure.
b. Beta-carotene. 60 mg TID × 2 weeks before starting sun exposure.
c. Antimalarial drugs. Hydroxychloroquine 400 mg daily (maximum 6.5 mg/kg lean body weight daily). Given ocular toxicity of the drug, baseline testing of visual acuity with close follow-up is recommended.
d. Omega-3 polyunsaturated fatty acids (PUFAs). Dietary supplementation with fish oil capsules totaling 10 g daily of mixed omega-3 PUFAs.
e. Antioxidants. Topical preparations containing vitamin E may be helpful, and can boost the efficacy of sunscreen use.

COURSE AND COMPLICATIONS

• The course of PMLE is chronic and recurrent. Eruptions tend to recur annually in early spring or summer, with resolution by late summer. Severity may increase or decrease with each year, and symptoms may spontaneously disappear. In a study following 114 PMLE patients over 7 years, 57% experienced relief of symptoms over that period, and 11% were asymptomatic throughout the final 2 years of the study.

• Typical PMLE lesions tend to resolve without scarring. Complications arise from side effects of treatment, and can include skin cancer with phototherapy, or skin atrophy and systemic side effects with corticosteroids.

ICD9 Code

692.72   *Acute dermatitis due to solar radiation*

Suggested Reading

Brown TT, Quain RD, Troxel AB, et al. The epidemiology of sunburn in the US population in 2003. *J Am Acad Dermatol.* 2006;55:577–583.

Han A, Maibach HI. Management of acute sunburn. *Am J Clin Dermatol.* 2004;5:39–47.

Khoo SW, Tay YK, Tham SN. Photodermatoses in a Singapore skin referral centre. *Clin Exp Dermatol.* 1996;21(4):263–268.

Lee PA, Freeman S. Photosensitivity: The 9-year experience at a Sydney contact dermatitis clinic. *Australas J Dermatol.* 2002;43(4):289–292.

Ling TC, Gibbs NK, Rhodes LE. Treatment of polymorphic light eruption. *Photodermatol Photoimmunol Photomed.* 2003;19(5):217–227.

Magnus IA. Studies with a monochromator in the common idiopathic photodermatoses. *Br J Dermatol.* 1964;76:245–264.

Mastalier U, Kerl H, Wolf P. Clinical, laboratory, phototest and phototherapy findings in polymorphic light eruptions: A retrospective study of 133 patients. *Eur J Dermatol.* 1998;8(8):554–559.

Morison W, Marwaha S, Beck L. PUVA-induced phototoxicity: Incidence and causes. *J Am Acad Dermatol.* 1997;36(2):183–186.

Ofori, AO. Polymorphous light eruption. In: *UpToDate,* Basow, DS (Ed), UpToDate, Waltham, MA, 2009.

Saraiya M, Hall HI, Uhler RJ. Sunburn prevalence among adults in the United States, 1999. *Am J Prev Med.* 2002;23:91–97.

Sunburn prevalence among adults—United States, 1999, 2003, and 2004. *MMWR Morb Mortal Wkly Rep.* 2007;56:524–528.

23 Bullous Diseases

Ilka A. Netravali and James Y.T. Wang

The skin has adhesion molecules that anchor keratinocytes to one another and to the underlying basement membrane, partly to resist mechanical trauma. Many of these molecules are targets of autoantibodies in blistering skin diseases. These autoimmune bullous diseases are divided into two major categories, depending on whether the blistering is intraepidermal (pemphigus) or subepidermal (pemphigoid). Blistering reactions also occur as a reaction to infection or drug exposure, with the most concerning presentation being that of fulminant toxic epidermal necrolysis (TEN).

While these disorders have been of the target of intense laboratory research, and mechanisms of their pathogenesis have become clearer, these conditions remain difficult to manage as their treatment necessitates the use of relatively high doses of systemic corticosteroids and immunosuppressive agents. From the perspective of a primary health care provider, these dermatoses have three unique and critical dimensions. First, they are exceedingly rare, and the diagnosis can be easily missed without a high index of suspicion. Second, access to the required diagnostic tests is readily available in the United States, and any delay in assessment and management is unjustified. This is particularly important because early diagnosis customarily results in rapid improvement and better prognosis. Third, these diseases are often better handled by specialized dermatologists with extensive experience in their diagnosis and management. The treating clinician may perform a great service by referring the patient to the closest immunodermatology expert who has a focused interest in vesiculobullous diseases.

A wide variety of autoimmune bullous dermatoses exists, but this section will focus on the two most etiologically relevant members of the pemphigus and pemphigoid classes of diseases, respectively: pemphigus vulgaris and bullous pemphigoid. Erythema multiforme and the Stevens-Johnson syndrome/toxic epidermal necrolysis spectrum will also be covered in separate sections.

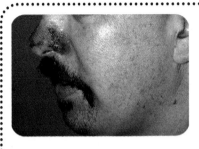

A 49-year-old white man was referred to a dermatologist with a 5-month history of a bullous disorder. The patient initially presented to his internist with gingival and buccal erosions; occasional flaccid blisters, crusted papules, and plaques involving the scalp, back, face, and chest were also noted (Fig. 23-1). A diagnosis of pemphigus vulgaris was made when indirect immunofluorescence testing revealed IgG deposits on the surface of keratinocytes. The patient initially failed to respond to systemic prednisone and azathioprine but ultimately responded to cyclophosphamide. Metastatic carcinoma (primary unknown) was diagnosed 6 months later (approximately 18 months after presentation) and, despite chemotherapy, the patient died.

Pemphigus Vulgaris

BACKGROUND

Pemphigus comprises a group of chronic, progressive autoimmune diseases that cause blistering and ulceration of the skin, mucous membranes, or both, loss of normal epithelial cell–cell adhesion (acantholysis), and the presence of pathogenic IgG autoantibodies directed against transmembrane desmosomal proteins termed desmogleins. There are two basic forms of pemphigus—vulgaris and foliaceus—that affect different layers of the skin, have unique symptoms, and target distinct antigens. In the "deep" pemphigus vulgaris, blisters develop just above the basal-cell layer and are associated with autoantibodies to desmoglein 3, a keratinocyte cell-surface adhesion molecule. In the "superficial" pemphigus foliaceus, the blisters are high in the epidermis, just below the stratum corneum, and are associated with antibodies against desmoglein 1, another cell-surface adhesion molecule. Several subtypes of each form exist.

EPIDEMIOLOGY

Pemphigus is a rare disease with an annual incidence of 0.75 to 5 cases per million. Incidence of the different forms, however, varies across the globe: pemphigus vulgaris (PV) is most common in the United States and Europe. PV can develop at any age, but is typically diagnosed in the fourth to sixth decades of life. The disease can affect anyone, occurring in equal frequency for both sexes; however, it is most prevalent in those of Mediterranean or Jewish descent. Individuals with certain human leukocyte antigen (HLA) allotypes are predisposed to the disease, though the susceptibility gene varies according to ethnic origin. PV rarely affects more than one family member and patients are of various HLA types; it is therefore not considered a hereditary disease.

Pemphigus foliaceus (PF) is more prevalent in Africa and in certain rural areas in underdeveloped nations, where it afflicts up to 3% of the population. Sporadic and endemic forms of PF exist. The sporadic form is most frequent in the United States and Europe, where its incidence ranges from 0.1 to 0.2 of PV. Endemic PF (also termed *fogo selvagem* and Brazilian PF) is a variant that is usually diagnosed in certain regions of Brazil, Tunisia, and Colombia. Clinically and histologically, the disease is similar to sporadic PF. The endemic form, however, typically afflicts individuals in late adolescence and early adulthood. Importantly, it often affects multiple members of the same family. The epidemiology of the endemic form suggests an environmental cause, which remains unidentified, although an insect vector is suspected. Endemic PF typically arises at the border between developing and undeveloped areas; as an area becomes industrialized, the disease disappears.

PV and PF are associated with myasthenia gravis and thymic abnormalities, including benign or malignant thymomas and thymic hyperplasia. Although irradiation of the thymus or thymectomy is helpful in management of myasthenia gravis, they do not necessarily reduce pemphigus disease activity.

KEY FEATURES

- Epidemiology: rare; equal in men and women; onset 40 to 60 years of age; more common in Jewish or Mediterranean descendants.

- Clinical features:
  - Generalized flaccid blisters or crushed erosions, located on head, upper trunk, intertriginous areas, and mucosa; often begins on oral mucosa, may lead to hoarseness; skin is usually painful and Nikolsky sign is positive.
  - Extracutaneous manifestations: oral mucosal erosions; rarely, thymoma and myasthenia gravis.

- Caused by autoantigens: desmoglein 3.

- Diagnosis:
  - Light microscopy: suprabasilar blister with acantholysis and vesicle formation, eosinophilic infiltrate.
  - Direct immunofluorescence: intercellular IgG and/or C3 on keratinocyte cell surface.
  - Indirect immunofluorescence: IgG against keratinocyte cell surface.

(Continued)

KEY FEATURES (*Continued*)

- Therapy: Corticosteroids (prednisone 1 mg/kg/d) taper to maintenance; may add azathioprine, methotrexate, cyclophosphamide, mycophenolate mofetil, plasmapheresis.

- Note: May be fatal if untreated; risk of infection in treated and untreated cases.

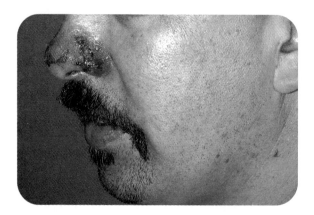

Figure 23-1 Pemphigus vulgaris on the nose. There are no remaining bullae, only erosion and crust (Photo courtesy of Lynne Morrison, MD).

CLINICAL PRESENTATION

Pemphigus Vulgaris ("Deep Pemphigus")

Virtually all patients with this deep form of pemphigus first present with painful, nonhealing ulcerations in the mouth. Blisters are rare (Fig. 23-2), as they rupture soon after forming to leave an ulcerated area (Fig. 23-3). Ulcerations are usually multiple, superficial, and irregular in shape, and arise from mucosa of healthy appearance. Although any surface can be involved, the most common sites are the buccal and labial mucosa, the palate, and the tongue (Fig. 23-4). The ulcers of PV do not heal, in contrast to the oral lesions of aphthous stomatitis or viral infections that heal over days to weeks. Ulcers are also multiple, which differentiates them from an ulcerated tumor, which is single.

Because the disease is rare, PV is not often diagnosed at a first examination, but rather considered only after lesions have been present for weeks to months and the patient has not responded to antibiotic, antifungal, or antiviral therapy. PV should be considered in anyone who has multiple, nonhealing oral ulcers that persist for longer than a month.

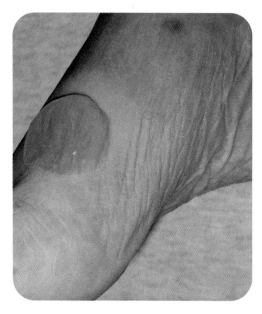

Figure 23-2 An intact flaccid bulla of pemphigus vulgaris. From Berg D, Worzala K. *Atlas of Adult Physical Diagnosis.* Philadelphia: Lippincott Williams & Wilkins, 2006.

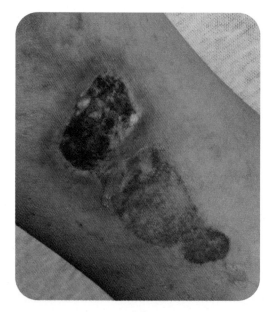

Figure 23-3 Erosions and ulcerations from pemphigus vulgaris. From Berg D, Worzala K. *Atlas of Adult Physical Diagnosis.* Philadelphia: Lippincott Williams & Wilkins, 2006.

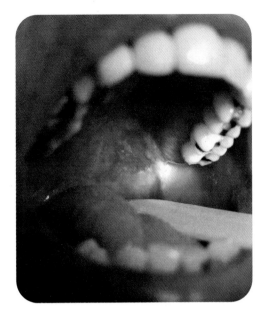

Figure 23-4 Oral erosion on the posterior palate from pemphigus vulgaris.

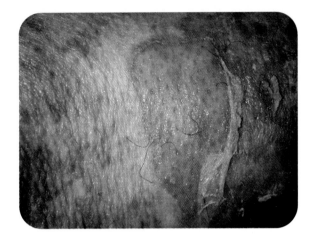

Figure 23-5 Pemphigus foliaceus on the chest.

The condition progresses over weeks to months with lesions developing on the skin and symptoms indicating nasal and esophageal involvement. Occasionally, such skin lesions are the initial manifestations. They usually begin as small blisters filled with a clear fluid, arising from normal-appearing skin. The blisters are typically flaccid because the overlying epidermis is thin and cannot sustain much pressure. Because they are thin, the blisters rupture in several days, and are replaced by well-demarcated, coin-sized, superficial erosions with a surrounding collar of loose epidermis (Fig. 23-1). Lesions appear most often on the scalp, upper chest, and back and have predilection for the medial portion of the torso rather than the sides. The face and neck are also commonly involved, but any surface covered by stratified squamous epithelium can be affected.

Sites that are often missed on examination include the periungual areas; the pharynx and larynx, indicated by pain on swallowing food and by hoarseness; the nasal cavity, manifested by nasal congestion and morning mucous discharge; and the cervix.

Nikolsky sign: a characteristic mechanical feature of all forms of active and severe pemphigus is the Nikolsky sign, in which firm, sliding pressure on normal-appearing skin causes separation of the epidermis from the underlying dermis. This sign is elicited most easily adjacent to an active lesion.

Pemphigus Foliaceus ("Superficial Pemphigus")

In this superficial form of pemphigus, there is insufficient overlying tissue to trap fluid and cause blister formation. Lesions typically start with multiple, pruritic, crusted, coin-sized patches on the upper torso, face, and scalp (Fig. 23-5). They arise from healthy-looking skin and are likened to cornflakes. The crusts can be removed easily, leaving superficial erosions. Untreated lesions do not heal, and increase in number over weeks to months. Lesions can become confluent to resemble exfoliative dermatitis in severe cases. Notably, oral involvement in PF is rare, in contrast to that seen in deep PV.

Drug-induced Pemphigus (DIP)

Certain drugs can trigger both PV and PF (Table 23-1). Though uncommon, this possibility should be excluded in all patients with newly diagnosed disease.

Table 23-1   Medications Implicated in Pemphigus

THIOLS	ANGIOTENSIN-CONVERTING ENZYME INHIBITORS	OTHERS
Penicillamine	Enalapril	Aspirin
Benzylpenicillin	Cilazapril	Nonsteroidal anti-inflammatory drugs (NSAIDs)
Captopril	Fosinopril	Rifampicin
Tiopronin	Ramipril	Levodopa
Cephalosporin		Phenobarbital
Pyritinol		Pentachlorophenol
		Interferon
		Interleukin
		Propranolol
		Nifedipine

The clinical, histological, and immunofluorescence abnormalities of drug-induced and idiopathic pemphigus are similar. The most commonly implicated drugs contain sulfhydryl groups and include penicillamine and the angiotensin-converting enzyme inhibitors, such as captopril. In contrast to other drug-induced eruptions, DIP may not develop for up to several months after initiation of treatment with the offending agent. Most patients with DIP have a good prognosis and clear with adequate therapy and discontinuing of the causative agent.

PATHOGENESIS

The basic abnormality in all forms of pemphigus is acantholysis, or the separation of keratinocytes from one another. The primary event is the dissolution of the intercellular substance (ICS), followed by separation of desmosomes. This process leads to the formation of a cleft within the epidermis, which subsequently enlarges into a bulla. All forms of pemphigus are characterized by circulating and skin-fixed autoantibodies, referred to as intercellular antibodies, against keratinocyte cell-surface antigens. Circulating intercellular antibodies are present in about 80% of patients with active disease, and their titers usually correlate with disease activity. Tissue-fixed intercellular antibodies are present in lesions and in adjacent healthy skin in about 90% of patients. They are usually IgG, although IgM, IgA, and the complement protein C3 may also be deposited.

Intercellular antibodies are directed against multiple keratinocyte cell-surface antigens, of which the adhesion molecules, desmogleins 1 and 3, are best characterized. The antigens targeted in the two forms of pemphigus differ. In PV, intercellular antibodies are predominantly directed against desmoglein 3 and less often against desmoglein 1; in PF, they are predominantly directed against desmoglein 1.

Scant knowledge exists regarding the generation of the intercellular antibodies. The disease is idiopathic in most individuals, although it is triggered in some by an external cause, such as a drug (Table 23-1). Different drugs cause different forms of pemphigus. Many of the frequently associated medications contain sulfhydryl groups that may interact with sulfhydryl groups found in desmogleins 1 and 3 to increase the antigenicity of these adhesion molecules. Importantly, significant inflammatory cell infiltrate is not observed in pemphigus lesions, suggesting that cellular immune mechanisms are not directly involved in the pathogenesis. It remains possible, however, that T-cell responses play a role in regulating the formation of the pathogenic autoantibodies.

DIAGNOSIS

Diagnostic Methods

Diagnosis is based on three independent sets of criteria: clinical features, histology, and immunologic tests.

Clinical features
- PV: classic findings include multiple flaccid blisters arising from healthy skin that have a tendency to extend at their periphery, multiple chronic oral ulcers, and a positive Nikolsky sign.
- PF: distinguishing characteristics include easily rupturing blisters leaving superficial erosions that are usually confined to the face, neck, and upper trunk.

Histology
- PV: intraepidermal blisters characterized by suprabasal acantholysis of keratinocytes.
- PF: acantholytic skin cleavage occurs just at the level of the stratum granulosum.

Immunologic tests
- These assays are used to detect the circulating and tissue-fixed intercellular antibodies against keratinocyte surface antigens that are encountered in all forms of pemphigus.
- Indirect immunofluorescence (IIF) and direct immunofluorescence (DIF): circulating intercellular antibodies are detected by IIF assays on patient serum (with monkey esophagus serving as an ideal substrate for PV and guinea pig for PF). Tissue-fixed intercellular antibodies are identified by DIF assays on skin biopsies.
- Enzyme-linked immunosorbent assay (ELISA): ELISA is also available to detect antibodies to desmoglein 1 and desmoglein 3. The presence of antibodies against desmoglein 3, sometimes together with those against desmoglein 1, is associated with PV, whereas antibodies to desmoglein 1 alone are associated with PF. ELISA is more specific and somewhat more sensitive than IIF.
- The presence and concentration of the intercellular autoantibodies relate to disease activity. Increases in titers may precede clinical flares, and they usually disappear in patients in remission.

Differential Diagnosis

Pemphigus must be differentiated from the many other conditions that also cause skin blisters or oral ulcers and erosions (Table 23-2) (Figs. 23-6 to 23-10). Blisters arise as a sign of many other autoimmune, genetic, and metabolic diseases:

- Blisters in most of these cases occur within or below the dermal-epidermal junction (DEJ) and can be readily excluded by skin biopsy.
- Biopsy: for maximal information, a deep shave or 4-mm punch biopsy should be performed for routine light microscopy at the edge of an active

Table 23-2 Differential Diagnosis of Pemphigus

INTRAEPIDERMAL BLISTERING DISEASES WITHOUT AUTOANTIBODIES

- Familial benign pemphigus (Hailey-Hailey disease) (Fig. 23-6)
- Bullous impetigo, staphylococcal scalded skin syndrome
- Blisters of herpes simplex and zoster
- Allergic contact dermatitis (Fig. 23-7)
- Epidermolysis bullosa simplex
- Incontinentia pigmenti

MOUTH ULCERS/EROSIONS WITHOUT AUTOANTIBODIES

- Aphthous ulcers
- Candidiasis
- Behçet disease

SUBEPIDERMAL BLISTERING DISEASES WITH AUTOANTIBODIES

- Bullous pemphigoid
- Herpes gestationis
- Cicatricial pemphigoid (Figs. 23-8, 23-9)
- Epidermolysis bullosa acquisita
- Linear IgA disease and chronic bullous disease of childhood
- Dermatitis herpetiformis (Fig. 23-10)
- Bullous lupus erythematosus

SUBEPIDERMAL BLISTERING DISEASES WITHOUT AUTOANTIBODIES

- Erythema multiforme
- Toxic epidermal necrolysis
- Porphyria
- Epidermolysis bullosa

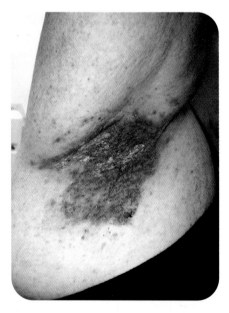

Figure 23-6 Hailey-Hailey disease in the axilla.

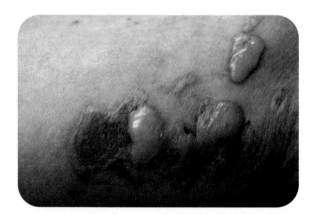

Figure 23-7 Bullous allergic contact dermatitis from poison ivy.

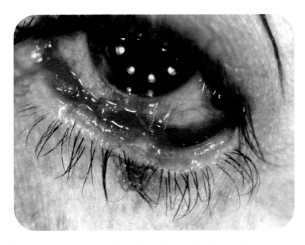

Figure 23-8 Cicatricial pemphigoid. Symblepharon formation.

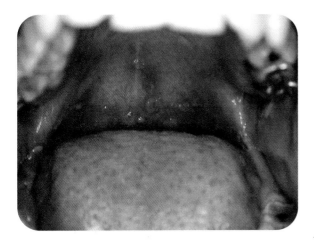

Figure 23-9 Oral cicatricial pemphigoid. Note intact bulla in posterior pharynx.

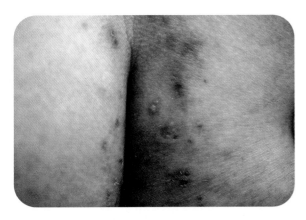

Figure 23-10 Dermatitis herpetiformis. Intact bullae and erosions/ulcerations from scratching on the buttocks.

lesion. Adjacent healthy skin should also be included so that the level of the blister can be accurately identified.

Paraneoplastic Pemphigus (PNP)

PNP is sometimes judged as a variant of pemphigus because it is associated with acantholysis and with antibodies against desmoglein 1 and 3; it is usually associated with an occult lymphoproliferative neoplasm (especially B-cell lymphoma/leukemias, thymomas, and Castleman tumors), however, and may be considered a separate disease:

- As with PV, the skin lesions in PNP can arise both in the oral mucosa and skin, and there is histologic acantholysis and intercellular antibodies on both DIF and IIF.
- PNP has certain features that differentiate it from other forms of pemphigus:
  - Clinical: extensive, recalcitrant oral lesions characteristically involve the vermillion border of the lips and the polymorphic skin lesions often resemble those of erythema multiforme or toxic epidermal necrolysis.
  - Histologic: in addition to suprabasal clefting and acantholysis, interface changes (i.e., inflammation) occur at the DEJ.
  - Immunologic: on DIF, abnormal deposits of Ig, complement, or both, are also present at the DEJ (in addition to on the surfaces of keratinocytes). Intercellular antibodies also react against columnar and transitional epithelia. Most importantly, the antibodies are also directed against plakin proteins (e.g., envoplakin and periplakin). None of these abnormalities occur in pemphigus.

This disease is generally progressive and often fatal within 2 years if associated with a malignant neoplasm. Treatment of the underlying malignancy does not influence the skin disease, although treatment of associated benign neoplasms does lead to resolution of PNP.

TREATMENT

Treatment modalities used to control pemphigus are categorized into those that act rapidly, and those with a delayed effect that are used in chronic management to reduce the requirement for systemic corticosteroids. The goal of treatment is to achieve a complete remission with the least side effects. The three phases of treatment are control, consolidation, and maintenance.

- Control phase: in this period, treatment is swiftly intensified until disease activity is suppressed, as confirmed by a major reduction of new lesion formation, lack of itching, and the start of healing of established lesions. Pemphigus typically responds to treatment within 2 weeks if the correct dose of medication is used; continued disease activity implies insufficient treatment or a complicating factor.

- The initial treatment is chosen according to the extent and rate of progression of lesions. If lesions are few and progressing gradually, they can be treated individually with topical, high-potency corticosteroid ointments or with intralesional injections of corticosteroids. New lesions that incessantly appear at rapid rates should be managed with a low dose of oral prednisone (20 to 40 mg/d).
- Patients who do not respond, or have initially extensive disease are treated with a moderately high dose (70 to 90 mg/d). The dose is increased in 50% increments every 1 to 2 weeks until disease activity is controlled. Importantly, if only corticosteroids are used, this dose may rise to over 240 mg/d in resistant cases.
- If a response is not seen with prednisone at 120 mg/d or more, other treatment options should be attempted, such as plasmapheresis, intravenous immunoglobulins (IVIg), or intravenous methylprednisolone at 1 g/d for 5 days. If no improvement is observed to any of the presented options, there may be secondary bacterial, fungal, or viral (herpes simplex) contamination of skin lesions, which must be treated. Appropriate culture of skin lesions can exclude this possibility.
- Consolidation phase: the objective of this phase is to maintain the type and dose of treatment(s) needed to control disease activity until the majority of lesions have healed. Like the control phase, this period usually lasts for weeks. If lesions are observed to heal slowly, the strength of therapy is inadequate, and needs to be increased. To prevent future flares, medications should not be tapered until about 80% of lesions have healed.
- Maintenance phase: this period begins when most lesions have healed and represents the gradual tapering of medication doses to the lowest levels required to prevent the appearance of new lesions. The long-term goal here is to ultimately discontinue all systemic treatments and this can be achieved in most patients. If multiple drugs are being used, these should be tapered one at a time. Importantly, tapering too rapidly will increase the chance of a flare, while tapering too slowly may lead to unnecessary side effects.
- Adjuvant therapies: although systemic corticosteroids are the mainline treatment for pemphigus, the side effects that are associated with the required high and prolonged doses can be severe. Adjuvant therapies should be considered in the presence of contraindications to the use of systemic corticosteroids, development of serious side effects to corticosteroids, or the inability to reduce corticosteroid doses without repeated flares in disease activity.
  - Consider immunosuppressive such as cyclophosphamide, azathioprine, cyclosporine, methotrexate, and mycophenolate mofetil, anti-inflammatory drugs including gold, dapsone, and antimalarials, and antibiotics such as tetracycline and minocycline.
  - Most of these agents are characterized by a 4- to 6-week lag phase before becoming effective.
- Topical treatments: these modalities are used to alleviate pain and prevent and treat secondary infections, which can delay the response to therapy.
  - Pain and the sticking of clothing to lesions can be lessened with petrolatum-based ointments.
  - Normal saline compresses or diluted bacteriostatic solutions, such as silver nitrate or potassium permanganate, can be used to keep lesions clean.
  - Stubborn lesions can be treated with topical high-potency corticosteroids like clobetasol, or with intralesional corticosteroid injections. Intralesional corticosteroids are more successful in high doses (e.g., 20 µg/L triamcinolone acetonide).
  - Unresponsive lesions should be cultured to exclude secondary infection.

- Oral lesions: oral lesions respond significantly slower to therapy than their skin counterparts and as such, pose a treatment challenge. Successful strategies include the use of high-potency topical corticosteroids such as clobetasol and steroids in an adherent base such as triamcinolone acetonide in gelatin; allowing corticosteroid tablets to dissolve in the oral cavity rather than swallowing, and rinsing with dexamethasone solution may also be effective. The best results, however, are achieved with intralesional injections of triamcinolone acetonide at 20 μg/L. Secondary candidiasis commonly occurs, but is managed with antifungals. Laryngoscopy should be employed to evaluate throat pain on swallowing to differentiate pemphigus and secondary candidiasis. As emphasized above, patients should be followed closely and regular monitoring of side effects should continue throughout therapy duration.

Prevention of Disease Flares

Many factors that aggravate pemphigus should be avoided. These include dental work, sun exposure, radiographs, stress, and trauma. Disease flares following dental work are common enough to merit prophylactic administration of 20 mg/d prednisone (in addition to the patient's normal requirement) for 5 to 7 days, for each dental procedure associated with trauma to the gums. Patients should also be instructed to avoid unnecessary exposure to the sun and to use broad-spectrum sun-protective creams and clothing.

COURSE AND COMPLICATIONS

Pemphigus Vulgaris (PV)

The clinical course of PV is rather unpredictable, but invariably chronic. Several factors direct the clinical outcome: age of onset, severity of disease, response to systemic corticosteroids, and disease progression. Typically, however, bullae and erosions will spread if left untreated (Fig. 23-1). As with burns, these lesions when widespread can be complicated by metabolic disturbances or severe infection and sepsis, which are leading causes of death. Before the advent of systemic corticosteroids, about 75% of patients who developed PV died within a year. With treatment, however, lesions heal with crusting followed by re-epithelialization. There is no scarring, although transient residual hyperpigmentation can occur at sites of former lesions. Most patients with PV eventually enter a phase of partial remission in which they can be maintained, lesion-free, with minimum (<15 mg/d prednisone) doses of corticosteroids, or achieve complete remission in which they are lesion-free and require no therapy. Unfortunately, the immunosuppressive therapy is also a major contributor to the development of infections of the denuded epithelium and the resultant fatal sepsis that often claims the lives of PV patients.

Pemphigus Foliaceus (PF)

The prognosis of untreated PF is better than that of PV, mostly due to the superficial nature of the lesions, and because of the lower risk of infection, fluid loss, and metabolic disturbance. The treatment, however, is no easier, because the doses of drugs needed to control PF are similar to those used for PV.

WHEN TO REFER ⊘

- Referral to a dermatologist, especially one interested in bullous disorders, may be helpful in initial workup and management.
- Consider ear, nose, and throat examination if pharyngeal or esophageal involvement is present.
- Ophthalmologic consultation may be helpful for ocular disease and topical therapy.

NOT TO BE MISSED

- Secondary HSV or bacterial infection.
- Consider the patient's medications as a potential cause and stop potentially offending families of drugs.

ICD9 Codes

694.4	Pemphigus
757.39	Other specified congenital anomalies of skin

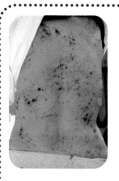

A 67-year-old woman noted onset of erythematous urticarial plaques and vesicles on her waist, back, arms, and legs (Fig. 23-11), and the associated pruritus interfered with her sleep. Her internist prescribed topical glucocorticoids that provided only minimal improvement. The patient went to a dermatologist 6 months later who performed biopsies of lesional and normal-appearing perilesional skin for light and immunofluorescence microscopy studies, respectively. The former revealed a subepidermal blister with an associated eosinophil-rich leukocytic infiltrate; the latter identified continuous linear deposits of C3 in the epidermal basement membrane (BM). These clinical and laboratory findings were consistent with a diagnosis of bullous pemphigoid.

The patient was initially treated with systemic glucocorticoids alone but was eventually placed on a combination regimen of prednisone (20 mg/d), azathioprine, calcium carbonate, and cholecalciferol. Over the next 6 months, the patient's glucocorticoid regimen was reduced to 10 mg/d; repeated attempts at further reduction were met with disease flares. Five years later, her bullous pemphigoid remains active yet controlled.

Bullous Pemphigoid

Ilka A. Netravali

BACKGROUND

Epidemiology

Bullous pemphigoid (BP) is the most common autoimmune blistering disease, with an annual incidence of 6.1 to 7.0/million. The incidence increases with age. When controlling for age-related population gender, BP is almost twice as prevalent in men as it is in women. The disease tends to last between a few months to up to 10 years, and the mortality stems from age-related causes and treatment complications, rather than the disease process itself.

Association with Systemic Diseases

The coexistence of autoimmune diseases is a well-recognized phenomenon of which BP is no exception. Numerous case reports reveal BP in association with rheumatoid arthritis, systemic lupus erythematosus, Sjögren syndrome, multiple sclerosis, myasthenia gravis, primary biliary cirrhosis, autoimmune glomerulonephritis, factor V inhibitor, ulcerative colitis, Crohn disease, and other autoimmune skin diseases including pemphigus vulgaris and pemphigus foliaceus. Among the skin disorders, psoriasis may be more prevalent in patients with BP than in the general population. The incidence of malignancy does not appear to be elevated in patients with BP.

KEY FEATURES

- Epidemiology: more prevalent in men; onset in elderly (60 to 80 years of age), rare in children.

- Clinical features: tense bullae with clear fluid or erosions; may begin as erythematous urticarial, pruritic plaques, localized or generalized on the lower legs, forearms, thighs, groin, abdomen, but rarely on the mucosa.

- Extracutaneous manifestations: typically none.

- Autoantigens: BP antigen 1 and 2.

(Continued)

CLINICAL PRESENTATION

The hallmark of BP is widespread tense blisters arising on normal ("noninflammatory bullae") or erythematous skin ("inflammatory bullae") in an elderly person (Figs. 23-11, 23-12), often with marked pruritus. As the blisters rupture, the eroded bases do not spread further (i.e., Nikolsky negative). Lesions can appear anywhere, but show preference for the lower abdomen, groin, and flexor surfaces of the extremities. Two-thirds of patients present with pruritic urticarial plaques or localized erythema that becomes more edematous before bullae formation. This may last from months (urticarial type) to 6 years (eczematous type). If this phase occurs over extended periods of time the lesions are referred to as the variants, "nonbullous," "urticarial," or "eczematous" pemphigoid. Mucous membrane involvement is seen up to one-third of BP patients and is usually mild—often unnoticed by the patient, with nonscarring lesions limited to the oral mucosa, but sparing the lips (Table 23-3).

Drug-induced Bullous Pemphigoid (DIBP)

Several medications have been implicated in precipitating a clinically heterogeneous group of bullous disorders with similarities to BP (Table 23-4). Most of

KEY FEATURES (*Continued*)

- Diagnosis:
  - Light microscopy: subepidermal blister with mixed superficial infiltrate of eosinophils ± neutrophils.
  - Direct immunofluorescence: IgG and/or C3 in linear arrangement at the basement membrane along dermal-epidermal junction.
  - Indirect immunofluorescence: IgG against epithelial basement membrane zone.
- Therapy: corticosteroids (prednisone) alone or with azathioprine, mycophenolate mofetil, or a tetracycline.
- Note: BP is self-limited, rarely fatal even if untreated.

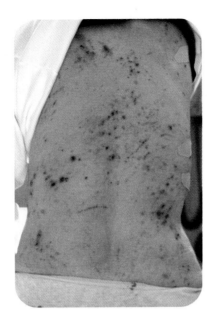

Figure 23-11 Multiple excoriations and bullae on the back of an elderly woman.

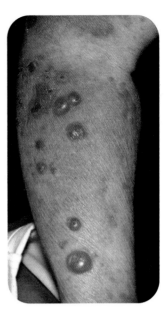

Figure 23-12 Tense bullae and ulcerations on the leg of a man with bullous pemphigoid.

Table 23-3 Clinical Variants of Bullous Pemphigoid

Classical pemphigoid (generalized)	Includes nonbullous, urticarial, and eczematous pemphigoid; see text for details
Localized pemphigoid	Recurrent localized lesions that never go on to a generalized stage (Figure 23-1B); can also occur in sites of trauma or following radiation treatment; most common locations are pretibial region and hands/feet
Nodular pemphigoid	Pruritic, hyperkeratotic papular/nodular eruption with preference for the trunk and extremities in elderly women, resembling prurigo nodularis; presence of bullae within hyperkeratotic lesions may precede, coincide with, or follow the nodular eruption; mechanical trauma may cause lesions to scar, resulting in "hyperkeratotic scarring" pemphigoid
Pemphigoid vegetans	Extremely rare variant; characterized by well-circumscribed, erythematous, erosive, purulent vegetating plaques with peripheral vesicles and pustules, typically located in intertriginous regions; lesions are reminiscent of pemphigus vulgaris, but histopathology and immunofluorescence are consistent with BP
Erythrodermic bullous pemphigoid	Generalized exfoliative dermatitis with subsequent onset of tense blisters, concomitant presentation of both types of lesions, or blisters followed by erythroderma
Vesicular pemphigoid	Small, tense pruritic vesicles grouped on trunk and extremities; presentation reminiscent of dermatitis herpetiformis (DH), but both histopathology and immunofluorescence confirm BP
Erosive BP	Extremely rare variant; characterized by large eroded areas of skin on the trunk, buttocks, and flexor surfaces of the extremities; lesions are resistant to therapy and patients may die from septicemia; immunofluorescence studies compatible with BP
Lichen planus (LP) pemphigoides (LPP)	Describes coexistence of bullous lesions with immunohistochemistry consistent with BP on both LP lesions and previously unaffected skin
Childhood bullous pemphigoid	Extremely rare variant; occur as early as 2 months of age, with most patients younger than 8 years; present with pronounced involvement of mucous membranes, and of the hands, feet, and face.
Drug-induced bullous pemphigoid (DIBP)	See text for details

Table 23-4 Medications and Treatments Associated with the Onset of Bullous Pemphigoid (BP) and Drug-induced BP		
LIKELY ASSOCIATION[a]	**PROBABLE ASSOCIATION**[b]	**QUESTIONABLE ASSOCIATION**[c]
Furosemide	Penicillamine	Chloroquine
Phenacetin	Ampicillin	Topical fluorouracil
Enalapril	Penicillin	UVA with psoralen
Ibuprofen	Sulfapyridine	UVB
Influenza vaccine	Cephalexin	Electron beam
	Bone marrow transplant (with graft vs. host disease)	Captopril
	Fluoxetine	Tetanus toxoid
	Spironolactone	Risperidone
	Bumetanide	Interleukin-2
		Omeprazole
		Sulfonamide
		Amiodarone

[a] Likely association, rechallenge evidence supports association.
[b] Probable association, young age group with BP and temporally associated with medication, or spontaneous resolution of BP after drug withdrawal alone (without topical or systemic corticosteroid therapy).
[c] Questionable association, elderly age group and temporally associated with medication.

these agents contain free sulfhydryl groups, in either the parent compound or a catabolized metabolite. Of note, the rash can appear between 24 hours to 3 months after consumption of the offending agent. DIBP can mirror the clinical findings of idiopathic BP, but many reports suggest more severe nonscarring mucosal or palm and sole involvement. Some cases have also been reported with negative immunofluorescence in the face of a subepidermal blister, which may be more suggestive of a bullous drug reaction than DIBP. It is important to note that once the offending drug has been withdrawn, the treatment of DIBP is identical to BP.

PATHOGENESIS

Hemidesmosomes are specialized multiprotein junctional complexes located on the ventral surfaces of basal keratinocytes that attach the epithelial cells to the underlying basement membrane (BM). Research has shown that autoantibodies against two independent antigens localized to the hemidesmosomes, BP230 and BP180, are associated with BP. Significantly, autoantibody deposition along the BMZ alone does not induce disease. Subsequent complement deposition and activation through the classical pathway is required for lesion formation. Mast cells also play an early pivotal and subsequent amplification role in the disease process.

DIAGNOSIS

Differential Diagnosis

Other autoimmune subepidermal blistering disorders included in the differential diagnosis of BP are: linear IgA bullous dermatosis (LABD); dermatitis herpetiformis (DH), bullous systemic lupus erythematosus (BSLE), cicatricial pemphigoid (CP), epidermolysis bullosa acquisita (EBA), and pemphigoid gestationis (PG).

- Clinical, histological, and immunopathological techniques readily distinguish LABD, DH, and BSLE from BP.
- CP: whereas CP predominantly affects the mucous membranes BP more commonly affects the skin. Both disorders recognize the same target antigen (NC16A site of BP180), but have subtle differences in antibody restriction, prevalent immunoglobulin class, and the concentration of complement versus IgG deposited in the BMZ.
- EBA: skin fragility, trauma-induced lesions, absence of inflammation, healing with milia and scarring, and lesions localized to extensor surfaces are characteristic of EBA. A subset of patients exists, however, who present with a generalized inflammatory skin blister phenotype. As such, clinical overlap between EBP and BP occurs. It is suggested that up to 10% of patients initially diagnosed as BP were actually EBA cases. With this in mind, further studies, including special immunohistochemical techniques may be necessary for correct diagnosis in specific cases.
- PG: while PG is associated with pregnancy, hydatiform moles, choriocarcinoma, and trophoblastic tumors, BP does not have these associations. Despite these findings, some cases that presented initially as PG, subsequently transformed into classic BP, questioning the distinction between these two entities.

Other blistering disorders including bullous erythema multiforme, generalized fixed drug eruption, impetigo, porphyria cutanea tarda, bullous LP, pemphigus vulgaris, and paraneoplastic pemphigus may also be considered in the differential diagnosis of BP. Each of these entities and the aforementioned autoimmune disorders, however, commonly has unique clinical and histological presentations in a context distinct from BP, aiding in differentiation.

Among rare cases in the childhood groups, the differential diagnosis of BP includes congenital causes of tense blisters such as variants of epidermolysis bullosa and other genodermatoses including incontentia pigmenti.

Diagnostic Methods

Clinical features

- Although the clinical presentation of BP can vary widely with the variants discussed above, the majority of patients present with large tense blisters on either erythematous or clinically normal skin.
- Labs are nondiagnostic for BP, but may reveal the presence of peripheral eosinophilia in approximately 22% to 50% of patients. Associated elevation of serum IgE and erythrocyte sedimentation rate (ESR) may occur. When present, the level of peripheral eosinophilia may correspond to disease activity and treatment response.

Histology. Routine histology of a blister in BP demonstrates subepidermal bulla formation that is either infiltrate-poor (taken from a bulla on clinically normal skin) or infiltrate-rich (taken from a bulla on clinically erythematous skin). Biopsies of bullae from inflamed skin are preferable as the large numbers of eosinophils in the dermis and bulla cavity, and the possible presence of papillary microabscesses containing eosinophils, are highly suggestive of BP (Table 23-5).

Table 23-5 An Approach to the Diagnosis of Bullous Pemphigoid (BP)

SCENARIO 1: CLASSIC BP

- Clinical context: tense blisters on normal skin or erythematous bases located on the body or extremities of an elderly person in the absence of atrophy or scarring
- Histopathology (perilesional erythematous skin from upper body preferred): subepidermal bulla with predominant eosinophilic infiltrate ± lymphocytes, neutrophils, fibrin, papillary eosinophilic/neutrophilic abscesses or eosinophilic spongiosis
- Direct or indirect immunofluorescence: showing C3 ± IgG in linear deposition along basement membrane zone

SCENARIO 2: BP VARIANT OR UNRESPONSIVE TO STANDARD THERAPY

- Direct immunofluorescence on salt-split skin or
- Indirect immunofluorescence on salt-split skin (e.g., guinea pig or monkey esophagus, human tissue) or
- Direct or indirect immune electron microscopy (gold standard)

Immunofluorescence

- *Direct immunofluorescence (DIF):* to confirm that bullae are due to antibody deposition at the DEJ, DIF for IgG, IgM, IgA, and C3 is performed. The biopsy site should be either perilesional skin on the upper body within 2 cm of a bulla, or clinically uninvolved skin from the flexor aspect of a forearm or anterior thigh. Biopsy specimens from the lower legs should be avoided because of false-negative results in up to one-third of samples from this region.
- *Indirect immunofluorescence (IIF):* using various substrates can detect circulating IgG to BMZ antigens in 48% to 88% of cases.
- The vast majority of patients with BP can be diagnosed on the basis of clinical scenario, histological pattern, and immunologic criteria with deposition of C3 and/or IgG along the BMZ on DIF. DIF and IIF, however, do not distinguish the precise locations of the antigens that are being recognized by IgG, and thus cannot distinguish between immunohistologically related disorders such as EBA, BSLE, CP, and PG, with immunoreactants that bind to the BMZ. In order to distinguish among these entities, several different techniques can be performed, including: direct or indirect immune electron microscopy; DIF or IIF on salt-split skin (SSS); immunoprecipitation, immunoblotting, and Western detection; or immunoperoxidase staining of type IV collagen on a histologic sample of a blister.

TREATMENT

Initial Considerations

BP is usually regarded as a benign, self-limited disease of 2- to 5-year duration with rare cases lasting up to 10 years. Exacerbations and remissions are common and tend to be milder than the initial episode. Although a benign disease, morbidity can be considerable. The mortality rate averages approximately 27% across different studies of between 3 months and 3 years follow-up, and is often due to factors related to treatment and age. In fact, present-day conventional therapy with corticosteroids produces a mortality rate similar to that observed in untreated patients in the past. As the majority of BP patients are elderly, have multiple disease comorbidities, and are taking multiple medications, they are also at high risk for both drug interactions and adverse effects

Table 23-6 Treatment Algorithm for Bullous Pemphigoid (BP)

MILD-TO-MODERATE DISEASE

First-line
- Topical clobetasol propionate BID

Second-line
- Tetracycline (1–2 g divided BID) or erythromycin (400 mg TID) or minocycline (50–100 mg/day)
  ± Nicotinamide (2 g divided QID)
- Prednisone (0.5–0.75 mg/kg/day)

Third-line
- Methotrexate, azathioprine, mycophenolate mofetil, dapsone, IVIg

MODERATE-TO-SEVERE DISEASE

First-line
- Prednisone (0.5–0.75 mg/kg/day)
  ± Topical clobetasol propionate BID ± tetracycline/erythromycin/minocycline
  ± nicotinamide (2 g divided BID)

Second-line
- Methotrexate (5 mg/week increasing by 2.5 mg/week)
- Azathioprine (administered according to TPMT levels)
- Mycophenolate mofetil (2–3 g divided BID)
- IVIg (2 g/kg/cycle)

Third-line
- Dapsone (50–100 mg/day)
- Chlorambucil (0.1 mg/kg/day)
- Cyclophosphamide (pulsed or oral)
- Leflunomide (20 mg/day)
- Plasmapheresis/photophoresis

SPECIFIC INDICATIONS

Localized pemphigoid: topical clobetasol propionate BID

Neutrophil-heavy infiltrate on biopsy: dapsone 50–100 mg/day

BP with concomitant psoriasis (>15% total body surface area): methotrexate 5–15 mg/week

IVIg, intravenous immunoglobulin; TPMT, thiopurine methyl transferase.

of therapy. Therapy should thus be directed toward suppressing disease activity with the minimum amount of treatment.

Management

Table 23-6 presents an approach to the treatment of BP. Treatment options include:

- Topical corticosteroids: localized disease is generally self-limited and responds to potent topical corticosteroids such as clobetasol propionate. Studies also demonstrate that such medication applied twice daily to hospitalized BP patients successfully controls even moderate and extensive disease in the majority of patients.
- Systemic corticosteroids: standard treatment has classically relied on systemic corticosteroids. Many investigations have revealed that prednisone,

prednisolone, and methylprednisolone are similarly efficacious for BP treatment. Experts recommend maximum starting doses of ≤0.75 mg/kg/d. Twelve percent to 24% of BP patients are resistant to such treatment.

- Antibacterials: tetracycline (1 to 2 g at four times per day), erythromycin (400 mg at three times per day), or minocycline (50 to 100 mg once daily) may control disease activity alone or with nicotinamide (2 g divided four times daily). Addition as adjuvant therapy with oral or topical corticosteroids may be helpful.
- Corticosteroid-sparing adjuvants:
  - The classic corticosteroid-sparing adjuvant, although controversial, is azathioprine. Low-dose azathioprine (1.5 mg/kg/d) with prednisone can shorten both the length of therapy and the total prednisone dose by 30% in comparison with prednisone alone. Current guidelines suggest that the addition of azathioprine should be considered only if the corticosteroid dose cannot be reduced to an acceptable level without reemergence of disease activity due to potential severe medication complications.
  - Methotrexate in combination with potent topical corticosteroids, or as an oral corticosteroid-sparing agent may be used. Typical starting dose is 5 mg/week and increased by 2.5 mg/week until control of disease activity is achieved (total 5 to 12.5 mg/week). Response occurs within days to a maximum of 1 month.
  - Mycophenolate mofetil is used as either a corticosteroid-sparing or as a second-line monotherapy agent in corticosteroid-resistant disease. The typical dosage range is between 2 to 3 g/d divided twice daily.
  - Dapsone has been successful as either sole treatment or as an adjunct to systemic or topical corticosteroids in a small subset of patients. Remission is seen in 14% to 44% of patients and is generally apparent within 2 weeks from the start of therapy. Glucose-6-phosphate dehydrogenase levels must be assessed before commencing therapy.

WHEN TO REFER

- Nonresponsive cases of BP should be managed by a dermatologist.
- Referral for skin biopsy and immunofluorescence is essential.

NOT TO BE MISSED

- BP is self-limited though quality of life may be significantly compromised due to pruritus and skin breakdown. Aggressive therapy should be balanced by the potential side effects of the medication.

COURSE AND COMPLICATIONS

BP is considered to have a better prognosis than other blistering diseases. The clinical course can vary considerably. Some patients have a self-limiting illness, and may achieve spontaneous early remission without treatment; others require treatment for only a finite time. Individuals may also harbor a protracted chronic course over months to years; exacerbations often occur, although recurrences can be milder than the initial episode. Most patients achieve a long-term clinical remission and approximately half of treated cases will remit between 2.5 and 6 years of disease onset. Importantly, untreated BP can be fatal, especially in the active phase, because the blisters can become easily infected. As mentioned above, age-related causes and treatment (i.e., corticosteroid) complications, as opposed to the disease itself, are the major contributors to mortality in BP patients. In addition, recent studies illustrate that poor outcome with BP is associated with advanced age, low serum albumin levels reflecting poor physical conditioning, elevated erythrocyte sedimentation rate (ESR), and high doses of systemic corticosteroids required to control disease.

ICD9 Code	
694.5	Pemphigoid

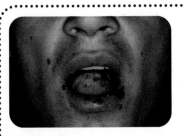

A 22-year-old man presents with a 5-day history of a "cold sore" on the lateral lower lip (Fig. 23-13) and a 2-day history of oral pain, blistering, and ulceration. He noted new targetoid plaques (Fig. 23-14)

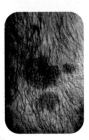

on his hands/feet/arms and legs yesterday. He relates having similar lesions in the past year in relation to a cold sore outbreak, but never this severe. What is the cause of his oral ulcerations and skin lesions? How should he be treated?

Erythema Multiforme

James Y.T. Wang

BACKGROUND/EPIDEMIOLOGY

Erythema multiforme (EM) was historically divided into EM minor and EM major. EM as discussed in this section will refer exclusively to the less severe form of EM, namely EM minor with little or no extracutaneous findings. The more severe form, EM major (Stevens-Johnson syndrome/toxic epidermal necrolysis), involves severe mucosal necrosis in addition to cutaneous target lesions. SJS/TEN is discussed in detail in the following section. The cutaneous lesions of EM minor arise in temporally clustered fashion, indicating infection as the most likely culprit. After an initial manifestation of EM, it will recur in 30% of patients. Although there may be a large proportion of body surface covered, mucous membrane involvement is limited. Infrequently, there will be a low-grade fever.

Disease prevalence is slightly skewed toward males, who account for around 60% of cases. There does not seem to be a racial bias. Although it is uncommon in childhood, there have been some cases due to *M. pneumoniae* in children. Most commonly, EM is caused by HSV infection in young adults. EM is not rare, but is relatively uncommon, with less than 1% of new dermatology patients manifesting with this condition.

PATHOGENESIS

The most common cause is herpes virus outbreak, which can be directly linked in half of EM cases. EM eruptions begin an average of 7 days after herpes flare. The most common strain is HSV type 1, most likely because it is the most common type found in humans. However, HSV type 2-induced EM has been reported. The second most common cause, and likely most common in children, is *M. pneumoniae* infection. EM manifestation from *Mycoplasma* is less typical and more severe than HSV infection. Other likely causes include the Orf virus, histoplasmosis, and Epstein-Barr virus. Although EM has been linked with Varicella-zoster virus, parvovirus B19, hepatitis B virus, hepatitis C virus, medications, immunizations, and other fungal infections, these are not as clearly associated and have not been proved to have a direct causation.

The targetoid lesions seen in EM are a result of immune complex formation and deposition in cutaneous microvasculature. Staining for C3, IgM, and fibrin have revealed these elements in upper dermal blood vessels in a majority of EM patients. Histologically, mononuclear cell infiltrate can be found in the upper dermal blood vessels.

CLINICAL PRESENTATION

EM can have prodromal symptoms with malaise, fever, itching, and burning at the site where lesions will appear. In the weeks prior, some may have had signs of herpes virus infection or outbreak, such as cold sores or fever (Fig. 23-13). Other may have had mild cough from *M. pneumoniae*.

When cutaneous lesions arise, they often appear suddenly as dusky red, round papules on the back of the hands and on the feet, as well as on the extensor

KEY FEATURES

- Epidemiology: uncommon; slight preponderance in adolescent males; no racial biases; associated with herpes simplex virus (HSV) and *Mycoplasma pneumoniae* infection.

- Clinical features: recent history of HSV lesions or respiratory symptoms; viral prodrome (mild fever); "target lesions" on extremities.

- Extracutaneous manifestations: few oral mucosal lesions in some cases.

- Pathogenesis: deposit of C3, IgM, and fibrin around dermal vasculature.

- Diagnosis:
  - Chest radiograph: mild atypical pneumonia.
  - Serology: IgM Ab/elev. IgG Ab for *M. pneumoniae*, elev. ESR, mod. leukocytosis.
  - Direct immunofluorescence: IgG and/or C3 at dermal-epidermal junction.
  - Tzanck preparation: detect HSV.

(Continued)

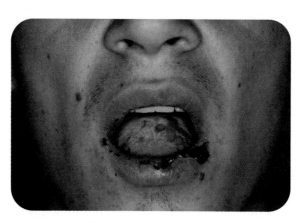

Figure 23-13 Herpes simplex-1 infection on the lip and oral erosions secondary to erythema multiforme.

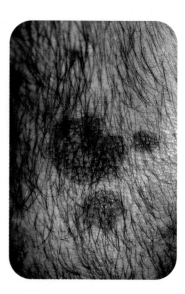

Figure 23-14 Target lesions of erythema multiforme.

surfaces of the forearms and legs (Fig. 23-14). There is a propensity for the upper extremities and they tend to be either asymptomatic or itch and burn. Within 24 to 48 hours, they usually develop into the classic lesions, called target lesions, resulting from centrifugal spread of the red papules to a circumference of 1 to 3 cm. The center of the target is cyanotic, purpuric, or vesicular, indicating a zone of acute epidermal injury or necrosis. The next concentric zone going outward is one of pale edema. The outermost zone has erythema.

Partially formed target lesions on the palms and soles can resemble urticaria. Lesions heal in 1 to 2 weeks without scarring but often lead to transient hypo- or hyper-pigmentation. New lesions can also occur in crops.

In up to 70% of cases, mucosal lesions occur, most commonly on the lip and buccal mucosa, but also on the gingiva and palate. In EM minor, mucosal lesions are mild and do not constitute serious infection risks. The lesions are painful and can cause the patient distress.

DIAGNOSIS

Differential Diagnosis

The most common condition misdiagnosed as EM is annular urticaria, which can produce similar-looking lesions to EM. However, there are distinctive qualities of urticaria that are not present in EM, such as its transient nature and association with allergies. Other common conditions misdiagnosed as EM are contact dermatitis, drug eruptions, lupus erythematosus flare, and viral exanthems (Table 23-7). Diseases that produce cutaneous manifestations that can be mistaken for targetoid lesions include pityriasis rosea, leukocytoclastic vasculitis, dermatitis herpetiformis, mycosis fungoides, bullous pemphigoid, and more severe forms of EM such as Stevens-Johnson syndrome/toxic epidermal necrolysis.

History

Obtain a complete drug history (penicillins, barbiturates, hydantoin, sulfonamides) to rule out potentially more serious conditions. Look for signs of *M. pneumoniae* infections, such as fever, malaise, cough, or other respiratory symptoms. Pathognomonic are HSV lesions 1 week before the onset of cutaneous lesions. Most of the herpetic lesions may be healed by the time the

KEY FEATURES (Continued)

- Therapy:
  - Treat underlying infection; prednisone (40 mg daily) for severe cases; for recurrent cases, consider HSV prophylactic acyclovir (400 mg twice daily).
  - No treatment is necessary for mild cases, but can administer HSV prophylaxis in frequently recurring erythema multiforme.

- Note: Look out for more serious forms of erythema multiforme (EM), such as Stevens-Johnson syndrome/toxic epidermal necrolysis (SJS/TEN).

Table 23-7 Differential Diagnoses of Erythema Multiforme

CONDITION	CUTANEOUS LESIONS	MUCOSAL LESIONS
Urticaria	Transient, raised; two zones of color	None
Drug eruption	Widespread macules/papules, polymorphous	Lips (severe cases)
Lupus	Annular plaques, usually localized to face and chest	Mouth
Pemphigoid	Circinate erythematous patches	Rare
SJS	Widespread targetoid blisters	Persistent
Erythema migrans	Expanding annular macules	None
Viral exanthems	Monomorphous confluent papules, centrally distributed	Rare

patient presents with target lesions. Because herpetic flares can be relatively asymptomatic, the only indicator may be fever and malaise.

Physical Findings

On physical exam, distinctive morphologic target lesions are classic for EM. Immediately look for mucosal lesions, commonly found on oral labia and buccal mucosa. A pulmonary exam listening for signs of pneumonia, as well as looking closely around the lips and genital area for signs of a recent herpetic flare, can be helpful. Remember that EM is clinically diagnosed and that tests may not be necessary for confirmation.

Tests

EM is diagnosed by clinically apparent targetoid lesions. If cutaneous lesions are ambiguous, tests may be helpful to look for underlying causes associated with EM. Because the two most common causes are HSV and *M. pneumoniae*, first perform a Tzanck preparation or HSV PCR from cutaneous lesion, then obtain a chest radiograph to look for atypical pneumonia. *Mycoplasma* PCR testing is the most sensitive assay for detecting *M. pneumoniae* infection.

Serology may also be helpful to look for cold agglutinins (IgM Antibodies) or increased IgG Antibodies to *M. pneumoniae*. Elevated ESR and moderate leukocytosis are seen in severe cases of EM.

A biopsy is only indicated in atypical cases and is usually not required for diagnosis because clinical manifestations are apparent. Immunofluorescence studies (IgG at D/E interface) can differentiate pemphigoid from EM in unclear cases.

THERAPY

There is no evidence that mild EM requires any treatment. The best therapy is to discontinue the responsible medication or to treat the precipitating infection. In the case of:

- HSV
  - First-line: oral acyclovir (400 mg BID)
  - Second-line: 5-day course of oral valacyclovir (500 mg BID) or famciclovir (125 mg BID)
  - Third-line: dapsone (100 to 150 mg daily)
  - Last resort: azathioprine (100 to 150 mg daily)

WHEN TO REFER

EM is a self-limited and usually mild disease. However, some causes for concern include lesions that do not disappear after 3 to 6 weeks or the patient continues to have constitutional symptoms. Patients who do not respond to HSV antiviral therapy, have lesions that look atypical, or have many mucosal lesions should be referred. If there is concern for Stevens-Johnson syndrome or severe drug reactions, send patient to the emergency room immediately.

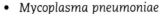

- *Mycoplasma pneumoniae*
  - Short course of azithromycin (500 mg PO on day 1, 250 mg PO QD for 4 more days), erythromycin, or clarithromycin

In cases where EM is more severe and there are many target lesions, a 1- to 3-week course of prednisone (40 to 80 mg daily) with rapid taper in 1 week has been shown to be effective. Prophylaxis is appropriate in patients with chronically recurrent EM. Maintenance herpes antiviral therapy is expensive, but may prevent disruption to patient's lifestyle.

COURSE AND COMPLICATIONS

Cutaneous lesions usually resolve in 2 to 3 weeks, but can last up to 6 weeks. Although hypo- or hyper-pigmentation may occur where lesions arose, these are mostly transient and will not result in scarring. Patients on chronic corticosteroids have longer, more frequent episodes of EM. The frequency and severity of EM is variable. One study showed average number of six episodes per year and 33% of patients have persistence of outbreaks for more than 10 years, although the episodes tend to decrease in both frequency and severity over time (2+ years).

NOT TO BE MISSED

- Recently taken medications.
- Recent viral infections or flares.
- Pneumonia.
- Mucosal ulcerations.

ICD9 Codes

695.10	Erythema multiforme, unspecified
695.11	Erythema multiforme minor
695.12	Erythema multiforme major
695.13	Stevens-Johnson syndrome
695.14	Stevens-Johnson syndrome-toxic epidermal necrolysis overlap syndrome
695.15	Toxic epidermal necrolysis
695.19	Other erythema multiforme
054.9	Herpes simplex without mention of complication
486	Pneumonia, organism unspecified

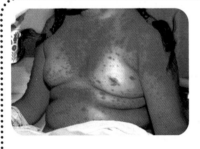

A 13-year-old girl is seen in the emergency department with a sudden onset "rash," fever, and fatigue. She was otherwise healthy before to this illness other than a recent course of TMP/SMX DS for an uncomplicated urinary tract infection. On exam, she has flat, two to three zone target lesions on her hands/feet, arms, and legs. Her trunk has confluent erythema with oval dusky purple plaques especially on her mid-back (Fig. 23-15). Her conjunctivae are injected, and she has genital and oral ulcerations. What is your diagnosis? What further tests should be done emergently? How should this be treated?

Stevens-Johnson Syndrome/Toxic Epidermal Necrolysis

James Y.T. Wang

BACKGROUND/EPIDEMIOLOGY

Stevens-Johnson syndrome (SJS) and toxic epidermal necrolysis (TEN) are similar to each other but distinct from erythema multiforme minor. The two conditions are characterized by severe purulent conjunctivitis, severe stomatitis with extensive mucosal necrosis, with varying degrees of "EM-like" cutaneous lesions. Some distinctions can be made between SJS and TENS, but there is also significant clinical and histological overlap, making diagnosis difficult and controversial.

The primary signature of SJS is significant mucosal ulcerations with some cutaneous involvement (<10%), while in TEN, the distinguishing characteristic

KEY FEATURES

- Epidemiology: rare; no racial or gender biases; most cases caused by reaction to medication; average mortality rate ranging from 5% to over 30% depending on body surface area involvement.

- SJS and TEN differ primarily in percent of body surface area involved and whether more than two mucosal sites are involved.

- For SJS, prodrome of respiratory illness, fever, and lymphadenopathy is followed by 1 to 14 days of severe erosions of at least two mucosal surfaces with extensive superficial necrosis of oral mucosa and hemorrhagic crusts on lips, purulent conjunctivitis, and cutaneous target-like lesions in most cases.

- Red macules develop within hours become bullae, and large areas of skin necrosis and denudation develop rapidly.

- For SJS, <10% body surface area involved, while up to 70% to 80% for TEN.

- Extracutaneous manifestations: severe mucosal necrosis in upper gastrointestinal/respiratory tracts as well as eyelids, resulting in inability to swallow, airway obstruction/pneumonia, and ocular scarring; high fever, pain, weakness.

- SJS/TEN has significant mortality rate and prolonged course, lasting longer with often long-term sequelae.

- In most cases, SJS is caused by a drug reaction while it is almost always the cause of TEN.

- Therapy: immediately withdraw offending medication and admit to a burn unit or ICU for supportive care; offer nutritional support; consult ophthalmology for ocular complications; consider plasmapheresis or immunosuppressants.

is widespread skin necrosis (>30%) with mucosal ulcerations. However, the area of controversy is when skin involvement is between 10% and 30%. In addition, TEN has some additional differences from SJS. It begins with an SJS-like mucous membrane disease, but additionally has generalized detachment of epidermis at the level of the DEJ. The full-thickness loss leads to high rates of sepsis, which is the leading cause of mortalities. SJS has a mortality rate of 5% to 12% while TEN's is greater than 30%. While EM-minor is generally caused by infections, SJS/TEN is caused by drug-related reactions. Around 95% of TEN cases and 50% of SJS cases are believed to be drug-related. Of the drug-related TEN cases, 40% are caused by antibiotics, 11% by anticonvulsants, and 5% to 23% caused by analgesics.

In contrast to EM, SJS/TEN has a prolonged course with a significant mortality rate. The exact incidence is unknown, but it is suspected that for SJS, there are between 1.2 and 6 cases per million per year while there are between 0.4 and 1.2 cases per million per year for TEN. Development of SJS/TEN seems to depend on both genetic predisposition (slow acetylators and certain HLA variations) and exposure to particular drug classes, especially NSAIDs, anticonvulsants, and antibiotics.

PATHOGENESIS

Drugs are the major cause of SJS/TEN, with the primary culprits being NSAIDs (ibuprofen, naproxen), anticonvulsants (hydantoins, barbiturates), and antibiotics (sulfonamides, penicillins, tetracycline, doxycycline). The causal link can be established in about 70% of cases. In contrast to EM, SJS/TEN is not commonly associated with infections in general although a few cases of SJS/TEN induced by bacterial (especially *M. pneumoniae*), fungal, and viral infections have been reported. Other less common causes include recent irradiation from cancer treatments, inflammatory bowel disease, and vaccines (BCG) (Table 23-8).

CHAPTER 23 Bullous Diseases

Table 23-8 Known Precipitants of SJS and TEN

DRUGS	INFECTIONS	OTHERS
NSAIDs Ibuprofen Naproxen	Bacterial *Mycoplasma pneumoniae* *Yersinia* *Mycobacterium tuberculosis* *Treponema pallidum* *Chlamydia trachomatis* *Streptococcus* *Pneumococcus* *Salmonella typhi* *Enterobacteria*	Irradiation Inflammatory bowel disease Vaccines (BCG)
Sulfonamides		
Anticonvulsants Carbamazapine Phenytoin Phenobarbital Lamotrigine Valproate		
Penicillins	Fungal Coccidioidomycosis Histoplasmosis	
Chloramphenicol		
Macrolides Tetracyclines Doxycycline	Viral Enterovirus Adenovirus Measles Mumps Influenza	
Quinolones		
Allopurinol		

Medications are believed to elicit a cytotoxic immune reaction after the original compounds or metabolites bind to proteins in the DEJ, causing rapid necrosis of skin or mucous membrane. Drug-associated mucosal lesions appear in SJS 2 to 5 weeks after drug ingestion. In cases of SJS not associated with medications, the pathogenesis is unknown, although there has been some associated with certain HLA subtypes (i.e., HLA-B12) to SJS susceptibility.

Independent of the cause, the cutaneous and mucosal damage is due to cytotoxic T-killer CD8+ cells, which are believed to activate Fas ligand and induce apoptosis in keratinocytes. There may be a possible role for autoantibodies to Desmoplakin I and II in patients with SJS, which have been shown to induce apoptosis in mouse models. However, it is unclear whether this phenomenon is a primary cause of skin necrosis or whether it helps to amplify an initial response. As symptoms of SJS/TEN progress, there is relative paucity of immune cells found in the skin.

CLINICAL PRESENTATION

Patients have a distinctive prodrome of upper respiratory illness, fever, cough, rhinitis, sore throat, headache, vomiting, diarrhea, and malaise. Patients often complain of fever, stinging eyes, and pain with swallowing. These symptoms usually precede cutaneous manifestations by 1 to 3 days in SJS/TEN, but can precede the appearance of symmetrical red macules by up to 2 weeks. The mucosal lesions, which are characteristic of SJS, appear within 2 weeks of prodromal symptoms. Multi-organ signs can also arise from this condition. The diagnosis of SJS/TEN requires immediate attention and hospitalization, but especially concerning signs include rapid progression of symptoms, new signs, severe pain, and constitutional symptoms.

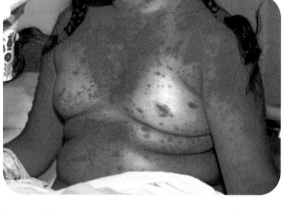

Figure 23-15 Stevens-Johnson syndrome from a sulfonamide medication. From Fleisher GR, Ludwig S, Baskin MN. *Atlas of Pediatric Emergency Medicine.* Philadelphia: Lippincott Williams & Wilkins, 2004.

Cutaneous Lesions

SJS lesions are atypical targets or purpuric maculae, described as red or dusky, that often appear first on the palms and soles. As the condition progresses, lesions may become confluent or distributed on the trunk initially before spreading to the neck, face, and proximal upper extremities (Fig. 23-15). Preceding the cutaneous eruptions, patients may experience pruritus. In EM, lesions are typical target lesions (papular) that appear on the extremities or face. The maculae in SJS/TEN rapidly develop into blisters with clear areas of epidermal necrosis.

The diagnosis of SJS requires cutaneous lesions and should not be diagnosed without their presence. Mucous membranes are involved most of the time and the number of sites is irrelevant to diagnosis. In cases of severe mucosal erosion with no skin findings, consider *M. pneumoniae*-associated mucositis. This condition may be severe, but does not have the morbidity and mortality associated with SJS/TEN.

TEN must have significant cutaneous involvement. In TEN, diffuse hot erythema develops over a large portion of body area. Within hours, the skin becomes painful and signs of epidermal detachment from the dermis appear (Nikolsky sign). The skin wrinkles and slides laterally with applied pressure (Fig. 23-16). Small blisters to large bullae appear. However, nonerythematous skin remains intact and the scalp is spared.

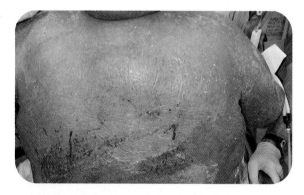

Figure 23-16 Toxic epidermal necrolysis on the back. Note the dusky purple areas centrally. These areas will denude within the next 24 hours. From Mulholland MW, Maier RV, et al. *Greenfield's Surgery Scientific Principles and Practice,* 4th ed. Philadelphia: Lippincott Williams & Wilkins, 2006.

Mucosal Lesions

In SJS, there are almost always mucosal sites involved. Bullae appear abruptly within 2 weeks after prodromal symptoms on the conjunctivae and mucous membranes of the nares, mouth, anorectal junction, vulvovaginal region, and urethral meatus. Ulcerative stomatitis with hemorrhagic crusting is the most distinctive feature. Because mucosal lesions can extend to the esophagus, patients are often unable to eat or drink and are dehydrated on presentation. The oral mucosa is involved 90% of the time with severe stomatitis, hemorrhagic crusting, and denudation of the mucosa.

Ocular mucosal involvement occurs 85% of the time with symptoms of purulent conjunctivitis and photophobia. Long-term sequelae include decreased visual acuity, corneal scarring, pseudomembrane and adhesion formation with immobility of the eyelids, entropion, trichiasis, conjunctival erosions with revascularization, and blindness.

Involvement of respiratory epithelium can lead to pneumonia and pneumonitis, primarily from sloughing of the epithelium. Bronchial epithelium is involved in 27% of cases, where patients present with dyspnea from bronchial hypersecretion. They have a normal chest radiograph, but exhibit marked hypoxemia. Bronchopneumonia will develop in 30% of cases, requiring ventilator support. If sufficient sloughing of the epithelium leads to airway obstruction, patients can even develop a pneumothorax.

Genital and anal involvement is common and can cause complications. In women, erosions leading to vaginal bleeding are sometimes associated with severe pain. In women with TEN and genital involvement, gynecologic consultation and continued care is recommended to prevent vaginal stenosis as the mucous membranes heal.

Systemic Involvement

Generalized lymphadenopathy, arthritis, and arthralgias can develop and, in some cases, enlargement of the liver and spleen can be palpated. Rarely, myocarditis or nephritis will develop. Leukocytosis, eosinophilia, anemia, hepatitis, microscopic hematuria, and proteinuria can be detected in many cases of SJS/TEN.

DIFFERENTIAL DIAGNOSIS

SJS and TEN are at opposite ends of the spectrum, but describe presumably the same condition and pathophysiologic process. Distinguishing between SJS and TEN is difficult in many instances since the two conditions have significant overlap.

Other diseases that may mimic some characteristics of SJS/TEN include EM minor, Kawasaki disease, staphylococcal scalded skin syndrome (SSSS), paraneoplastic pemphigus, and drug eruptions/poisonings/overdoses. However, they can generally be distinguished based on a few features. In Kawasaki disease, the lips are red and chapped, but there are no hemorrhagic crusts and mucosal denudation. The conjunctivae are red, but no exudates are present. Cutaneous lesions are transient red macules, not targetoid. There is often coronary artery involvement as well. In paraneoplastic pemphigus, severe necrosis of lips, eyes, and oral mucosa can occur but is rare. There are distinctive features via histology on direct/indirect immunofluorescence. Associated are lymphomas, Castleman tumor, or other malignancy. Generalized bullous fixed-drug eruption, colchicine poisoning, and methotrexate overdose may lead to similar-appearing skin lesions, but the rash usually is not macular. TEN appears similar to SSSS, but SSSS causes separation below the stratum corneum, not below the epidermis. Therefore, SSSS has a lower infection risk.

DIAGNOSIS

Typical clinical characteristics, such as prodrome of fever with eruption of mucosal ulcers and cutaneous target lesions, if present, help confirm the diagnosis of SJS or TEN. Further differentiation between the two conditions can usually be made. However, a significant portion of the time, there is overlap and the diagnosis becomes less clear. For SJS/TEN classification, there are three possible grades. In Grade 1 (SJS), mucosal erosions and epidermal detachment are less than 10% of body surface area. In Grade 2, there is overlap between SJS/TEN, where epidermal detachment is between 10% and 30%. In Grade 3 (TEN), epidermal detachment is more than 30%.

In cases where typical target lesions are not present or atypical body areas are involved, the most useful diagnostic technique is skin biopsy with frozen section processing immediately following biopsy. Frozen sections can quickly identify SJS, EM minor, or SSSS (separation below stratum corneum, not entire epidermis) from the characteristic pathology found in TEN (described previously). Additional specimens for routine pathology also are recommended. In addition, direct immunofluorescence may be helpful in detecting reactions at the DEJ and help rule out other bullous diseases such as pemphigoid. *M. pneumoniae* PCR may be helpful, as infection by this bacteria may induce mucositis with similar initial features to SJS and may cause actual SJS in about 5% of cases. Challenge tests are dangerous, possibly leading to further progression of disease, and are therefore contraindicated.

Once a clear diagnosis of TEN has been established, TEN can be graded according to SCORTEN, a system that predicts mortality rate in patients with the condition. It is based on the patient's age, history of malignancy, heart rate, severity of epidermal detachment, serum urea, serum glucose, and serum bicarbonate levels (Table 23-9).

THERAPY

Beyond identifying the offending agent and immediately discontinuing its usage, the next step should be to obtain inpatient placement for the patient at a burn unit or an ICU. Early inpatient supportive care has been shown to decrease morbidity and mortality. Because SJS/TEN is life threatening, most of the care will be delivered in a hospital setting. The foremost tasks are caloric replacement if the patient has been unable to eat or drink due to esophageal and pharyngeal ulcerations, protection from secondary infection of denuded skin, ophthalmologic care to prevent long-term sequelae, and pulmonary toilet to prevent obstruction from necrotic bronchial mucosa.

Table 23-9 SCORTEN Scoring for TEN

PARAMETER	TOTAL SCORE	MORTALITY (%)
Age >40 y/o		
Heart rate >120 bpm	0–1	3.2
Malignancy	2	12.1
Body surface area >10%	3	35.8
Serum urea >27 mg/dL	4	58.3
Serum bicarbonate <20 mEq/L	>5	90
Serum glucose >250 mg/dL		

Adapted from Bastuji-Garin S, Fouchard N, Bertocchi M, et al. SCORTEN: A severity-of-illness score for toxic epidermal necrolysis. *J Invest Dermatol.* 2000;149–153.

Upon admission, the patient will need a full set of laboratory tests with serum osmolarity and monitoring of urine output. Fluid and electrolyte abnormalities should be corrected promptly, although dehydration is rarely a cause of death in patients with SJS/TEN. An attempt to decrease the severity of skin denudation is controversial because many of the treatments currently given are not based on sufficient empirical evidence.

The most common therapies are corticosteroids or intravenous immunoglobulin G (IVIg). Some studies suggest that systemic corticosteroid use actually leads to harm by making patients more susceptible to wound infections and sepsis (in one study in children); other studies claim that steroid use is beneficial and potentially life-saving and not using them was "unethical." Other forms of immunosuppressants used are cyclosporin A (3 to 4 mg/kg/day); cyclophosphamide (100 to 300 mg/day IV for 5 days); and plasmapheresis. However, these compounds have not yet been determined to have a significant effect on disease course. Usage of IVIg had recently shown promise as therapy but the data supporting its use is not definitive. In the opinion of this editor (PCS), usage of IVIg early in the course of SJS/TEN is warranted as it is has few potential side effects and some patients seem to have dramatic responses from its use. If future long-term studies support other best practices, then those should be followed.

Wound care is best performed with the help of a dermatologist and burn specialist/surgeon in a burn center. Early supportive skin care can prevent significant scarring and contractures over joints. Physical therapy can help prevent contractures. Cutaneous blisters should be treated with cool, wet compresses. Silver sulfadiazine and mafenide acetate delay epithelialization and are not recommended. Topical steroid usage can increase chance for wound infection and should therefore not be used. Because septicemia from wounds and gram-negative pneumonia are the most common causes of death in SJS/TEN, catheters and central lines should be avoided if possible. In addition, oral antibiotics can be prescribed if risk of sepsis or severe wound infection is high.

Eye care is equally crucial, as serious long-term sequelae often result from this condition. In addition to designating an ophthalmologist as part of the care team, the patient may receive antiseptic eye drops for conjunctivitis as well as topical and systemic vitamin A for lacrimal hyposecretion due to scarring. For pharyngeal mucosal ulcers, lidocaine hydrochloride may ease the patient's discomfort. In addition, patient should be placed on a liquid or soft diet. For severe pruritus, patients may be prescribed antihistamines such as hydroxyzine or doxepin.

In patients with SJS/TEN whose onset is not caused by drug ingestion, but rather by infection, the underlying infection should be treated.

WHEN TO REFER

- Patients should be referred to burn center or ICU once diagnosis of SJS or TEN is reasonably certain.

- Outpatient treatment of this condition is not recommended and leads to poorer outcome.

- Especially concerning symptoms include rapid progression of symptoms, new signs, severe pain, and constitutional symptoms.

COURSE AND COMPLICATIONS

The disease course is highly variable, but generally begins with prodrome followed within 2 weeks with cutaneous and/or mucosal symptoms. Epidermal detachment progresses over 5 to 7 days, followed by a plateau phase when re-epithelialization occurs, lasting days to weeks. Mucosal ulcerations can also last for weeks, affecting the pharynx, anogenital regions, airways, and eyes. The disease course usually lasts for months before complete recovery.

In patients with SJS, renal involvement occurs in 50% of patients, who show signs of hematuria, proteinuria, and elevated serum creatinine levels. Renal failure ensues in 15% of those affected. Thirty percent of patients experience multi-organ failure. The mortality rate is ~5% for patients with SJS.

In patients with TEN, the mortality is greater than 30% mainly due to wound infection and resultant septicemia. Most commonly, *Staphylococcus aureus* and *Pseudomonas aeruginosa* are responsible. Late ophthalmic complications arise in 20% to 75% of SJS/TEN patients. If initial complications do not lead to total visual loss, decreased visual acuity from ocular ulcerations may

NOT TO BE MISSED

- It is essential to take a medication history within the prior 4 weeks.
- Patient's ability to swallow and ingest food and water should be assessed.
- Signs of serious systemic illness.

last for years. Permanent sequelae are common. Damage to the skin leads to permanent dyspigmentation of large areas of skin, scarring, contracture of peri-articular skin, and shedding of the nails resulting in anonychia. Ulcerations in the airways can cause dead mucosa to shed and obstruct parts of the pulmonary tree, leading to severe pneumonitis and pneumothorax. This phenomenon tends to occur 2 or more weeks into disease progression.

ICD9 Codes

695.10	Erythema multiforme, unspecified
695.11	Erythema multiforme minor
695.12	Erythema multiforme major
695.13	Stevens-Johnson syndrome
695.14	Stevens-Johnson syndrome-toxic epidermal necrolysis overlap syndrome
695.15	Toxic epidermal necrolysis
695.19	Other erythema multiforme
695.15	Toxic epidermal necrolysis

Suggested Reading

Auquier-Dunant A, Mockenhaupt M, Naldi L, et al. Correlation between clinical patterns and causes of erythema multiforme major, Stevens Johnson and toxic epidermal necrolysis. *Arch Dermatol.* 2002;138:1019.

Bastuji-Garin S, et al. A clinical classification of cases of toxic epidermal necrolysis, Stevens-Johnson syndrome and erythema multiforme. *Arch Dermatol.* 1993;129:92.

Bastuji-Garin S, Fouchard N, Bertocchi M, et al. SCORTEN: A severity-of-illness score for toxic epidermal necrolysis. *J Invest Dermatol.* 2000;115:149–153.

Forman R, Koren G, Shear NH. Erythema multiforme, Stevens-Johnson syndrome and toxic epidermal necrolysis in children: A review of 10 years' experience. *Drug Saf.* 2002;25:965.

Kazmierowski JA, Peizner DS, Wuepper KD. Herpes simplex antigen in immune complexes of patients with erythema multiforme: Presence following recurrent herpes simplex infection. *JAMA.* 1982;247: 2547–2550.

Paul C, Wolkenstein P, Adle H, et al. Apoptosis as a mechanism of keratinocyte death in toxic epidermal necrolysis. *Br J Dermatol.* 1996;134:710–714.

Roujeau JC, Kelly JP, Naldi L, et al. Medication use and the risk of Stevens-Johnson syndrome or toxic epidermal necrolysis. *N Engl J Med.* 1995;333:1600–1607.

Roujeau JC, Kelly JP, Naldi L, et al. Medication use and the risk of Stevens-Johnson syndrome, not erythema multiforme (von Hebra). *J Am Acad Dermatol.* 1996;35:757–760.

Schalock PC, Dinulos JG, Pace N, et al. Erythema multiforme due to *Mycoplasma pneumoniae* infection in two children. *Ped Dermatol.* 2006;23:6 546–555.

Schalock PC, Dinulos JGH. *Mycoplasma pneumoniae* induced Stevens-Johnson syndrome without skin lesions: Fact or fiction? *J Am Acad Dermatol.* 2005;52:312–315.

Schofield JK, Tatnall FM, Leigh IM. Recurrent erythema multiform: Clinical features and treatment in a large series of patients. *Br J Dermatol.* 1993;128:542.

Tatnall FM, Schofield JK, Leigh IM. A double-blind, placebo-controlled trial of continuous acyclovir therapy in recurrent erythema multiforme. *Br J Dermatol.* 1995;132:267.

Wolkenstein P, Charue D, Laurent P, et al. Metabolic predisposition to cutaneous adverse drug reactions: Role in toxic epidermal necrolysis caused by sulfonamides and anticonvulsants. *Arch Dermatol.* 1995;131:544–551.

CHAPTER

24 Hair Loss

Lilla Landeck and Nina Otberg

Overview of Hair Physiology and Anatomy

HAIR TYPES

The human body exhibits three different types of hair: terminal, vellus, and lanugo hair. Fine hair on the fetal body is shed in utero or during the first weeks of life and is called lanugo hair. Terminal hairs are pigmented, thick, and visible, with a shaft diameter of greater than 60 μm, and are located over the scalp, armpits, pubic area, and in men, the androgen-dependent body areas (for example, beard, leg, and chest). In contrast, vellus hair is fine, soft, short, colorless, and has a shaft diameter of less than 30 μm. Except for the palms and soles, vellus hair can be found on the entire body although density varies considerably in different body sites.

GROWTH CYCLE

Hair growth occurs cyclically, alternating periods of growth (anagen phase, 85% of hair follicles) with rest (telogen phase, 10% to 15%). The short regression phase between the former and the latter is the catagen phase (<1%). The length of each phase is characteristic for each anatomic site. For example, scalp hair is characterized by a 2- to 6-year anagen phase, and a 3-month telogen phase. The growth cycle of the 100,000 scalp hair is asynchronous. The daily growth rate is approximately 0.3 mm (1 cm per month), and 50 to 200 hairs are physiologically shed per day. Resulting hair length is determined by the lengths of the anagen and telogen phases.

HAIR FOLLICLE STRUCTURE

The hair follicle is a specialized skin appendage, which can be seen as an invagination of the epidermis that forms the outer root sheath and, in anagen hair, the inner root sheath. The epithelial root sheath is surrounded by connective tissue, the fibrous root sheath. Hair follicles are a reservoir for epithelial and melanocytic stem cells, contain a pigmentary unit for hair shaft pigmentation, and display special immunologic and anti-infection defenses. The hair follicle is comprised of an upper segment consisting of the follicular infundibulum, the isthmus, the sebaceous gland, and the arrector pili muscle, and an impermanent lower segment consisting of the bulb and the suprabulbar area (Fig. 24-1). The impermanent part is present only during anagen. The bulb is the thickest part of the follicle and contains the proliferating pool of undifferentiated cells, which give rise to the various layers. The majority of cell divisions can be found in the lower part of the bulb. At the constriction

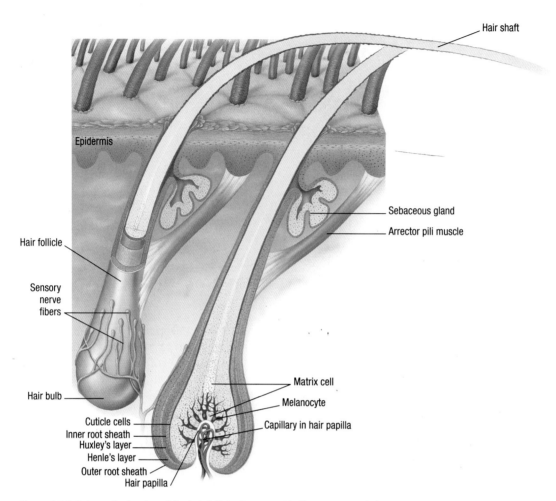

Figure 24-1 Schematic drawing of the hair follicle. Asset provided by Anatomical Chart Co.

above the bulb, the differentiation process begins and about halfway up the follicle the cells begin to die and cornify. The hair is fully hardened as it emerges from the follicle.

Hair Loss (Alopecia)

The importance of human hair in view of social communication and sexual attraction is enormous. Thus, diseases that lead to hair loss may be accompanied by a diminished sense of self-esteem, anxiety, depressive mood, and social withdrawal.

Disorders resulting in hair loss can be grouped into scarring (synonym: cicatricial) and nonscarring forms. Scarring forms are characterized by a pathophysiologic pathway leading to permanent destruction of hair follicular stem cell structure with loss of hair-producing attribute. In contrast, in nonscarring alopecia the hair follicle is not destroyed and hair regrowth generally follows periods of hair shedding. In both scarring and nonscarring alopecia, the distribution of hair loss can occur in a diffuse pattern over the whole scalp or in circumscribed patterns, affecting only a few well-demarcated areas.

The terms "effluvium" and "alopecia" are commonly used when describing hair loss. While effluvium typifies the process of hair shedding, alopecia is the final result of this hair loss. Both terms are not disease specific and do not give etiologic information regarding underlying hair loss. The following section is an introduction to the classification of hair loss. A summary of the major non-scarring alopecias will be followed by a brief overview of scarring alopecia.

Evaluation of Hair Problems

Evaluation of hair problems in the physician's office includes the patient's history, physical examination of the entire skin surface with its appendages (hairs and nails), and, if necessary, special procedures.

PATIENT'S HISTORY

Before starting the physical exam, it is helpful to have patients fill out a detailed history form. This should be reviewed with them during the consultation. As shown in Table 24-1, details of the patient's hair problem, personal health history, hair care, and the family history must be carefully considered.

Table 24-1 Questionnaire for Evaluation of Hair Problems

RECENT HAIR PROBLEMS

What is the nature of the problem?

What body areas are affected?

If the scalp is affected, which areas of the scalp?

When did the hair loss begin? Did you have similar experience in the past?

Was the course stable or did you recognize worsening/improvement?

Does the hair come out at the roots or is it breaking off?

Have you counted the hairs you are losing on a daily basis?

Have you recognized associated symptoms affecting the skin or the nails?

Do you pull or twist your hair?

HAIR CARE PRACTICES

What are your hair care practices? List brands and application frequency of shampoos, conditioners, hair sprays, and other styling products.

Do you use hair colors/bleaches or hot combs/brushes or straighteners?

Have you changed any of these in the past year?

Are elastics used in the hair? Are you wearing hair tightly up (braids, plaits)?

MEDICAL HISTORY

Do you have current health problems, particularly thyroid disease or iron deficiency?

Do you have allergies?

Did you suffer from severe illness or emotional problems in the past?

Have you recently undergone any surgery?

Have you been treated with chemotherapeutics, x-rays, or other forms of radiation?

List all drugs taken before the hair loss.

Have you experienced any significant life change during the past 6 months?

What are your dietary habits?

Are you exposed to children or pets that have unusual hair loss as well?

For females: Have you been pregnant? Date of last pregnancy? Was there hair loss following childbirth? Do you take or have you recently taken birth control pills?

PHYSICAL EXAMINATION

Physical examination should include the entire scalp and the rest of the cutaneous surface if appropriate. Important information includes hair distribution and density, color, length, thickness, curliness, and texture. The shape and location of the frontal line should be noted. Furthermore, pathologic findings with regard to the appearance and texture of both skin and nails should be recorded. Any primary and secondary cutaneous lesions in their relationship to the follicles must be noted.

SPECIAL PROCEDURES

Pull Test

The examiner grasps approximately 50 to 60 hairs and tugs at them from proximal to distal end. Removal of six hairs indicates a positive pull test and active shedding. However, the test can be considered positive if three hairs can be pulled out in several different areas of the scalp. The proximal ends can be examined against a white background for dark hair, or a black background for light hair. A blunt tip indicates hair breakage; a tapered tip can indicate regrowth or miniaturized hairs. The proximal end of the hair shafts may also be examined with a light microscope to determine if the hairs broke off (blunt ends) or came out as club hairs (telogen hair).

Biopsy

A scalp biopsy is necessary when confirming the diagnosis of scarring alopecia. Recommendations developed at the consensus meeting on cicatricial alopecia in 2001 are given here. One 4-mm punch biopsy including subcutaneous tissue should be taken from a clinically active area, processed for horizontal sections. A second 4-mm punch biopsy from a clinically active disease-affected area should be cut vertically into two equal pieces. One half provides tissue for transverse cut routine histologic sections; the other half can be used for direct immunofluorescence (DIF) studies (requires special transport media). Usually only one biopsy from the affected area is necessary for the diagnosis of a nonscarring alopecia; the samples are preferably processed with horizontal sections.

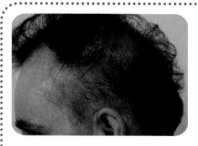

A 44-year-old man presents with a complaint of "I'm losing hair all over my scalp. It's just falling out over the past several months" (Fig. 24-2). He has severe atopic dermatitis, which is currently well controlled with topical corticosteroids and is otherwise healthy. He has recently had significant stressors in his life. Which alopecia would you diagnose his hair loss as?

Nonscarring Alopecia (Telogen Effluvium)

BACKGROUND

Telogen effluvium is a form of hair loss resulting from the sudden conversion of large numbers of anagen hair into telogen hair. A subsequent shedding that can last for several months indicates that the conversion did not occur all at once. Telogen effluvium is followed by an initiation of a new hair cycle 3 to 6 months later if the initiating trigger is eliminated. The molecular mechanisms and signals that switch the hair into a resting phase are still unknown.

PATHOGENESIS

Detailed information of molecular mechanisms and signals that switch the hair follicle apparatus from actively growing anagen stage to the resting

KEY FEATURES

KEY FEATURES

- Telogen effluvium is a non-scarring alopecia.

- It results from a sudden conversion of large numbers of actively growing anagen follicles to telogen due to a yet not completely understood molecular signal which leads to diffuse hair shedding.

- It is seen following severe illness, surgery, nutritional deficiency, iron deficiency, childbirth, in association with certain medications, and in patients with thyroid disease.

- The process is reversible once the initiating factor is eliminated.

Table 24-2 Causes of Telogen Effluvium

EXTERNAL TRIGGERS	MEDICATIONS
Childbirth	Heparin
Administration of new medication	Coumarins
High fever	Allopurinol
Surgery	Amitriptyline
Metabolic problems including hypothyroidism	Carbamazepine
Major weight loss	Doxepin
Iron deficiency	Oral retinoids (isotretinoin/etretinate)
	Haloperidol
Accidents and traumatic life events	Indomethacin
	Levodopa
	Lithium carbonate
	Metoprolol
	Probenecid
	Propranolol Sulfasalazine Valproic acid Vitamin A (high dose)

telogen are still not known. On the basis of clinical observations that telogen effluvium followed severe illness or emotional stress and was sometimes seen in association with thyroid dysfunction, it is believed that systemic signals, such as endocrine, neural, or nutritional signals, may play a role in the initiation of apoptosis in the anagen follicle (Table 24-2).

CLINICAL PRESENTATION

Telogen effluvium is characterized by moderate or massive shedding of telogen hair (Fig. 24-2). The patients usually report that they find hair all over the house, on the pillow, on the floor, or in their food. Oftentimes, patients bring in a bag of collected hair ("bag sign"). It is important to ask the patient for how long they collected the hair to get an idea about the activity of the condition. A decrease in hair density is often difficult to appreciate, especially during the first visit. Thinning occurs on the entire scalp; however, it is most noticeable in the frontotemporal and lateral parietal areas. Patients may report a 20% to 50% decrease of their ponytail diameter. The shedding usually starts 2 to 3 months after the initiating trigger. The severity of drug-induced hair loss tends to be dose-related.

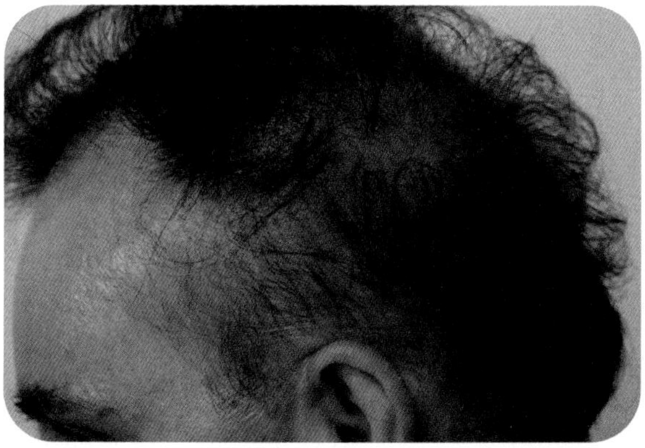

DIAGNOSIS

Diagnosis of telogen effluvium is based on patient history and a clinical picture of diffuse hair thinning. Patient history should include questions about the duration of effluvium, distribution of hair loss, and whether severe life events/illness occurred 2 to 3 months before the shedding. A thorough drug history can reveal triggering medications. To rule out iron deficiency and thyroid

Figure 24-2 Severe telogen effluvium in a man with atopic dermatitis.

WHEN TO REFER

- Patients should be referred to a specialist when telogen effluvium seems to be associated with therapy-resistant thyroid dysfunction or iron deficiency.
- The primary care physician or internist should be involved if patients are exposed to drugs that are associated with telogen effluvium.

dysfunction, ferritin and thyroid-stimulating hormone (TSH) should be ordered. A hair pull test should be performed on every patient. If three or more hairs can be pulled out in different areas of the scalp, telogen effluvium can be suspected. A scalp biopsy may help to confirm the diagnosis and should be performed if the diagnosis is in question.

Differential Diagnosis

- Male and female pattern hair loss
- Diffuse alopecia areata

THERAPY

Telogen effluvium can be a very distressing experience for the patient. It is important to reassure the patient that he or she will not go bald and that the condition will likely resolve once the trigger is found and eliminated. In cases of iron deficiency or thyroid dysfunction, iron or thyroid hormone replacement therapy usually results in a reversal of the alopecia. When recognizing a connection of telogen hair loss and the use of a possibly triggering medication, a switch to another drug is indicated, if possible. Minoxidil 2% for women and 5% for men can be considered for treatment as well, especially if the patient is not able to eliminate the triggering medication or if the trigger cannot be identified.

"AT A GLANCE" TREATMENT

- If iron deficiency or thyroid dysfunction is identified, appropriate supplementation in most cases will resolve the hair loss
- TE caused by acute stress or illness will resolve once the trigger is resolved/eliminated
- Identify offending medications and discontinue
- Consider minoxidil 2% for women and 5% for men

COURSE AND COMPLICATIONS

Telogen effluvium is usually a self-limited form of hair loss, with initiation of a new hair cycle 3 to 6 months later once the causing trigger is eliminated. Chronic telogen effluvium may be caused by multiple triggers; however, in many patients with prolonged hair loss, the triggers are difficult to identify.

ICD9 Codes	
704.00	Alopecia, unspecified
704.02	Telogen effluvium

NOT TO BE MISSED

- Hair loss related to iron deficiency or thyroid dysfunction.
- Drug-related telogen effluvium.

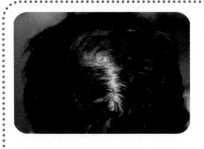

A 22-year-old man presents for evaluation, accompanied by his father. He noticed a frontoparietal recession of his hairline, as well as thinning at the crown in the past year (Fig. 24-3). His 45-year-old father presents with baldness in the parietal areas and remaining hair in a horseshoe-shaped rim around the scalp.

Androgenetic Alopecia (Syn. Male and Female Pattern Hair Loss)

BACKGROUND

Androgenetic alopecia has a postpubescent onset and can be seen as a genetically determined event in the lives of 50% of all men and around 38% of all women. It is the most common form of alopecia. The development and occurrence of androgenetic alopecia depends on the genetic predisposition and an interaction of endocrine factors.

Clinical hallmarks are the reduction of scalp hair density due to conversion of terminal to vellus-like hair and an increase of telogen hair under the influence of androgens (DHT). Severity and distribution among individuals with androgenetic alopecia varies considerably from slight scalp hair thinning to complete baldness in the parietal areas with a remaining horseshoe pattern. Distribution and amount of androgen-stimulated hair in other body areas is not related to the degree of hair loss on the scalp.

PATHOGENESIS

The complete pathogenesis of male pattern hair loss has still not been completely established, though contributing risk factors such as genes, hormones, and other environmental aspects have been widely investigated. On the basis of clinical, chemical, and histopathologic studies, it was found that follicles became progressively smaller in size (miniaturization) and have shorter periods of growth. This process is androgen dependent and androgen-converting enzymes seem to play a crucial role. 5-Alpha-reductase converts testosterone to dihydrotestosterone (DHT). Two enzyme subtypes are known, of which type II predominates in the hair follicles of the scalp, beard, and chest hair as well as the liver and prostate. Increased enzyme activity is followed by elevated levels of DHT. Female pattern hair loss is believed to be androgen-mediated as well, but with modified clinical presentation due to female genetic factors and converting enzymes and aromatase concentration in the frontal hairline. Even though androgens are essential for the process of male pattern hair loss, there is no difference in the excretion of ketosteroids or the blood levels of testosterone between balding and nonbalding individuals.

With regard to the modus of inheritance, it has been suggested that this is polygenic with a variable level of penetrance; however, recent publications also described a gene locus on chromosome 20 that has been associated with hair loss. The gene for the androgen receptor is known to be on the X-chromosome.

CLINICAL PRESENTATION

Androgenetic alopecia describes a nonscarring form of scalp hair effluvium that occurs in a well-defined pattern. There is great inter-individual variation in the amount of hair loss and also with regard to concerns about it.

In men, the hair loss usually starts in the frontal region with recession of the hairline, followed by involvement of the crown with further progress (Fig. 24-3). In final stages, a horseshoe-shaped rim of hair around the scalp is characteristic. In addition to the pattern of loss, there is a decrease in length that can be observed along with a decreased thickness of the hair shafts in balding areas; follicular openings remain intact. Fine vellus-like hair can still be seen in balding areas. In the course of years to decades severe hair loss may occur, but there is always some remaining hair growth in a horseshoe-like pattern in the temporal and occipital areas. Body hair is not affected. In the 1950s, Hamilton classified the patterns of baldness based on frontal and frontotemporal recession and vertex thinning, later revised by Norwood, creating seven categories that are shown in Fig. 4A (Fig. 24-4).

Women presenting with female pattern hair loss complain of increased hair shedding and generally decreased amount of hair, of which both have been progressive. Clinical findings in female pattern alopecia include usually a decrease in terminal hair density in the frontal and parietal areas and a well-preserved frontal hairline. Other clinical variations of female pattern hair loss include diffuse thinning or thinning on the lateral scalp. Moreover, hair loss in

KEY FEATURES

- Androgenetic alopecia (AGA) is the most common form of hair loss.

- AGA presents as a nonscarring hair loss condition under the influence of androgens (dihydrotestosterone; DHT).

- Clinical characteristics include a reduction of terminal hair density on the scalp, following a typical pattern in both genders, with a conversion of terminal to vellus-like hairs and an increase of telogen hair.

- FDA-approved therapeutic options are topical minoxidil 2% (women), 5% (men) and oral finasteride 1 mg daily (men). Hair restoration surgery and low-level laser light may be considered as well.

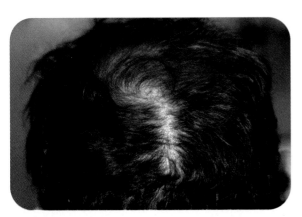

Figure 24-3 Androgenetic alopecia of the vertex scalp.

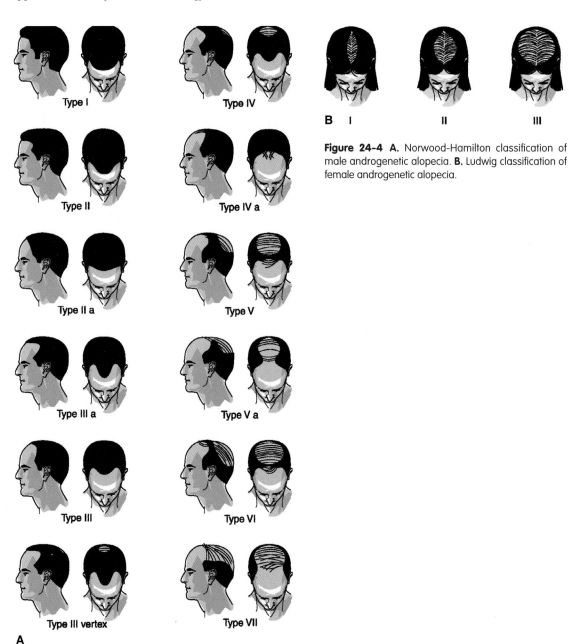

Figure 24-4 A. Norwood-Hamilton classification of male androgenetic alopecia. **B.** Ludwig classification of female androgenetic alopecia.

women can present in male patterns involving complete frontotemporal recession and vertex thinning. Ludwig in 1977 described the presentation of the "female type of androgenetic alopecia" and divided it into three clinical stages (Fig. 24-4B). He also emphasized the progression of hair loss with aging.

COURSE AND COMPLICATIONS

Female patients presenting with hair loss, hirsutism, irregular periods, and abnormal serum hormone levels of free and total testosterone and dehydroepiandrosterone sulfate should be checked by an endocrinologist and gynecologist to detect diseases associated with increased androgen production. Those include particularly adrenal cortex diseases (adrenal hyperplasia, adrenal adenoma or carcinoma) and ovary diseases (Leydig cell hyperplasia, Stein-Leventhal syndrome, hyperthecosis, ovarian tumors, polycystic ovary syndrome [PCOS]).

Table 24-3 The Norwood-Hamilton Classification of Male Androgenetic Alopecia (Fig. 24-4A)

- **Type I:** no recession or very minimal recession along the anterior border of the hairline in the frontotemporal region
- **Type II:** triangular areas of recession along the anterior border of the frontotemporal region that tend to be symmetrical and extend no further than 2 cm back from the natural hairline; hair is also lost to a lesser extent along the midfrontal border of the scalp
- **Type III:** minimal extent of hair loss sufficient to define baldness; commonly symmetrical, frontotemporal recessions are bare or very sparsely covered with hair
- **Type IV:** involves a frontal and frontotemporal recession which is more severe than type III with sparseness or absence of hair in the vertex area; areas of recession are separated from each other by a band of moderately dense hair that extends across the top of the scalp
- **Type V:** essentially an extension of type VI
- **Type VI:** hair loss has increased to lateral and posterior scalp
- **Type VII:** horseshoe-shaped pattern

DIAGNOSIS

The diagnosis of male pattern hair loss is usually easily made on the basis of the clinical picture. Similarly, female pattern hair loss is diagnosed on the basis of clinical grounds as well. A trichogram of the scalp can show up to 25% telogen hair. Scalp dermoscopy can help to identify variations in hair shaft diameter as a sign of the miniaturization process. A scalp biopsy can confirm the diagnosis if noninvasive diagnostic tools leave doubts. Positive family history is often seen in both male and female pattern hair loss and is supportive for diagnoses of these entities. For monitoring and communicating with other physicians, the patient should be classified with the Norwood-Hamilton scale (Table 24-3) and the Ludwig scale (Table 24-4) for males and females, respectively.

Diagnostic Methods

In general, telogen effluvium should be ruled out, as both conditions can occur together. Tests of thyroid function (T3, T4, TSH) are recommended to rule out hypothyroidism even in the absence of obvious disease. Similarly, serum levels of free and bound testosterone and dehydroepiandrosterone sulfate (DHEAS) should be determined for exclusion of diseases associated with increased androgen production. This is necessary in women with irregular periods, hirsutism, or other signs of masculinization.

Table 24-4 The Ludwig Classification for Female Androgenetic Alopecia (Fig. 24-4B)

- **Grade I:** perceptible hair thinning on the crown, limited in the front by a line situated 1–3 cm behind the frontal hair line
- **Grade II:** pronounced rarefaction of the hair on the crown within the area seen in grade I
- **Grade III:** full baldness (total denudation) within the area seen in grades I and II

Differential Diagnosis

- Secondary syphilis
- Tinea capitis
- Other forms of hair loss such as telogen effluvium and alopecia areata

THERAPY

It is important for patients that the physician explains the nature of the process and advises about treatment options. Currently there are several FDA-approved treatment options used for male pattern alopecia that include topical application of minoxidil and oral administration of finasteride. Minoxidil is an established drug for the treatment of hypertension. For its positive effects on hair growth it has been suggested to have an antiapoptotic and microcirculation-enhancing effect. Minoxidil (Rogaine 5% 1 mL) has to be applied twice daily to the affected scalp sites. In many cases, treatment for at least 6 months is necessary before regrowth (or stability of the current amount of hair) is achieved. Continued treatment is necessary for continued effect.

In contrast, finasteride (Propecia) is given orally in a daily dosage of 1 mg. It inhibits 5-alpha-reductase that converts testosterone into DHT. By intervention of hormone conversion, less hair loss-triggering hormone is available. For both minoxidil and finasteride, treatment has to be pursued continuously to maintain hair regrowth and prevent further hair loss. First treatment results may be seen after 4 to 6 months. To date there is no curative treatment available.

Low-level laser light has been suggested to promote hair regrowth in male and female pattern hair loss. A comb device is approved by the FDA; however, more evidence on the efficacy of low-level laser light is needed.

Female pattern hair loss is receptive to minoxidil as well, but is used in a decreased concentration of 2% twice daily. In contrast to males, 5-alpha–reductase-inhibitors seem to be less effective in female patients because of different precursors and converting enzymes in dihydrotestosterone (DHT) synthesis. However, studies with 2.5 mg finasteride daily have shown improvement in hair density in women. Finasteride has significant teratogenic potential; therefore, use of birth control is mandatory in premenopausal women. Finasteride is not approved by the FDA for use in women.

Moreover, hair transplantation can be considered. Good candidates for hair transplant surgery are those individuals with sufficient donor hair density and Norwood-Hamilton types III-V or Ludwig II. Best results are seen from a combination of medical and surgical therapy.

If hair loss progresses or surgical hair restoration is not possible, management of baldness with wigs and hairpieces may be considered.

"AT A GLANCE" TREATMENT

- No treatment is curative for either gender
- Male pattern androgenetic alopecia:
  - Minoxidil 5% (OTC) BID for at least 6 months
  - Finasteride 1 mg PO qd
  - Hair prostheses
  - Hair transplantation may be considered
- Female pattern androgenetic alopecia:
  - Minoxidil 2% (OTC) BID for at least 6 months
  - Hair prostheses
  - Hair transplantation may be considered

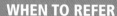

WHEN TO REFER

- Hair transplantation is an option for both men and women if they do not have contraindications and have realistic expectations and a good donor area.

- Female patients with hair loss associated with abnormal serum hormone levels of testosterone and dehydroepiandrosterone sulfate and/or other signs of masculinization should be referred to an endocrinologist and/or gynecologist.

- Female patients desiring treatment with non–FDA–approved medications should be managed by a dermatologist experienced in treating patients with alopecia.

COURSE AND COMPLICATIONS

The course of AGA is difficult to predict. Family history and age of onset can be helpful to make a rough estimate of the possible course. Positive family history and early age of onset are predictors for a more severe process.

ICD9 Codes

704.00   Alopecia, unspecified

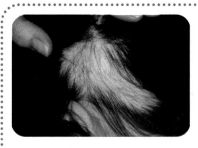

Three months ago, a mother noticed a single large round bald spot on her 10-year-old daughter's scalp (Fig. 24-5). In the course of the past weeks new spots have appeared. The original area of hair loss persists, but they note small hairs are growing back. Clinical investigation and patient's history reveals vitiligo on both hands. The patient is otherwise healthy. What is the most likely diagnosis?

Alopecia Areata

BACKGROUND

Alopecia areata (AA) has an estimated lifetime risk of 1.7%; it is a common cause of abrupt-onset hair loss, but it occurs less frequently than androgenetic alopecia or telogen effluvium. Both sexes are equally affected. Although it may occur at any age, incidence is more common at younger age. AA is the most common form of alopecia seen in children. The familial occurrence is around 15%, but expression of the disorder is variable between different family members. Bald, round, or oval spots in a diffuse distribution most frequently located at the scalp characterize the clinical appearance. Alopecia totalis results in the loss of the entire scalp hair and may occur suddenly or follow partial alopecia. Partial alopecia may be observed in other areas of the body as well. Loss of total body hair is called AA universalis and may also occur suddenly or follow longstanding partial alopecia.

KEY FEATURES

- Alopecia areata is a non-scarring hair disorder.

- It occurs in both genders equally and can affect every age group, though incidence at younger age is higher. It is the most common form of hair loss in children.

- Clinically it presents with well-demarcated round or oval bald spots on the scalp or other parts of the body.

(Continued)

PATHOGENESIS

Detailed mechanisms and signals that lead to hair loss in AA are not completely understood. It has been suggested that AA is an autoimmune disease with inappropriate immune response to hair follicle-associated antigens. Moreover a genetic basis may be discussed, based on the observation of occurrence in other family members. Many patients report the experience of major emotional stress before onset of alopecia.

CLINICAL PRESENTATION

AA is characterized by an acute onset. Typically it presents with oval- or round-shaped, well-circumscribed patches with a smooth surface (Fig. 24-5). Characteristic hallmarks of AA include so-called "black dots," resulting from hair that breaks off by the time it reaches the skin surface. Exclamation point hairs, with a blunt distal end and proximally tapered, appear when the broken hairs (black dots) are pushed out of the follicle. The locus of the initial patch is most frequently seen on the scalp, but may occur on any hair-bearing part of the body. Patches are usually without further symptoms, but may show mild itching and erythema in some cases. Besides this well-demarcated localized form, AA can also present in a diffuse generalized pattern that resembles androgenetic alopecia or

Figure 24-5 Alopecia areata.

Table 24-5 Systemic Diseases Associated with Alopecia Areata

Cataracts	Psoriasis
Thyroid disease	Cronkhite-Canada syndrome
Vitiligo	Down syndrome
Atopic dermatitis	

telogen effluvium. In the acute stages, gentle pulling from the periphery of bald areas may yield more than 10 hairs. Involvement of nails is common with pitting and a sandpaper-like appearance. The disease has been described in association with a variety of other disorders (Table 24-5).

COMPLICATIONS

Relapsing course and progress of hair loss to severe forms of alopecia totalis or universalis are dreaded complications. Missing hair on the scalp and face, including nasal hair and eye lashes/brows can increase incidence of sunburns and skin cancers, but also of nasopharyngeal and ophthalmologic inflammation. Although the condition is not life threatening, changes in appearance frequently cause a diminished sense of personal well-being and self-esteem, leading to severe depressive mood and withdrawal from social interims.

DIAGNOSIS

In many patients the physical findings are characteristic and the diagnosis is obvious. Moreover positive family history and/or the presence of associated diseases may give further evidence in cases of doubt.

Diagnostic Methods

Clinical characteristics, such as shape and look of the patches, presence of exclamation point hair, and nail changes (pitting or sandpaper nails) are seen in AA. Scalp biopsy may support diagnosis. Screening for thyroid disease is necessary.

DIFFERENTIAL DIAGNOSES

Localized hair losses that may mimic AA include tinea capitis, secondary syphilis, lupus erythematodes, lichen planus, and traction alopecia. These can be generally excluded by history and physical examination. Diffuse AA may resemble telogen effluvium because of hair shedding in large quantities, but only in the former are dystrophic hairs present. Androgenic alopecia should be considered as a differential diagnosis as well.

THERAPY

At this time there is no single therapy that can alter the natural course of the disease. Established treatment for patchy alopecia includes intralesional and topical corticosteroids (i.e., clobetasol propionate solution). Injection of corticosteroid suspension (triamcinolone acetonide, 3 mg/mL) in multiple sites may be useful for limited lesions, but repeated treatment in 4- to 6-week cycles may, over months and years, cause skin atrophy. In more severe cases topical corticosteroids applied under occlusion and topical immunotherapy with contact sensitizers such as diphenylcyclopropenone (DPCP) or anthralin expand the therapeutic spectrum. Sensitization and local application of DPCP and other chemicals that have been suggested to block the autoimmune mechanism causing the disease, have been proven to be effective in inducing hair growth. Further therapeutic options include Psoralen+UVA therapy and oral

KEY FEATURES (Continued)

- Five percent of alopecia areata patients develop hair loss over their entire scalp (alopecia areata totalis), 1% of patients develop alopecia areata universalis (total loss of body hair).

- Nail changes include pitting or sandpaper nails.

- Alopecia areata is thought to be an autoimmune disease with a possible hereditary component.

- In general, alopecia areata is a medically benign condition, but it can coexist with other autoimmune disorders such as Hashimoto thyroiditis or vitiligo.

corticosteroids. When, despite treatment, alopecia is progressive and there no hope for hair regrowth, permanent adaptation to the disease is necessary. Extensive AA of the scalp can be camouflaged with hairpieces. In women with AA of the eyebrows, permanent make-up may be considered.

"AT A GLANCE" TREATMENT

- Topical corticosteroids: use superpotent topical steroid solution such as clobetasol propionate or betamethasone dipropionate for the scalp. Adjust the steroid class based on body location
- Intralesional triamcinolone acetonide, 3 mg/mL, repeated PRN q4 to 6 weeks
- Severe/Nonresponsive cases: consider short contact anthralin, Psoralen+UVA or oral corticosteroids
- In some countries, DPCP is available for use as described in the text

COURSE AND COMPLICATIONS

The course of the disease is highly variable and characterized by an irregular relapsing progression, with about 25% of affected individuals having a solitary episode. Spontaneous regrowth of hair is common. Different body areas appear to regrow hair independently. About 60% of patients have at least a partial regrowth by 1 year, but this is often followed by repeated episodes of hair loss. About 40% of the relapses occur within the first year, but a large percentage of patients may relapse after 5 years. Hair can regrow white but may change to the patient's natural color over time. Poor prognosis is linked to involvement of the occiput and/or hairline, to chronic-relapsing course, to presence of nail changes, and when onset is in childhood.

Patients with AA have a 5% risk to lose their entire scalp hair (AA totalis) and an estimated 1% risk for progressing to AA universalis, characterized by total body and scalp hair loss. The number of patients progressing to AA totalis is higher in the younger age groups, and in patients with hair loss from the trunk and extremities.

ICD9 Codes

704.01	*Alopecia areata*
704.09	*Other alopecia*

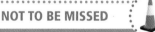

WHEN TO REFER

- For mild to moderate disease, referral is not necessary if a provider is comfortable with treatment techniques and medications.
- Severe alopecia totalis/universalis should be treated by a specialist such as a dermatologist.
- Psychological care and integration of patients in support groups is desirable in many cases.

NOT TO BE MISSED

- Screen all AA patients for thyroid and possibly other autoimmune disease.
- Telogen effluvium may mimic AA.

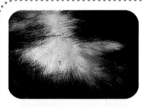

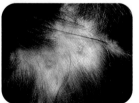

A 56-year-old woman noticed painful skin lesions on her face and scalp (Figs. 24-6, 24-7) for 5 months. The lesions became more symptomatic and extensive during the summer, when she spent a lot of time outdoors. Upon examination she presented with erythematous, well-demarcated plaques with follicular hyperkeratosis on the forehead, cheeks, nose, ears, and frontal scalp region. The lesions on the scalp presented with atrophy, lack of follicular ostia, and hyperpigmentation.

Scarring Alopecias (Syn. Cicatricial Alopecias)

BACKGROUND

Scarring alopecias, which are also known by the term cicatricial alopecia, represent a heterogeneous group of different conditions resulting in permanent hair loss as a consequence of destruction and replacement of the hair follicle with fibrous tissue. With the destruction of the hair follicle, follicular ostia disappear and the lesion may present with a smooth, shiny surface. Primary cicatricial alopecia refers to a group of idiopathic inflammatory diseases, characterized by a folliculocentric

CHAPTER 24 Hair Loss

KEY FEATURES

- Scarring alopecia occurs in a heterogeneous etiologic group of various disorders.

- The inflammatory process leads to permanent destruction of hair follicular stem cell structure and subsequent replacement with fibrous tissue.

- Loss of hair-producing attribute finalizes this process and results clinically in permanent alopecia.

Table 24-6 Proposed Working Classification of Primary Scarring Alopecia

LYMPHOCYTIC

- Chronic cutaneous lupus erythematosus (discoid lupus erythematosus)
- Lichen planopilaris (LP)
  - Classic LP
  - Frontal fibrosing alopecia
  - Graham-Little-Syndrome
- Classic pseudopelade of Brocq
- Central centrifugal cicatricial alopecia
- Alopecia mucinosa
- Keratosis follicularis spinulosa decalvans

NEUTROPHILIC

- Folliculitis decalvans
- Perifolliculitis abscendens et suffodiens

MIXED

- Folliculitis acne keloidalis nuchae
- Folliculitis acne necrotica
- Erosive pustular dermatoses

NONSPECIFIC

inflammatory process that ultimately destroys the hair follicle. Secondary cicatricial alopecias can be caused by almost any cutaneous inflammatory process of the scalp skin or by physical trauma, which injures the skin and skin appendages. Regardless of underlying etiology, scarring alopecias are psychosocially highly distressing for the affected patient and a medico-surgical challenge for the treating physician.

Little is known about most of the etiologies. Hence exact mechanisms causing the follicle stem cell destruction are not completely understood; there is no cure to date. A working classification on the basis of pathology seen in scalp biopsy was suggested by the North American Hair Research Society in 2001 and is listed in Table 24-6.

CLINICAL PRESENTATION

Clinical features are pursuant to the variety of underlying causes and conditions are broad. Scarring areas on the scalp may occur in a diffuse or well-demarcated pattern, and can be accompanied by inflammation of the subjacent epidermis. Examples of the most common entities associated with scarring alopecia are briefly described below.

Lymphocytic

Chronic cutaneous lupus erythematosus (a. k. a. discoid lupus erythematosus) Chronic cutaneous lupus erythematosus (CCLE), together with lichen planopilaris, are the most common causes of inflammatory cicatricial alopecia (Figs. 24-6, 24-7). Women are more often affected than men and the disease is more common in adults than in children. Clinically, CCLE usually presents with one or more erythematous atrophic alopecic patches, mainly

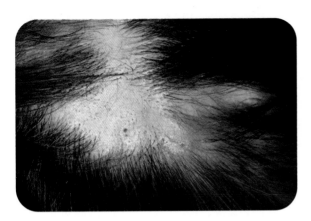

Figure 24-6 Chronic cutaneous lupus erythematosus (DLE) scarring alopecia. This lesion is minimally active.

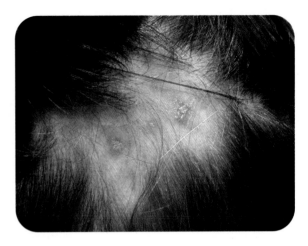

Figure 24-7 Chronic cutaneous lupus erythematosus (DLE) scarring alopecia. This plaque has active lupus; note scale and erythema.

affecting convex areas of the scalp. Follicular hyperkeratosis, hyperpigmentation, hypopigmentation, and telangiectasia can be present. Hyperpigmentation is frequently found in the center of the lesion. Active lesions can be sensitive and pruritic, and the patient may report a worsening after UV exposure. Diagnosis of CCLE is based on medical history, clinical examination of the scalp, and confirmed by biopsy. Laboratory tests should include analysis of serum antinuclear antibody titer, complete blood count (CBC), and urine analysis to rule out a possible systemic involvement. Two biopsies, according to the consensus meeting on cicatricial alopecia, are needed to confidently confirm the diagnosis. Longstanding CCLE lesions are prone to develop squamous cell carcinomas with a high occurrence of metastasis; therefore, every hyperkeratotic or ulcerated lesion in a CCLE patch should be biopsied early. Effective treatment in this condition is hydroxychloroquine (200 to 400 mg daily dose in adults, 4 to 6 mg/kg in children) with therapeutic baseline ophthalmologic examination and CBC. Bridge therapy with oral prednisone (1 mg/kg) tapered over the first 8 weeks of treatment may be helpful in adult patients with rapidly progressing disease. Local therapeutic options are intralesional triamcinolone acetonide injections and topical corticosteroids, alone or in combination.

Lichen Planopilaris (LPP)

Lichen planopilaris (LPP) has three clinical forms: classic lichen planopilaris, frontal fibrosing alopecia, and Graham-Little syndrome. Lichen planopilaris represents a manifestation of lichen planus (LP) of scalp hair follicles. Further changes due to LP on the skin, the mucous membranes, or nail changes may be seen. Clinically LPP is characterized by follicular hyperkeratosis, patchy hair loss, perifollicular erythema, and scarring (Fig. 24-8). Distribution may be localized in the crown area or can occur in a more reticulated pattern. Symptoms such as itching, burning, or pain are often present. The process may extend slowly over a number of years, with a spontaneous healing and limited degree of alopecia. However, the hair loss can be extensive and at times rapid. Management of LPP is difficult, and disfiguring scarring hair loss is a frequent outcome. Injection of corticosteroid solutions in combination with topical corticosteroids are first-line treatment options. Further treatment options include antibiotics, antimalarial medications, oral retinoids, and in severe courses, cyclosporine.

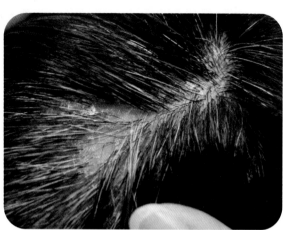

Figure 24–8 Lichen planopilaris.

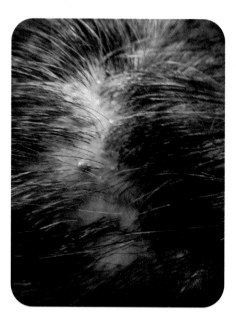

Figure 24-9 Pseudopelade type scarring alopecia.

Classic Pseudopelade

The etiology of this disorder is unknown, but has been described as an end stage of discoid lupus erythematosus, lichen planus, or other scarring diseases such as scleroderma and keratosis pilaris atrophicans. Lesions are usually asymptomatic, beginning with small, white depressed bald spots devoid of follicles located on the vertex, temporal, and parietal regions of the scalp. Typically there is no visible erythema present. This appearance has been likened to footprints in the snow. Clinical overlap with LPP is common.

Over the course of several years, patches spread, forming irregular bald zones that appear with a glossy skin surface and islands of normal hair (Fig. 24-9). Treatment options include those for discoid lupus erythematosus.

Neutrophilic

Folliculitis decalvans. One-tenth of patients diagnosed with primary scarring alopecia have folliculitis decalvans. Folliculitis decalvans predominantly occurs in young- to middle-aged adults with a slight preference toward the male gender. Folliculitis decalvans seems to occur more frequently in African Americans. A bacterial infection involving *Staphylococcus aureus* (*S. aureus*) in combination with hypersensitivity reaction to "superantigens" and a defect in host cell–mediated immunity have been suspected as a possible pathogenetic factor. The clinical presentation is characterized by erythematous alopecic patches, follicular pustules, and hyperkeratosis (Fig. 24-10). A typical finding in folliculitis decalvans is "tufted folliculitis" (multiple hairs emerging from one single dilated follicular orifice) (Fig. 24-11). In older lesions pustules can be absent but progressive scarring may still continue. An overlap with acne keloidalis is possible as some patients with acne keloidalis not only develop cicatricial lesions on the nape of the neck but also develop progressive cicatricial alopecia that resembles folliculitis decalvans in other areas of the scalp. Patients frequently complain about pain, itching, and/or burning sensations. Bacterial cultures with the testing of antibiotic sensitivities are recommended. Oral eradication therapy of *S. aureus* should be combined with topical antibiotics such as mupirocin, 1.5% fusidic acid, and 2% erythromycin and antibacterial cleansers. Intralesional triamcinolone acetonide at a concentration of 10 mg/cc every 4 to 6 weeks might help to reduce the inflammation and reduce symptoms such as itching, burning, and pain. Treatment of folliculitis decalvans

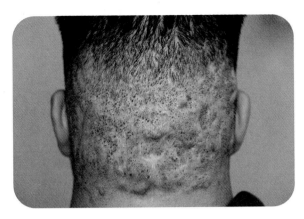

Figure 24-10 Folliculitis decalvans of the occipital scalp. This patient has only mild activity; note few crusts/erosions on the lower hairline.

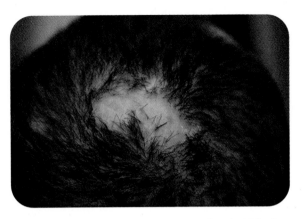

Figure 24-11 End-stage scarring alopecia with "tufted folliculitis" ("doll's hair").

in general is difficult and disease activity can frequently be noted over many years. Flare-ups of the condition and first manifestation of folliculitis decalvans are known to have occurred after scalp and hair restoration surgery.

COURSE AND COMPLICATIONS

Possible complications depend on the underlying cause. Due to the process of scarring, scalp skin is dominated by fibrous tissue. Cicatricial tissue does have decreased physiologic qualities, such as impaired barrier function. In addition, it is more vulnerable to trauma due to decreased elasticity.

DIAGNOSIS

The diagnosis is made on the basis of the patient's history, clinical picture, and histopathologic assessment of biopsies. Baseline clinical evaluation should address issues of age at onset; total duration of the condition; history of lupus erythematosus, lichen planus, or other autoimmune disease; severe forms of acne, keloids, or recurrent infections; and family history of similar hair loss. In addition, hair care practices (using relaxers, styling products, hair color, hot comb) should be investigated.

Diagnostic Methods

For histopathologic assessment, two deep scalp biopsies taken from clinically active areas are necessary, each measuring 6 mm. One biopsy specimen provides for a horizontal section (hematoxylin/eosin stain) and a further one for vertical slicing and direct immunofluorescence. Microbiologic cultures should be taken at baseline visits especially when pustules or crusting are seen. Optional laboratory assessments include hemoglobin, WBC, platelets, AST, ALT, bilirubin, alkaline phosphatase, ANA, creatinine, urinalysis, erythrocyte sedimentation rate, and VDLR.

Differential Diagnosis

Differential diagnoses include tinea capitis (KOH, culture), secondary syphilis (serology), trichotillomania (history), traction alopecia (history, habits), and alopecia areata (history, clinical examination, histopathology).

THERAPY

Treatment is related to the underlying etiology and includes antibiotics (e.g., cephalosporin, minocycline, doxycycline, erythromycin, rifampicin); immunosuppressants (e.g., corticosteroids, topical calcineurin inhibitors, oral cyclosporine,

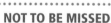

WHEN TO REFER

Because scarring alopecia may result from a wide range of very different etiologies, and disease activity can lead to further disfiguring scarring hair loss, referral to a dermatologist in all cases is helpful.

azathioprine, imiquimod); antimalarials (hydroxychloroquine, chloroquine); and others (e.g., isotretinoin, dapsone, thalidomide, topical minoxidil solution).

"AT A GLANCE" TREATMENT

- For burned out, inactive areas of scarring alopecia: no treatment will restore hair growth
- CCLE:
  - Local therapeutic options are intralesional triamcinolone acetonide injections and topical corticosteroids (i.e., clobetasol propionate solution), alone or in combination
  - Hydroxychloroquine (200 to 400 mg daily dose in adults, 4 to 6 mg/kg in children)
  - Oral prednisone (1 mg/kg) tapered over the first 8 weeks of treatment may be helpful in adult patients with rapidly progressing disease
- Lichen planopilaris:
  - Intralesional triamcinolone in combination with topical corticosteroids are first-line treatment options
  - Further treatment options include oral antibiotics (minocycline), antimalarial medications (hydroxychloroquine), and oral retinoids (acitretin)
  - In severe cases, cyclosporine
- Classic pseudopelade:
  - Treatment options include those for discoid lupus erythematosus
- Folliculitis decalvans and mixed scarring alopecia:
  - Oral eradication therapy of *S. aureus* should be combined with topical antibiotics such as mupirocin or clindamycin and antibacterial cleansers.
  - Intralesional triamcinolone acetonide 10 mg/cc every 4 to 6 weeks

COURSE AND COMPLICATIONS

Tissue scarring is an irreversible process, without possibility of hair regrowth in this area. Detailed course is depending on the specific condition.

NOT TO BE MISSED

- Scarring alopecia, regardless of the cause, should not be missed. Progression leads to permanent, irreversible hair loss.

ICD 9 Codes

704.09	*Other alopecia*
697.0	*Lichen planus*

Suggested Reading

Abeck D KH, Braun-Falco O. Folliculitis decalvans. Long-lasting response to combined therapy with fusidic acid and zinc. *Acta Derm Venereol.* 1992;72:143–145.

Barman J, Astore I, Pecoraro V. The normal trichogram of the adult. *J Invest Dermatol.* 1965; 44:233–236.

Birch MP, Messenger JF, Ag M. Hair density, hair diameter and the prevalence of female pattern hair loss. *Br J Dermatol.* 2001;144:297–304.

Brozena SJ CL, Fenske NA. Folliculitis decalvans: response to rifampin. *Cutis.* 1988;42:512–515.

Callen JP. Chronic cutaneous lupus erythematosus. Clinical, laboratory, therapeutic, and prognostic examination of 62 patients. *Arch Dermatol.* 1982;118:412–416.

Garrett AB. Multiple squamous cell carcinomas in lesions of discoid lupus erythematosus. *Cutis.* 1985;36:313–314.

George PM TWJ. Childhood discoid lupus erythematosus. *Arch Dermatol.* 1993;129:613–617.

Hanneken S, Ritzmann S, Nöthen MM, et al. Androgenetic alopecia. Current aspects of a common phenotype. *Der Hautarzt.* 2003;54:703–712.

Headington JT. Cicatricial alopecia. *Dermatol Clin.* 1996;14:773–782.

Lu W, Shapiro J, Yu M, et al. Alopecia areata: pathogenesis and potential for therapy. *Expert Rev Mol Med.* 2006;8:1–19.

McElwee KJ, Yu M, Park SW, et al. What can we learn from animal models of Alopecia areata? *Dermatology.* 2005;211:47–53.

Messenger AG. The control of hair growth and pigmentation. In: *Disorders of Hair Growth - Diagnosis and Treatment* (Olsen EA, ed.), Vol. 1. New York: McGraw-Hill Companies, Inc., 2003:49–69.

Olsen E, Stenn K, Bergfeld W, et al. Update on cicatricial alopecia. *J Investig Dermatol Symp Proc.* 2003;8:18–19.

Olsen EA, Bergfeld WF, Cotsarelis G, et al. Summary of North American Hair Research Society (NAHRS)-sponsored Workshop on Cicatricial Alopecia, Duke University Medical Center, February 10 and 11, 2001. *J Am Acad Dermatol.* 2003;48:103–110.

Olsen EA. Pattern Hair Loss in Men and Women. In: *Disorders of Hair Growth - Diagnosis and Treatment* (Olsen EA, ed.), Vol. 1. New York: McGraw-Hill, 2003:321–362.

Otberg N, Richter H, Schaefer H, et al. Variations of hair follicle size and distribution in different body sites. *J Invest Dermatol.* 2004;122:14–19.

Otberg N, Wu WY, McElwee KJ, et al. Diagnosis and management of primary cicatricial alopecia: part I. *Skinmed.* 2008;7:19–26.

Peters EM, Liotiri S, Bodó E, et al. Probing the effects of stress mediators on the human hair follicle: Substance P holds central position. *Am J Pathol.* 2007;171:1872–1886.

Piraccini BM, Iorizzo M, Rech G, et al. Drug-induced hair disorders. *Curr Drug Saf.* 2006;3: 301–305.

Powell J DR. Successful treatment regime for folliculitis decalvans despite uncertainty of all aetiological factors. *Br J Dermatol.* 2001;144: 28–429.

Powell JJ DR, Gatter K. Folliculitis decalvans including tufted folliculitis: Clinical, histological and therapeutic findings. *Br J Dermatol.* 1999;140:328–333.

Richards JB, Yuan X, Geller F, et al. Male-pattern baldness susceptibility locus at 20p11. *Nat Genet.* 2008;40:1282–1284.

Ross EK TE, Shapiro J. Update on primary cicatricial alopecias. *J Am Acad Dermatol.* 2005;53:1–37.

Rushton DH, Norris MJ, Dover R, et al. Causes of hair loss and the developments in hair rejuvenation. *Int J Cosmet Sci.* 2002;24:17–23.

Shapiro J. Clinical practice. Hair loss in women. *N Engl J Med.* 2007;18:1620–1630.

Shapiro J. *Hair Loss: Principles of Diagnosis and Management of Alopecia*, 1st ed., Vol. 1. London: Martin Dunitz, 2002.

Sulica VI KG. Squamous-cell carcinoma of the scalp arising in lesions of discoid lupus erythematosus. *Am J Dermatopathol.* 1988;10:137–141.

Tan E MM, Ball N, Shapiro J. Primary cicatricial alopecias: Clinicopathology of 112 cases. *J Am Acad Dermatol.* 2004;50:25–32.

Tebbe B MU, Wollina U, Auer-Grumbach P, et al. Markers in cutaneous lupus erythematosus indicating systemic involvement. A multicenter study on 296 patients. *Acta Derm Venereol.* 1997;77:305–308.

Whiting D. Chronic telogen effluvium: Increased scalp hair shedding in middle-aged women. *J Am Acad Dermatol.* 1996; 35: 899–906.

Whiting D. The *Structure of the Human Hair Follicle - Light Microscopy of Vertical and Horizontal Sections of Scalp Biopsies*, Vol. 1. Fairfield: Canfield Publishing, 2004.

Whiting DA. Cicatricial alopecia: Clinico-pathological findings and treatment. *Clin Dermatol.* 2001;19: 211–225.

Wilson CL BS, Dean D, Dawber RP. Scarring alopecia in discoid lupus erythematosus. *Br J Dermatol.* 1992; 126:307–314.

Wu WY, Otberg N, McElwee KJ, et al. Diagnosis and management of primary cicatricial alopecia: Part II. *Skinmed.* 2008;7:78–83.

CHAPTER 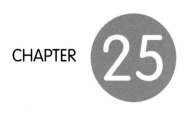 Common Disorders of the Nail Apparatus

Chao Li

Human nails are both aesthetic and functional. Not only do they complete the healthy appearance of hands and feet, they also protect the distal phalanges, allow interaction with small objects, and serve as a natural weapon and grooming tool. Additionally, their appearance, composition, and state of health can hold a wealth of diagnostic information to the careful clinical observer. This chapter endeavors to address common diseases that afflict the nails as well as illuminate the various signs of systemic illnesses that can be seen in the nails.

Normal Nail Biology

The nail apparatus is comprised of the nail plate and four types of supporting soft tissue: the nail matrix, the proximal nail fold, the nail bed, and the hyponychium. The various anatomic regions of the nail are displayed in Figure 25-1. The nail plate is the hard, protective product of the nail apparatus; it derives strength from matrix proteins high in sulfur and its shape relates to the shape of the underlying bone. The nail matrix contains a proliferating layer of basal cells that produce keratinocytes that differentiate, harden, die, and become the building blocks of the nail plate. Nail matrix melanocytes are also found in the lower layers of the nail matrix and remain quiescent unless activated by certain pathologic conditions in which case they can cause nail pigmentation. The proximal nail fold is a fold of skin that closely adheres to and covers one-fourth of the nail plate. It also forms the cuticle, which prevents separation of the nail plate from the nail fold and protects the region from foreign infection. The dermis of the proximal nail fold contains many longitudinally oriented capillaries that run parallel to the skin surface; the organization of these capillaries are disrupted or become more prominent (see Fig. 25-21) in connective tissue diseases such as lupus or dermatomyositis. The lunula region (Fig. 25-2) underlies the proximal nail fold and is the most distal region of the nail matrix; it normally appears white. The nail bed contains a network of elastic fibers, fat cells, lymphatics, and blood vessels, which contribute to its normal pink appearance through the translucent nail plate. The hyponychium describes the space from the point of separation between the nail plate and the nail bed to the distal edge of the nail plate. Fingernails have a mean growth rate of 3 mm/month and toenails have a mean growth rate of 1 mm/month; this rate varies between individual as well as between different digits of the same individual. Total regeneration of fingernails can take between 3 to 6 months and toenails require 12 to 18 months. Conditions that

Nail

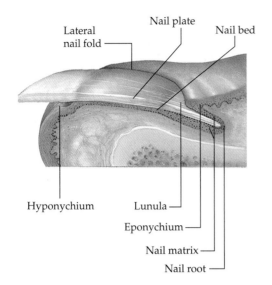

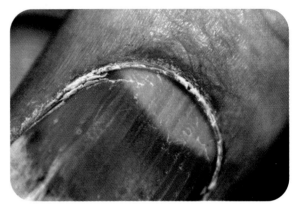

Figure 25-1 Anatomic terms for the nail. Asset provided by Anatomical Chart Co.

Figure 25-2 The white lunula region, which is the most distal region of the nail matrix.

slow growth rate include infection, malnutrition, peripheral vascular and neurologic diseases, systemic diseases, and treatment with antimitotic drugs. Pregnancy, trauma, psoriasis, and antifungal drugs can also lead to accelerated nail growth.

Nomenclature of Nail Abnormalities

Leukonychia	White opacification of nail plate associated with distal nail matrix damage, commonly caused by trauma (Fig. 25-3).
Melanonychia	Pigmentation of the nail plate by melanin, can either appear as single or multiple dark longitudinal bands, or color the entire nail plate (Fig. 25-4).
Onycholysis	Separation of the nail plate from the nail bed usually beginning at the free margin and progressing proximally (Fig. 25-5). Common in psoriasis, trauma, distal subungual onychomycosis.
Onychomadesis	Shedding of the nail plate due to growth arrest of the nail matrix. Involvement of a single nail is typically traumatic. Multiple nail involvement points to a systemic source (Fig. 25-6; see also Beau's lines [Fig. 25-17]).
Onychorrhexis	Longitudinal ridges and fissures in the nail plate. Usually caused by defective keratinization of the proximal nail matrix.
Paronychia	Inflammation of the proximal nail fold. Typically accompanied by periungual tenderness, erythema, and purulence.
Pitting	Punctate depression in the surface of the nail plate. See section 5 of this chapter for disease associations (Fig. 25-7).

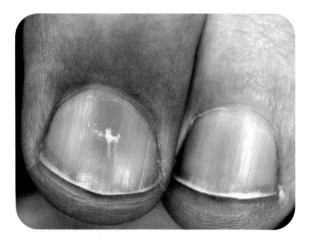

Figure 25-3 Leukonychia.

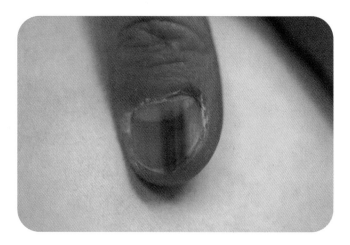

Figure 25-4 Melanonychia.

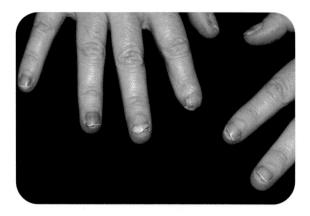

Figure 25-5 Onycholysis: separation of the nail plate from the nailbed.

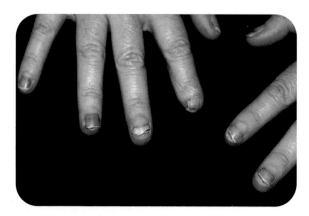

Figure 25-6 Onychomadesis secondary to chemotherapy with docetaxel.

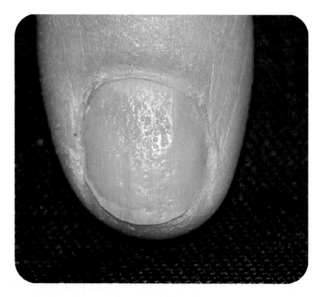

Figure 25-7 Nail pitting from psoriasis. From Goodheart HP. *Goodheart's Photoguide of Common Skin Disorders*, 3rd ed. Philadelphia: Lippincott Williams & Wilkins, 2009.

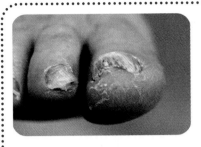

A 75-year-old man presents to your clinic complaining of yellowing and thickening of his toenails on both feet (Fig. 25-8), as well as an itchy and scaly rash in the interdigital spaces of the same foot. He works out daily at his local gym and uses communal showers, though he relates having slowly thickening toenails "since I was overseas in military service." What is the most likely diagnosis? Is this condition curable?

NAIL INFECTIONS
Fungal Nail Infections: Onychomycosis

Onychomycosis is a broad term that describes an infection of the nail apparatus typically caused by dermatophyte fungi, less frequently by nondermatophyte fungi and yeasts (Fig. 25-8). Onychomycosis is the most common disease of the nail, and its incidence increases with age. Fungal infections of the nail are transmitted by fomite or direct contact, commonly among family members. Therefore, it is believed that tight shoes and use of communal locker rooms are risk factors. Individuals who suffer from atopy, diabetes mellitus, immunosuppression, or human immunodeficiency virus (HIV) disease are also at an increased risk. Onychomycosis is discussed in detail in Chapter 9.

CHAPTER 25 Common Nail Disorders

KEY FEATURES

- Onychomycosis is the most common disease of the nail; incidence increases with age.

- It commonly presents with areas of nail opacification and discoloration with intermittent paronychia with periungual tenderness, erythema, and pus. Toenails are more commonly involved, with associated tinea pedis.

- The diagnosis can be made by light microscopy of nail scrapings in a potassium hydroxide solution, nail biopsy, and fungal culture. Confirmation of diagnosis is recommended before initiating oral antifungal agents.

- A combination of topical and oral antifungal agents is most effective.

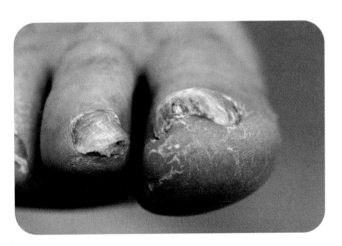

Figure 25-8 Total dystrophic onychomycosis.

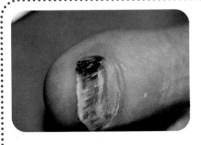

A 48-year-old attorney who swims in a communal pool for exercise four to five times weekly presents with black-green discoloration of the right great toe (Fig. 25-9). He has a history of chronic onycholysis and onychomycosis of that toe. He is worried that he might have a melanoma. What is the most likely diagnosis? How is this condition treated?

BACTERIAL NAIL INFECTIONS
Green Nail Syndrome (Chloronychia)

BACKGROUND

Bacteria are not typically able to invade or infect under the nail plate. However, patients with chronic onycholysis or paronychia of the fingernails/toenails who endure prolonged immersion of the affected hand or feet in fresh water may develop a secondary *P. aeruginosa* infection of diseased nail plate.

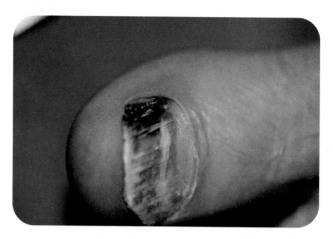

Figure 25-9 Subungual *Pseudomonas aeruginosa* infection with characteristic green/black color.

PATHOGENESIS

Green nail syndrome or chloronychia is a secondary infection of an oncholytic nail plate by incidental or chronic environmental exposure to *P. aeruginosa*-contaminated water. This organism produces a pyocyanin pigment, which adheres to the surfaces of the nail plate and stains it a green-black color.

CLINICAL PRESENTATION

Patients typically present with green-black discoloration of one to two nail plates (Fig. 25-9). These nail changes often occur in nail plate that already suffer from chronic onycholysis, onychomycosis, or paronychia.

DIAGNOSIS

Differential Diagnosis

Common: onychomycosis. Stain from lacquers, dyes, or paints. Uncommon: subungual melanoma.

Clinical diagnosis consists of observing a typical triad of: green discoloration of the nail plate, chronic proximal nail paronychia, and distolateral onycholysis. Rule out fungal infections by potassium hydroxide (KOH) exam and fungal culture of nail scrapings. In recalcitrant cases, subungual melanoma should be suspected.

TREATMENT

Patients should be counseled to avoid prolonged immersion of nails in water, even when gloves are worn. Care should be taken to dry the nail thoroughly after washing; a hair dryer can help. Topical therapy is usually successful. Oral antibiotics are not necessary or effective in most cases. Over-the-counter remedies such as vinegar (acetic acid 1%) or solutions of 2% sodium hypochlorite may help. Prescription chlorhexidine solution soaks twice daily for 3 to 4 weeks will suppress bacterial growth. Another topical option is ciprofloxacin 0.2% otic solution BID to the affected nail for 2 to 4 weeks. In some cases, it may take up to 12 months for clearance of the green-black pigmentation as normal nail grows out. Oral antibiotic treatment is not necessary.

KEY FEATURES

- *Pseudomonas aeruginosa* infection of the nail produces a green-black discoloration of the nail bed, associated with chronic onycholysis and exposure to water.

- The affected nail can also suffer from concurrent fungal infection.

- The diagnosis consists of visual observation, history of prolonged nail exposure to water, and exclusion of green dyes and fungal infection.

- It is treated with topical bleach, vinegar, or chlorhexidine drops combined with reduced water exposure.

CHAPTER 25 Common Nail Disorders

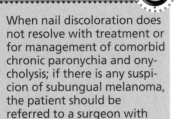

"AT A GLANCE" TREATMENT

- OTC:
  - Acetic acid (vinegar) 1% or sodium hypochlorite 2% soaks
- Prescription:
  - Chlorhexidine solution BID × 3 to 4 weeks
  - Ciprofloxacin 0.2% otic solution BID to the affected nail for 2 to 4 weeks

COURSE AND COMPLICATIONS

In general, chloronychia is self-limited and resolves with therapy. Avoiding excess water immersion is essential. This condition can also present with a concomitant fungal infection of the same nail. In these cases, treatment of concurrent onychomycosis is indicated.

ICD9 Code

041.7   *Pseudomonas infection in conditions classified elsewhere and of unspecified site*

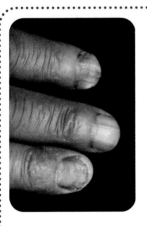

A 45-year-old African American man presents with multiple dark longitudinal bands in his thumb and fingernails, bilaterally (Fig. 25-10). Upon closer inspection of his fingernails, pigmented bands are found in the thumbnails bilaterally as well as the index and middle fingernails of his dominant hand. The bands are straight with distinct borders. He says that he remembers having the bands in his fingers for many years but he has grown more concerned because the other bands have appeared more recently, within the last few months. He also has had psoriasis for many years. What may be causing the recent development of additional longitudinal bands in his fingernails? What questions may help better evaluate his condition? Would you refer this patient to be evaluated by dermatology? Would you still refer this patient to dermatology if he says he began azidothymidine (AZT) for recently diagnosed HIV disease?

PIGMENTED LESIONS
Longitudinal Melanonychia
BACKGROUND

Pigmented lesions of the nail usually present as longitudinal pigmentation of the nail or longitudinal melanonychia. It appears as a brown to black band that runs longitudinally in the nail plate from the proximal nail fold to the free edge. These bands can be congenital or acquired later in life and they can be common in African American, Latino, or Asian patients. Many different conditions can cause this feature, including early subungual melanoma.

PATHOGENESIS

Longitudinal melanonychia is either caused by activation of normally dormant nail matrix melanocytes or from benign or malignant nail matrix melanocyte hyperplasia.

CLINICAL PRESENTATION

Typically a brown or black longitudinal band in the nail plate; however, the width of the band is variable between nails (but uniform within a given band) (Fig. 25-10). There may be more than one band per nail plate. Full-width melanonychia presents as pigment involvement of the entire nail plate.

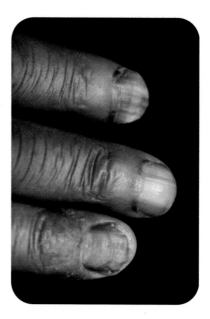

Figure 25-10 Longitudinal melanonychia and nail dystrophy secondary to psoriasis.

DIAGNOSIS

The diagnosis of this condition is largely clinical. In the appropriate patient with a stable lesion, a biopsy is not needed. There are many exogenous causes of nail pigmentation which are summarized in Table 25-1.

It is important to elicit a clear history of the lesion; most importantly, ascertaining whether it is congenital or acquired, its duration, changes over

KEY FEATURES

- Longitudinal melanonychia presents as longitudinal pigmentation of the nail and generates a broad differential that ranges from nail trauma to benign nevi to malignancy.

- It is common among ethnicities with darker skin types and appears to increase in prevalence with age.

- Because nail pigmentation carries the possibility of melanoma, patients with changing lesions should be referred for evaluation by a dermatologist.

Table 25-1 Exogenous Causes of Nail Pigmentation
• Ethnic nail pigmentation: can be physiologic in dark-skinned individuals and features multiple pigmented longitudinal bands on multiple fingernails or toenails.
• Nail matrix nevus: appears either as brown-colored linear bands that can become deeply pigmented or as homogenous pigmentation of the nail plate. Can be congenital or acquired, often seen in children and young adults. Dermoscopy will reveal parallel longitudinal brown lines with regular spacing and width.
• Traumatic longitudinal melanonychia: can be caused by repeated trauma such as repeated nail biting, picking, or friction; typically associated with overt nail plate abnormalities. Resolves after trauma stops.
• Radiation or drug-induced nail pigmentation: affects one or more digits and features gray-colored straight linear streaks. More common in patients with darker skin types, and typically appears 1–2 months after beginning treatment. It is estimated two thirds of patients using AZT will develop drug-related nail pigmentation. This pigmentation may fade over several months after AZT is stopped.
• Vitamin B12 or folate deficiency: nail pigment tends to be blue-black, and pigmentation on the skin can also be found over the knuckles and fingers. This is reversible with B12 or folate repletion.
• Subungual hematoma (see Fig. 25-13): usually contain black to reddish hues, are usually confined to the nail matrix and nail bed, and will grow out distally with the nail plate. However, subungual hematoma that does not grow out with the nail or recurs at the same place are suspicious for neovascularization of a tumor.

Table 25-2 Differential Diagnosis of Longitudinal Melanonychia

- Endogenous
  - Nail matrix nevus
  - Traumatic focal activation of nail matrix
  - Radiation-induced
  - Drug-induced (AZT, hydroxyurea, minocycline)
  - Vitamin B12 or folate deficiency
  - Endocrine (Addison disease, Cushing syndrome, acromegaly)
  - Peutz-Jeghers or Laugier-Hunziker syndrome
  - Subungual melanoma

- Exogenous origin
  - Exposure to cosmetic, therapeutic, or occupational chemical agents such as henna, hair dyes, silver nitrate, tobacco
  - Subungual hematoma
  - Fungal infections can resemble melanonychia but often do not form a linear streak

time, and personal or family history of melanoma. Current and past medications can also uncover drug-induced nail pigmentation. On physical exam, the oral and genital mucosa can identify the multiple lentigines associated with Peutz-Jeghers syndrome or Laugier-Hunziker syndrome. Nail longitudinal melanonychia and macular buccal pigmentation frequently occur in association with these conditions.

The coloration and dimensions of the pigmented lesion at both the distal and proximal ends of the nail should be recorded.

Differentiation between the various pigmented lesions can be challenging (Table 25-2). Lesions are usually evaluated using dermoscopy. If subungual melanoma is suspected, definitive diagnosis is made by nail matrix biopsy.

WHEN TO REFER

Prompt referral to dermatology should be made for further evaluation of pigmented nail lesions. Investigation of systemic or other benign causes of longitudinal melanonychia should not delay referral.

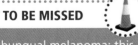

NOT TO BE MISSED

- Subungual melanoma: this is a rare malignancy of the nail apparatus that carries a grave prognosis. To make matters worse, it is often misdiagnosed in the early stages due to its initial resemblance to the plethora of benign pigmented nail lesions. More details of this disease will be discussed below.

TREATMENT

Treatment will be based on the individual cause of longitudinal melanonychia. Treatment of subungual melanoma will be covered in the next section.

"AT A GLANCE" TREATMENT

- In general, treatment is not necessary for stable lesions. Any changing pigmented lesion or questionable lesion should be referred for biopsy.

COURSE AND COMPLICATIONS

Longitudinal melanonychia is usually a stable condition. When caused by exogenous sources, identification and avoidance of the offending agent or replacement of the vitamin deficiency is helpful. Nail biopsies can lead to permanent nail dystrophy.

ICD9 Code

703.8   *Other specified diseases of nail*

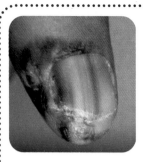

A 57-year-old African American woman presents with spreading black pigment under the nail and on the right index finger (Fig. 25-11). She says she has had a brown longitudinal streak in the nail of the affected finger that appeared several years prior. The pigment began spreading several months ago. On examination of the affected finger, there is spreading black irregular pigmentation subungually with spreading onto the cuticle and adjacent finger. What is the most likely diagnosis? What should be the next step in the care of this patient?

KEY FEATURES

- Subungual melanoma is a rare variant of acral lentiginous melanoma; it comprises 2% to 3% of all melanoma cases in whites and 15% to 20% of all melanoma cases in blacks.

- It typically first appears as longitudinal melanonychia. Distinguished from benign pigmented lesions by eventual extension of pigment to periungual folds (Hutchinson sign) with or without nail dysplasia.

- Individuals presenting with sudden development of longitudinal melanonychia should be referred for evaluation by a dermatologist.

(Continued)

Subungual Melanoma

BACKGROUND

Subungual melanoma, also called nail matrix melanoma is a variant of acral lentiginous melanoma. It is a rare disease with a reported incidence of 2% to 3% among of all melanoma cases in whites and comprises 15% to 20% of all melanoma cases in blacks. It was first called "Melanotic Whitlow" by Sir Johnathan Hutchinson in 1886 in which he described a rare malignant disease of the nail bed that appears as "a little border of coal-black colour at the edge of the inflamed nail." Today, this finding of periungually extending melanin pigmentation from longitudinal melanonychia is referred to as Hutchinson sign and is an important indication of a subungual melanoma in its radial growth phase. Because of delay in presentation and diagnosis, subungual melanoma is often associated with advanced stage at diagnosis.

PATHOGENESIS

The pathogenesis of subungual melanoma is largely unclear. It arises from neoplastic melanocytes present in the nail matrix. Due to its typical location in the thumbs and toes, the role of preceding trauma in pathogenesis has been suggested but remains unproven. Also, an association between subungual melanoma and exposure to ultraviolet (UV) light has not been demonstrated. The nail plate has been shown to be a protective barrier against UVB radiation.

CLINICAL PRESENTATION

Subungual melanoma is usually first seen as a brown or black longitudinal band in the nail plate that may or may not be associated with proximal nail plate dystrophy (Fig. 25-11). An example of a suspicious nail change is seen in Fig. 25-12. One-fourth of subungual melanomas can be amelanotic, when pigmentation is not particularly obvious or prominent. Table 25-3 highlights features of malignancy.

DIAGNOSIS

Dermoscopy is a noninvasive technique that enables dermatologists to more closely evaluate nail pigmentation and is helpful in reducing unnecessary biopsies and surgeries. Biopsy is indicated for lesions with irregular patterns on dermoscopy and accompanying clinical findings (listed above). While definitive diagnosis is made by nail matrix biopsy, the procedure is painful and can cause permanent nail damage. Appropriate staging should be performed on this and all types of melanoma based on the histopathology.

Differential Diagnosis

The differential diagnosis for subungual melanoma is very broad. Because it has a variable presentation it is often misdiagnosed and inappropriately treated.

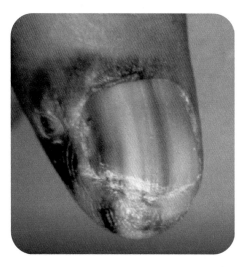

Figure 25-11 Subungual melanoma (acral lentiginous type). Note the strikingly positive Hutchinson sign. From Goodheart HP. *Goodheart's Photoguide of Common Skin Disorders,* 3rd ed. Philadelphia: Lippincott Williams & Wilkins, 2009.

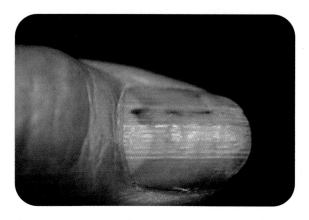

Figure 25-12 Irregular nail pigmentation suspicious for an evolving melanoma.

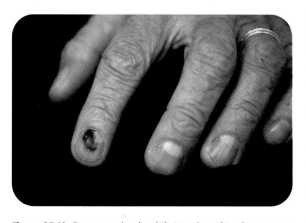

Figure 25-13 Trauma to the distal digit and resulting hematoma.

This leads to delays in proper management and increased morbidity and mortality. Trauma to the distal digit and/or nail may cause a hematoma, which in some cases may be concerning (Fig. 25-13). These lesions should grow out with the nail and otherwise be stable in size and shape.

Early Stage: ethnic pigmentation; nail matrix nevus; trauma; traumatic focal activation of nail matrix; radiation-induced; drug-induced (AZT, hydroxyurea, minocycline); exposure to cosmetic, therapeutic, or occupational chemical agents.

Later Stage with Ulceration: trauma, pyogenic granuloma, paronychia, osteomyelitis, onychotillomania, squamous cell carcinoma, Bowen disease, basal cell carcinoma, bony metastases with secondary nail ulceration.

KEY FEATURES (*Continued*)

- This is commonly misdiagnosed, causing delay in treatment with poorer prognosis than cutaneous melanoma; 5-year survival rate ranges from 16% to 87%.

- Definitive diagnosis is established by nail bed biopsy and tissue histology.

- Treatment involves amputation of affected digit.

Table 25-3	ABCDE Criteria for Acral Lentiginous (Subungual) Melanoma
A	Age: Peak 4th to 7th decades. African American, Native American, Latino, or Asian descent.
B	Sudden development of isolated brown-black pigmented longitudinal band in previously normal nail plate. Breadth of band >3 mm. Border of band blurred/irregular. Bleeding mass or ulcer.
C	Change: rapid growth of pigmented band. Nail dysplasia unchanged despite treatment.
D	Digits involved include: Thumb > Toe > Index finger. Dominant hand.
E	Extension of brown pigment from the nail bed, matrix, and plate onto proximal or lateral nail folds (Hutchinson sign). Lesions positive for Hutchinson sign should be viewed as malignant until proven otherwise.
F	Family or personal history of melanoma.

CHAPTER 25 Common Nail Disorders

WHEN TO REFER ?

- Patients with pigmented lesions suspicious for subungual melanoma should be referred to dermatology as soon as possible, as this diagnosis carries a grave prognosis and is often misdiagnosed in its early stages.

- Confirmed melanoma should be evaluated by surgical and medical oncologists.

- Patients (as well as first-degree family members) with melanoma should be referred to a dermatologist for regular full-body skin exams.

NOT TO BE MISSED

- A skin biopsy should always be obtained for changing melanocytic lesions (nail and cutaneous).

- Ulcerated lesions may require biopsy to differentiate and diagnose appropriately.

TREATMENT

Management of confirmed melanoma is surgical. For melanoma in situ, complete removal of the nail apparatus will be necessary. The excision can be later repaired with a skin graft. Treatment of invasive melanoma of the nail apparatus requires partial or full amputation of the digit. The level of amputation is determined by the thickness of the tumor and the functional importance of the affected digit. Several studies have found that more distal amputation of the affected digit with achievement of clear margins does not compromise survival while preserving more limb function.

"AT A GLANCE" TREATMENT

- An early appropriate biopsy of changing nail lesions is necessary.
- Treatment of subungual melanoma is surgical. Excision with appropriate margins, including digit amputation, is essential.

COURSE AND COMPLICATIONS

Nail biopsies can lead to permanent nail dystrophy, especially when the proximal nail matrix is involved. However, if the lesion of interest is located in the upper nail plate, biopsy of the proximal nail matrix may be unavoidable. Recurrence of the tumor may also occur if excision does not obtain clear margins.

As with other types of melanoma, tumor thickness and ulceration are associated with worse prognosis. In one study of patients with subungual melanoma, 5-year survival rate was 74% for stage I melanoma and 40% for stage II melanoma. In another study, 5-year survival rate was 80% for lesions without ulceration and 39% for lesions with ulceration.

ICD9 Code

172.6   *Malignant melanoma of skin of upper limb, including shoulder*

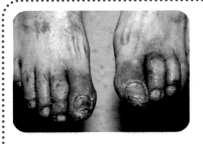

A 55-year-old woman with a medical history of skin psoriasis presents with complaints of nail changes in multiple fingers in both feet. They are not painful or particularly uncomfortable, but she finds these changes cosmetically troubling. On exam, her affected nails have numerous pits and ridges scattered on the surface and appear thickened. There is active rash on the toes and dorsal feet (Fig. 25-14). The patient asks if the changes in the appearance of her nails and feet can be reversed, as she would like to look her best at her daughter's wedding in the summer. What is the most likely diagnosis? What else could it be? What treatments are most appropriate for reversing her nail changes?

CUTANEOUS DISEASES INVOLVING THE NAIL
Nail Psoriasis

BACKGROUND

Psoriasis is a common skin condition, affecting up to 5% of the population. In its common form, it is marked by thick white or silvery scale (often called micaceous) on top of scaling erythematous plaques. It may or may not be accompanied by pruritus. Common areas of involvement are the elbows, knees, umbilicus, upper gluteal cleft, and nails. Almost all individuals with psoriasis develop nail psoriasis at some point during their lifetime. Rarely, psoriasis can be limited solely to the nails. The manifestations of nail psoriasis can be functionally and cosmetically troubling to patients. Nail psoriasis is

KEY FEATURES

- Nail psoriasis is found in >50% of patients afflicted with skin psoriasis, and is even more prevalent in patients with psoriatic arthritis.

- Nail psoriasis commonly affects the nail matrix and the nail bed, causing nail thickening, detachment from nail bed, pitting, and salmon patches.

- Multiple nails are involved at one time, but isolated nail psoriasis is not rare.

- Systemic psoriasis treatments are generally effective for nail psoriasis.

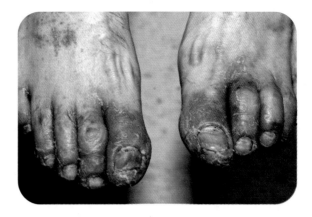

Figure 25-14 Plantar psoriasis with prominent nail involvement.

challenging to diagnose in the setting of minimal cutaneous changes because of its resemblance to many other causes of abnormal-appearing nails.

PATHOGENESIS

Psoriasis is a chronic inflammatory disease with a strong genetic component that causes abnormal epidermal development. Studies have shown that between 36% and 91% of patients with psoriasis have positive family histories. Furthermore, certain HLA types including HLA-B13, B17, B37, Bw16, and DR7 are more common among those with psoriasis. Exacerbating factors: streptococcal infections, viral exanthems, life stressors, direct cutaneous trauma, medications such as lithium, beta-blockers, NSAIDs, and steroid tapers have all been reported to trigger psoriasis.

CLINICAL PRESENTATION

Nail psoriasis causes onycholysis, pitting, ridging, subungual hyperkeratosis, periungual psoriatic plaque, and salmon patches (Figs. 25-5, 25-7, 25-14). Onycholysis is the most common feature of this condition and can affect both fingernails and toenails. Psoriatic nail pits are large, deep, irregular, and only found in the fingernails; this indicates involvement of the proximal nail matrix. Salmon patches, or the oil drop sign, appear as spots of orange discoloration in the center of the nail or at the proximal fringes of onycholysis. Salmon patches indicate involvement of the nail bed. Figure 25-15 demonstrates nail pits, salmon patches, and onycholysis. Subungual hyperkeratosis describes thickening of the nail plate, and is typically found in combination with onycholytic toenails that are afflicted with psoriasis. Occasionally psoriatic nails can crumble or develop splinter hemorrhages.

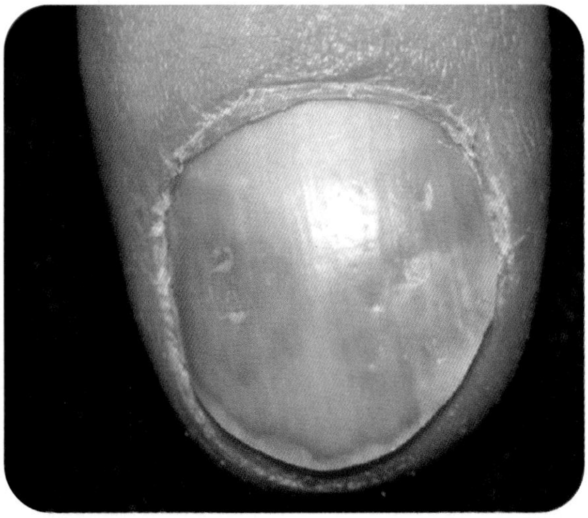

Figure 25-15 Nail psoriasis. Note the findings of onycholysis, nail pitting, and salmon patches (oil spots). From Goodheart HP. *Goodheart's Photoguide of Common Skin Disorders,* 3rd ed. Philadelphia: Lippincott Williams & Wilkins, 2009.

DIAGNOSIS

Diagnosis can be made based on history and physical findings. While nail biopsies carry a risk of permanent nail dystrophy, histopathology can be a useful aid in difficult cases. In particular, periodic acid-Schiff (PAS)-staining of nail samples helps differentiate between nail psoriasis and onychomycosis. The nail changes produced by nail psoriasis can resemble a vast number of other nail disorders. However, salmon patches or erythema at proximal borders of onycholysis are diagnostic for nail psoriasis.

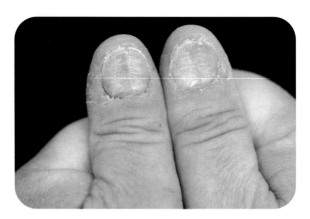

Figure 25-16 Median nail dystrophy can be mistaken for psoriatic nail changes.

Alopecia areata of the nail can also cause nail pitting, but unlike the deep and irregular pitting in nail psoriasis, it features vertical and horizontal rows of small, shallow pits in a grid-like pattern.

Differential Diagnosis

Onycholysis, onychomycosis, alopecia areata, trauma, atopic dermatitis (look for periungual scaling), or median nail dystrophy (Fig. 25-16).

TREATMENT

In general, topical therapy for nail psoriasis is unsuccessful. Several subtypes may improve with topical therapy. Nail matrix psoriasis (indicated by pitting) is best treated by intralesional triamcinolone acetonide 2.5 to 5.0 mg/mL every 4 to 8 weeks. Topical calcipotriene or tazarotene may reduce subungual hyperkeratosis found in nail bed psoriasis. Therapy of cutaneous psoriasis is discussed in Chapter 12.

Generally, systemic treatments for psoriasis are effective for nail psoriasis. First-line therapy for severe nail involvement would include acitretin 0.3 mg/kg/day for 4 to 6 months or oral methotrexate. In recalcitrant cases, cyclosporine A may be useful. Phototherapy is not helpful.

"AT A GLANCE" TREATMENT

- Topical therapy: rarely successful:
  - Nail matrix psoriasis: intralesional triamcinolone acetonide 2.5 to 5.0 mg/mL every 4 to 8 weeks
  - Subungual hyperkeratosis: calcipotriene 0.005% solution BID or tazarotene 0.1% gel QD may reduce subungual hyperkeratosis
- Systemic therapy:
  - First-line therapy: acitretin 0.3 mg/kg/day for 4 to 6 months or
  - Other options: oral methotrexate or cyclosporine A

COURSE AND COMPLICATIONS

Diagnostic nail biopsies can lead to permanent nail dystrophy. Nails affected by psoriasis are more prone to secondary fungal infection. Severe nail psoriasis can lead to diminished manual dexterity.

ICD9 Code

696.1   *Other psoriasis and similar disorders*

WHEN TO REFER

Patients with nail psoriasis who experience functional or severe cosmetic impairment should be referred to dermatology for further treatment options including systemic retinoids or methotrexate. Patients who describe digital arthritis and stiffness should be evaluated by rheumatology.

NOT TO BE MISSED

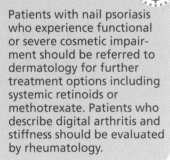

- 21% of psoriatic nails have secondary onychomycosis.
- Concurrent complaint of digit pain can indicate psoriatic arthritis.

Nail Signs of Systemic Diseases

Patients complain about the appearance of their nails to their health care providers. Like the appearance of the skin, nail morphology can be an insightful window into an individual's state of health. Therefore, inspection of the nails should be a part of any complete physical exam. Nail findings associated with systemic disease are discussed in Table 25-4 (Figs. 25-17 to 25-23).

Table 25-4 Nail Findings Associated With Systemic Disease	
CONDITION/PHYSICAL EXAM	**IMPORTANT ASSOCIATIONS**
Beau's Lines (See Fig. 25-17): A type of horizontal nail ridging that is characterized by transverse depressions in nail plate surface caused by transient arrest of nail proliferation. These ridges can move distally along with nail growth. Timing of the nail proliferation arrest can be estimated in months by measuring the distance of Beau's lines from the cuticle in millimeters and dividing by 3 for fingernails and 1 for toenails. Onychomadesis is the severe endpoint of this nail plate growth arrest.	Multiple lines in the same nail plate suggest proliferation was stopped multiple times. Beau's lines at the same levels in multiple nails suggest a severe systemic insult to all nail proliferation. This is commonly caused by chemotherapy, organ transplantation, surgery, peripheral ischemia, Raynaud disease, viral illness, chronic renal failure, pemphigus, and even deep dives or high altitude.
Clubbing (Fig. 25-18): Describes the convexity of the proximal nail fold with thickening of the distal finger; these changes are accompanied by increased sponginess of the nail bed and loss of the normally <180° angle between the nail bed and the cuticle. Schamroth's test is helpful for clinical determination of clubbing (Fig. 25-19).	Clubbing is associated with chronic obstructive pulmonary disease, idiopathic pulmonary fibrosis, asbestosis, cystic fibrosis, pulmonary malignancy, cirrhosis, cyanotic heart disease, endocarditis, and inflammatory bowel disease.
Koilonychia (Fig. 25-20): Features loss of normal nail convexity, and flattening or concavity of the nail plate. Also known as "spoon nails."	This variation in nail shape can be normal in children. In adults, it is commonly associated with nail trauma but can indicate iron deficiency anemia, hemochromatosis, systemic lupus (SLE), and Raynaud disease.
Periungual Telangiectasia (Fig. 25-21): Examination of eponychium with a magnifying glass would reveal irregular, tortuous, and dilated vessels. When viewed with the naked eye, this area may appear erythematous.	Associated with rheumatoid arthritis, SLE, dermato-myositis, and scleroderma.
Pitting (Fig. 25-7): Punctate divots in the surface of the nail plate caused by disruption of normal nail formation at the proximal nail matrix.	Typically seen in psoriasis, eczema, and local chemical dermatitis. Can also be associated with Reiter syndrome, sarcoidosis, pemphigus, alopecia areata, and connective tissue disorders.
Nail Ridging: Vertical nail surface ridging typically results from defective keratinization of the proximal nail matrix, causing bands of depression in the nail plate that are bordered by ridges and fissures (Fig. 25-22).	Vertical nail surface ridging can occur as a normal part of aging. If accompanied by bands of nail thinning, it can indicate nail manifestations of alopecia areata, lichen planus, and nail matrix compression by a myxoid cyst in the proximal nail fold.
Splinter Hemorrhage: Describes thin red or brown lines seen in the nail plate. They are caused by leakage of subungual capillaries.	Caused by trauma, psoriasis, and classically, endocarditis. This sign is more specific for endocarditis if it is found in the proximal nail plate and is accompanied by a heart murmur, Roth's spots, Osler's nodes and Janeway's lesions.
Yellow Nail Syndrome (Fig. 25-23): First described in 1964 as slowed or arrested nail growth with yellowing and thickening of the nail plate, increased convexity of the lateral edges and disappearance of the cuticle. Periorbital edema and orbital hypertelorism have also been observed.	Seen in individuals with chronic respiratory tract disease such as: pneumonia, bronchiectasis, sinusitis, and pleural effusions. Also associated with lymphedema, nephrotic syndrome, tuberculosis, thyroiditis, syndromes of immunodeficiency, internal malignancies, and rheumatoid arthritis patients treated with thiol drugs.

CHAPTER 25 Common Nail Disorders

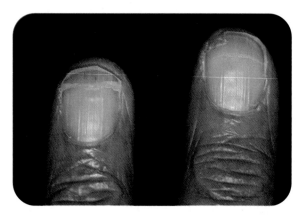

Figure 25-17 Onychomadesis: in this photo, Beau's lines from a woman with bullous pemphgoid.

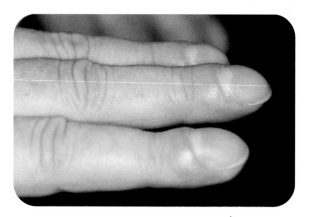

Figure 25-18 Nail clubbing secondary to pulmonary disease.

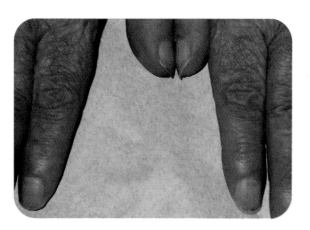

Figure 25-19 Schamroth's sign shows flattening of the plate to fold angle. From Berg D, Worzala K. *Atlas of Adult Physical Diagnosis*. Philadelphia: Lippincott Williams & Wilkins, 2006.

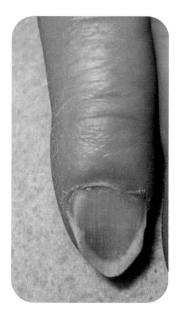

Figure 25-20 Koilonychia. In this case the patient was iron deficient. Image provided by Stedman's Medical Dictionary.

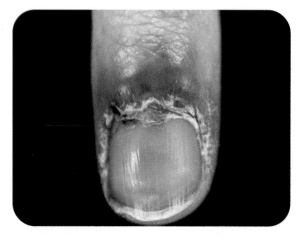

Figure 25-21 Periungual telangiectasias seen in dermatomyositis.

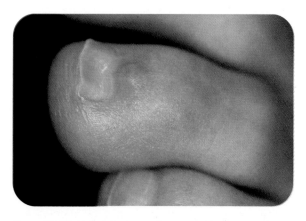

Figure 25-22 Nail plate depression caused by compression on the nail matrix from a digital mucous cyst (note papule proximal to cuticle).

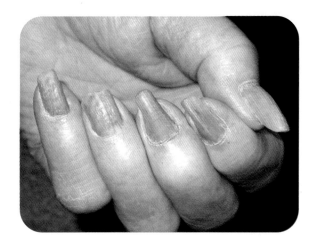

Figure 25-23 Yellow nail syndrome.

Suggested Reading

Agger WA, Mardan A. Pseudomonas aeruginosa infections of intact skin. *Clin Infect Dis.* 1995 Feb;20(2): 302–308.

Ayata A, Unal M, Ersanli D, et al. Ocular findings in yellow nail syndrome. *Can J Ophthalmol.* 2008;43(4): 493–494.

Baran R, Kechijian P. Hutchinson's sign: A reappraisal. *J Am Acad Dermatol.* 1996;34(1):87–90.

Bellis F, Nickol A. Everest nails: A prospective study on the incidence of Beau's lines after time spent at high altitude. *High Alt Med Biol.* 2005;6(2):178–180.

Braun RP, Baran R, Le Gal FA, et al. Diagnosis and management of nail pigmentations. *J Am Acad Dermatol.* 2007;56(5):835–847. Epub 2007 Feb 22.

Brazzelli V, Martinoli S, Prestinari F, et al. An impressive therapeutic result of nail psoriasis to acitretin. *J Eur Acad Dermatol Venereol.* 2004;18(2):229–230.

Dominguez-Cherit J, Roldan-Marin R, Pichardo-Velazquez P, et al. Melanonychia, melanocytic hyperplasia, and nail melanoma in a Hispanic population. *J Am Acad Dermatol.* 2008;18.

Elewski BE. Bacterial infection in a patient with onychomycosis. *J Am Acad Dermatol.* 1997;37(3 Pt 1):493–494.

Fawcett RS, Linford S, Stulberg DL. Nail abnormalities: Clues to systemic disease. *Am Fam Physician.* 2004;69(6):1417–1424.

Finley RK 3rd, Driscoll DL, Blumenson LE, et al. Subungual melanoma: An eighteen-year review. *Surgery.* 1994;116(1):96–100.

Grover C, Reddy BS, Uma Chaturvedi K. Diagnosis of nail psoriasis: Importance of biopsy and histopathology. *Br J Dermatol.* 2005;153(6):1153–1158.

Haneke E, Baran R. Longitudinal melanonychia. *Dermatol Surg.* 2001;27(6):580–584.

Levit EK, Kagen MH, Scher RK, et al. The ABC rule for clinical detection of subungual melanoma. *J Am Acad Dermatol.* 2000;42(2 Pt 1):269–274.

Maes M, Richert B, de la Brassinne M. Green nail syndrome or chloronychia. *Rev Med Liege.* 2002;57(4): 233–235.

Mazereeuw-Hautier J, Bonafé JL. Bilateral Beau's lines and pyogenic granulomas following Guillain-Barré syndrome. *Dermatology.* 2004;209(3):237–238.

Murray HE, Anhalt AW, Lessard R, et al. A 12-month treatment of severe psoriasis with acitretin: Results of a Canadian open multicenter study. *J Am Acad Dermatol.* 1991;24(4):598–602.

Sakata S, Howard A. Pseudomonas chloronychia in a patient with nail psoriasis. *Med J Aust.* 2007;186(8):424.

Salem A, Al Mokadem S, Attwa E, et al. Nail changes in chronic renal failure patients under haemodialysis. *J Eur Acad Dermatol Venereol.* 2008;22:1326–1331.

Scher RK, Stiller M, Zhu YI. Tazarotene 0.1% gel in the treatment of fingernail psoriasis: A double-blind, randomized, vehicle-controlled study. *Cutis.* 2001;68(5):355–358.

Schwartz H. Clinical observation: Beau's lines on fingernails after deep saturation dives. *Undersea Hyperb Med.* 2006;33(1):5–10.

Tan KB, Moncrieff M, Thompson JF, et al. Subungual melanoma: A study of 124 cases highlighting features of early lesions, potential pitfalls in diagnosis, and guidelines for histologic reporting. *Am J Surg Pathol.* 2007;31(12):1902–1912.

Wolff K, Johnson RA, Suurmond D. "Section 30. Disorders of the Nail Apparatus" In Wolff K, Johnson RA, Suurmond D. *Fitzpatrick's Color Atlas & Synopsis of Clinical Dermatology,* 5th ed: http://www.accessmedicine.com.ezp-prod1.hul.harvard.edu/content.aspx?aID=761727.

Connective Tissue Disease and Vasculitis-Related Dermatoses

Stephanie Hu and Peter C. Schalock

Autoimmunity is the state of the immune system erroneously attacking self—antigens such as cellular DNA or dermal collagen. The diseases caused by this state are dependent upon the target antigen and the antibody(s) involved. In the case of immune-related dermatoses, some primarily affect the skin, such as chronic cutaneous lupus erythematosus or capillaritis/small vessel vasculitis. Others involve the skin secondarily to other systemic disease (e.g., systemic lupus, dermatomyositis). Vasculitis as a topic is exceedingly broad. Causes range from infections to autoimmune disease to systemic hypersensitivity reactions. In this chapter, the discussion of vasculitis will be limited to Henoch-Schönlein purpura.

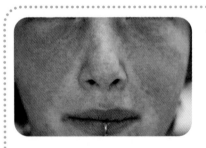

A 21-year-old woman presents with diffuse polyarticular arthralgias, unable to walk due to pain, hematuria, proteinuria, severe mouth/tongue pain, and striking macular erythema on the central face/cheeks with sparing of the upper eyelids (Fig. 26-1). Erythrocyte sedimentation rate (ESR) is 102, antinuclear antibody (ANA) reveals a 1:2,320 positive with speckled pattern, and the double-stranded DNA test is positive. What is the most likely diagnosis?

Systemic Lupus Erythematosus

BACKGROUND/EPIDEMIOLOGY

Systemic lupus erythematosus (SLE) is a serious multi-system disease arising from polyclonal B-cell autoimmunity, which involves connective tissue and blood vessels. The age of onset of SLE is typically around age 30 in females and age 40 in males. The disease is more common in women (with a female to male ratio of 8:1) and blacks, and less than 5% of patients report a positive family history of SLE. An SLE syndrome can be induced by drugs (i.e., hydralazine, certain anticonvulsants and antibiotics, and procainamide), but rash is a relatively uncommon feature of drug-induced SLE. Clinical manifestations of SLE include fever (90%); fatigue (100%); weight loss; malaise; skin lesions (85%); arthralgia or arthritis; abdominal pain; and CNS, renal, cardiac, and pulmonary disease.

PATHOGENESIS

Lupus erythematosus (LE) encompasses a spectrum of diseases that share systemic clinical findings and distinct patterns of cellular and humoral autoimmunity. Skin lesions that are directly related to the LE autoimmune process can

KEY FEATURES

- Systemic lupus erythematosus (SLE) is a serious multi-system disease arising from polyclonal B-cell autoimmunity.

- SLE syndrome can be induced by drugs (i.e., hydralazine, certain anticonvulsants and antibiotics, and procainamide).

- Clinical manifestations of SLE include fever (90%); fatigue (100%); weight loss; malaise; skin lesions (85%); arthralgia or arthritis; abdominal pain; and central nervous system (CNS), renal, cardiac, and pulmonary disease.

- The butterfly rash is the classic acute cutaneous finding in SLE. It is characterized by erythema in a sharply-defined malar distribution over the cheeks and bridge of the nose that appears in approximately one-half of patients, usually after UV exposure.

- Treatment is with topical and oral corticosteroids, antimalarials, and in severe cases immunosuppressives such as azathioprine.

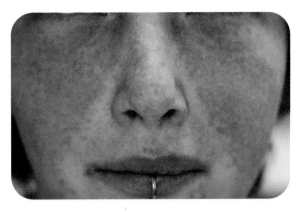

Figure 26-1 Facial dermatitis seen in systemic lupus erythematosus.

be divided into LE-specific skin disease and LE–nonspecific skin disease. Within the LE-specific skin diseases, three clinical subtypes exist: acute cutaneous LE (ACLE); subacute cutaneous LE (SCLE); and chronic cutaneous LE (CCLE, also known as discoid LE or DLE) (see Figure 26-2 for classification). Some forms of LE-specific skin disease (i.e., ACLE) often occur in the clinical context of active underlying SLE, whereas other forms are usually associated with only mild or minor degrees of SLE activity (i.e., SCLE) or no SLE activity at all (i.e., CCLE, with localized DLE being the most common variety).

CLINICAL PRESENTATION

Skin and mucous membranes are symptomatically involved at some point in over 80% of patients with SLE, although there is great variability and diversity in the type of involvement. Lesions in ACLE are typically precipitated by sunlight and are present for several weeks. Such lesions include the butterfly rash (Fig. 26-1), or localized ACLE, which is an erythematous, confluent, macular eruption on the face. This rash may precede other symptoms of lupus by months or even years or may be accompanied by other symptoms and signs of acute SLE. It often recurs. Application of alcohol (found in many sunscreens)

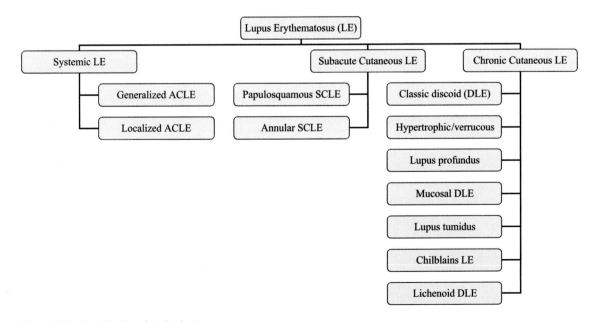

Figure 26-2 Classification of LE skin lesions.

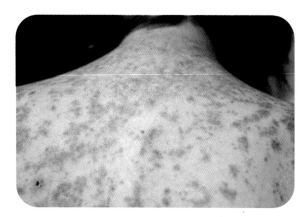

Figure 26-3 Systemic lupus erythematosus on the upper back and posterior neck.

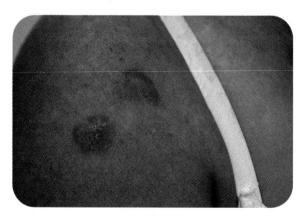

Figure 26-4 Subacute cutaneous lupus erythematosus.

can enhance the redness, due to vasodilation in the skin. The SLE rash or generalized ACLE, may also be observed, which manifests as erythematous, discrete, papular, or urticarial lesions on the face, dorsa of hands, arms, and the V of the neck (Fig. 26-3).

Vasculitis is a rare but important feature of SLE. Finding a cutaneous vasculitis often occurs in conjunction with a disease flare and is considered a poor prognostic factor. Commonly seen manifestations include livedo reticularis, microinfarcts on digital tips, palpable purpura, and urticaria.

Subacute cutaneous lupus erythematosus (SCLE) is a distinct entity and is frequently, but not uniformly, associated with SLE. Lesions are often nonscarring, nonindurated, erythematous, and papulosquamous (psoriasis-like), and/or annular and occur in a symmetrical pattern (Fig. 26-4). A subset of SCLE which presents with erythematous, nonscaling indurated plaques is tumid lupus. Approximately 50% of affected patients have SLE, and about 10% of patients with SLE have this type of skin lesion. The male to female ratio is 4:1. Cytopenia, serositis, and the presence of antinuclear antibodies (ANA) are significantly less frequent among those with SCLE than SLE, while photosensitivity is nearly twice as prevalent in those with SCLE as those with SLE (86% vs. 46%, respectively). The prevalence of renal disease in those with SCLE and SLE are not significantly different. Anti-Ro/SS-A antibodies are often found in SCLE. Medications (Table 26-1) may be responsible for initiating or exacerbating the skin disease.

General photosensitivity develops in 60% to 100% of patients with SLE, in which patients develop a rash after exposure to the UVB radiation found in sunlight or fluorescent lights. Some patients are also sensitive to UVA (as from a photocopier), and may even be sensitive to the visible light spectrum. Glass protects individuals sensitive to UVB, but only partially protects those sensitive

Table 26-1 **Medications Commonly Causing SCLE**	
• Docetaxel	• Statin family medications
• Hydrochlorothiazide	• Terbinafine
• Interferons	• Tumor necrosis factor inhibitors
• Minocycline	
• Other antihypertensive medications (calcium channel blocker and ACE inhibitor classes)	

CHAPTER 26 Autoimmune Dermatoses

to UVA. Blond, blue-eyed, fair-skinned individuals are much more photosensitive than brunettes or individuals with pigmented skin; the incidence is also great in those with anti-Ro antibodies.

Other cutaneous lesions in SLE include bullae, which can be hemorrhagic in acute flares; papules and scaly plaques as in SCLE; discoid plaques in CCLE, predominantly on the face, arms, and scalp; and erythematous, sometimes violaceous, slightly scaling, densely set and confluent papules on the dorsa of the finger, usually sparing the articular regions (different from dermatomyositis, in which the rash overlies joint regions). Palmar erythema, mostly on fingertips, nail fold telangiectasias, "palpable" purpura (vasculitis), and urticarial lesions with purpura (urticarial vasculitis) are also seen. These vascular lesions occur in approximately 50% of patients. Diffuse alopecia or discoid lesions with patchy alopecia may be present, occurring in a majority of patients with SLE at some time during their illness. In some cases, alopecia can precede other manifestations of lupus. Mucous membrane involvement occurs in 12% to 45% of patients with SLE. This may manifest in painless ulcers arising in purpuric necrotic lesions on the palate (80%), buccal mucosa, or gums, in characteristic discoid lesions with erythema, atrophy, and depigmentation of the lips, or in gingivitis that is more common in individuals with xerostomia. There is no apparent association between the presence of oral involvement and systemic activity; oral lesions may be the first sign of lupus.

Physical Findings

The butterfly rash is the classic acute cutaneous finding in SLE. It is characterized by erythema in a sharply defined malar distribution over the cheeks and bridge of the nose that appears in approximately one-half of patients, usually after UV exposure. Fine scaling, erosions (in acute flares), and crusts may be present. The involved skin feels warm and appears slightly edematous. Generalized ACLE may occur as erythematous, discrete, papular, or urticarial lesions on photodistributed areas of the body, including the face, dorsa of hands, arms, and the V of the neck.

SCLE lesions begin as small, erythematous, slightly scaly papules that evolve into either a psoriasiform (papulosquamous) or annular rash. The latter often coalesces to form polycyclic or figurative patterns. The lesions typically have erythematous, and sometimes crusted, margins. In contrast to CCLE/DLE, follicular plugging, hyperkeratosis, dermal atrophy, permanent pigment changes, and scarring do not occur, although telangiectasia may be seen. The most commonly affected areas in SCLE are those exposed to sunlight: the shoulders, forearms, neck, and upper torso, with frequent sparing of the face.

Subepidermal bullous skin lesions may occur as a result of toxic necrolysis of the skin. In addition, SLE is rarely associated with bullous pemphigoid, dermatitis herpetiformis, or epidermolysis bullosa acquisitum.

Lichen planus (LP)-LE overlap syndrome is a rare skin disorder that demonstrates findings of both LE and LP. The cutaneous lesions consist of atrophic red to violaceous plaque and patches that are most often present on the acral portions of the extremities. The nails are commonly involved and there may be anonychia (absence of the nail). These lesions are persistent and resistant to treatment. Photosensitivity, pruritus, and follicular plugging (characteristics of discoid lupus) are generally absent. Some patients with this overlap develop SLE.

Nail lesions, particularly pitting, ridging, and onycholysis, have been noted in 25% of patients. About 20% of patients have redness of the lunula, a finding nearly always associated with periungual erythema.

Lupus alopecia may be scarring or nonscarring and can involve the scalp, eyebrows, eyelashes, beard, and/or body hair. Early lesions of scarring alopecia are characterized by well-circumscribed, erythematous, infiltrative patches with adherent follicular hyperkeratosis. Later, the lesion progresses toward an atrophic, smooth, depressed, white–ivory-colored plaque. In nonscarring alopecia caused by premature hair loss (telogen effluvium), a diffuse thinning of the scalp is seen 3 months after a stressful event, emotional upset, pregnancy, or the use of glucocorticoids. During exacerbations of SLE the hair is thin, unruly, and easily fractures. It usually occurs along the frontal hairline and grows back normally when the disease activity subsides.

DIAGNOSIS

The diagnosis is made on the basis of clinical findings, histopathology of the skin biopsy specimen, the lupus band test using immunofluorescence, and serology within the framework of the revised American Rheumatism Association (ARA) criteria for classification of SLE (see Table 26-2). The lupus band test (LBT, direct immunofluorescence demonstrating IgG, IgM, and C3) is positive in lesional skin in 90% of patients, in clinically normal sun-exposed skin in 70% to 80% patients and in clinically normal non–sun-exposed skin in 50% of patients.

ANA is positive in greater than 95% of patients, with a peripheral pattern of nuclear fluorescence. Anti–double-stranded DNA antibodies, anti-Sm antibodies, and rRNP antibodies are specific for SLE. Low levels of complement are seen, particularly in patients with renal involvement. Anticardiolipin autoanti-

Table 26-2 ARA Criteria for Diagnosis of Systemic Lupus Erythematosus

CRITERION	DEFINITION
Malar rash	Fixed erythema, flat or raised, over the malar eminences, tending to spare the nasolabial folds
Discoid rash	Erythematosus raised patches with adherent keratotic scaling and follicular plugging; atrophic scarring may occur in older lesions
Photosensitivity	Skin rash as a result of unusual reaction to sunlight, by patient history or physician observation
Oral ulcers	Oral or nasopharyngeal ulceration, usually painless, observed by a physician
Arthritis	Nonerosive arthritis involving two or more peripheral joints, characterized by tenderness, swelling, or effusion
Serositis	Pleuritis: convincing history of pleuritic pain or rub heard by a physician or evidence of pleural effusion **OR** Pericarditis: documented by EKG, rub or evidence of pericardial effusion
Renal disorder	Persistent proteinuria greater than 0.5 g/d or greater than 3+ if quantitation not performed **OR** Cellular casts: may be red cell, hemoglobin, granular, tubular, or mixed
Neurologic disorder	Seizures **OR** psychosis: in the absence of offending drugs or known metabolic derangements (uremia, ketoacidosis, or electrolyte imbalance)
Hematologic disorder	Hemolytic anemia: with reticulocytosis **OR** Leukopenia: less than 4,000/mm^3 total on two or more occasions **OR** Lymphopenia: less than 1,500/mm^3 on two or more occasions **OR** Thrombocytopenia: less than 100,000/mm^3 in the absence of offending drugs
Immunologic disorders	Positive antiphospholipid antibody **OR** Anti-DNA: antibody to native DNA in abnormal titer **OR** Anti-Sm: presence of antibody to Sm nuclear antigen **OR** False-positive serologic test for syphilis known to be positive for at least 6 months and confirmed by *Treponema pallidum* immobilization or fluorescent treponemal antibody absorption test
Antinuclear antibody	An abnormal titer of antinuclear antibody by immunofluorescence or an equivalent assay at any point in time and in the absence of drugs known to be associated with "drug-induced lupus" syndrome

From Tan EM, Cohen AS, Fries JF, et al. The 1982 revised criteria for the classification of systemic lupus erythematosus. *Arthritis Rheum.* 1982;25:1271–1277.

bodies (lupus anticoagulant) are present in the specific subset of patients with the anticardiolipin syndrome, and anti-Ro/SS-A autoantibodies have a low specificity for SLE but are specific in the subset of patients with SCLE lesions.

Hematologic findings in SLE include anemia (usually normocytic, normochromic, or rarely, hemolytic Coombs-positive); leukopenia ($<$4,000/μL); lymphopenia; thrombocytopenia; and elevated ESR (which can be a useful guide to monitoring disease activity). Urinalysis can demonstrate persistent hematuria, proteinuria, and casts with the development of lupus nephritis.

THERAPY

General measures in the treatment of SLE include rest, avoidance of sun exposure and photosensitizing medications, and liberal use of daily sunscreen. A lupus rash should initially be treated with topical glucocorticoids. Hydrocortisone may suffice for early, superficial involvement, but more potent steroids (particularly the fluorinated preparations) should be used for thicker lesions.

Antimalarials are useful for treatment of the skin lesions in subacute and chronic LE but do not reduce the need for prednisone. Precautions need to be observed in its use; adverse events include precipitation of flares of psoriasis and porphyria cutanea tarda, hemolytic anemia in patients with G6PD deficiency and ocular changes such as macular degeneration. Currently, the most commonly used antimalarial in SLE is hydroxychloroquine, dosed by weight (less than 6.5 mg/kg per day to a maximum of 400 mg/day, and less than 400 mg/day for patients weighing less than 61 kg). Chloroquine 250 to 500 mg/day is somewhat more potent but has a higher risk of eye damage. Quinacrine 50 to 100 mg/day is even more effective and has a much lower risk of eye damage, but the skin turns yellow in many patients and bone marrow suppression is a rare complication. Improvement with antimalarials may not be seen until 6 to 12 weeks of use.

Indications for prednisone (60 mg/day in divided doses) include a) CNS involvement; b) renal involvement; c) severely ill patients without CNS involvement; d) hemolytic crisis; and e) thrombocytopenia. Concomitant immunosuppressive drugs, i.e., azathioprine or cyclophosphamide, can be added, with the choice of the agent depending on organ involvement and disease activity. In renal disease, intravenous cyclophosphamide bolus therapy may be beneficial. Systemic steroids and immunosuppressive agents are rarely needed to clear skin lesions except for bullous lesions, although local injections of resistant lesions with glucocorticoids may be effective for resistant skin lesions.

Hair loss in active SLE usually responds well to treatment of the lupus, while hair loss due to glucocorticoids recovers as the steroid dose is lowered. The hair loss is usually permanent when associated with scarring, as with discoid lesions of the scalp. Intralesional triamcinolone injection (3 to 10 mg/cc) may be useful for treatment of localized areas of alopecia, especially early in the course before scarring has occurred to a significant extent. Topical minoxidil may be beneficial in a limited number of patients with acute, nonscarring alopecia.

Mucous membrane lesions respond well to topical glucocorticoids (usually Orabase mixed with either 0.1% triamcinolone or 0.05% clobetasol), 0.1% tacrolimus ointment, intralesional glucocorticoids, and systemic antimalarial drugs. The response to topical steroids takes a few days to weeks, while the response to hydroxychloroquine takes weeks to months.

"AT A GLANCE" TREATMENT

- General Measures:
  - Rest, avoidance of sun exposure and photosensitizing medications, and liberal use of daily sunscreen.

CHAPTER 26 Autoimmune Dermatoses

NOT TO BE MISSED

- Sun protection, both in the form of sun avoidance and sun protection, is mandatory for all lupus patients. Sunlight exposure alone may activate cutaneous or systemic lupus.

- Cutaneous SLE: initially treated with topical glucocorticoids:
  - Hydrocortisone 2.5% cream BID for early, superficial involvement
  - Clobetasol propionate 0.05% cream/ointment should be used for thicker lesions.
- Oral prednisone (60 mg/day in divided doses) for:
  - a) CNS involvement, b) renal involvement, c) severely ill patients without CNS involvement, d) hemolytic crisis, and e) thrombocytopenia
- Antimalarials treat skin lesions in subacute and chronic LE but do not reduce the need for prednisone for systemic therapy:
  - Hydroxychloroquine, dosed by weight (less than 6.5 mg/kg per day to a maximum of 400 mg/day, and less than 400 mg/day for patients weighing less than 61 kg).
  - Chloroquine 250 to 500 mg/day is somewhat more potent but has a higher risk of eye damage.
  - Quinacrine 50 to 100 mg/day is even more effective and has a much lower risk of eye damage, but the skin turns yellow in many patients and bone marrow suppression is a rare complication.
  - Improvement with antimalarials may not be seen until 6 to 12 weeks of use.

COURSE AND COMPLICATIONS

The 5-year survival rate for SLE is currently 93% and has increased dramatically over the last several decades due to increased disease recognition with more sensitive diagnostic tests, earlier diagnosis or treatment, the inclusion of milder cases, and increasingly judicious therapy and prompt treatment of complications. Most patients have a relapsing and remitting course, which may be associated with the use of high-dose steroids during the treatment of severe flares.

Factors that may be associated with a shorter delay between disease onset and organ damage include Hispanic ethnicity, greater disease activity, a history of thrombotic events, and glucocorticoid use of less than 10 mg per day.

ICD9 Code	
710.0	Systemic lupus erythematosus

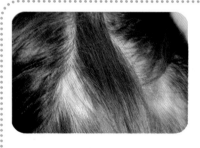

A 47-year-old woman presents with the complaint of hair loss. She reports having slowly progressive hair loss associated with focal erythematous, scaling plaques in her scalp (Fig. 26-5). She has also had similar lesions on her skin which were slightly pruritic. They healed spontaneously after months to years with residual scarring and hyperpigmentation. What is her diagnosis and what is the best therapy to initiate?

Chronic Cutaneous Lupus

Stephanie Hu

BACKGROUND/EPIDEMIOLOGY

Chronic discoid lesions develop in up to 25% of patients with SLE but may also occur in the absence of any other clinical feature of SLE. Patients with only cutaneous discoid lupus generally have a negative or low-titer antinuclear antibody (ANA), and rarely have low titers of anti-Ro antibodies. Patients with cutaneous discoid lupus have approximately 5% to 10% risk of eventually developing SLE, which tends to be mild. Patients with more numerous and widespread lesions appear to be more likely to develop SLE. The disease is possibly more severe in Africans or African Americans. DLE lesions can be precipitated by sunlight, but to a lesser extent than ACLE or SCLE. Lesions last for months to years and are usually asymptomatic, although they can sometimes be slightly pruritic or painful.

Less common cutaneous lesions of CCLE include lupus panniculitis/profundus, lupus tumidus, and chilblains (pernio). Patients with lupus panniculitis/profundus present with firm, circumscribed subcutaneous nodules that occur before or following the typical lesions of DLE but also in their absence. Some patients with lupus panniculitis/profundus exhibit no other manifestations of SLE; only 10% to 25% of such patients eventually develop SLE.

Lupus tumidus is a rare variant of CCLE/DLE. Patients are photosensitive and generally lack ANA, and it is rare for patients presenting with this form of cutaneous LE to develop clinically significant SLE later.

Chilblains lesions (pernio) can occur as a benign isolated clinical phenomenon (idiopathic chilblains) or as a cutaneous manifestation of an evolving underlying autoimmune disease such as LE (i.e., chilblains LE). Lesions tend to occur after cold exposure. Patients having chilblains associated with SLE are more often female and tend to exhibit persistent lesions beyond the cold season. Lesions resemble old lesions of DLE both histologically and clinically, and most patients with this variant have Raynaud phenomenon and DLE elsewhere; individuals presenting with chilblains skin lesions should be carefully evaluated and followed for the development of SLE.

PATHOGENESIS

The pathogenesis of CCLE is the same as that of all types of lupus. See the SLE section for a detailed discussion.

CLINICAL PRESENTATION

Discoid lesions are characterized by brightly erythematous papules that evolve into discrete, slightly infiltrated plaques covered by a well-formed adherent scale that extends into dilated hair follicles (follicular plugging). Scales are difficult to remove and show spines (upon magnification) on the undersurface resembling carpet tacks. Discoid lesions are most often seen on the face, neck, and scalp, but also occur on the ears, dorsa of forearms, hands, fingers, toes, and infrequently on the upper torso. They tend to slowly expand with active inflammation at the periphery, and then to heal, leaving depressed central scars, atrophy, telangiectasia, and hyperpigmentation/depigmentation. Some discoid lesions are hyperkeratotic. Scarring alopecia can be seen with residual inflammation and follicular plugging (Fig. 26-5).

Lupus panniculitis/profundus manifests as a firm, nodular lesion or a platelike infiltration with or without an overlying surface cutaneous lesion. The nodules, which are often painful and may be better felt than seen, may appear on the scalp, face, arms, chest (especially the breasts), back, thighs, and buttocks. The nodules usually resolve but may leave a depressed area. Subcutaneous calcification can result, which may produce considerable disability from secondary overlying cutaneous ulceration and infection.

Lupus tumidus is a rare variant of CCLE/DLE characterized by photodistributed, succulent lesions consisting of chronic pink to violaceous papules, nonscarring urticarial plaques, and/or nodules, in the absence of surface changes (i.e., overlying scale or follicular hyperkeratosis), which is in contrast to classic DLE lesions. They typically present over the face, neck, upper trunk, and proximal upper extremities.

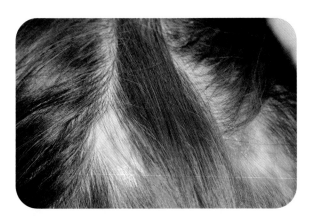

Figure 26-5 Scarring alopecia due to chronic cutaneous lupus erythematosus.

Chilblains skin lesions (pernio) are cold-induced violaceous papules, nodules, and plaques typically distributed over the face and acral aspects of the extremities. As these lesions evolve, they usually assume the appearance of scarred atrophic plaques with associated telangiectasia; persistent lesions can develop a verrucous surface change.

DIAGNOSIS

Diagnosis of CCLE lesions requires correlation of clinical and histopathological findings. Immunofluorescence in the form of the lupus band test is positive in 90% of active lesions at least 6 weeks old and not recently treated with topical glucocorticoids. The lupus band test is negative in burned-out (scarred) lesions and in the normal skin, both sun-exposed and nonexposed. Serology may show a low incidence of ANA in a titer greater than 1:16. Patients are also occasionally leukopenic with white blood cell counts of typically less than 4,500/μL.

THERAPY

Classic CCLE/DLE lesions may be treated with topical glucocorticoids. Intralesional triamcinolone acetonide, 3 to 10 mg/mL, may also be injected. Administration of antimalarials, such as hydroxychloroquine, equal to or less than 6.5 mg/kg body weight per day, is another option. If this is ineffective, quinacrine, 100 mg TID may be added. Appropriate ophthalmologic evaluation is needed for patients on antimalarial agents. Hyperkeratotic DLE lesions respond well to systemic acitretin at 1 mg/kg body weight. Topical sunscreens (SPF >45 with broad UVA coverage) should be used routinely to prevent further development of lesions.

Lupus panniculitis/profundus may be treated with antimalarials or a short course of systemic glucocorticoids. Lupus tumidus also responds to antimalarial therapy.

Newer treatments showing promise in the treatment of chronic LE include mycophenolate mofetil, anti-TNF therapy, thalidomide, B-cell targeted therapy (i.e., rituximab, epratuzumab), and costimulatory blockade (i.e., abatacept and leflunomide).

"AT A GLANCE" TREATMENT

- CCLE/DLE/tumid lupus lesions:
  - Topical corticosteroids: clobetasol propionate 0.05% cream/ointment BID to AA for nonfacial/genital skin
  - Intralesional triamcinolone acetonide, 3 to 10 mg/mL
  - Hydroxychloroquine, equal to or less than 6.5 mg/kg body weight per day, quinacrine, 100 mg TID may be added as necessary:
    - Appropriate ophthalmologic evaluation is needed for patients on antimalarial agents. Hyperkeratotic DLE: acitretin at 1 mg/kg body weight.
  - Topical sunscreens (SPF >45 with broad UVA coverage) are essential

COURSE AND COMPLICATIONS

Overall, only 1% to 5% of patients with CCLE develop SLE. With localized lesions, complete remission occurs in 50% of patients, whereas remission is less frequent (<10%) with generalized lesions. CCLE lesions may be the presenting cutaneous sign of SLE.

ICD9 Code	
695.4	*Lupus erythematosus*

WHEN TO REFER

Patients with recalcitrant symptomatic lesions may benefit from a dermatology consultation. For those with symptoms suggestive of transformation to active systemic lupus, a rheumatology consultation may facilitate further diagnosis and care.

NOT TO BE MISSED

- Sun protection and sunscreen is essential for preventing new lesions and progression of established lesions.

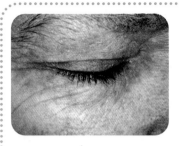

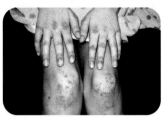

A 52-year-old woman presents for a recalcitrant facial, eyelid, and hand dermatitis (Figs. 26-6, 26-7) that has been present for several months. She has never had a similar rash in the past, is not atopic. She is feeling well other than a vague complaint of abdominal enlargement. On further questioning, she reports having new onset problems standing up from a chair and with combing her hair. What is the most likely diagnosis? What further screening exams should be performed?

Dermatomyositis
Stephanie Hu

BACKGROUND/EPIDEMIOLOGY

Dermatomyositis (DM) is a systemic disease classified with the idiopathic inflammatory myopathy, a heterogeneous group of genetically determined autoimmune diseases targeting the skin and/or skeletal muscles. Defined clinically, the prevalence rate of DM is estimated at approximately one per 100,000 in the general population. There is a female to male predominance of about 2:1. Although the peak incidence in adults occurs between the ages of 50 and 60, individuals of any age may be affected, and both juvenile and adult (>40 years) onset variants of the disease have been described.

KEY FEATURES

- Dermatomyositis is an idiopathic inflammatory myopathy commonly involving skin and muscle.

- Pathogenesis is unknown. Drug-induced DM is uncommon. In some cases, this is a paraneoplastic condition.

- This is most commonly a disease of adults, but juvenile variants exist (which are not paraneoplastic in etiology).

- Diagnosis is through characteristic skin biopsies and serologies including an anti-Jo1, anti-SRP and anti-Mi2 antibody.

- Treatment is with oral corticosteroids or other immunomodulatory agents. Diagnosis and treatment of underlying malignancy is essential.

PATHOGENESIS

The etiology of DM remains unknown. The disease is considered to be a humorally mediated disorder in which the cellular infiltrate, located principally in perifascicular regions of muscle, is often focused around blood vessels. The inflammatory infiltrate is composed of B cells and plasmacytoid CD4+dendritic cells. Other typical features include perifascicular atrophy and fibrosis. Abnormal muscle fibers are usually grouped in one portion of the fascicle, suggestive of microinfarction mediated by blood vessel dysfunction. Drug-induced DM is uncommon, but hydroxyurea is the most frequently implicated agent.

CLINICAL PRESENTATION

In persons over 55 years of age, this disease is often associated with malignancy. The clinical spectrum ranges from DM with only cutaneous inflammation (amyopathic DM) to polymyositis (PM) with only muscle inflammation. Cutaneous involvement occurs in 30% to 40% of adults and 95% of children with DM/PM. Table 26-3 shows the classification of DM. Muscle weakness is the most common presenting feature of DM. This usually occurs with an insidious onset and gradual worsening over a period of several months before medical attention is sought. Patients typically describe difficulty in rising from the

Table 26-3 Classification of Dermatomyositis (DM)	
ADULT ONSET	**JUVENILE ONSET**
• Classic DM alone	• Classic DM
• Classic DM with malignancy	• Amyopathic DM
• Classic DM of an overlap connective tissue disorder	• Hypomyopathic DM
• Amyopathic DM	

From Kovacs SO, Kovacs SC. Dermatomyositis. *J Am Acad Dermatol.* 1998;39:899.

CHAPTER 26 Autoimmune Dermatoses

supine position, climbing stairs, raising arms over the head (such as when combing hair), and turning in bed. The distribution of weakness is typically symmetric and proximal. Distal muscle weakness, if present, tends to be mild and usually does not cause significant functional impairment. Myalgias and muscle tenderness occur in 25% to 50% of cases, and these symptoms tend to be mild, unlike the more prominent muscle pain that occurs in polymyalgia rheumatica, fibromyalgia, and viral or bacterial myositis. Muscle atrophy is generally not seen in early cases, even in patients with marked weakness, but may occur in severe, long-standing disease.

The skin lesions in DM include the characteristic violaceous, highly pruritic, periorbital heliotrope rash, usually associated with some degree of edema of the eyelids and periorbital area (Fig. 26-6). This may extend to involve the scalp, entire face, upper chest, and arms. The shawl sign or V sign is a diffuse, flat erythematous lesion occurring over the chest and shoulders or in a V-shaped distribution over the anterior neck and chest. This rash may be exacerbated by exposure to ultraviolet light. Erythroderma may be seen in the DM patient, manifesting as extensive areas of cutaneous erythema that may include the malar region and the forehead. In addition, flat-topped, violaceous papules (Gottron sign) often occur, with various degrees of atrophy on the nape of the neck and shoulders and over the knuckles (Gottron papules) and interphalangeal joints (Fig. 26-7). (Note: in lupus, the lesions usually occur in the interarticular region of the fingers and do not involve skin overlying knuckles.) Lesions over the elbows and knuckles may evolve into erosions and ulcers that heal with stellate scarring (particularly in juvenile DM with vasculitis). Calcifications in subcutaneous/fascial tissues are common later in the course of juvenile DM, particularly about the elbows, trochanteric, and iliac regions. These lesions may also develop into calcinosis universalis. In addition, periungual erythema, thrombosis of capillary loops, and infarctions are also seen. Pruritus and skin burning are frequently experienced by DM patients. The combination of Gottron papules, periungual telangiectasia, and dystrophic cuticles represent a diagnostic/pathognomonic cutaneous constellation of DM skin change.

Systemically, esophageal involvement can be seen in elderly patients and may underlie the increased incidence of bacterial pneumonia. Dysphagia, nasal regurgitation, and/or aspiration can occur in DM due to weakness of the striated muscle of the upper one-third of the esophagus and/or the oropharyngeal muscles. Cardiac involvement with conduction defects or histologic evidence of myocarditis is well-described in DM, but myocardial injury severe enough to cause heart failure is unusual. Those with severe disease may present with a variety of other manifestations, including fever, weight loss, Raynaud phenomenon, and a nonerosive inflammatory polyarthritis.

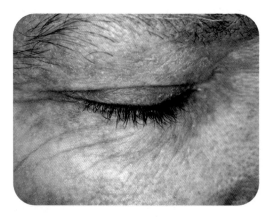

Figure 26-6 "Heliotrope" rash on the upper eyelids associated with dermatomyositis.

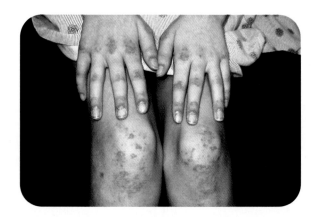

Figure 26-7 Skin involvement of the hands, arms, legs, and body due to dermatomyositis. Note Gottron papules above the joints.

Up to 30% of patients with DM have a constellation of clinical findings termed "the antisynthetase syndrome." These findings include a relatively acute disease onset; constitutional symptoms (i.e., fever); Raynaud phenomenon; "mechanic's hands" (a roughening and cracking of the skin of the tips and lateral aspects of the fingers, resulting in irregular, dirty-appearing lines that resemble those of a manual laborer); arthritis; and interstitial lung disease (ILD). However, not all patients with antisynthetase antibodies or even those classified as having this syndrome have all manifestations of this syndrome, and this group of clinical findings is not specific for the presence of antisynthetase antibodies.

When patients harbor the typical rash and the dermatopathologic findings of DM but no clinical evidence of myopathy, they are said to have "amyopathic dermatomyositis" or "dermatomyositis sine myositis." Most of these patients eventually develop clinical, histologic, or radiologic evidence of myositis, but muscle involvement may not be seen for as long as 6 years after disease onset.

DM and its related condition, polymyositis (PM) may both overlap with features of other connective tissue diseases, particularly scleroderma, systemic lupus erythematosus, mixed connective tissue disease, and, less often, rheumatoid arthritis and Sjögren syndrome. The myopathy associated with the other connective tissue diseases varies from clinically insignificant (with minimal muscle enzyme elevations and minimal inflammatory changes on muscle biopsy) to severe DM or PM in which myopathy dominates the clinical picture.

Patients with DM have a higher than expected risk for malignancy, particularly ovarian cancer in females. Patients greater than 50 years of age should be investigated for associated malignancy carcinoma of the ovary, breast, bronchopulmonary system, and gastrointestinal (GI) tract. Most cancers are detected within 2 years of diagnosis of DM.

DIAGNOSIS

The diagnosis of DM is suggested by the above clinical findings and correlated with laboratory test results. The medical history can help to eliminate use of prescription and illicit drugs as a cause of muscle damage (i.e., colchicine, statins, hydroxychloroquine, alcohol, cocaine). In addition, risk factors for human immunodeficiency virus (HIV) infection and features of connective tissue diseases should also be sought.

During the acute active phase of DM, elevation of creatine phosphokinase (CPK) can be seen in 65% of patients, which is most specific for muscle disease. In addition, elevations in aldolase (40%), lactate dehydrogenase (LDH), and alanine and aspartate aminotransaminases (ALT and AST) are also seen. Elevated 24-hour creatine excretion (>200 mg/24 hours) may be seen in the urine.

Antinuclear antibodies (ANA) detected by standard immunofluorescence methods are present in up to 80% of patients with DM. The detection of anti-Ro, anti-La, anti-Sm, or anti-ribonucleoprotein (RNP) antibodies strongly suggests a diagnosis of myositis associated or overlapping with another connective tissue disease. Thirty percent of patients with DM have myositis-specific autoantibodies, three major categories of which are antibodies to aminoacyl-tRNA synthetases (i.e., antisynthetase antibodies like anti-Jo-1), antibodies to signal recognition particle (anti-SRP antibodies), and antibodies to Mi-2, a nuclear helicase. Anti-Jo-1 antibodies are the most common myositis-specific autoantibody and are strongly associated with ILD, Raynaud phenomenon, arthritis, and "mechanic's hands." Anti-SRP antibodies occur almost exclusively in PM and are associated with severe myopathy and aggressive disease that is difficult to control, even with high-dose glucocorticoids and adjunct immunosuppressive agents. Anti-Mi-2 antibodies are associated with the relatively acute onset of classic DM with erythroderma and the shawl sign. Serologic abnormalities are common, but their routine use for diagnosis is not presently helpful for diagnosis or prognostic prediction.

In addition to laboratory testing for muscle enzyme, electromyography (EMG) and tissue biopsies of skin and/or muscle may be important tools in evaluating a patient with possible DM. While EMG abnormalities are not diagnostic of DM, the EMG can show features that are characteristic of inflammatory myopathies and exclude neuromyopathy. The EMG is also of value in directing the site of muscle biopsy. In recent years, magnetic resonance imaging of muscular tissue has emerged as an important technique because it can demonstrate large areas of involvement, unlike muscle biopsy. It may also be useful in defining the response to therapy as it is noninvasive and lends itself to serial assessments.

A histopathologic confirmation of the diagnosis of DM should be obtained whenever possible. Skin biopsy often reveals an interface dermatitis that is difficult to differentiate from lupus erythematosus. For the majority of myositis cases, then, muscle biopsy is the definitive test for establishing the diagnosis of inflammatory myopathy and excluding the myriad other causes of muscle weakness.

A systemic evaluation should be conducted in all patients at the time of diagnosis and should include a chest X-ray, esophageal motility, pulmonary function tests, and an electrocardiogram. An age-appropriate evaluation for a possible malignancy should also be performed at the time of diagnosis and annually for at least 3 years. Female patients should be screened for ovarian cancer.

THERAPY

An important concept in the treatment of DM is that therapy should be guided primarily by patients' strength and not the concentration of their muscle enzymes, which may not accurately reflect and correlate with the degree of muscle dysfunction.

Skin disease is treated in a similar manner to cutaneous LE with slight modifications. Topical corticosteroids or nonsteroidal topical immunomodulators can be effective. Antimalarial agents and other systemic agents such as thalidomide, methotrexate, mycophenolate mofetil, dapsone, retinoids, intravenous immunoglobulin (IVIg), and biologic agents are also options.

Muscle disease is treated with systemic therapies. DM is typically treated with prednisone 0.5 to 1 mg/kg body weight per day, increasing to 1.5 mg/kg if lower doses are ineffective but not exceeding 80 mg/day. The dose is tapered when CPK levels approach normal. For patients who are severely ill, initiating glucocorticoid therapy with an intravenous methylprednisolone pulse (1,000 mg/day for 3 days) may be beneficial. The regimen is most effective if combined with azathioprine, 2 to 3 mg/kg per day, with an attempt to discontinue immunosuppressive therapy after the first round of treatment and careful follow-up for possible disease recurrence. Alternatives include methotrexate, cyclosporine, mycophenolate mofetil, and systemic tacrolimus.

High-dose IVIg bolus therapy (1,000 mg/kg/day for 2 days each month for at least six months) may spare glucocorticoid doses to achieve or maintain remissions. Of note, steroid myopathy may occur after 4 to 6 weeks of therapy. DM has also been treated successfully with the use of biologic TNF-α inhibitors.

In general, it is also critical to initiate physical therapy and rehabilitation early as part of the treatment regimen, as well as measures to avoid ultraviolet light and address osteoporosis as an adverse effect of prolonged steroid therapy.

"AT A GLANCE" TREATMENT

- Skin disease is treated with potent topical corticosteroids (clobetasol or mometasone) or nonsteroidal topical immunomodulators (tacrolimus ointment):
  - Antimalarial agents and other systemic agents such as thalidomide, methotrexate, mycophenolate mofetil, dapsone, retinoids, intravenous immunoglobulin (IVIg), and biologic agents are also options.

- Muscle disease is treated with systemic therapies:
  - DM is typically treated with prednisone 0.5 to 1 mg/kg body weight per day, increasing to 1.5 mg/kg if lower doses are ineffective but not exceeding 80 mg/day. The dose is tapered when CPK levels approach normal.
  - For severely ill patients: methylprednisolone pulse (1,000 mg/day for 3 days) may be beneficial.
    - +/− addition of azathioprine, 2 to 3 mg/kg per day
    - Alternatives include methotrexate, cyclosporine, mycophenolate mofetil, and systemic tacrolimus.
  - High-dose IVIg bolus therapy (1,000 mg/kg/day for 2 days each month for at least 6 months) may spare glucocorticoid doses to achieve or maintain remissions.

COURSE AND COMPLICATIONS

Determinants of prognosis in DM include disease severity, time to diagnosis, the presence of selected extramuscular disease features, and autoantibody profile (antisynthetase antibodies are often associated with ILD and a worse long-term prognosis). With treatment, the prognosis for DM is relatively good except in patients with malignancy and those with pulmonary involvement. With aggressive immunosuppressive therapy, the 8-year survival rate is 70% to 80%. However, the majority of DM patients require ongoing treatment.

A better prognosis is seen in individuals who receive early systemic treatment. The early and aggressive use of glucocorticoids has reduced the mortality rates in children to less than 10%, although contractures can develop in children with severe disease if they do not receive physical therapy. The most common causes of death are malignancy, infection, cardiac, and pulmonary disease. Successful treatment of an associated neoplasm is often followed by improvement in or resolution of DM.

ICD9 Code

710.3   Dermatomyositis

CHAPTER 26 Autoimmune Dermatoses

WHEN TO REFER

Referral to a dermatologist is helpful for further workup of dermatitis. The differential diagnosis of many conditions would include DM and skin biopsy is often helpful.

NOT TO BE MISSED

- Ovarian cancer is associated with DM in some female patients.
- All newly diagnosed DM patients should have age-appropriate malignancy screening.

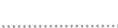

A 57–year-old man presents with a single 3-cm mobile subcutaneous nodule on his lateral right olecranon process (Fig. 26-8). He has a 15-year history of untreated rheumatoid arthritis. He wonders what this growth could be and if it is something about which he should be concerned.

Rheumatoid Nodules/Arthritis

Stephanie Hu

BACKGROUND/EPIDEMIOLOGY

Rheumatoid arthritis (RA) is a chronic, systemic, inflammatory disorder of unknown etiology that primarily involves joints. The arthritis is symmetrical and may be remitting, but if uncontrolled, may lead to destruction of joints due to erosion of cartilage and bone, and ultimately, deformity of involved structures. The disease usually progresses from the periphery to more proximal joints, and in patients who do not fully respond to treatment, results in significant locomotor disability within 10 to 20 years.

Table 26-4 is a summary of the clinical features that are useful for diagnostic and classification purposes.

The annual incidence of RA has been reported to be around 30 per 100,000 in the population, and it may affect any age group from children to the elderly. Women are affected two to three times as often as men. The disease prevalence

- Rheumatoid arthritis (RA) is a chronic, systemic, inflammatory disorder of unknown etiology that primarily involves joints.

- Extraarticular features of RA include subcutaneous ("rheumatoid") nodules, anemia, fatigue, pleuropericarditis, neuropathy, episcleritis, scleritis, splenomegaly, Sjögren syndrome, vasculitis, and renal disease.

- Rheumatoid nodules are the most common of the cutaneous manifestations of RA. These are skin-colored, nontender, subcutaneous lesions that develop at sites of trauma or at pressure points.

- Rheumatoid nodules have been shown to signal more severe systemic extraarticular manifestations in some studies, which subsequently led to clinically poorer outcomes.

- Treatment of rheumatoid nodules is supportive.

Table 26-4 Clinical Criteria for the Diagnosis of Rheumatoid Arthritis

- Morning stiffness for at least 1 hour and present for at least 6 weeks
- Swelling of three or more joints for at least 6 weeks
- Swelling of wrist, metacarpophalangeal, or proximal interphalangeal joints for at least 6 weeks
- Symmetric joint swelling
- Hand X-ray changes typical of RA that must include erosions or unequivocal bony calcification
- Rheumatoid subcutaneous nodules
- Rheumatoid factor

From Arnett FC, Edworthy SM, Bloch DA, et al. The American Rheumatism Association 1987 revised criteria for the classification of rheumatoid arthritis. *Arthritis Rheum*. 1988;31:315–324.

is about 1% in whites, but varies between 0.1% (in rural Africans) and 5% (in Pima and Chippewa Indians). The peak onset is between the ages of 30 and 55 and, because of the consistently higher rates in females, the prevalence of RA in females over 65 years is up to 5%.

PATHOGENESIS

Although RA develops its central pathology within the synovium of diarthrodial joints, many nonarticular organs can become involved as well, particularly in patients with severe joint disease. In fact, it has become clear in recent years that the same cytokines that drive synovial pathology are also responsible for generating pathology in extraarticular tissues. The extraarticular features of RA include anemia, fatigue, subcutaneous ("rheumatoid") nodules, pleuropericarditis, neuropathy, episcleritis, scleritis, splenomegaly, Sjögren syndrome, vasculitis, and renal disease. Most patients with such extraarticular manifestations also have the classic joint symptoms of RA. It is a rare patient who presents with extraarticular disease in the absence of clinical arthritis.

CLINICAL PRESENTATION

The key features of early rheumatoid inflammation are pain and swelling of the affected joints. Painful inflammation is demonstrated either by local tenderness from pressure applied on the joint, or by pain on moving the joint. Swelling may be due to synovial hypertrophy or effusion. Synovial thickening is detected by a "boggy" feel to a swollen joint, and effusion by demonstrating fluctuation. Heat and redness are not prominent features of RA, although an involved joint is often perceptibly warmer on careful examination. The characteristic joint deformities are late manifestations of disease that result from the physical stresses and local anatomy of involved joints.

Rheumatoid nodules are the most common of the cutaneous manifestations of RA (Fig. 26-8). Palpable rheumatoid nodules are present in 20% to 35% of patients with RA, and they are more commonly found in patients with severe RA and a high titer of rheumatoid factor (90% of patients have positive tests for rheumatoid factor), joint erosions, and an increased incidence of rheumatoid vasculitis. These are skin-colored, usually nontender, subcutaneous lesions that develop at sites of trauma or at pressure

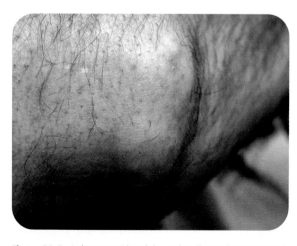

Figure 26-8 A rheumatoid nodule on the elbow of a patient with rheumatoid arthritis.

points. They typically measure from several millimeters to more than 5 cm in diameter, and their numbers may vary from 1 to over 100 in a single patient. The nodules are most commonly found on the extensor aspect of the forearms and elbows (particularly the olecranon process), the feet, knees, fingers and knuckles (metacarpophalangeal and proximal interphalangeal joints), buttocks, scalp, and back. They have also been described involving a wide variety of other sites, including the abdominal wall, heart (pericardium, myocardium, and valves), larynx, lungs, pleura, splenic capsule, peritoneum, eye, bridge of nose, pinna, ischial tuberosity, and Achilles tendon. They are often moveable, but can also be fixed to the underlying periosteum or deep fascia and present as firm, asymptomatic, dome-shaped masses in the subcutaneous fat or deeper tissues.

In many cases, rheumatoid nodules are neither symptomatic nor a cosmetic concern. However, they can be painful, disfiguring, interfere with function, or cause compressive neuropathies. Some patients find the nodules more distressing than the arthritis. The nodules may also ulcerate and thus serve as a site for local infection, or other distant infectious complications by hematogenous spread of bacteria.

Other cutaneous manifestations may arise when rheumatoid vasculitis is present or due to dermal infiltration of neutrophils. Atrophic skin over involved joints is sometimes present. Cold or stress-induced skin color change, suggestive of true Raynaud phenomenon, is found so infrequently in RA, that if present, the diagnosis of RA should be reconsidered.

Ulcerative lesions may result from venous stasis, arterial insufficiency, neutrophilic infiltration, and/or vasculitis. Dermal manifestations associated with sterile infiltration of neutrophils are uncommon, and include Sweet syndrome, pyoderma gangrenosum, and rheumatoid neutrophilic dermatitis.

DIAGNOSIS

In a patient with RA and high rheumatoid factor titers, a slowly developing firm, painless, subcutaneous nodule located at a pressure point is almost certainly a rheumatoid nodule. These can be movable or bound down to underlying fascia or periosteum. In the absence of symptoms related to the presence of the nodule, no additional diagnostic testing is necessary.

Rheumatoid nodules in viscera may be more difficult to diagnose with confidence. As an example, a rheumatoid nodule in the lung may not be definitely diagnosed until lung cancer has been excluded by biopsy or excision.

The finding of a nodule with the appropriate histologic characteristics is nearly pathognomonic of RA. However, nodules with a similar histologic pattern of palisading necrobiotic granuloma rarely occur in some patients with SLE and in otherwise healthy children without arthritis (pseudorheumatoid nodules). In the latter case, the nodules most frequently arise when the children are between the ages of 8 and 10 years. They represent nontender nodules of undetermined cause and self-limited course, and are found at sites uncharacteristic of true rheumatoid nodules (i.e., prepatellar areas, pretibial areas, feet, scalp, and malleoli).

THERAPY

Most rheumatoid nodules are asymptomatic and require no specific treatment. In fact, drainage, injection, or excision of nodules is to be avoided due to a high risk of infection or recurrence with such interventions. Nodules usually improve or resolve with conventional treatment for RA, although they may persist or even worsen in some instances (i.e., in accelerated rheumatoid nodulosis).

However, for painful nodules or those that interfere with joint motion or impinge upon nerves, local injection with a mixture of a potent glucocorticoid and local anesthetic may be beneficial and is recommended. Surgical excision

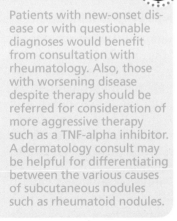

WHEN TO REFER

Patients with new-onset disease or with questionable diagnoses would benefit from consultation with rheumatology. Also, those with worsening disease despite therapy should be referred for consideration of more aggressive therapy such as a TNF-alpha inhibitor. A dermatology consult may be helpful for differentiating between the various causes of subcutaneous nodules such as rheumatoid nodules.

CHAPTER 26 Autoimmune Dermatoses

of skin nodules is rarely indicated but may be necessary for nodules that are causing serious complications, including skin erosion and infection, pain or neurologic dysfunction arising from pressure on a peripheral nerve, and limitation of motion due to the location of the lesion. Nodules often recur within scar tissue in zones subjected to repetitive trauma.

Discontinuing treatment with methotrexate can be considered when the formation of rheumatoid nodules is suspected to be caused by its use in accelerated nodulosis. This decision depends on several factors, including how successfully RA disease activity other than nodulosis has been controlled by methotrexate, the availability of other DMARDs and biologic response modifying agents (i.e., anti-TNF-α agents such as anakinra), safety of alternative drugs, and cost concerns. Regression of nodules has been noted in patients who received various DMARDS or colchicines, however, there is insufficient evidence to conclude that any specific treatment was beneficial for methotrexate-associated nodulosis.

"AT A GLANCE" TREATMENT

- Most rheumatoid nodules are asymptomatic and require no specific treatment.

COURSE AND COMPLICATIONS

Rheumatoid nodules can enlarge or regress, recur, or persist indefinitely. Although they are mostly benign, complications can occur. Infection, ulceration, and even gangrene can follow the rupture of skin overlying subcutaneous nodules. Such lesions may require surgical excision. Occasionally, internal nodules in the synovium track up to the skin, creating a fistula. This condition is known as fistulous rheumatism and requires extensive synovectomy. Acute synovial rupture in RA patients may present with a cutaneous hemorrhagic (ecchymotic) crescent sign, due to synovial fluid enzymatic damage that causes capillary permeability. Nodules also may contain significant amounts of lipids and cholesterol that are released into adjacent bursae and lead to milky bursal effusions, known as rheumatoid chyliform bursitis.

ICD9 Codes

714.0	Rheumatoid arthritis

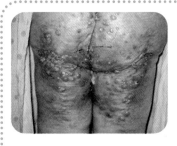

A 57-year-old woman presents for evaluation of new red areas on her face. She reports also having recently retired from her job as a word processor due to scarring and stiffness of her fingers. On further questioning, she has difficulties swallowing at times. On exam, there are many hard white papules on her buttocks and thighs (Fig. 26-9). She has a history of a positive anticentromere antibody. What is your diagnosis?

Morphea/Scleroderma/CREST Syndrome

Stephanie Hu

BACKGROUND/EPIDEMIOLOGY

Scleroderma is a multi-system, chronic autoimmune disease characterized by inflammatory, vascular, and sclerotic change of the skin and various internal organs, especially the lungs, heart, and GI tract. In the United States, the prevalence of systemic sclerosis is about 240 per million in adults with evidence of increasing incidence.

Systemic scleroderma can be divided into two subsets: localized scleroderma and diffuse systemic scleroderma (Table 26-5). Localized scleroderma patients comprise 60% of all patients with the disease. These patients are

Table 26-5 **Classification of Primary Cutaneous Sclerosis (Scleroderma)**

I. Systemic sclerosis (SSc)
   A. SSc with diffuse cutaneous scleroderma (*i.e., systemic scleroderma, proximal scleroderma*)
   B. SSc with limited cutaneous scleroderma (*i.e., CREST syndrome, acrosclerosis*)

II. Localized cutaneous sclerosis (*localized scleroderma, circumscribed scleroderma*)
   A. Morphea (localized and generalized forms)
      1. Plaque, subcutaneous/profunda, guttate, keloidal, superficial, generalized
   B. Linear scleroderma
      1. Craniofacial
         a. En coup de sabre
         b. Facial hemiatrophy (*Parry-Romberg syndrome*)
      2. Extremities

III. Cutaneous sclerosis as a component of an overlap syndrome
   A. Mixed connective tissue disease
   B. Undifferentiated connective tissue disease
   C. Sclerodermatomyositis

IV. Cutaneous sclerosis as a component of eosinophilic fasciitis (*Shulman's syndrome*)

From LeRoy EC, Black CM, Fleischmajer R, et al. Scleroderma (systemic sclerosis): Classification, subsets and pathogenesis. *J Rheumatol.* 1988;15:202.

usually female and older than those with diffuse systemic scleroderma. They have a long history of Raynaud phenomenon with skin involvement limited to the hands, feet, face, and forearms (acrosclerosis) and a high incidence of anti-centromere antibodies. Diffuse systemic scleroderma patients have a relatively rapid onset and diffuse involvement, not only of hands and feet but also of the trunk and face, synovitis, tendosynovitis, and early onset of internal involvement. Anticentromere antibodies are uncommon, but Scl-70 (antitopoisomerase I) antibodies are present in 33% of these patients.

PATHOGENESIS

The etiology and pathogenesis of this disease remains unknown. The primary event might be endothelial cell injury in blood vessels, the cause of which is unknown. Early in the course of the disease, target organ edema occurs, followed by fibrosis; cutaneous capillaries are reduced in number, and the remainder dilate and proliferate, becoming visible telangiectasia. Fibrosis occurs due to overproduction of collagen by fibroblasts.

KEY FEATURES

- Scleroderma is a multi-system, chronic autoimmune disease characterized by inflammatory, vascular, and sclerotic change of the skin and various internal organs, especially the lungs, heart, and gastrointestinal (GI) tract.

- Localized scleroderma comprises 60% of all patients.

- The pathogenesis is unknown.

- No serologic test absolutely confirms the diagnosis. Antinuclear antibodies are common, anti-centromere autoantibodies occur in 21% of patients with diffuse disease and 71% of CREST syndrome patients, and anti-DNA topoisomerase I (Scl-70) antibodies occur in 33% of diffuse disease and 18% of CREST patients.

- Treatment is guided by severity of disease and systems involved.

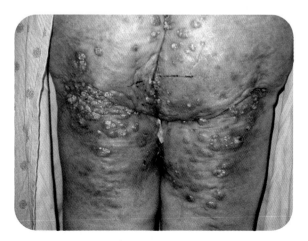

Figure 26-9 Calcinosis cutis on the buttocks and thighs of a woman with CREST syndrome.

CLINICAL PRESENTATION

Localized scleroderma can be further divided into linear scleroderma, *en coup de sabre,* and localized and generalized morphea. Linear scleroderma (most commonly occurring in childhood) causes abnormalities of the skin and subcutaneous tissues that often follow a dermatomal distribution and are found predominantly on one side of the body. *En coup de sabre* describes a type of linear scleroderma that resembles the consequences of a saber blow. In this variant, the face or scalp lesion is accompanied by marked abnormalities of underlying mesenchymally-derived tissues, including the skull. Parry-Romberg facial hemiatrophy is another form of linear scleroderma. Ipsilateral neurologic abnormalities can occur in both Parry-Romberg facial hemiatrophy and *en coup de sabre* (to a lesser extent).

Morphea can be divided into localized (circumscribed) or generalized disease, and is characterized by patches of sclerotic skin that develop on the trunk and limbs at sites of previously normal texture. Localized morphea refers to the presence of one or more circumscribed isolated plaques of sclerotic skin (Fig. 26-10). Plaque-type morphea is the most common clinical form of localized scleroderma in adults. Plaque-type morphea begins as asymmetrical, circumscribed, indurated plaques on the trunk or proximal extremities. During the early active phase, the plaques are often surrounded by halos of violaceous erythema. Both hyperpigmentation and hypopigmentation of the overlying skin can be seen. By comparison, skin changes are much more widespread in generalized morphea. These lesions often symmetrically involve the trunk and limbs, and can lead to widespread skin sclerosis (Fig. 26-11). Severe generalized morphea is distinguished from diffuse systemic sclerosis by noting the sparing of the hands and face and the lack of associated major vascular symptoms or visceral disease including restrictive lung defects from chest wall involvement. However, both entities have widespread skin involvement, and generalized morphea may require the use of the same immunosuppressive and antifibrotic regimens as used in diffuse systemic sclerosis.

Other variants of localized scleroderma include guttate and profunda morphea. Guttate morphea frequently involves the shoulders and chest with multiple, small (2 to 10 mm), hypopigmented and pigmented papules, with minimal sclerosis. Morphea profunda is a subcutaneous variant with a significant inflammatory component and poorly defined skin borders. Bullous disease is rare.

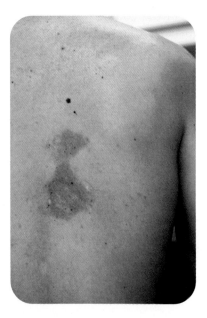

Figure 26-10 Morphea on the back.

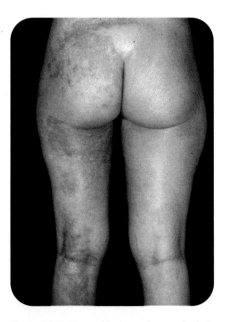

Figure 26-11 Generalized morphea on the buttocks and thighs of a woman (slide courtesy of Dartmouth Hitchcock Section of Dermatology slide collection).

The principal subsets of diffuse systemic sclerosis (SSc) include diffuse cutaneous SSc and limited cutaneous SSc. Limited cutaneous SSc (lcSSc) and diffuse cutaneous SSc (dcSSc) are distinguished principally by the extent of skin sclerosis and the forms of organ involvement. Patients with lcSSc typically have skin sclerosis restricted to the hands, and to a lesser extent, the face and neck. They also have prominent vascular manifestations and may suffer from the CREST syndrome (calcinosis cutis) (Fig. 26-9), Raynaud phenomenon, esophageal dysmotility, sclerodactyly (Fig. 26-12), and telangiectasia (Fig. 26-13). The presence of severe vascular abnormalities on nailfold capillary microscopy may be another sensitive indicator of the presence of lcSSc. Patients with dcSSc (one-third of SSc patients) have extensive skin sclerosis and are at a greater risk for developing significant renal, lung, and cardiac disease. The central criterion for the diagnosis of dcSSc is the extension of skin sclerosis proximal to the wrists (especially over the proximal limbs and trunk but commonly sparing the upper back).

Environmentally induced scleroderma is characterized by the generally diffuse distribution of skin sclerosis in addition to a history of exposure to an agent suspected of precipitating scleroderma (i.e., vinyl chloride, epoxy resins, pesticides, and a number of organic solvents used in paints). Patients who demonstrate some features of SSc (or, uncommonly, localized scleroderma) in combination with manifestations of other rheumatic diseases, such as SLE, DM, or RA, are considered to have an overlap syndrome.

Raynaud phenomenon is a frequent finding in early stages of diffuse systemic sclerosis, manifesting with triphasic color changes from pallor to cyanosis to rubor. This can precede the sclerosis by months to years. Nonpitting edema of the hands and feet can also occur at this early stage, along with painful ulcerations at the fingertips ("rat-bite necrosis") and knuckles; healing may be accompanied by pitted scars. In later stages, sclerodactyly with tapering of fingers (Madonna fingers) and waxy, shiny, hardened skin is seen. Flexion contractures can occur, as well as periungual telangiectasia, and claw-like nails that grow over shortened distal phalanges. Bony resorption and ulceration results in the loss of the distal phalanges. As sclerosis proceeds proximally, there are loss of sweat glands with anhidrosis and thinning and complete loss of hair on distal extremities.

On the face, periorbital edema may be the initial sign. Edema and fibrosis may result in the loss of normal facial lines with the progression of disease (patients look younger than their age), with thinning of the lips, microstomia, radial perioral furrowing, and a beak-like sharp nose. Telangiectasia and diffuse hyperpigmentation can also occur.

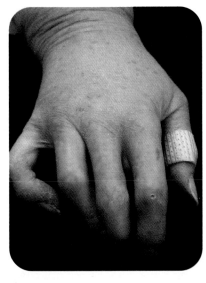

Figure 26-12 Sclerodactyly due to CREST syndrome.

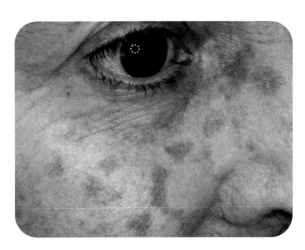

Figure 26-13 Mat telangiectasias on the face of a CREST syndrome patient.

In diffuse systemic sclerosis, the chest and proximal upper and lower extremities are involved early. Tense, stiff, and waxy-appearing skin that cannot be folded is observed, with impairment of respiratory movement of chest wall and of joint mobility. Cutaneous calcification may be seen on fingertips or over bony prominences or any sclerodermatous site. These lesions may ulcerate and exude white paste. Hyperpigmentation (generalized or on the extremities) may be accompanied by perifollicular hypopigmentation. Sclerosis of sublingual ligaments may occur, with rare, painful induration of the gum and tongue.

Other systemic findings in the diffuse type can involve the esophagus (dysphagia, diminished peristalsis, reflux esophagitis); gastrointestinal system (constipation, diarrhea, bloating, and malabsorption); lung (pulmonary fibrosis and alveolitis, restricted movement of the chest wall); heart (cardiac conduction defects, heart failure, pericarditis); kidney (slowly progressive uremia, malignant hypertension); and musculoskeletal system (carpal tunnel syndrome, muscle weakness).

DIAGNOSIS

Clinical findings and histopathologic manifestations on skin biopsy help to pinpoint the diagnosis. Serology is also useful. Patients with diffuse disease have circulating autoantibodies by ANA testing. Autoantibodies react with centromere proteins or DNA topoisomerase I; fewer patients have antinucleolar antibodies. Anticentromere autoantibodies occur in 21% of patients with diffuse disease and 71% of CREST patients, and anti-DNA topoisomerase I (Scl-70) antibodies occur in 33% of diffuse disease and 18% of CREST patients.

Unfortunately, there are no tests that confirm the diagnosis of morphea. Frequent abnormalities include an eosinophilia, positive ANA, positive antissDNA antibodies, and positive antihistone antibodies. Radiographic studies may be abnormal if deeper tissues are involved.

THERAPY

Systemic glucocorticoids may be of benefit for limited periods early in the diffuse form of the disease. All other systemic treatments (EDTA, aminocaproic acid, D-penicillamine, *para*-aminobenzoate, colchicines, immunosuppressive drugs) have not been shown to be of lasting benefit. Currently, interferon-γ is being tested clinically, as is photopheresis.

For localized scleroderma, including morphea, UVA-1 light therapy appears to soften the lesions in preliminary studies. Other options include highly potent topical glucocorticoids, topical calcipotriene, systemic methotrexate, and systemic vitamin D_3. The combination of high-dose systemic glucocorticoid and low-dose methotrexate has also been used. Therapies being investigated for treatment of skin thickening include the use of a humanized anti-TGF-β-1 monoclonal antibody, the plant alkaloid halofuginone that interferes with TGF-β induced type I collagen production, and thalidomide.

Intense pruritus can occur in the earliest stages of diffuse disease, although it usually decreases as the disease plateaus. Maintaining adequate hydration of the skin with creams (particularly those that are lanolin-based) and minimizing contact with water should not be overlooked, and low-dose oral glucocorticoids can be effective for severe pruritus.

Telangiectasia can be a cosmetic problem, especially if it occurs on the face, especially in CREST syndrome. These lesions can be covered with green foundation make-up. Larger lesions and multiple lesions can be treated quite successfully with laser therapy.

Diltiazem has shown marked clinical efficacy in the treatment of calcinosis of the skin (previous attempts to dissolve or prevent new lesions using probenecid, colchicines, and/or warfarin have failed). Calcium channel blockers may also help symptoms of Raynaud phenomenon.

WHEN TO REFER

- Treatment of the scleroderma spectrum requires the coordination of many specialties, depending on the severity of disease. For localized, nonprogressive disease, such as morphea, a dermatologic consultation may be useful for biopsy to confirm diagnosis.

- CREST patients may benefit from gastroenterologic consultation if they are having swallowing issues.

- For systemic disease, involvement of the appropriate specialist for each involved system may be necessary (rheumatology, nephrology, pulmonology, etc.).

"AT A GLANCE" TREATMENT

- Localized disease:
  - UVA1 phototherapy is very effective but challenging to get coverage and find a center with a UVA-1 machine.
  - Highly potent topical glucocorticoids (clobetasol), topical calcipotriene (Dovonex), systemic methotrexate, and systemic vitamin D_3 may be helpful.
- Systemic disease:
  - Systemic glucocorticoids may be of benefit for limited periods early in the diffuse form of the disease. All other systemic treatments are not particularly effective.
  - Diltiazem: helpful in preventing Raynaud phenomenon and for reversing calcinosis cutis in some cases.

COURSE AND COMPLICATIONS

Diffuse systemic sclerosis is characterized by slow, relentless progression of skin and/or visceral sclerosis, with an overall mortality rate about five- to eightfold higher than that of the general population, when adjusted for age and gender. Most deaths among patients with diffuse disease are due to pulmonary fibrosis and/or pulmonary hypertension rather than to scleroderma renal crisis, which had been the most common cause of death for several decades. Spontaneous remissions do occur, however.

Limited systemic sclerosis, which includes the CREST syndrome, progresses more slowly and has a more favorable prognosis; some cases do not develop visceral involvement. The increase in mortality rate is about twofold. However, patients with the presence of anti-Th/To antibodies (rather than anticentromere antibodies) have a worse prognosis, owing to the association of these antibodies with pulmonary hypertension in limited systemic sclerosis.

NOT TO BE MISSED

- Most deaths among patients with diffuse disease are due to pulmonary fibrosis and/or pulmonary hypertension, not scleroderma.

ICD9 Codes

710.1	*Systemic sclerosis*
443.0	*Raynaud's syndrome*
701.0	*Circumscribed scleroderma*

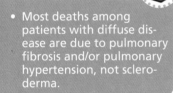

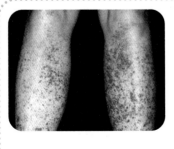

A 19-year-old woman presents with diffuse and confluent palpable purpuric plaques on the lower legs (Fig. 26-14) and thighs. She has had a cough for 2 weeks as well as a fever of 101 degrees F. She has a diffuse "atypical" pneumonia on chest x-ray. In addition, she has diffuse abdominal pain and positive stool guaiac test. A skin biopsy shows leukocytoclastic vasculitis and direct immunofluorescence testing shows clumped perivascular IgA at the basement membrane. What is the most likely diagnosis and what would be the most likely cause?

Henoch-Schönlein Purpura

Peter C. Schalock

BACKGROUND/EPIDEMIOLOGY

Vasculitis is a vast topic, with many etiologies from autoimmune to infectious to idiopathic. Many, but not all, types have prominent skin manifestations which can aid in the diagnosis through appearance and/or skin biopsy. It is the goal of this section to introduce one of the more commonly seen small vessel vasculitides (Henoch-Schönlein purpura) and also give a brief overview of other vessel inflammations (Table 26-6).

Table 26-6 Definitions of Vasculitis*

	CHCC DEFINITION	ACR CRITERION
Large-vessel vasculitis		
Giant cell (temporal) arteritis	Granulomatous arteritis of the aorta and its major branches, with a predilection for the extracranial branches of the carotid artery; *often involves the temporal artery; usually occurs in patients older than 50 years. Associated with polymyalgia rheumatica*	1. Age >50 years at onset 2. New type of headache 3. Abnormal temporal artery on clinical examination (tenderness to palpation or decreased pulsation) 4. Elevated erythrocyte sedimentation rate 5. Temporal artery biopsy showing vasculitis Three criteria classify GCA with sensitivity of 93.5% and specificity of 91.2%
Takayasu arteritis	Granulomatous inflammation of the aorta and its major branches; *usually occurs in patients younger than 50 years*	1. Age less than 40 years at onset 2. Limb claudication 3. Decreased brachial artery pulses 4. BP >10 mm Hg difference between two arms 5. Bruits 6. Arteriogram abnormal Three criteria classify TA with sensitivity of 90.5% and specificity of 97.8%
Medium-sized vessel vasculitis		
Polyarteritis nodosa (classic PAN)	Necrotizing inflammation of medium-sized or small arteries without glomerulonephritis or vasculitis in arterioles, capillaries, or venules	1. Weight loss >4 kg 2. Livedo reticularis 3. Testicular pain or tenderness 4. Myalgias, myopathy, or tenderness 5. Neuropathy 6. Hypertension (diastolic BP >90 mm Hg) 7. Renal impairment (elevated BUN or creatinine) 8. Hepatitis B virus 9. Abnormal arteriography 10. Biopsy of artery showing PMN Three criteria classify PAN with sensitivity of 82.2% and specificity of 86.6%
Kawasaki disease	Arteritis involving large, medium-sized or small arteries and associated with mucocutaneous lymph node syndrome; *coronary arteries are often involved; aorta and veins may be involved; usually occurs in children*	
Small-vessel vasculitis		
Wegener granulomatosis	Granulomatous inflammation involving the respiratory tract, and necrotizing vasculitis affecting small to medium-sized vessels (e.g., capillaries, venules, arterioles, and arteries); *necrotizing glomerulonephritis is common*	1. Nasal or oral inflammation 2. Chest x-ray showing nodules, infiltrates (fixed) or cavities 3. Microscopic hematuria or red cell casts in urine 4. Granulomatous inflammation on biopsy (within vessel wall or perivascular) Two criteria classify WG with sensitivity of 88.2% and specificity of 92.0%

(Continued)

CHAPTER 26 Autoimmune Dermatoses

Table 26-6 Definitions of Vasculitis* *(Continued)*

	CHCC DEFINITION	ACR CRITERION
Small-vessel vasculitis		
Churg-Strauss syndrome	Eosinophil-rich and granulomatous inflammation involving the respiratory tract, necrotizing vasculitis affecting small to medium-sized vessels, and associated with asthma and eosinophilia	1. Asthma 2. Eosinophilia (10%) 3. Neuropathy 4. Pulmonary infiltrates (nonfixed) 5. Sinusitis 6. Extravascular eosinophils on biopsy Four criteria classify CSS with sensitivity of 85% and specificity of 99.7%
Microscopic polyangiitis	Necrotizing vasculitis, with few or no immune deposits, affecting small vessels (i.e., capillaries, venules, or arterioles); *necrotizing arteritis involving small and medium-sized arteries may be present; necrotizing glomerulonephritis is very common; pulmonary capillaritis often occurs*	
Henoch-Schönlein purpura	Vasculitis, with IgA-dominant immune deposits, affecting small vessels (i.e., capillaries, venules, or arterioles); *typically involves skin, gut, and glomeruli and is associated with arthralgias or arthritis*	1. Palpable purpura 2. Age at onset <20 years 3. Bowel angina 4. Vessel wall granulocytes on biopsy Two criteria classify HSP with sensitivity of 87% and specificity of 88%
Essential cryoglobulinemic vasculitis	Vasculitis, with cryoglobulin immune deposits, affecting small vessels (i.e., capillaries, venules, or arterioles), and associated with cryoglobulins in serum; *skin and glomeruli are often involved*	
Cutaneous leukocytoclastic angiitis	Isolated cutaneous leukocytoclastic angiitis without systemic vasculitis or glomerulonephritis	
Hypersensitivity vasculitis		1. Age >16 years at onset 2. Medications that may have precipitated event 3. Palpable purpura 4. Cutaneous eruption 5. Positive biopsy results Three criteria classify HSV with sensitivity of 71.0% and specificity of 83.9%

*Modified from Fiorentino DF. Cutaneous vasculitis *J Am Acad Dermatol.* 2003;48:311–340.

CHAPTER 26 Autoimmune Dermatoses

KEY FEATURES

- Henoch-Schönlein purpura is the most common pediatric vasculitis.

- It is often associated with viral or bacterial upper/lower respiratory infections, especially streptococcal infections (30% of cases).

(Continued)

Henoch-Schönlein purpura (HSP) is described in the case above. It is an uncommon vasculitis presenting most commonly in the pediatric population, although adults may also be affected. It occurs in approximately 14:100,000 school-aged children.

PATHOGENESIS

The pathogenesis of vasculitis is broad. HSP is thought to be caused by environmental and genetic factors in addition to exposures/infections. Seventy-five percent of affected patients exhibit signs of an upper or lower respiratory infection before presentation with vasculitis. HSP is an IgA (almost specifically IgA1)

KEY FEATURES (Continued)

- HSP is associated with a triad of palpable purpura, abdominal pain, and arthritis.

- 90% of cases are in children <10 years old.

- In general, the course is self-limited; oral prednisone may be helpful in cases of systemic involvement.

- Monitor renal function for at least 3 months following resolution to rule out late glomerulonephritis.

Table 26-7   Causes of HSP*

INFECTIONS	MEDICATIONS	VACCINATIONS
Streptococcus species (especially group A)	Penicillin	Typhoid
Yersinia species	Ampicillin	Paratyphoid A and B
Legionella species	Erythromycin	Measles
Parvovirus	Quinidine	Yellow fever
Adenovirus	Quinine	Cholera
Mycoplasma species (especially *pneumoniae*)		
Epstein-Barr virus		
Varicella		

*Modified from Dyne PL, Sawtelle S, DeVore HK. Pediatrics, Henoch-Schönlein Purpura. Available online at: http://emedicine.medscape.com/article/804681-overview. Accessed December 7, 2009.

condition, but the antigenic stimulus is unknown. Clinical symptoms/disease occurs due to circulating antigen-antibody complexes which are deposited in organs/vessels resulting in inflammation and induction of vascular prostaglandins. Infections, medications, and vaccinations have been associated with development of HSP (Table 26-7).

CLINICAL PRESENTATION

The characteristic triad of HSP is cutaneous palpable purpura, abdominal pain, and arthritis. These findings may occur in any order and abdominal pain and arthritis may not occur. The skin findings begin as discrete erythematous papules and urticarial plaques which progress to palpable purpura. The most commonly involved area is the lower extremities and buttocks. The most common skin findings in HSP are palpable purpura, both discrete and confluent, most often on the calves, thighs, and outer buttocks (see Fig. 26-14). Other clinical findings include: migratory arthralgias, abdominal cramping, and hematuria.

The arthritis which may occur in up to 75% of cases is migratory. The most commonly affected joints are the knees and ankles, with rare involvement of the small joints such as the hands. This is a nondestructive arthritis which resolves as the condition resolves.

Abdominal pain is secondary to bowel wall angina due to deposited immune complexes. This finding is present in ~65% of all HSP patients. The pain is colicky in quality and may be similar in intensity to an acute abdomen. Thirty percent of patients will have occult or frank gastrointestinal (GI) bleeding and vomiting. Another potential complication is intussusception.

The most severe complication of HSP is renal disease, which occurs in 40% to 50% of patients. Hematuria may be present and microscopic hematuria and red cell casts may be seen on urinalysis. Patients older than 10 years of age and those with chronic proteinuria are at greatest risk for progressive renal disease (progressive glomerulonephritis).

Other manifestations of HSP-related vasculitis less commonly seen include central nervous system disease (aphasia, ataxia, cerebral hemorrhage, chorea, cortical

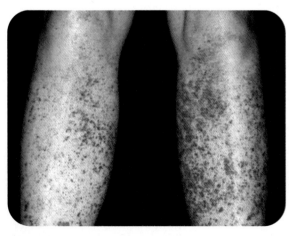

Figure 26-14 Leukocytoclastic vasculitis on the lower legs of a woman with new *Mycoplasma pneumoniae* infection and related Henoch-Schönlein purpura.

Table 26-8 Suggested Initial Workup for Suspected HSP

Complete blood count

Basic metabolic panel (electrolytes, BUN/Cr)

Antistreptolysin O titer

Mycoplasma pneumoniae titer

IgA level

Stool guaiac

PT/aPTT

Urinalysis

Skin biopsy (routine and DIF processing)

Routine imaging studies are indicated for specific symptomatic workup (i.e., barium enema to rule out intussusception or abdominal computed tomography (CT) scan or ultrasound for abdominal pain)

blindness, neuropathy, paresis, seizure), anterior uveitis, myocarditis, myositis, orchitis, scrotal edema, and testicular torsion.

DIAGNOSIS

There are no specific serologic tests which can be used to confirm diagnosis of HSP. Diagnostic criteria are summarized in Table 26-8. In the process of evaluating a patient with suspected HSP, multiple serologic and imaging studies may be helpful. Some suggestions for workup are presented in Table 26-8. A skin biopsy for both routine pathology and for direct immunofluorescence (DIF) is often quite helpful as the characteristic leukocytoclastic vasculitis on routine pathology and IgA deposition in the skin is found in the DIF.

THERAPY

Therapeutic recommendations are based on the severity of disease. For minimal disease, supportive care only is recommended. Mild abdominal pain and arthritis is managed with ibuprofen or acetaminophen as necessary. For moderate disease (considerable arthritis, abdominal pain, or early renal involvement), early administration of oral corticosteroids should be considered. Early oral prednisone therapy (1 to 2 mg/kg for 2 weeks) does not prevent renal disease, but is effective in treating renal involvement and helps prevent long-term disease. Also, it has been shown to shorten the resolution time of GI pain in children. For severe disease (progressive renal disease or pulmonary hemorrhage), prednisone, in addition to an adjunctive immunosuppressant such azathioprine, cyclophosphamide, intravenous immunoglobulin, or plasmapheresis may be considered.

"AT A GLANCE" TREATMENT

- Minimal disease: supportive care only
- Moderate disease: early oral prednisone therapy (1 to 2 mg/kg for 2 weeks)
- Severe skin and systemic disease: prednisone in addition to a adjunctive immunosuppressant such azathioprine, cyclophosphamide, intravenous immunoglobulin, or plasmapheresis

COURSE AND COMPLICATIONS

- Most patients recover fully, without long-term sequelae, within 4 to 6 weeks.
- The most common long term complication of HSP is chronic progressive glomerulonephritis, occurring in 1% to 5% of affected individuals.

WHEN TO REFER

- Minimal or mild HSP disease, not requiring systemic therapy and without renal involvement is unlikely to require referral.

- For moderate or severe disease, referrals are recommended based on the symptom profile and organ system(s) involved. Some consultations that may be necessary are: nephrology, gastroenterology, dermatology, general surgery, and/or rheumatology.

NOT TO BE MISSED

• Renal involvement is common and not to be missed. The patient should be followed for at least 6 months following resolution to ensure chronic progressive glomerulonephritis is not present.

• Following a urinalysis for at least 6 months following resolution of the condition is recommended to ensure any late renal disease is found.
• Ninety-seven percent of patients developing late renal disease were found within 6 months following their HSP. Approximately 30% of HSP patients may have a recurrence within the first 3 months following resolution, especially those with renal disease.

ICD9 Codes

287.0	*Allergic purpura*
582.4	*Chronic glomerulonephritis with lesion of rapidly progressive glomerulonephritis*

Suggested Reading

Arnett FC, Edworthy SM, Bloch DA, et al. The American Rheumatism Association 1987 revised criteria for the classification of rheumatoid arthritis. *Arthritis Rheum.* 1988;31:315–324.

Black CM. Scleroderma and fasciitis in children. *Curr Opin Rheumatol.* 1995;7:442.

Callen JP. Collagen vascular diseases. *J Am Acad Dermatol.* 2004;51:427–439.

Callen JP. Update on the management of cutaneous lupus erythematosus. *Br J Dermatol.* 2004; 151:731.

Costner MI, Grau RH. Update on connective tissue diseases in dermatology. *Semin Cutan Med Surg.* 2006;25:207–220.

Dillon MJ, Ozen S. A new international classification of childhood vasculitis. *Pediatr Nephrol.* 2006;21(9):1219–1222.

Drake LA, Dinehart SM, Farmer ER, et al. Guidelines of care for dermatomyositis. *J Am Acad Dermatol.* 1996;34:824.

Dutz J. Treatment options for localized scleroderma. *Skin Therapy Lett.* 2000;5:3.

Dyne PL, Sawtelle S, DeVore HK. Pediatrics, Henoch-Schönlein Purpura. Available online at: http://emedicine.medscape.com/article/804681-overview. Accessed December 7, 2009.

Falanga V, Medsger TA Jr, Reichlin M, et al. Linear scleroderma: Clinical spectrum and laboratory abnormalities. *Ann Intern Med.* 1986;104:849.

Falanga V. Localized scleroderma. *Med Clin North Am.* 1989;73:1143.

Garcia-Patos V. Rheumatoid nodule. *Semin Cutan Med Surg.* 2007;26:100–107.

Gerami P, Schope JM, McDonald L, et al. A systematic review of adult-onset clinically amyopathic dermatomyositis (dermatomyositis sine myositis): A missing link within the spectrum of the idiopathic inflammatory myopathies. *J Am Acad Dermatol.* 2006;54:597.

Gilliam JN, Sontheimer RD. Skin manifestations of SLE. *Clin Rheum Dis.* 1982;8:207.

Ginsberg MH, Genant HK, Yu TF, et al. Rheumatoid nodulosis: An unusual variant of rheumatoid disease. *Arthritis Rheum.* 1975;18:49.

Kovacs SO, Kovacs SC. Dermatomyositis. *J Am Acad Dermatol.* 1998;39:899.

Laman SD, Provost TT. Cutaneous manifestations of lupus erythematosus. *Rheum Dis Clin North Am.* 1994;20:195.

LeRoy EC, Black CM, Fleischmajer R, et al. Scleroderma (systemic sclerosis): Classification, subsets and pathogenesis. *J Rheumatol.* 1988; 5:202.

Lonzetti LS, Joyal F, Raynauld JP, et al. Updating the American College of Rheumatology preliminary classification criteria for systemic sclerosis: Addition of severe nailfold capillaroscopy abnormalities markedly increases the sensitivity for limited scleroderma. *Arthritis Rheum.* 2001;44:735.

Mastboom WJ, van der Staak FH, Festen C, et al. Subcutaneous rheumatoid nodules. *Arch Dis Child.* 1988;63:662.

McCauliffe DP, Sontheimer RD. Cutaneous Lupus Erythematosus. In: *The Clinical Management of Systemic Lupus Erythematosus,* 2nd ed., Schur, PH (ed.); Philadelphia: JB Lippincott, 1996.

McGrath MH, Fleischer A. The subcutaneous rheumatoid nodule. *Hand Clin.* 1989;5:127.

Mills JA, Michel BA, Bloch DA, et al. The American College of Rheumatology 1990 criteria for the classification of Henoch-Schönlein purpura. *Arthritis Rheum.*1990;33(8):1114–1121.

Patatanian E, Thompson DF. A review of methotrexate-induced accelerated nodulosis. *Pharmacotherapy.* 2002;22:1157.

Patel P, Werth V. Cutaneous lupus erythematosus: A review. *Dermatol Clin.* 2002;20:373.

Petri M. Dermatologic lupus: Hopkins Lupus Cohort. *Semin Cutan Med Surg.* 1998;17:219.

Reamy BV, Williams PM, Lindsay TJ. Henoch-Schönlein Purpura. *Am Fam Physician.* 2009;80(7):697–704.

Rencic A, Goyal S, Mofid M, et al. Bullous lesions in scleroderma. *Int J Dermatol.* 2002;41:335.

Sayah A, English JC. Rheumatoid arthritis: A review of the cutaneous manifestations. *J Am Acad Dermatol.* 2005;53:191–209.

Sontheimer RD, McCauliffe DP. Cutaneous manifestations of lupus erythematosus. In: *Dubois' Lupus Erythematosus,* 6th ed., Wallace DJ, Hahn BH (eds), Philadelphia: JB Lippincott, 2002, 573.

Sontheimer RD. Skin manifestations of systemic autoimmune connective tissue disease: Diagnostics and therapeutics. *Best Pract Res Clin Rheumatol.* 2004;18:429–462.

Tan EM, Cohen AS, Fries JF, et al. The 1982 revised criteria for the classification of systemic lupus erythematosus. *Arthritis Rheum.* 1982;25:1271–1277.

Targoff IN. Myositis specific autoantibodies. *Curr Rheumatol Rep.* 2006;8:196.

Wolff K, Johnson RA, Suurmond D. *Fitzpatrick's Color Atlas and Synopsis of Clinical Dermatology.* 2005. New York: McGraw-Hill, 356–431.

CHAPTER 27 Other Dermatologic Conditions

Jennifer L. Greenman

This chapter will review six common dermatologic conditions that do not neatly fit into the previous chapters. All of the conditions discussed are benign, but it is important to distinguish them from malignancy and infection, as well as offering appropriate treatment when indicated.

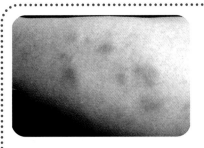

A 26-year-old woman presents with a 5-day history of painful, red plaques and nodules distributed over her shins (Fig. 27-1). The lesions are moderately well demarcated with dusky erythema.

She complains of mild generalized aching that began at the onset of the eruption. Her only routine medication is an oral contraceptive, which she has used for the past 8 years. She denies any history of fever, fatigue, cough, gastrointestinal (GI) symptoms, malaise, mucosal ulcerations, foreign travel, or illicit drug use. She has never developed similar lesions in the past.

Erythema Nodosum

BACKGROUND/EPIDEMIOLOGY

Panniculitis refers to a group of disorders involving inflammation of the subcutaneous fat. Erythema nodosum (EN) is the most common form of panniculitis and in most cases represents a hypersensitivity response to a remote focus of infection or inflammation. Overall, the prevalence of EN in the United States is approximately 1 to 5 per 100,000 persons, with peak incidence occurring between the ages of 20 and 30 years. In adults, it is more common among women, with a female to male ratio of 6:1. In children, the sex ratio is 1:1.

PATHOGENESIS

Although most often idiopathic, EN has been associated with a wide variety of disease processes, including bacterial or deep fungal infections, tuberculosis, sarcoidosis, inflammatory bowel disease, and cancer. Medications including oral contraceptives and some antibiotics have also been implicated as triggers (Table 27-1). When a patient presents with EN, it is imperative to search for its etiology, because management of underlying disease is often the most definitive means of alleviating symptoms.

CLINICAL PRESENTATION

Clinically, EN appears as symmetrically distributed, erythematous, deep nodules located on the shins, ankles, and knees. The skin nodules are usually painful or tender. Patients may describe nonspecific flu-like symptoms occurring

KEY FEATURES

- Erythema nodosum (EN) is the most common form of panniculitis.
- Reactions are mostly in young women, often from oral contraceptive medications.
- Other associations with EN include bacterial or deep fungal infections, tuberculosis, sarcoidosis, inflammatory bowel disease, and cancer.

(Continued)

KEY FEATURES (Continued)

- Erythematous nodules on shins are the most common presentation.

- First-line treatment is with nonsteroidal anti-inflammatory agents (ibuprofen).

- The course is usually self limiting, typically lasting 3 to 6 weeks.

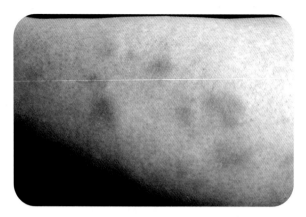

Figure 27-1 Erythema nodosum on the shins of a young woman.

1 to 2 weeks before the eruption. Fever with generalized aching sometimes accompanies the onset of skin lesions and arthralgias are reported by a majority of patients. EN may also appear as traumatic bruises, but the patient's history should discriminate between these two conditions. Superficial thrombophlebitis produces tender lesions on the lower legs, but these lesions are usually located on the lateral aspect of the lower legs. In addition, they consist of hard, irregular, and fibrotic cords or plaques, rather than the erythematous nodules seen in EN.

Usually, EN is diagnosed clinically, but the physician should consider alternative diagnoses (Table 27-2). Lesions of EN appear as erythematous, well localized, deep nodules that are 1 to 5 cm in diameter (Fig. 27-1). Nodules may coalesce to produce larger plaques. Typically, multiple lesions are present and are distributed symmetrically. Pretibial involvement is most common, although the extensor surfaces of the forearms, thighs, and trunk may also be affected. Lesions begin bright red in color, but become deeper red or purple within several days. Ultimately, they evolve into brownish-yellow, bruise-like discolorations with indistinct borders. Lesions typically regress spontaneously without ulceration, scarring, or atrophy.

DIAGNOSIS

Because EN has an extensive list of etiologies (Table 27-3), a rational, cost-effective diagnostic approach is desirable. A complete clinical history should be

Table 27-1 **Causes of EN**
Idiopathic (up to 55%)
Infections (28%–48%) streptococcal pharyngitis, *Yersinia* spp., *Mycoplasma pneumoniae*, *Chlamydia*, histoplasmosis, coccidioidomycosis, mycobacteria, tuberculosis
Sarcoidosis (11%–25%)
Medications (3%–10%) antibiotics (sulfonamides, amoxicillin), oral contraceptives
Pregnancy (2%–5%)
Enteropathies (1%–4%) regional enteritis, ulcerative colitis
Malignancies lymphoma, leukemia, others

Table 27-2 Differential Diagnosis of EN

DIAGNOSIS	FINDINGS/HISTORY
Nodular panniculitis	Ulcerative lesions over calves, atrophic scars
Traumatic bruises	History of recent injury
Superficial thrombophlebitis	Hard, irregular, and fibrotic cords or plaques on lower extremities
Cutaneous B-cell lymphoma	Erythematous nodules on lower extremities often in elderly females
Subcutaneous fat necrosis	Pancreatitis, pancreatic carcinoma, raised serum amylase and lipase levels

elicited in all patients, with reference to previous diseases, recent infection, current medications, foreign travel, pets, as well as familial cases. Suggestions for initial evaluation are summarized in Table 27-3.

Beta-hemolytic streptococcal infection is the most common identifiable cause of EN, accounting for up to 44% of cases in adults and 48% of cases in children. Nodules tend to develop within 3 weeks of streptococcal pharyngitis. Patients should undergo throat culture for group A streptococci and have anti-streptolysin-O (ASO) titers drawn or a polymerase chain reaction (PCR) analysis performed. Recent streptococcal infection is likely when ASO titers change by at least 30% in two consecutive determinations performed in a 2- to 4-week interval. PCR assays more rapidly evaluate for viral infection and have been considered an effective stand-alone alternative to rapid antigen immunoassays for the identification of streptococcal infection.

A chest radiograph should be performed in all patients with EN to rule out pulmonary diseases as the cause of the cutaneous eruption. EN in combination with radiographically demonstrable bilateral hilar lymphadenopathy, arthritis, and no evidence of tuberculosis characterize Lofgren syndrome. In most cases, this represents an acute variant of pulmonary sarcoidosis with a benign course. This condition is more frequent in females, specifically during pregnancy and puerperium. All patients with EN should also be stratified by risk for tuberculosis exposure.

The patient's geographic location and recent travel history may also be relevant when considering disease etiology. In western and south-western areas of the United States, approximately 5% of patients infected with

Table 27-3 Key Diagnostic Studies for EN

Complete blood count with differential

Erythrocyte sedimentation rate

C-reactive protein levels

Evaluation for streptococcal infection:
• Consider throat culture for group A streptococci, rapid antigen test, antistreptolysin-O titer, or polymerase chain reaction assay

Clinical suspicion of sarcoidosis or tuberculosis:
• Chest radiograph, purified protein derivative test

Patients with diarrhea or gastrointestinal symptoms:
• Stool culture and evaluation for ova and parasites; consider workup for inflammatory bowel disease, if history indicates

Excisional biopsy when clinical diagnosis is in doubt

coccidioidomycosis, also known as San Joaquin Valley fever, develop EN. Prevalence of EN increases to 15% to 40% in patients with acute respiratory symptoms. Because resolution of fungal infection often coincides with the resolution of EN, patients who present with relevant physical findings and travel history should be evaluated for coccidioidomycosis and treated, if applicable. Diagnosing coccidioidomycosis involves either the recovery of *Coccidioides* species from clinical specimens or the detection of specific anticoccidioidal antibodies in serum or other body fluids. The diagnosis is most often made by serologic testing for antibodies. A commercial immunodiffusion kit is currently available.

In patients who present with diarrhea or gastrointestinal (GI) symptoms, practitioners should obtain a stool culture, evaluate for ova and parasites, and consider a workup for inflammatory bowel disease. In adults, EN is more often associated with ulcerative colitis than Crohn disease. EN often parallels disease course: cutaneous eruptions often coincide with GI disease flares, while lesion resolution often occurs with bowel disease calming.

Medications are often implicated as the cause of EN. Antibiotics, especially sulfonamides, have been cited as one the most common drugs responsible for outbreaks. If patients develop EN while taking antibiotics; however, it is often difficult to determine if the medication or the initial infection is responsible for the cutaneous lesions. Oral contraceptives (OCPs) may also cause EN, although these drugs are becoming less frequently implicated. Presumably, the much lower amounts of hormones in newer OCP preparations account for this decline.

EN is often diagnosed clinically, but a tissue biopsy can be useful when a patient presents atypically. If lesions persist beyond 6 to 8 weeks, become ulcerated, or are not located on the shins, a deep incisional or excisional biopsy should be performed for histologic evaluation. Small punch biopsies should be avoided as they often produce inadequate samples.

THERAPY

Initial therapy should be aimed at treating any underlying disease, if one has been identified. Resolution of an underlying process often leads to resolution of EN.

- For exquisitely tender lesions, pain can be managed conservatively with nonsteroidal anti-inflammatory drugs (aspirin 325 to 650 mg PO every 4 to 6 hours, ibuprofen 400 to 800 mg PO every 6 to 8 hours, naproxen 275 mg PO every 6 to 8 hours, or indomethacin 25 to 50 mg PO three times daily).
- Bed rest and avoidance of contact irritation of affected areas is also helpful.
- Oral potassium iodide prepared as a supersaturated solution in a dosage of 400 to 900 mg per day for 1 month is another therapeutic option. This treatment is most effective in providing symptomatic relief when initiated at the onset of lesion eruption:
  - Prolonged use should be avoided to minimize the risk of hyperthyroidism, and this treatment is contraindicated in pregnancy as it may produce goiter in the fetus.
- Intralesional, topical, or systemic corticosteroids can be therapeutic as well. Injection of triamcinolone acetonide (Kenalog), in a dosage of 5 mg/mL, into the center of the nodules may cause them to resolve. Applying topical corticosteroids with kitchen-grade plastic wrap occlusion at night may also help to reduce inflammation.
- Systemic steroids should be reserved for cases that become recurrent or prolonged, or in patients with significant discomfort:
  - Prednisone 40 to 60 mg per day in a tapering dose has yielded nodule resolution within a few days.
  - Although a short course of systemic corticosteroids can provide dramatic relief, steroids should only be offered as a therapeutic option if underlying infection, risk of bacterial dissemination, or sepsis and malignancy has been excluded through thorough evaluation.

"AT A GLANCE" TREATMENT

- Identify underlying cause
- First-line: nonsteroidal anti-inflammatory drugs:
  - Aspirin 325 to 650 mg PO every 4 to 6 hours, ibuprofen 400 to 800 mg PO every 6 to 8 hours, naproxen 275 mg PO every 6 to 8 hours, or indomethacin 25 to 50 mg PO three times daily
- Bed rest and avoidance of contact irritation:
  - Oral potassium iodide supersaturated 400 to 900 mg per day for 1 month
- Intralesional triamcinolone acetonide (Kenalog) 5 mg/mL, into the center of the nodules may cause them to resolve
- Systemic steroids should be reserved for cases that become recurrent or prolonged, or in patients with significant discomfort:
  - Prednisone 40 to 60 mg per day in a tapering dose

WHEN TO REFER

Patients with persistent or extremely painful lesions, or those that appear in atypical locations should be referred to a dermatologist for evaluation.

NOT TO BE MISSED

- Consider systemic fungal or mycobacterial infection in appropriate cases.
- The most common cause is strep or medications, exclude those first.

COURSE AND COMPLICATIONS

EN is usually self-limiting, typically lasting 3 to 6 weeks. More severe cases require about 6 weeks to resolve. Lesions do not scar. Relapses are exceptional, but they are more common in patients with idiopathic EN and EN associated with upper respiratory tract infections. When associated with inflammatory bowel disease, EN may parallel GI disease course, recurring with bowel flares and regressing between episodes. Finally, in elderly patients, especially those with severe venous insufficiency and gravitational edema of the lower extremities, an acute episode of EN may be followed by a persistent erythematous swelling of the ankles.

ICD9 Code	
695.2	*Erythema nodosum*

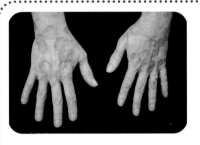

A 32-year-old woman presents with an annular, pinkish lesion on the dorsum of her right foot, lateral ankle region, and dorsal hands (Fig. 27-2). The lesion was first noticed approximately 1 month ago. Although it has not bothered the patient, she is concerned because this pinkish ring had slowly expanded in size. On examination, the lesion has slightly elevated peripheral borders with palpable and mobile subcutaneous granules. What is the most likely diagnosis?

KEY FEATURES

- Granuloma annulare (GA) is a benign, self-limited, papular eruption most often distributed on the dorsal aspect of the hands and feet.

(Continued)

Granuloma Annulare

BACKGROUND/EPIDEMIOLOGY

Granuloma annulare (GA) is a benign, self-limited, papular eruption most often distributed on the dorsal aspect of the hands and feet (Fig. 27-2). Usually, it is asymptomatic and comes to the physician's attention because of cosmetic concerns. Its name derives from its histological and clinical appearances. Clinically, lesions present as ringlike or annular groups of papules. GA may affect patients at any age, but most cases are diagnosed during the first three decades of life. Incidence is highest in women, with a ratio of 2:1. It is also seen more frequently in atopic individuals.

PATHOGENESIS

Although the etiology of GA remains unclear, some studies have shown it to follow viral infections, insect bites, tuberculin skin tests, cell-mediated hypersensitivity reactions, and trauma. In children, GA has not been associated with any systemic illness. In adults, several reports have also documented cases of

KEY FEATURES (Continued)

- It may affect patients at any age, but most cases are diagnosed during the first three decades of life.

- Etiology is unknown and diagnosis is clinical. Rigorous studies are unnecessary.

- GA resolves between 2 months and 2 years after initial presentation in 75% of patients.

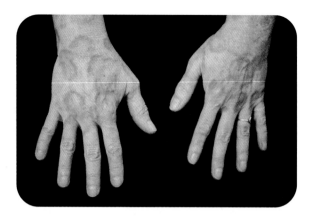

Figure 27-2 Granuloma annulare on the dorsal hands.

GA occurring in patients with acquired immunodeficiency syndrome, specifically at the site of a previous herpes zoster infection.

CLINICAL PRESENTATION

GA can take many clinical forms. The four main variants are localized (Fig. 27-3), disseminated (Fig. 27-4), subcutaneous, and perforating (Table 27-4). Seventy-five percent of patients present with localized GA. Each subtype is discussed below.

Localized Type

Localized GA typically begins as a small, expanding ring or arc of 2- to 4-mm papules that are usually flesh-colored but sometimes erythematous, violaceous, or brown (Fig. 27-4). These papules are closely set and often give the ring's border a "beaded" appearance. Although overlying epidermal markings may be distorted, they are intact. Scaling, vesicles, erosions, and pustules are absent. As the condition progresses, ring centers may become slightly depressed and hyperpigmented. Lesion borders remain distinct and feel slightly indurated on palpation. Several lesions may become confluent and merge to form larger annular plaques. In general, lesions are asymptomatic, nontender, and nonpruritic. Most often, localized GA is found on the dorsal aspects of the hands and feet. More than 50% of patients will have spontaneous resolution within 2 years.

Disseminated Type

Disseminated or generalized GA is similar in appearance to the localized variant, but is more widespread. Multiple flesh-colored or erythematous papules may fuse

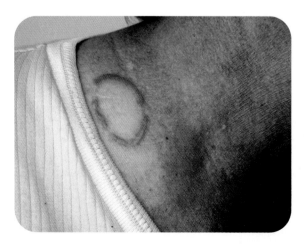

Figure 27-3 Localized granuloma annulare.

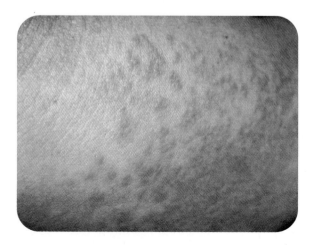

Figure 27-4 Disseminated granuloma annulare.

Table 27-4 Types of GA
Localized (75%): Expanding ring or arc of 2–4-mm papules; asymptomatic; spontaneous resolution in 50%
Disseminated: Widespread annular lesions; more persistent
Subcutaneous (rare): Asymptomatic, rapidly growing soft-tissue nodules in children; tends to resolve
Perforating (rare): 1–4 mm umbilicated, crusted, or scaly papules on the extremities in children and young adults; more persistent

to form annular rings on the extremities, trunk, and neck. These lesions occur almost exclusively in adults and tend to persist longer than localized lesions.

Subcutaneous Type

Subcutaneous GA is rare and mostly diagnosed in children between the ages of 2 to 5 years. Lesions are asymptomatic, rapidly growing soft-tissue nodules on the extremities, hands, scalp, buttocks, and pretibial and perioral areas. On palpation, the lumps are firm, nontender, and nonmobile and vary in size from 1 to 5 cm. Subcutaneous nodules are often solitary, but they may also occur in clusters. Lesions may resolve spontaneously or recur after excision.

Perforating Type

Perforating GA is another rare variant most commonly seen in children and young adults. It is characterized by 1- to 4-mm umbilicated, crusted, or scaly papules on the extremities. Most patients are asymptomatic, although 25% reported pruritus, and 25% complained of pain in at least one study.

Although GA is a common dermatologic condition in the pediatric and adult populations, it is frequently misdiagnosed. The ability to distinguish GA from other lesions is important, because it allows the clinician to counsel patients and parents appropriately and to avoid unnecessary and expensive medical evaluations. A number of common annular skin conditions, including tinea corporis, nummular eczema, psoriasis, erythema migrans, and pityriasis rosea can appear similar to GA (Table 27-5). The key feature that distinguishes GA from these other conditions is its lack of skin surface changes.

DIAGNOSIS

Often, the diagnosis of GA is clinical and rigorous studies are unnecessary. Potassium hydroxide preparations are simple and efficiently help rule out fungal infections, if scaling at lesion borders is subtle. In addition, a punch biopsy may be helpful in clinically confusing cases, especially with the subcutaneous variant of GA.

Imaging studies may also be helpful when evaluating for the subcutaneous variant of GA. Radiographs show a nonspecific soft-tissue mass without calcification or bone involvement. Ultrasonographic examination reveals a hypoechoic area in the subcutaneous tissues. Magnetic resonance imaging shows a mass with indistinct margins, isointense or slightly hyperintense to muscle with T1-weighted images.

THERAPY

In most cases, treatment is not necessary, and physicians should reassure their patient and his or her family about the good prognosis of this poorly understood entity. GA resolves between 2 months and 2 years after initial presentation in 75% of patients. However, 40% of children may have recurrent lesions,

Table 27-5 Differential Diagnosis for GA

DIAGNOSIS	FINDINGS/HISTORY
Tinea corporis	Well-demarcated annular lesion with scale across the entire erythematous border
Nummular eczema	Well-demarcated, coin-shaped plaques with vesicles and crusts; no central clearing; pruritus
Psoriasis	Well-demarcated, raised, erythematous plaques with thick micaceous scale; classic lesions distributed on the knees, elbows, scalp, and gluteal cleft
Pityriasis rosea	Herald lesion with collarette scale; subsequent rash of lightly scaling lesions in a truncal Christmas tree pattern
Erythema migrans	Erythematous papule expanding into an annular plaque with central clearing; patient history of viral-like symptoms; history of tick bite
Insect bite	Intense pruritus, blisters, crusting erosions
Urticaria	Circumscribed, raised, erythematous areas of edema lasting <24 hours
Erythema annulare centrifugum (EAC)	Annular expanding erythematous rings, which enlarge rapidly, fade, and then disappear as new lesions appear; scaling
Subacute cutaneous lupus erythematous	Bright red annular lesions with central regression and light scaling; ANA present in 60%–80%; antibodies to Ro (SS-A) positive in >80%, to La (SS-B) in 30%–50%
Necrobiosis lipoidica diabeticorum	Reddish yellow dermal plaques with shiny atrophic centers and overlying telangiectasias; history of diabetes
Rheumatoid nodules (Subcutaneous GA)	Deeply situated nodules with firm consistency and no changes on the skin surface; nodules at joints; localized or systemic signs of rheumatoid arthritis

often at the original eruption site. Above all, the physician should educate patients and family members on the natural course and benign nature of GA. Individuals should be reassured that GA is neither infectious nor contagious and usually resolves in several months to years.

Treatment is most often unnecessary unless symptoms, such as pruritus, are bothersome. Some patients, however, remain troubled by its appearance and persistently seek therapy. For adolescents and adults with disfiguring lesions, numerous treatments have been tried. In general, GA is difficult to treat.

Treatments include topical and intralesional corticosteroids, topical calcineurin inhibitors, cryotherapy, and surgical excision.

- Although intralesional steroids may be the most effective, associated pain and the risk of atrophy precludes their use in most children. 2.5 to 5.0 mg per mL triamcinolone acetonide (Kenalog) injected into the elevated lesion border is recommended.
- Topical corticosteroids are helpful for localized lesions. Clobetasol 0.05% ointment BID, under occlusion if possible for 4 to 6 weeks may clear localized lesions.
- Pimecrolimus or tacrolimus topically (Elidel or Protopic, respectively) applied twice daily may be helpful.
- Cryotherapy: one or two 3- to 4-second cycles may be helpful
- Oral Psoralen + ultraviolet A (PUVA) has been reported to be effective in some patients.
- In addition, systemic medications such as antibiotics, antimalarials, isotretinoin, alkylating agents, and immune modulators have all been used in the treatment of GA.

"AT A GLANCE" TREATMENT

- First-line: intralesional steroids may be the most effective; associated pain and the risk of atrophy preclude their use in most children. 2.5 to 5.0 mg per mL

triamcinolone acetonide (Kenalog) injected into the elevated lesion border is recommended.
- Second-line:
  - Topical corticosteroids: clobetasol 0.05% ointment BID, under occlusion if possible for 4 to 6 weeks.
  - Pimecrolimus or tacrolimus topically (Elidel or Protopic, respectively) applied twice daily may be helpful.
  - Cryotherapy: one or two 3- to 4-second cycles may be helpful
  - Oral Psoralen + ultraviolet A (PUVA) has been reported to be effective in some patients.

COURSE AND COMPLICATIONS

Most cases of localized GA are self-limited and resolve within 2 years, although some lesions may last for several decades. Patients should, therefore, be reassured of the benign course of their disorder and their excellent prognosis for recovery. Unfortunately, approximately 40% of cases recur, usually at the same location as the original lesion. Most recurrent lesions are smaller, however, and tend to resolve quickly with therapy. The subcutaneous type of GA may also spontaneously remiss but to a lesser degree. These lesions are also relatively responsive to steroid injection therapy. Generalized and perforating GA, in contrast, have a more chronic course with little reported spontaneous resolution. They are also poorly responsive to most therapies and have higher recurrence rates.

ICD9 Code

695.89   *Other specified erythematous conditions*

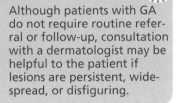

A 37-year-old man presents with a large, plugged "blackhead" on the upper back that has persisted for 4 years. The patient notes that years ago he had a large "boil" in the same location, which spontaneously ruptured, leaving the current lesion. Lately, he related increased pain and swelling of the lesion (Fig. 27-5). He is currently in good health and takes no medications.

Epidermal Inclusion Cysts

BACKGROUND/EPIDEMIOLOGY

Epidermal inclusion cysts (EIC) or epidermoid cysts are slowly enlarging, firm-to-fluctuant, flesh-colored nodules filled with expressible liquid or semisolid material. They are occasionally called "sebaceous cysts," although this is a misnomer, as epidermoid cysts have no sebaceous components. EICs are common and may occur at any age, but exact incidence is unknown because most are not brought to a physician's attention. Theses cysts are usually asymptomatic and frequently found incidentally by either the patient or examining physician. Occasionally, they are a patient's chief complaint if he or she is concerned about malignancy. Alternatively, patients may seek medical attention if cysts have ruptured, causing inflammation, pain, drainage of foul-smelling material, or secondary infection.

PATHOGENESIS

EICs often arise from a ruptured pilosebaceous follicle associated with acne. Duct obstruction of the hair follicle can result in a long, narrow channel opening in the surface comedo. Other causes include a developmental defect of the sebaceous duct or traumatic implantation of surface epithelium beneath the skin. The epidermal lining of these cysts is identical to that of the surface

KEY FEATURES (Continued)

- These lesions are discrete, flesh-colored, dome-shaped nodules that feel firm but not hard on palpation, often with a central pore.

- Treatment is not necessary, but surgical excision or drainage may be electively performed.

epidermis and produces keratin. Because there is no external surface from which the keratin can be shed, it accumulates internally, forming a cystic mass. The rancid odor often associated with these cysts relates to their relative content of fat, bacteria, and decomposing keratin. Spontaneous cyst rupture discharges the soft, yellow macerated keratin into the dermis. A tremendous inflammatory response ensues, which often produces a purulent material. If scarring occurs, subsequent cyst removal may become difficult.

CLINICAL PRESENTATION

In general, EICs present as solitary lesions. Multiple cysts in uncommon locations are a feature of Gardener syndrome, an uncommon, autosomal-dominant inherited disorder. Patients with this disorder may present with multiple epidermoid cysts (in uncommon locations especially such as the foot), fibromas, osteomas, lipomas, and intestinal polyps. Intestinal polyps undergo malignant degeneration, so referral to a gastroenterologist is recommended.

Lesions are discrete, flesh-colored, dome-shaped nodules that feel firm but not hard on palpation (Fig. 27-6). Their malleable texture is a helpful diagnostic aid as it suggests the semi-solid nature of their contents. Another useful diagnostic feature is the presence of a central pore, which represents the opening of the hair follicle from which the cyst originated. If this central pore is patent, the lesion can be gently squeezed to express the cyst's whitish, cheesy, and foul-smelling contents. Care should be taken when attempting to express such material. If the cyst pore is closed, pressure from squeezing may result in internal rupture, producing inflammation, pain, and potential infection (Fig. 27-5).

DIAGNOSIS

In general, EICs are diagnosed clinically, but the physician should rule out similar-appearing structures. EICs may be clinically indistinguishable from pilar/trichilemmal cysts. These cysts occur predominantly on the scalp as multiple lesions, are odorless and have less fat and more keratin than epidermoid cysts. In addition, 70% of cases have a familial component whereas epidermoid cysts are rarely inherited. The differential diagnosis is reviewed in Table 27-6.

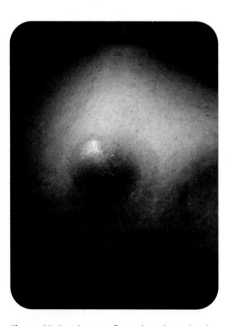

Figure 27-5 A large, inflamed epidermal inclusion cyst on the back.

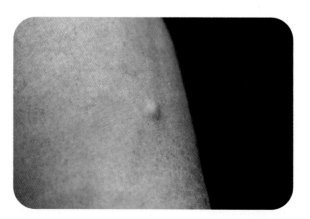

Figure 27-6 A small, noninflamed epidermal inclusion cyst.

Table 27-6 Differential Diagnosis of Epidermal Inclusion Cysts

DIAGNOSIS	FINDINGS/HISTORY
Pilar (trichilemmal) cysts	Occur on scalp as multiple odorless lesions with less fat and more keratin than epidermoid cysts; + family history
Dermoid cysts	Occur in the lines of cleavage and sublingually around the eyes and on the base of the nose; lesions can extend intracranially
Milia	Superficial 1–2-mm inclusion cysts containing keratin; located on face
Lipomas	Subcutaneous deep nodules that are freely movable and rubbery on palpation
Malignant tumor	Hard, fixed nodule; does not contain macerated keratin

In general, once the diagnosis of an EIC has been made, few if any studies are indicated. Because malignancy is very rarely associated with epidermoid cyst walls, most believe that it is not cost effective to send all walls for histologic evaluation. If any part of a lesion appears atypical or if any palpable irregularity is found in a cyst wall, the specimen should be sent for evaluation.

THERAPY

- Frequently, EICs require no treatment. Inflamed, uninfected lesions often resolve spontaneously, although they often recur:
  - Intralesional triamcinolone (Kenalog) 3 mg/mL for the face and 10 mg/mL for the trunk into the surrounding dermis may calm inflammation.
- EIC excision. When excising a lesion, the physician must take care to remove the entire cyst wall to prevent recurrence. Cyst walls become friable when inflamed, making complete removal challenging. If a cyst is inflamed, wait 4 to 6 weeks following inflammation resolution before excision.
  - Excision may be performed via conventional, punch, or minimal excision techniques:
    - Using the conventional technique, the physician makes an incision along the entire cyst diameter and removes the lesion without rupturing its wall. The length of the excision allows for ample cyst exposure, although closure may leave a noticeable scar.
    - The punch technique allows for extrusion with a curette of the cyst contents through a 3- to 4-mm opening in the skin created by a punch biopsy tool.
    - The minimal excision technique utilizes a 2- to 3-mm incision to excise the cyst in a similar manner. Although these two methods reduce the likelihood of scar formation, cyst recurrence rate is significant.
- EIC infection. When infected, cysts tend to be larger, more erythematous and more painful than sterile inflamed cysts. *Staphylococcus aureus* is the most common cause of infection. Drained contents should be sent for culture.
  - Incision and drainage is required. Make an incision the length of the cyst and then scrape out its contents using a curette. An iodoform gauze wick can be placed into the cyst cavity and left in place for 24 hours. If the cyst is not effectively draining after this duration, the wick should be replaced. It may be gradually withdrawn over a 1- to 3-week period.
  - Amoxicillin-clavulanate (Augmentin) 500 mg PO twice daily or cephalexin 500 mg PO QID is reasonable empiric therapy.

"AT A GLANCE" TREATMENT

- Frequently, EICs require no treatment:
  - Inflamed, uninfected lesions: intralesional triamcinolone (Kenalog) 3 mg/mL for the face and 10 mg/mL for the trunk

WHEN TO REFER

- For EICs that are unusually large or those in areas where scarring may have significant cosmetic impact, removal may be warranted.
- Patients presenting with multiple epidermoid cysts, especially if they are located on the extremities rather than the head, neck or trunk should be evaluated for Gardener syndrome and referred to a gastroenterologist for colonoscopy.
- If CT imaging shows a midline cyst to extend intracranially, referral to a neurosurgeon is recommended. A cyst that communicates with brain matter is most likely a congenital dermoid, not an epidermoid cyst.

• EIC excision: excision may be performed via conventional, punch or minimal excision techniques
• EIC infection: *Staphylococcus aureus* is the most common cause of infection. Drained contents should be sent for culture:
  • Incision and drainage is required
  • Amoxicillin-clavulanate (Augmentin) 500 mg PO twice daily or cephalexin 500 mg PO QID is reasonable empiric therapy

COURSE AND COMPLICATIONS

Untreated, most EICs reach a stable size between 1 and 3 cm, rarely larger. They may persist as asymptomatic nodules or spontaneously rupture. Complications are rare and usually limited to cyst rupture or infection, which results in erythema, tenderness, and increased fluctuance on examination. If a patient develops these symptoms, the lesion should be treated as an abscess with incision and drainage and oral antibiotics as necessary.

ICD9 Codes	
706.2	Sebaceous cyst
681.00	Unspecified cellulitis and abscess of finger
681.01	Felon
681.02	Onychia and paronychia of finger
681.10	Unspecified cellulitis and abscess of toe
681.11	Onychia and paronychia of toe
681.9	Cellulitis and abscess of unspecified digit
682.0	Cellulitis and abscess of face
682.1	Cellulitis and abscess of neck
682.2	Cellulitis and abscess of trunk
682.3	Cellulitis and abscess of upper arm and forearm
682.4	Cellulitis and abscess of hand, except fingers and thumb
682.5	Cellulitis and abscess of buttock
682.6	Cellulitis and abscess of leg, except foot
682.7	Cellulitis and abscess of foot, except toes
682.8	Cellulitis and abscess of other specified sites
682.9	Cellulitis and abscess of unspecified sites

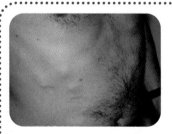

A 66-year-old man presents with multiple nodules on his abdomen (Fig. 27-7). He reports that the masses have been present for years that they have not changed in size and have not been bothersome. Recently, however, his wife was diagnosed with colon cancer, and she is concerned that these masses may also be malignant. He denies any symptoms of fatigue, malaise, or weight loss, although his appetite has diminished, since learning of his wife's condition. On examination, the mass is round, rubbery, and freely mobile with no evidence of overlying skin change. What is the most likely diagnosis?

Lipomas

BACKGROUND/EPIDEMIOLOGY

Lipomas, the most common form of benign soft-tissue neoplasms, are composed of fat cells with normal morphology and a connective tissue framework. They are characteristically soft, rounded, or lobulated, and are movable against the overlying skin. Although they affect individuals in a wide age range, they occur predominantly in adults between the ages of 40 and 60 years. Presentation in childhood is rare and there is no gender predilection. While these growths are common, their exact incidence is unknown, because most are not brought to a physician's attention.

KEY FEATURES

- Lipomas, the most common form of benign soft-tissue neoplasms, are composed of normal fat cells and a connective tissue framework.

- Treatment is not necessary unless lesions are painful or in a bothersome location.

- Excision for superficial lesions is treatment of choice.

PATHOGENESIS

Currently the etiology of these growths is unknown, although approximately 75% show karyotypic abnormalities. Cytogenetic findings are heterogeneous, but rearrangements of 12q13-15 are most common.

CLINICAL PRESENTATION

Superficial lipomas are typically small, measuring less than 5 cm. Infrequently, lipomas may be deep seated and grow up to 10 cm. These deeper lesions can affect a variety of anatomic locations, including the surface of bone (parosteal lipoma) and skeletal muscle. Intramuscular lipomas arise within skeletal muscle and may be circumscribed or infiltrative and most frequently appear on the trunk. In contrast, intermuscular lipomas develop between individual muscles and do not infiltrate skeletal muscle bundles. These are rare tumors with a predilection for the anterior abdominal wall. Lipomas of the forehead are frequently deep seated as well, usually presenting in a submuscular or subgaleal location.

Although most lipomas present as solitary masses, about 5% of cases involve multiple lipomas. Familial lipoma syndrome, an autosomal dominant disorder appearing in early adulthood, consists of hundreds of slowly growing nontender lesions. Adipositas dolorosa, or Dercum disease, occurs in middle-aged women who present with multiple tender, noncircumscribed diffuse fatty deposits. Benign symmetric lipomatosis, which affects middle-aged men, consists of many large nontender, coalescent, poorly circumscribed lipomas, located mostly on the trunk and upper extremities. On the neck, they may coalesce, forming a "horse-collar" appearance. The constellation of multiple lipomas, macrocephaly, lymphangiomas, and hemangiomas is known as Bannayan (Bannayan-Zonana) syndrome, an autosomal dominant disease caused by a mutation in the PTEN tumor suppressor gene. Lipomas may also be seen as a manifestation of Gardner syndrome, an autosomal dominant condition involving intestinal polyposis, desmoid fibromatosis, epidermal inclusion cysts, osteomas, and lipomas.

DIAGNOSIS

Lipomas usually present as painless, round, mobile masses that impart a slight elevation to normal-appearing over-lying skin (Figs. 27-7, 27-8). On palpation, they are characteristically freely movable and rubbery, but not hard.

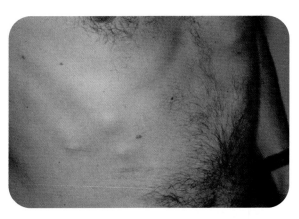

Figure 27-7 Multiple lipomas on the trunk. From Goodheart HP. *Goodheart's Photoguide to Common Skin Disorders,* 3rd ed. Philadelphia: Lippincott Williams & Wilkins, 2009.

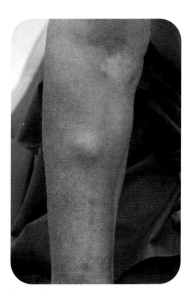

Figure 27-8 A large lipomas on the posterior leg.

Table 27-7 Differential Diagnosis of Lipoma

DIAGNOSIS	FINDINGS/HISTORY
Soft-tissue sarcoma	Fast growth; hard mass on palpation; often located on the retroperitoneum, shoulders, or lower extremities
Angiolipoma	Slightly reddish or purple raised nodule; painful
Epidermal inclusion cyst	Superficial mass filled with macerated keratin; central pore
Cutaneous metastasis (Fig. 27-9)	Single or multiple hard subcutaneous nodules, often in those with h/o carcinoma. Scalp is a common location but any location is possible.

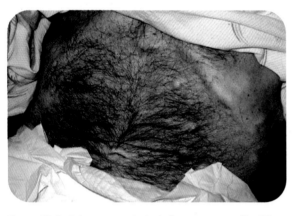

Figure 27-9 Cutaneous metastasis from a non–small cell lung carcinoma.

Lipomas range in size from 1 to 10 cm, rarely larger. They may occur anywhere, but are mostly found on the trunk, neck, and upper extremities. Involvement of the head, hands, and feet is uncommon.

Although lipomas are most often correctly diagnosed clinically, the physician should consider alternative disorders (Table 27-7) (Fig. 27-9). It is most important to distinguish these benign masses from malignant growths.

THERAPY

Lipomas are entirely benign tumors and unless lesions are large, disfiguring or painful, treatment is usually unnecessary. When pursued, treatment may be nonexcisional, including corticosteroid injections and liposuction, or excisional.

- Steroid injections cause local fat atrophy and tumor shrinkage:
  - They are best performed on lipomas less than 1 cm in diameter. A one-to-one mixture of 1% lidocaine (Xylocaine) and triamcinolone acetonide (Kenalog), in a dosage of 10 mg per mL, can be injected into the center of the lesion. The exact volume of steroid depends on the size of the lipoma, with an average of 1 to 3 mL of total volume administered. This procedure may be repeated several times at monthly intervals.
- Liposuction. This strategy is best suited for soft growths that have minimal connective tissue. A 16-gauge needle and large syringe may be used in the office, and diluted lidocaine usually provides adequate anesthesia. Complete elimination of the growth is often difficult to achieve.
- Surgical excision of lipomas often results in a cure:
  - Small lipomas can be removed by enucleation. This technique requires the physician to make a 3- to 4-mm incision over the lipoma and use a curette to free the mass from surrounding tissue. Once freed, the tumor is then enucleated through the incision with the curette. Sutures generally are not needed, and a pressure dressing is applied to prevent hematoma formation.
  - Larger lipomas are best removed through fusiform incisions made in the skin overlying the lipoma. To reduce the incidence of hematoma formation, a pressure dressing should be placed, as some lesions have ample blood supply (angiolipomas).
  - All specimens should be submitted for histologic analysis.

"AT A GLANCE" TREATMENT

- Steroid injections: a one-to-one mixture of 1% lidocaine (Xylocaine) and triamcinolone acetonide (Kenalog), in a dosage of 10 mg per mL, can be injected into the center of the lesion, 1 to 3 mL of total volume administered. This procedure may be repeated several times at monthly intervals.

- Liposuction: this strategy is best suited for soft growths that have minimal connective tissue.
- Surgical excision of lipomas often results in a cure:
  - Small lipomas can be removed by enucleation technique.
  - Larger lipomas are best removed through fusiform excision.
  - All specimens should be submitted for histologic analysis.

COURSE AND COMPLICATIONS

Common subcutaneous lipomas are benign growths that rarely require medical attention. Most lesions grow slowly to a stable size and persist. They are generally removed for cosmetic reasons or if their location causes pain or restricts movement. With the exception of intramuscular lipomas, local recurrence is rare. The infiltrative variant of intramuscular lipoma is associated with an approximately 19% chance of local recurrence. Rarely, lipomas may become more threatening if they present in internal organs. Lipomas growing in the GI tract can cause bleeding, ulceration, and painful obstructions. Malignant transformation into liposarcoma is very rare and most liposarcomas do not evolve from pre-existing benign lesions.

ICD9 Codes	
214.0	*Lipoma of skin and subcutaneous tissue of face*
214.1	*Lipoma of other skin and subcutaneous tissue*
214.2	*Lipoma of intrathoracic organs*
214.3	*Lipoma of intra-abdominal organs*
214.4	*Lipoma of spermatic cord*
214.8	*Lipoma of other specified sites*
214.9	*Lipoma, unspecified site*

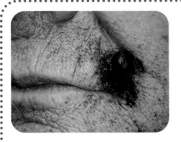

A 74-year-old man presents with a lesion on his upper lip of 1 month's duration (Fig. 27-10). He is bothered by its frequent bleeding, especially after shaving in the area and with minor trauma. He is otherwise feeling well. He is worried that this is a melanoma. On examination, the lesion is approximately 1 cm in diameter and glistening with an erosive surface. What is the most likely diagnosis?

Pyogenic Granuloma

BACKGROUND/EPIDEMIOLOGY

Pyogenic granuloma (PG), also known as lobular capillary hemangioma, is a benign vascular hyperplasia of the skin and mucous membranes. The name PG is a misnomer, because lesions are neither infectious in nature, nor macrophage-laden granulomatous entities. Clinically, PGs appear as solitary red nodules with smooth, glistening, or erosive surfaces that typically bleed easily. They most commonly occur in children and young adults. Cutaneous PGs have no gender predisposition and the mean age of onset is 6.7 years. Oral mucosal nodules occur in a 2:1 female to male ratio and incidence peaks in the second or third decade of life.

PATHOGENESIS

PG is associated with minor trauma, chronic irritation, hormonal factors, and infections. To date, however, no significant causative relationships have been verified. Local trauma to the affected area is reported in 50% of individuals. In these

---

WHEN TO REFER

- When a lipoma is very large, painful, restricts movement, or is in a location where scar formation has cosmetic impact, consultation with a surgeon may be helpful.

- If any lipomatous mass shows indication of malignant transformation on pathologic evaluation, referral to a surgeon is mandatory.

NOT TO BE MISSED

- Lipomas greater than 10 cm or lesions continuing to enlarge should be biopsied to rule out liposarcoma.

- Enucleation removal is quick and simple for most small, superficial lipomas.

KEY FEATURES

- Pyogenic granuloma (PG), also known as lobular capillary hemangioma is a benign vascular hyperplasia of the skin and mucous membranes.

(Continued)

KEY FEATURES *(Continued)*

- They often occur following local trauma, though pathogenesis is not known.

- Diagnosis is by clinical exam, but it is quite important to rule out amelanotic melanoma with a surgical biopsy.

- Treatment is with surgical biopsy/removal.

- Recurrences are common.

cases, excessive production of an angiogenic factor may be responsible for vascular hyperplasia. Female sex hormones may also play a role in the pathogenesis of PG. Although there is no relationship between sex hormones and cutaneous lesions, oral lesions occur at an increased frequency in pregnant women and in women taking oral contraceptives. Moreover, recurrence of excised nodules is not uncommon during pregnancy and lesions tend to resolve following parturition. Some researchers have suggested that an imbalance between angiogenic enhancers and inhibitors, driven by female sex hormones, might account for the vascular hyperplasia seen in PGs. Infection is another suspected, but unconfirmed cause of this condition. Although infectious organisms including *Bartonella* and human herpesvirus 8 have been identified in other vascular tumors, no etiologic agents have been repeatedly identified in PGs.

CLINICAL PRESENTATION

Patients typically present with a solitary red, glistening nodule located on the face, a finger, or the oral mucosa (Fig. 27-10). Because lesions often bleed easily, PGs are often accompanied by the "band aid sign," skin irritation often in a cross pattern due to the adhesive bandages a patient places over the lesion to absorb serosanguineous fluid. Cutaneous PGs often arise as painless, crusted or ulcerated papules with a mean diameter of 6.5 mm. Lesions develop over weeks, and growth typically stabilizes over several months. Eventually, PGs may shrink, becoming fibrotic "angiomas" (Fig. 27-11) or may spontaneously infarct and involute. Cutaneous lesions are most often located on the head, neck, trunk, or limbs, while oral lesions typically develop on the gingiva, lips, or buccal mucosa. Satellite PGs are rare, and usually occur after treatment or manipulation of a solitary nodule. Subcutaneous and intravenous PG are also uncommon and their diagnosis may be challenging, given their depth. Biopsy helps distinguish these varieties from other vascular entities.

DIAGNOSIS

When considering a differential diagnosis, it is most important for the physician to differentiate PG from amelanotic melanoma. Amelanotic melanoma is a subtype of malignant melanoma that is nonpigmented and appears pink or flesh-colored. Unlike PGs, these lesions rarely bleed, continue to evolve, and show more asymmetry and border irregularity. Other lesions appearing similar to PG are summarized in Table 27-8.

If any uncertainty around the diagnosis exists, especially if amelanotic melanoma is suspected, excisional biopsy is recommended.

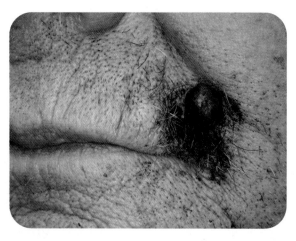

Figure 27-10 Pyogenic granuloma on the upper lip.

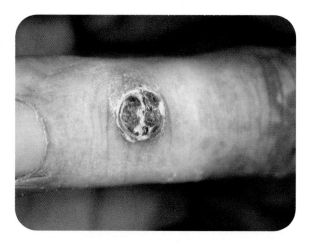

Figure 27-11 A fibrotic, regressing pyogenic granuloma.

Table 27-8 Differential Diagnosis of PG

DIAGNOSIS	FINDINGS/HISTORY
Amelanotic melanoma	Rarely bleeds, border asymmetry, evolving size
Angiosarcoma	Rarely bleeds, bluish purple color, in elderly white men, often on the scalp
Basal cell carcinoma	Pink or flesh-colored pearly papules with superimposed telangiectasia and possible ulceration; on sun-exposed skin; continued slow growth
Squamous cell carcinoma	Erythematous or skin-colored hyperkeratotic papule or nodule that may ulcerate
Kaposi sarcoma	Multiple deep-red, brown, or purple patches, plaques or nodules; history of HIV infection or Mediterranean heritage; HHV-8 infection
Hemangioma	Deep-red papules quickly enlarging to between 2 and 8 cm over a period of a year, appear during first few months of life; spontaneous regression
Bacillary angiomatosis	Painful lesions; history of scratches or bites by cats; history of HIV infection or immunocompromised state
Visceral metastasis	Multiple skin lesions; history of visceral malignancy or systemic symptoms, including malaise, chronic fatigue, and weight loss
Granulation tissue	History of recent skin injury

THERAPY

Although PGs often resolve independently, numerous treatment options are available, including surgical excision, shave excision, cryotherapy, electrodessication and curettage, laser surgery, ligation, or a combination of methods.

- Surgical excision with linear closure offers the lowest recurrence rate and allows histological examination of the tissue sample. Closure, however, results in a linear scar, which may be undesirable cosmetically.
- Shave excision followed by electrocautery is an effective alternative that minimizes scar tissue while preserving the ability to confirm the diagnosis with histologic evaluation. Recurrence rate with this method may be as high as 44%.
- Cryotherapy with liquid nitrogen or electrodessication and curettage:
  - Complete resolution can be expected after one to three treatments with these methods, and most patients do not develop scars or skin pigmentary changes.
  - Neither of these tissue-preserving methods allows for histologic evaluation, they are recommended for classically presenting lesions where the diagnosis is clear.

WHEN TO REFER

Large lesions located in areas with cosmetic impact may be best treated by a dermatologist experienced in surgical procedures or a plastic surgeon.

"AT A GLANCE" TREATMENT

- Surgical excision with linear closure
- Shave excision followed by electrocautery
- Cryotherapy with liquid nitrogen or electrodessication and curettage
- Neither of the tissue-preserving methods allows for histologic evaluation; they are recommended for classically presenting lesions where the diagnosis is clear.

CHAPTER 27 Other Dermatologic Conditions

COURSE AND COMPLICATIONS

PGs are benign lesions that typically develop over weeks, with growth stabilizing over several months. Medical attention is usually not necessary, but most patients typically seek treatment because of frequent bleeding or oozing. Lesions located on the fingers can greatly interfere with daily activities. Treatment is typically successful with surgical excision, cryotherapy, or electrodessication and curettage. Patients should be reassured of the benign nature of these lesions and their excellent prognosis.

ICD9 Codes	
686.1	Pyogenic granuloma of skin and subcutaneous tissue
172.0	Malignant melanoma of skin of lip
172.1	Malignant melanoma of skin of eyelid, including canthus
172.2	Malignant melanoma of skin of ear and external auditory canal
172.3	Malignant melanoma of skin of other and unspecified parts of face
172.4	Malignant melanoma of skin of scalp and neck
172.5	Malignant melanoma of skin of trunk, except scrotum
172.6	Malignant melanoma of skin of upper limb, including shoulder
172.7	Malignant melanoma of skin of lower limb, including hip
172.8	Malignant melanoma of other specified sites of skin
172.9	Melanoma of skin, site unspecified

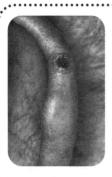

A 58-year-old white man presents with an exquisitely painful reddish bump on the helix of his right pinna (Fig. 27-12). The nodule developed spontaneously, has persisted at its current size for 6 to 8 months, and has not changed in appearance. He has no similar lesions elsewhere. The patient denies any associated symptoms but complains that if he rolls onto the affected side at night, pain awakens him. What is the most likely diagnosis? Would you biopsy this lesion?

Chondrodermatitis Nodularis Chronicus Helicis

BACKGROUND/EPIDEMIOLOGY

Chondrodermatitis nodularis chronicus helicis (CNH) describes a common, benign inflammatory condition of the external ear, characterized by an exquisitely tender small nodule or nodules involving the cartilage and overlying skin. Most cases occur in middle-aged or elderly white men who present with lesions on the outer rim of the helix. Women with the condition more often have nodules on the antihelix or antitragus.

PATHOGENESIS

Although the etiology of CNH is unknown, repeated trauma to ear cartilage, cold temperatures, actinic damage, and physical pressure especially during sleep may promote this condition. The lack of a thick, cushioning, subcutaneous layer in the auricle may predispose the underlying cartilage to pressure-induced ischemia and damage. The nodules are more commonly reported on the right ear, which is believed to be the preferred resting side during sleep. Moreover, many patients report that they tend to sleep on the side of affected ear.

CLINICAL PRESENTATION

The nodules of CNH are typically firm, dome-shaped, reddish gray with an erythematous rim, and range from 3 to 10 mm (Fig. 27-12). Lesions may be covered with superficial scale or crust and may be slightly depressed centrally. Ulceration is

KEY FEATURES

- Chondrodermatitis nodularis chronicus helicis (CNH) is characterized by an exquisitely tender small nodule or nodules involving the cartilage and overlying skin.

- CNH is caused by repeated pressure/trauma but the underlying pathophysiology is unknown.

- Multiple treatments exist; avoiding pressure on the affected ear often is helpful.

- Despite numerous treatments, lesion recurrence rates remain high.

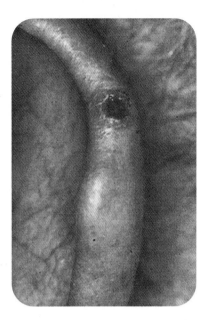

Figure 27-12 Chondrodermatitis nodularis helicis on the helix. A biopsy is necessary to rule out carcinoma. From Young EM Jr, Newcomer VD, Kligman AM. *Geriatric Dermatology: Color Atlas and Practitioner's Guide.* Philadelphia: Lea & Febiger, 1993.

common. Spontaneous remission is rare, but persistent nodules are not premalignant. Although these lesions typically appear unimpressive, pain is usually significant and patients often seek medical advice when pain interferes with sleep.

The characteristic location, appearance, and pain of these nodules usually allows for the correct diagnosis clinically. However, it is important for the physician to distinguish CNH from precancerous or malignant growths and other benign conditions (Table 27-9).

Table 27-9	**Differential Diagnosis of Chondrodermatitis Nodularis Chronicus Helicis**
DIAGNOSIS	**FINDINGS/HISTORY**
Actinic keratosis	Ill-defined, scaling, erythematous patches or plaques easier felt than seen, may be tender
Squamous cell carcinoma	Indurated or firm papules, plaques, or nodules with hyperkeratosis or ulceration; painless; enlarging; more common on auricle
Basal cell carcinoma	Pink or flesh-colored pearly papules with superimposed telangiectasia and possible ulceration; painless
Cutaneous horns	A conical hypertrophic protuberance emanating from a skin-colored to erythematous papular base; painless; refers to a reaction pattern and not a particular lesion
Keratoacanthoma	Rapid growth, achieving a size of 2.5 cm within a few weeks; central keratotic plug; painless
Wart	Firm papules, 1 to 10 mm, hyperkeratotic, clefted surface with vegetations; interruption of normal skin lines; continued slow growth
Elastotic nodules on the antihelix	Small pale papules or nodules on the crux of the antihelix; bilateral distribution, sun damage

DIAGNOSIS

In cases where the diagnosis of CNH is in question, especially if malignancy is under consideration, a biopsy with histologic evaluation should be performed. Differential diagnoses are discussed in Table 27-9.

THERAPY

Numerous treatment options have been suggested for CNH, ranging from excision and extensive resection of cartilage to curettage and electrocautery, carbon dioxide laser excision, and intralesional collagen or steroid therapy. Long-term follow-up, where described, has shown that none of these treatments is particularly effective. Given the numerous treatment options available and their variable success rates, it is reasonable to offer patients conservative therapy initially.

- Encourage the patient to sleep with the unaffected ear to the pillow and suggest using a protective device during sleep. Donut-shaped pillow prostheses are available at http://www.cnhpillow.com.
  - Home-made devices may prove equally therapeutic. Taping a cotton ball just below the nodule or surrounding the ear in a foam protector made by cutting a hole in a sponge are two methods that may relieve pressure over lesions.
- Surgical excision does not always yield high cure rates. Excision may only transfer pressure to an adjacent prominence of the ear, causing a new lesion.
- For patients desiring immediate pain relief, a corticosteroid injection of 0.1 to 0.2 mL of triamcinolone acetonide (Kenalog) (10 to 40 mg/mL) often offers dramatic improvement.
- Persistent lesions should be biopsied and treated surgically.

"AT A GLANCE" TREATMENT

- Encourage the patient to sleep with the unaffected ear to the pillow and suggest using a protective device during sleep.
- Surgical excision
- Corticosteroid injection of 0.1 to 0.2 mL of triamcinolone acetonide (Kenalog) (10 to 40 mg/mL) often offers dramatic improvement.
- Persistent lesions should be biopsied and treated surgically

COURSE AND COMPLICATIONS

CNH is a benign condition that may persist for years. Despite numerous treatment modalities, lesion recurrence rates remain high in many cases. This treatment failure combined with the exquisite pain associated with nodules makes this condition frustrating for both patients and clinicians. In general, it is reasonable to try conservative therapy, at least initially, as it may prove the best option in many cases.

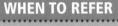

WHEN TO REFER

Patients with persistent, painful lesions should be referred for surgical excision of diseased cartilage.

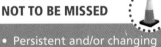

NOT TO BE MISSED

- Persistent and/or changing lesions should be biopsied to rule out malignancy.
- A pressure off-loading pillow often is helpful or curative.

ICD9 Code

380.02   *Chronic perichondritis of pinna*

Suggested reading

Argent JD, Fairhurst JJ, Clarke NMP. Subcutaneous granuloma annulare: Four cases and review of the literature. *Pediatr Radiol.* 1994;24:527–529.

Avakoff JC. Microincision for removing sebaceous cysts. *Plast Reconstr Surg.* 1989;84(1):173–174.

Dalal KM, Antonescu CR, Singer S. Diagnosis and management of lipomatous tumors. *J Surg Oncol.* 2008;97(4):298–313.

Earley CM Jr, Martens AJ. Adenomatosis of the colon associated with sebaceous cysts, osteomas, and fibrous tumors. *Dis Colon Rectum.* 1966;9(1):33–36.

Fang KS, Lawry M, Haas A. Papules on the hands. Granuloma annulare. *Arch Dermatol.* 2001;137:1647–1652.

Gamo VR, Sopena BJ, Guerra TA, et al. Pustular generalized perforating granuloma annulare. *Br J Dermatol.* 2003;149:866–868.

Goldstein B, Goldstein A. Cyst excision from dermatologic procedures. Accessed June 18, 2008 at http://utdol.com/online/content/topic.do?topicKey=pri_derm/7494#27.

Habif TP. *Clinical Dermatology: A Color Guide to Diagnosis and Therapy.* 3rd ed. St Louis: Mosby–Year Book Inc; 1996:643.

Harris MN, Desai R, Chuang TY, et al. Lobular capillary hemangiomas: an epidemiologic report, with emphasis on cutaneous lesions. *J Am Acad Dermatol.* 2000;42:1012–1016.

Hurwitz RM. Painful papule of the ear: A follicular disorder. *J Dermatol Surg Oncol.* 1987;13:270–274.

Kromann N, Hoyer H, Reymann F. Chondrodermatitis nodularis chronica helicis treated with curettage and electrocauterization: Follow-up of a 15-year material. *Acta Derm (Stockh).* 1983;63:85–87.

Kudejko J. Treatment of noninfectious sebaceous cysts by the pressing method. *Arch Dermatol.* 1970;101(3):370–371.

Lee J, Lynde C. Pyogenic granuloma: Pyogenic again? Association between pyogenic granuloma and *Bartonella. J Cutan Med Surg.* 2001;5:467–470.

Matsumoto K, Hukuda S, Ishizawa M, et al. MRI findings in intramuscular lipomas. *Skeletal Radiol* 1999;28:145–152.

Mehrabi D, Leonhardt JM, Brodell RT. Removal of keratinous and pilar cysts with the punch incision technique: analysis of surgical outcomes. *Dermatol Surg.* 2002;28(8):673–677.

Mert A, Ozaras R, Tabak F, et al. Erythema nodosum: An experience of 10 years. *Scan J Infect Dis.* 2004;36:424–427.

Munnoch DA, Herbert KJ, Morris AM. Chondrodermatitis nodularis chronica helicis et antihelicis. *Br J Plast Surg.* 1996;49:473–476.

Patrice SJ, Wiss K, Mulliken JB. Pyogenic granuloma (lobular capillary hemangioma): A clinicopathologic study of 178 cases. *Pediatr Dermatol.* 1991;8:267–276.

Requena L, Sangueza OP. Cutaneous vascular proliferations, part II: Hyperplasias and benign neoplasms. *J Am Acad Dermatol.* 1997;37:887–920.

Requena L, Yus ES. Panniculitis. Part I. Mostly septal panniculitis. *J Am Acad Dermatol.* 2001;45:163–183.

Ryan TJ. Cutaneous Vasculitis, in Champion RH, Burton JL, Burns, DA, et al. (eds): *Textbook of Dermatology,* 6th ed. Oxford: Blackwell Scientific Publications; 1998:2155–2225.

Sandberg AA. Updates on the cytogenetics and molecular genetics of bone and soft tissue tumors: Lipoma. *Cancer Genet Cytogenet.* 2004;150:93.

Smith MD, Downie JB, DiCostanxo D. Granuloma annulare. *Int J Dermatol.* 1997;36:326–322.

Yu GV, Farrar AK. (1994). Benign rheumatoid nodule versus subcutaneous granuloma annulare: A diagnostic dilemma. Are they the same entity? *J Foot Ankle Surg.* 1994;33:156–166.

CHAPTER 27 Other Dermatologic Conditions

Index

Page numbers in *italics* denote figures (*f*) and Tables (*t*).